Beyond Becquerel and Biology to
Precision Radiomolecular Oncology:
Festschrift in Honor of Richard P. Baum

Vikas Prasad

Editor

Beyond Becquerel and Biology to Precision Radiomolecular Oncology: Festschrift in Honor of Richard P. Baum

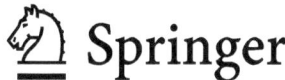 Springer

Editor
Vikas Prasad
Division of Nuclear Medicine
Mallinckrodt Institute of Radiology, Washington University in Saint Louis
Saint Louis, MO, USA

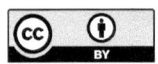

This book is an open access publication.

ISBN 978-3-031-33532-7   ISBN 978-3-031-33533-4   (eBook)
https://doi.org/10.1007/978-3-031-33533-4

This work was supported by Prof. Richard P. Baum

This Springer imprint is published by the registered company Springer Nature Switzerland AG
The registered company address is: Gewerbestrasse 11, 6330 Cham, Switzerland

Paper in this product is recyclable.

Contents

Vikas Prasad

1.1 The Beginning

Genius is 1 percent inspiration and 99 percent perspiration: Thomas Edison

There is one thing common among all those who have met and worked with Dr. Baum: their description of Prof. Baum's work ethics and dedication. His associates fondly describe him as a person with unmatched physical and mental strength, allowing him to work for 16–18 h every single day, 7 days a week.

Dr. Baum's passion for learning and making a difference in the lives of patients and their families was very much evident from the early days of his career. Many know Dr. Baum as a "Nuclear Medicine Physician" par excellence but only few are aware of his internal medicine and emergency medicine skills (see CV of Dr. Baum towards the end of this chapter). During some close interactions with Dr. Baum, he fondly remembers the time he spent providing emergency services. Armed with his special skill set, and his passion for targeted therapies using state-of-the-art radiolabeled antibodies and peptides, Dr. Baum made his presence felt in this special domain of cancer treatment in 1997 when he first introduced PRRT in Germany.

V. Prasad (✉)
Division of Nuclear Medicine, Mallinckrodt Institute of Radiology, Washington University in Saint Louis, St. Louis, MO, USA
e-mail: pvikas@wustl.edu

All great personalities and pioneers in this world always have someone whom they personally consider as their hero. Prof. Baum's personal hero is Prof. Paul Ehrlich, a nobel prize-winning German physician scientist, for providing the concept of amboceptors which ultimately paved the way to immunology. Spellbound, as all good ardent followers are when they speak about the enormity of a discovery which they personally feel pathbreaking, Dr. Baum often starts his lectures for students and audience of all ages and faculty with a slide showing his great admiration of Dr. Paul Ehrlich. It is important to understand why Dr. Baum liked what he saw in the concept of amboceptors. Based on his personal experience, he realized during the early stages of his medical career that chemotherapy, a generalized way of treating cancers without essential looking at the presence or absence of "targets'" on the cancer cells is only applicable to certain percentage of patients. This blanket treatment approach, still a mainstay of management in oncology, is more often than not associated with toxicity, which, sometimes can be extreme. Realizing that there has to be a better way for treating cancer patients, Dr. Baum started utilizing the concept of targeted radiopharmaceutical therapies in his early stages by using antibodies labeled with beta-emitting I-131 and Y-90. Dr Baum is one of the few physician scientists who strongly believed in "treating what you see" to maximize therapeutic efficacy

V. Prasad (ed.), *Beyond Becquerel and Biology to Precision Radiomolecular Oncology: Festschrift in Honor of Richard P. Baum*, https://doi.org/10.1007/978-3-031-33533-4_1

by minimizing toxicity. His patients' quality of life (now a central issue in almost all good clinical trials) centered approach is known to all. With the conviction and motivation only few people possess, Dr. Baum chooses to keep the following principle above all, even if that meant going against the "main streamline" oncology:

> "Aegroti salus supreme lex" which means "the health of the patient is the supreme law".

1.2   The Impedance

Both Galileo and Socrates were aware of the consequences of proposing and following an approach or scientific principle against the general accepted norms of the society in that particular era. Despite that, they continued their course as that was the right thing to do. Dr. Baum's approach using the principles of Theranostics was not really well understood among the oncologists in Germany in mid-nineties. Part of that was because those radiopharmaceuticals were not really tested in a rigorous clinical trial. In fact, there were practically no pharmaceutical companies interested in including radiopharmaceutical therapy in their portfolio in the late nineties and early 2000. However, that did not deter him from going ahead and treating patients with peptide receptor radionuclide therapy under the German medicinal product law described under the paragraph 13.2b. His conviction and motivation were rewarded when he successfully treated a child with debilitating metastases from paraganglioma/pheochromocytoma using PRRT in 1997. This child, who had exhausted all approved therapeutic options approved at that time, not only tolerated therapy with somatostatin receptor radioligand kindly provided by Dr. Helmut Maecke from Basel, but also showed dramatic improvement in his quality of life. The child who was on crutches and unable to walk started playing football. This might appear to be a "one-off" success but that was enough to drive Dr. Baum's conviction several notches higher. Finally, "the impedance" met its own "resistance" and a new

era started in the world of Theranostics which touched the life of several hundreds of patients from the world over, by one person!

1.3   The Fertilization

When "knowledge" marries a deserving hardworking person, offspring is a benevolent "success". Enriched by his enthusiasm and thirst for knowledge, multiplied by the success of his treatment approaches, Dr. Baum embarked on a journey few would have fathomed or dared to walk the path. It is important to remember that the time frame is roughly 25 years back, when in general in Germany, Nuclear Medicine was more diagnostic than therapeutic. It takes a visionary to do what he did: Dr. Baum left University Hospital in Frankfurt and joined a hospital in the eastern part of Germany. This hospital was so remotely placed in the middle of a jungle in the state of Thueringen, in a small town of 8000 people, that anybody else would have termed this step as insane. Well, people who are in love sometimes get infatuated, and there was no doubt that Dr. Baum was in love with "Theranostics". He needed a "Castle" to build the "Empire of Theranostics" And so came into existence, the Department of Nuclear Medicine at the Zentralklinik Bad Berka, Germany. A "Theranostics Empire" was rising under the governance of Dr. Baum: this empire was destined to lead various first in human Theranostics applications at the global stage.

1.4   Hard Yards

Sometimes it is not easy to appreciate what it takes to start a monumental project in Germany in a non-academic private hospital setting, with no "tax paid" money for research grants. Dr. Baum's tireless, almost inhumane efforts lead to the establishment of a GMP radiopharmacy with fully functional cyclotron, a PET/CT Centre, and 22 bedded radiopharmaceutical therapy ward within a space of 10 years of his joining. During all this time of continuous change in his department, one thing remained constant: his consultation time per patient referred for therapy. All his fellows, residents and attending who have accompanied him during the ward visit or patients have learned a lot from his communication skill and the art of patient consultation. Dr. Baum is methodical, his reports are elegant and as complete as they can ever be. During a personal communication with one other giant in the field of Theranostics, Dr. Helmut Maecke fondly remembers some of the patients' reports which he used to get from Dr. Baum as the best ever.

Methodology is central to science. Similarly, standardized operating procedures (SOP) are essential benchmarks of any Centre of Excellence. Prof. Baum's hand-picked team consisting of some excellent nursing staffs, radiochemists, medical physicists, and senior consultants contributed with great pleasure in writing SOPs for all procedures including PRRT. As his first research fellow, I am privy to the fact that several renowned centers who started doing PRRT in Europe, Asia, and USA have either directly or indirectly used his SOP. In this way, he democratized practical dissemination of knowledge for the ultimate benefit of patients.

Dissemination of knowledge is a great service for the enhancement of science. There was always a long list of researchers, clinicians, physicists, and chemists who wanted to visit Prof. Baum's Centre and profit from the freely available elixir of knowledge. It has never been disclosed before, but due to his open science policy and passion for theranostics, the quality of research in other academic centers around his empire started to increase and patients' advocacy groups became aware of the worthiness of this unique field of nuclear oncology. Hard yards in the field of radiopharmaceutical therapy, which started with PRRT in neuroendocrine tumors, started giving offshoots, slowly but continuously, and soon percolated in other areas of unmet clinical needs in oncology. Patients and their relatives, friends, and colleagues around the world were about to witness the expansion of the field of Theranostics.

1.5 Expansion of the Empire

Success of somatostatin receptor ligand therapy for neuroendocrine tumor patients has to thank few centers in the world, Dr. Baum's Centre was one of them. A passion and dedication for PRRT which started in 1997 took a real big turn when companies like Novartis and Advanced Accelerator Applications (AAA) started taking notice of the novel therapy. Prof. Baum started treating patients from all over the world, including, USA, India, and China, and his ward was always full, performing more than 1000 radiopharmaceutical therapy cycles every year. Managing such patients' data for research purposes was never going to be easy. As early as in 2004, he started thinking about 5, 10, and 15 years of follow-up of patients to generate sufficient data for proving the worthiness of theranostics approach. For that purpose, he developed an Access Databank which contributed to more than 40% of data in some national register studies for NET patients. At the same time, Rotterdam group paved the way to initiate a phase three clinical trial with the support of AAA. Dr. Baum's Centre contributed significantly to the trial and the rest is history. Lu-177 DOTATATE got approved for gastroenteropancreatic neuroendocrine tumor. But this was the beginning of next phase of expansion.

As soon as University Heidelberg, Germany, showed the diagnostic potential of prostate-specific membrane antigen, Dr. Baum was quick enough to grasp its potential and started treating patients with Lu-177 PSMA. His Centre had since then many firsts in the magnificent history of PSMA radioligands therapies, which included the first overall survival and response data published in the Journal of Nuclear Medicine. This was a major breakthrough, both at personal as well as scientific life of Dr. Baum.

Dr. Baum's close observational prowess together with excellent clinical skills made him soon realize that it is not always the dose of radiation which decides response to radiopharmaceutical therapies. This forced him to ask the basic question "why?"

That is when Dr Baum started diving more into the genetic and genomic make up of tumors to understand why some patients respond so quickly and achieve complete remission whereas others continue to progress despite achieving absorbed radiation dose of more than 100 Gy. At the same time, he expanded the use of alpha radiopharmaceutical therapies with Ac-225, as well as novel radioisotopes like Tb-161. One of the hallmarks of all great empires and good governance is that they are not limited to one place only. Embarkment on a new research path necessitated some changes, and change was about to come.

1.6   New Capital

Time is the fiercest competitor of the human race. After having spent more than 20 years in his empire at Bad Berka, it was time to move on. Another place was waiting for him, the "Advanced Center for Radiomolecular Precision Oncology (RPO) at Curanosticum Wiesbaden-Frankfurt, Germany" where he joined as Senior Consultant in 2020. Just like his move from Wolfgang Goethe University Medical Center, Frankfurt/Main to Bad Berka raised skepticism and eye-brows, this move was also seen as a "small step towards retirement". But great minds, dedicated doctors and good teachers never retire. Within an year of joining the Curanosticum, Prof. Baum got his GMP Radiopharmacy and a new PET/CT. Patients followed him from around the Germany and globe to Wiesbaden. Ony capital had changed, but the empire remained.

Teaching and expanding Theranostics worldwide has been Prof. Baum's passion. An academy was needed for this purpose. Dr. Baum's initiative resulted in the formation of International Centers for Precision Oncology (ICPO) Academy as well as the ICPO Scientific Committee. He was expanding fast. Sino-German collaboration was conceptualized. ICPO Academy produced its first "Teaching Module" and started teaching next-generation Theranostics enthusiasts, researchers, physicians, medical physicists, radiochemists, nurses, and technologists. Under the presidentship of Dr. Baum, ICPO Academy is armed to produce next-generation skilled, well-trained "Theranostics Experts". One man's dream and passion are transforming many hundreds of young brain. Hope for cancer patients around the world is increasing and many have to thank Dr. Baum for this.

RICHARD PAUL BAUM, CURRICULUM VITAE

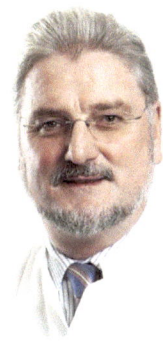

Living Principles: Rerum cognoscere causas and Carpe diem!

<u>Present Title and Affiliation</u>

Senior Consultant, Advanced Center for Radiomolecular Precision Oncology (RPO) at Curanosticum Wiesbaden-Frankfurt, Germany

President of the International Centers for Precision Oncology (ICPO) Academy and Chair of the ICPO Scientific Committee, member Board of Trustees of the ICPO and cofounder

<u>E-mail addresses:</u>
baum@curanosticum.de
richard.baum@icpo.foundation
baumrp@gmail.com

<u>Websites for information:</u>
www.curanosticum.de
www.icpo.foundation
www.linkedin.com/in/richard-p-baum-13045516//

<u>Academic Position</u>

Professor emeritus, Johann Wolfgang Goethe University of Frankfurt/Main, Germany

<u>Academic Titles</u>

Professor Dr. med.

<u>Education/Professional Experience</u>

1974-80	Johannes Gutenberg University, School of Medicine
1980-82	Internship/Residency in Internal Medicine/Cardiology, approbation 6th Nov. 1980
1985	Dr. med., magna cum laude (Dissertation)
1984-88	Fellow, Dept. of Nuclear Medicine Johann Wolfgang Goethe University Medical Center, Frankfurt/Main. Specialist in Nuclear Medicine (Facharzt) Oct. 1988
1990	Associate Professor of Nuclear Medicine, Johann Wolfgang Goethe University, Frankfurt/Main (Habilitation, PhD)
1994	Director, PET Unit, Dept. of Nuclear Medicine Johann Wolfgang Goethe University Medical Center, Frankfurt/Main
1996	Professor of Nuclear Medicine, University of Frankfurt/Main
1997-2019	Chairman and Clinical Director, THERANOSTICS Center for Molecular Radiotherapy and Molecular Imaging (previously Department of Nuclear Medicine, Center for PET/CT), Zentralklinik Bad Berka, Germany
2020-present	Senior Consultant, Advanced Center for Radiomolecular Precision Oncology (RPO) at Curanosticum Wiesbaden-Frankfurt, Germany

Honors and Awards/Service Professional Societies

1986   Board Election, Internatl. Research Group in Immunoscintigraphy/Immunotherapy (IRIST)

1986-   Consultant, International Atomic Energy Agency (IAEA)

1989   Election, President, International Research Group in Immunoscintigraphy and Immunotherapy

1989   Mallinckrodt Award (German Society of Nuclear Medicine)

1991   Election, Advisory Council of the EANM Chief Scientific Investigator of the IAEA

1996   Sharabai Memorial Oration Award, Society of Nuclear Medicine India

1999   EANM Committee Oncology

2001   Annual Lecture, British Nuclear Medicine Society

2003-   „Docente Especial de Professor Invitado" del Inst. Sup. de Ciencias Med. Habana/Cuba

2006   Member of the Executive Committee of the World Radiopharmaceutical Council (WRPTC) of the World Federation of Nuclear Medicine and Biology

2009   Key Note Speaker Canadian Nuclear Medicine Society Invited Lecturer, British Society of Nuclear Medicine for delivering "The Future Lecture", Manchester, UK

2009   Vice President World Association of Radionuclide and Molecular Therapy (WARMTH)

2010   F.Y. Khoo Lectureship and Medal, Academy of Medicine & Singapore Radiological Society

2010   Key Note Speaker Japanese Society of Nuclear Medicine Society (50th Anniversary)

2011   Founding Chair, First Theranostics World Congress, Bad Berka, Germany

2011-   Visiting Professor, FM Medical University (Tandu Hospital, Xi'an, Shaanxi, China

2011   Agasthiar Award by the Indian Society of Nuclear Medicine at the 43rd Annual Conference, Dec. 8, 2011 for "Life Time Contribution to The Field of Nuclear Medicine"

2012   Key Note Speaker Australian New Zealand Society of Nuclear Medicine (ANZSNM) Annual Scientific Meeting, Melbourne, Australia

2012-   Visiting Professor, Medical University Nanjing, China

2013   Co-Chair, Second Theranostics World Congress, Chandigarh, India

2013   Re-election as President of IRIST

2013   President, World Association of Radionuclide and Molecular Therapy (WARMTH)

2014-   Visiting Professor, Medical University Belgrade, Serbia

2014   GLORINET Award (NET Patients Support Group, Germany)

2015   Key Note Speaker, Royal Society of Medicine, London, UK

2015   Honorary Member of the Cuban Society of Oncology, Radiotherapy and Nuclear Medicine

2015   Co-chair, Third Theranostics World Congress, Baltimore, Ml, USA

2016   Editors' Choice Award The Journal of Nuclear Medicine for the three best clinical articles in 2015 (^{68}Ga- and ^{177}Lu-Labeled PSMA I&T: Optimization of a PSMA-Targeted Theranostic Concept and First Proof-of-Concept Human Studies. J Nucl Med. 2015 Aug;56(8):1169-76)

2016   Co-Chair, Fourth Theranostics World Congress, Melbourne, Australia

2017   Appointment by the European Society for Medical Oncology (ESMO) as Faculty Member for the CUP, Endocrine Tumours and Others for the period 2017-2018

2017   Invitation by the SNMMI to present the Henry Wagner, Jr. Lectureship at the Annual Meeting

2017   Visiting Professor invitation to McGill University, Montreal, Quebec

2018   Key Note Speaker, Taiwanese Society of Nuclear Medicine, Taipei, Taiwan

2019   Guest Professor, Peking University Health Science Center, China

2019   Saul Hertz Award (by SNNMI) – highest honor in the field of nuclear medicine therapy)

2019   President, ICPO Academy and Chairman of the Scientific Board

2022   Honorary membership, Society of Nuclear Medicine (Singapore)

2022   Keynote Lecture, WFNMB Congress Kyoto, Japan

2023   Honorary Fellow, Philippine Society of Nuclear Medicine (PSNM)

Memberships in Major Professional Societies

Member of the Society of Nuclear Medicine (SNMMI, USA), the European Association of Nuclear Medicine (EANM), European Society for Medical Oncology (ESMO), European Association for Cancer Research (EACR), Deutsche Krebsgesellschaft (German Cancer Society), World Association of Radionuclide and Molecular Therapy (WARMTH), International Research Group in Immunoscintigraphy and Immunotherapy (IRIST), International Society of Radiolabelled Blood Elements (ISORBE), and many others

Duties:

EANM: 1988 member of the Task Group CURA, Member, JETGURT (1990-1991), 1991 member of the EANM advisory board, 2000 Oncology Committee), Steering Committee Member, European PET Institute of the EANM, Lecturer, European School of Nuclear Medicine

SNMMI: Board Member of the Therapy Center of Excellence, Member of the Publication Committee

Member, Scientific Program Committee (since 1989), Faculty

DGN: 1990 Scientific Secretary of the Annual Congress; Member, Scientific Program Committee

WFNMB: Chairman Oncology Track, World Federation of Nuclear Medicine & Biology (WFNMB) Congress, Melbourne, Australia

WCI (World Council of Isotopes), Chairman of Medical Applications (2012-)

IRIST (International Research Group in Immunoscintigraphy and Immunotherapy), President 1989 and 2013

WARMTH (World Association of Radionuclide and Molecular Therapy), President 2013-2015

Patients' Groups: Scientific Board, Netzwerk Neuroendokrine Tumoren (NeT) e.V. (Germany), CNETS (Canada), CNETS (Singapore), mamazone (Germany)

ICPO (International Centers for Precision Oncology), cofounder, member Board of Trustees (2019-), President of the Academy and Chair of the ICPO Scientific Committee (2019-)

and many others…

Major Current Research Projects

- *THERANOSTICS and Precision Oncology (Personalized Radiomolecular Medicine)*
- *FAP Radio-Ligand Therapy (PTRT) and Tumor Microenvironment*
- *RadioVaccination (Radioligand Therapy and Adaptive Endoradio-Immuno-Therapy)*
- *PSMA Radio-Ligand Therapy (PRLT) of Prostate Cancer:*
- *Peptide-Receptor Radionuclide Therapy (PRRT) of Neuroendocrine Tumors:*

Lu-177, Y-90 and Ac-225 labeled molecules for therapy of malignant neoplasms

- *Individual Dosimetry after PRRT and PRLT*
- *Radioisotope Production*

Molecular Response Measurements in Solid Tumors

Assessment of metabolic and molecular response criteria, development of new software tools for automated, segmented images analysis (BBQ-MIT)

Molecular radiation treatment planning (MRTP)

- *Positron Emission Tomography:*

Total-body PET/CT (Explorer), neuroendocrine tumors, prostate cancer, lung cancer, breast cancer, new peptides for cancer imaging based on Ga-68 conjugates

Editorial and Journal Review Activities

Editorial Board Member

Journal of Nuclear Medicine, European Journal of Nuclear Medicine, Cancer Biotherapy and Radiopharmaceuticals, Quarterly Journal of Nuclear Medicine and Molecular Imaging, Thyroid Research, Clinical and Translational Imaging, Molecular Imaging, Nuclear Medicine and Molecular

Imaging (Korea), American Journal of Nuclear Medicine and Molecular Imaging International Journal of Biological Markers, Tumor Targeting, Radiation Oncology, Nuklearmediziner, Diagnostic Imaging Europe, Polish Journal of Nuclear Medicine, Austin Journal, Medical Oncology, Nuclear Medicine and Radiology Journal, Nuclear Medicine Review, and many others

Referee, Scientific Journals (selection)

Journal of Nuclear Medicine, European Journal of Nuclear Medicine, NuklearMedizin, Nuclear Medicine Communications, Journal of Immunological Methods, European Journal of Immunology, International Journal of Biological Markers, Tumor Targeting, Radiation Oncology, Journal of Cellular Biochemistry, European Radiology, Annals of Oncology, and many others

Publications/Lectures

Statistics

Research GATE H-Index: 73
Research Interest Score: 13,026
Reads: 135.528
Citations: 25,951
Publications: 729

Original Papers (in Peer Reviewed Journals)	739 (listed on Research Gate, 342 listed on PubMed)
Papers in Proceedings Books	>150
Invited Review Articles	>150
Books (Editor)	6
Handbook (Editor)	1
Chapters in Teaching Books	32
Chapters in Handbooks	36
Published Abstracts	>1000
Invited Scientific Lectures	>1000

1st of May 2023

Professor Dr. Richard P. Baum

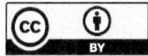

Mariela Agolti and Lucrecia Solari

2.1 Introduction

Immunotherapy is used to improve a patient's immune response to cancer cells, on the basis of the concept of immune surveillance, by activating both cell-mediated and humoral immunity to fight cancer. Immunomodulatory monoclonal antibody therapy utilizes preformed monoclonal antibodies directed against molecular targets to regulate T-cell activation. There are three main mechanisms involved in this kind of therapy: antibodies directed against the programmed death protein 1; (PD-1)/programmed death receptor ligand 1 (PD-L1). The mechanism is to block the PD1 receptor in the lymphocyte, while anti PDL1 is localized in the oncologic cell. The most common anti-PD1 and PDL1 drugs are: nivolumab, pembrolizumab, or atezolizumab.

The other involved mechanism is to block CTLA-4 in the T lymphocyte, and the main drug using this mechanism is imiliprumab (Fig. 2.1).

The number of these drugs are increasing exponentially during the last time and also the indications and combination with chemotherapy and radiotherapy. In below figures, we see the main drugs approved in the USA by FDA for immunotherapy up to December 2018.

M. Agolti (✉) · L. Solari
Centro de Medicina Nuclear de la Clinica Modelo,
Paraná, Entre Ríos, Argentina

V. Prasad (ed.), *Beyond Becquerel and Biology to Precision Radiomolecular Oncology: Festschrift in Honor of Richard P. Baum*, https://doi.org/10.1007/978-3-031-33533-4_2

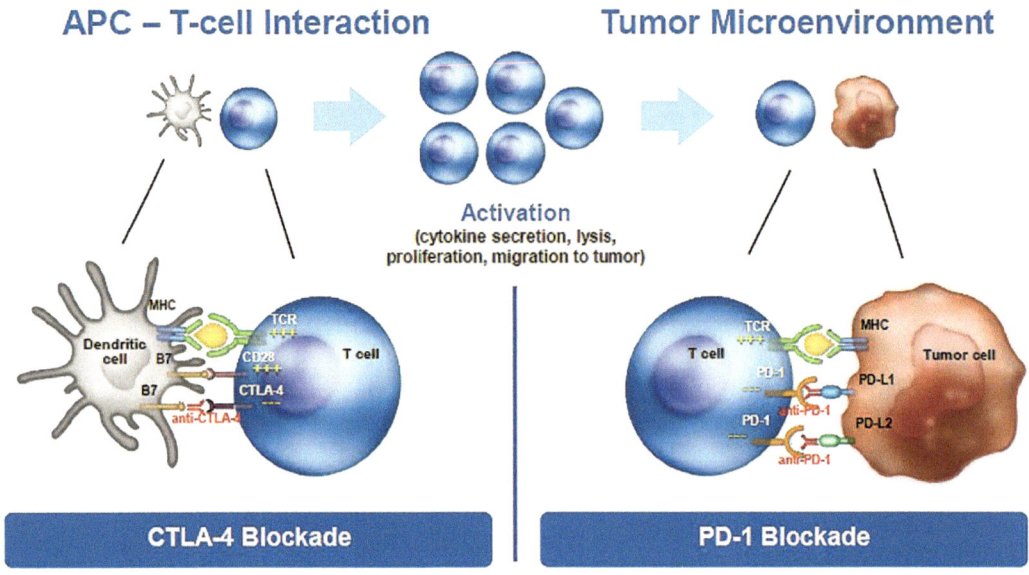

Fig. 2.1 Aleksandra Filipovic, 2017. Mechanism of action of immune-oncology agents. Recovered: https://cancer-world.net/e-grandround/the-role-of-immunotherapy-in-treating-solid-cancers

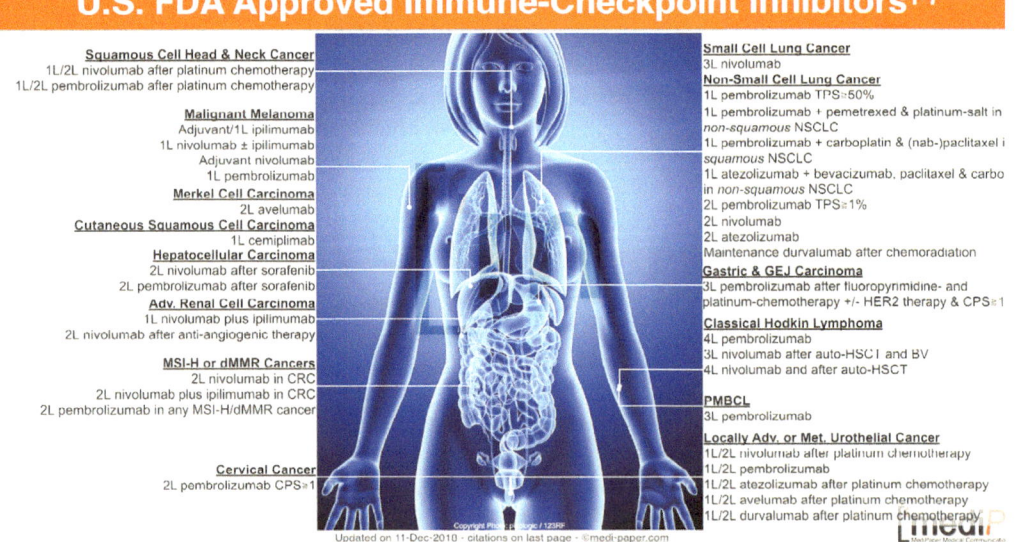

US approved immunotherapies brief overview of the approved immune-checkpoint inhibitors. The information on U.S. FDA approved immune-checkpoint inhibitors is based on the FDA approved package inserts (USPI) and is complete as of 9th March 2019. Countries other than the USA may have variations in approvals as to the overview in this article. Recovered: https://medi-paper.com/us-fda-approved-immune-checkpoint-inhibitors-approved-immunotherapies/

2.2   Patterns of Response

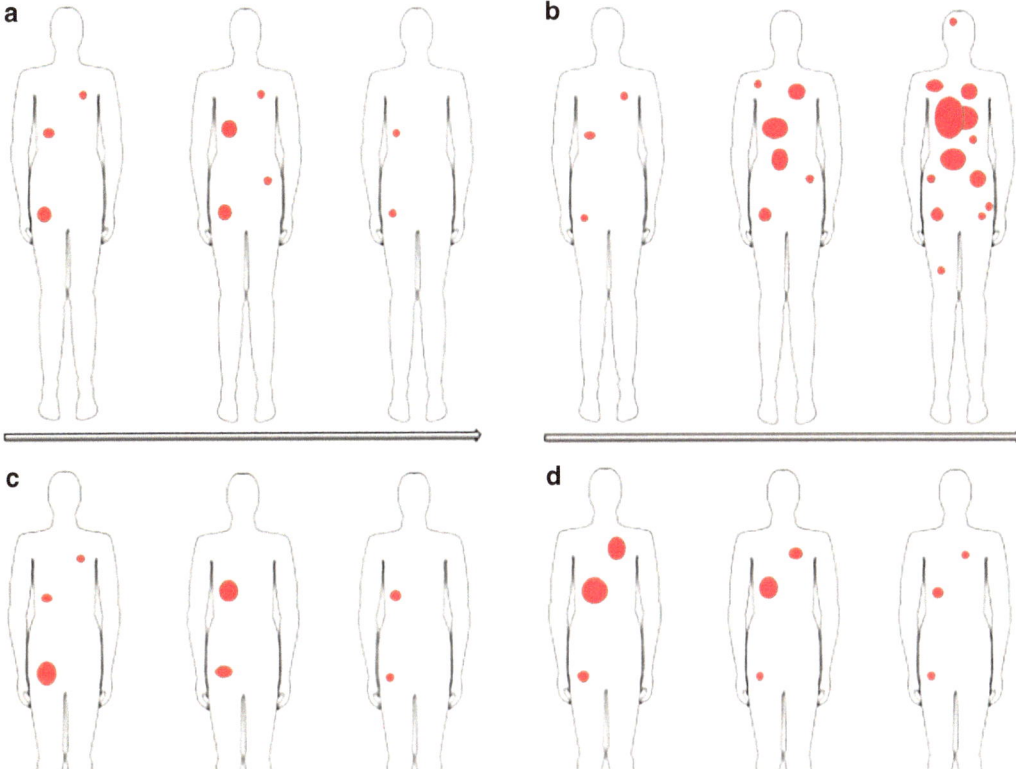

According to the Joint EANM/SNMMI/ANZSNM practice guidelines/procedure standards on recommended use of [18F]FDG PET/CT imaging during immunomodulatory treatments in patients with solid tumor, there are four patterns of interest: (a) pseudoprogression; (b) hyperprogression; (c) dissociated response; (d) durable response.

2.2.1   Pseudoprogression

Interpretative criteria in CT By restoring an efficient antitumor T-cell response, immunotherapy can be followed by pseudoprogression which is defined as an objective response following initial disease progression. For CT (computed tomography) based on these observations, new specific response criteria have been developed, a consensus guideline-iRECIST was developed by the RECIST working group for the use of modified Response Evaluation Criteria in Solid Tumors (RECIST version 1.1) in cancer immunotherapy trials, including immune-related response criteria (irRC); defining the concept of unconfirmed progressive disease (uPD) that may be confirmed by a new radiological evaluation up to 12 weeks later [1]. This concept can only be considered when there is a clear clinical benefit (CB) of the patient meaning that we can see transient enlargement of tumors or the presence of new lesions and after sometime the tumor will respond to therapy. This pseudoprogression is expected in 15% of the patients treated with Ipilimumab and in 10 % of the patients treated with pembrolizumab in NSCLC.

To evaluate response to treatment we have different articles published. Hodi et al. [2] conducted a study-wide analysis and found that 12% of patients (51 of 411 patients) with melanoma treated with pembrolizumab were classified as responders or as having stable disease by immune response criteria [3]. Basically, four different forms of treatment response have been reported.

1. Reduction in tumor size after treatment initiation in comparison to baseline.
2. Initial increase of tumor size and/or new lesions followed by a decrease that meets criteria for partial or complete response in comparison to baseline.
3. Initial increase in tumor size and/or new lesions followed by a stable course.
4. Almost stable tumor size without any significant changes.

This pattern of increasing size is confirmed by biopsy as inflammatory cell infiltrates or necrosis, with subsequent decreased tumor burden.

Interpretative criteria in PET CT An iconic publication in EJNMMI: "FDG PET/CT for assessing tumor response to immunotherapy: Report on the EANM symposium on immune modulation" [4] includes these response criteria including a new category of unconfirmed progression (iUPD) to be confirmed by a further follow-up scan. This can also include identification of new lesions. A good approach that I think is the best approach should consider these categories:

1. Complete metabolic response (CMR) when there are no more detectable tumoral lesions in the 18 FDG PET/CT.
2. Partial metabolic response (PMR) when there is a diminution of 15–25% of basal SUV after the first cycle and of 25% of the basal SUV after 2 cycles.
3. Stable metabolic disease (SMD) decreases in less than 15% in SUVmax values or a decrease in 25% of the uptake after at least 2 cycles.
4. Progressive metabolic disease (PMD) is defined as an increase in SUVmax of $\geq 25\%$ from baseline imaging or the appearance of new metastatic lesions.

A good correlation between metastatic and new hypermetabolic lesions could be the application of the Heidelberg criteria, they describe a sensitivity (correctly predicting CB) of 84% and a specificity (correctly predicting No-CB) of 100%; this group uses functional size (the size of the lesion (in centimeters) as measured on the fused PET/CT images). This cut-off was lower for lesions with larger functional diameters:

(a) Four new lesions of less than 1 cm
(b) three new lesions larger than 1.0 cm
(c) two new lesions larger than 1.5 cm

Although this approach is really practical, this work was done only for ipilimumab in melanoma, necessitating to validation for other drugs [5].

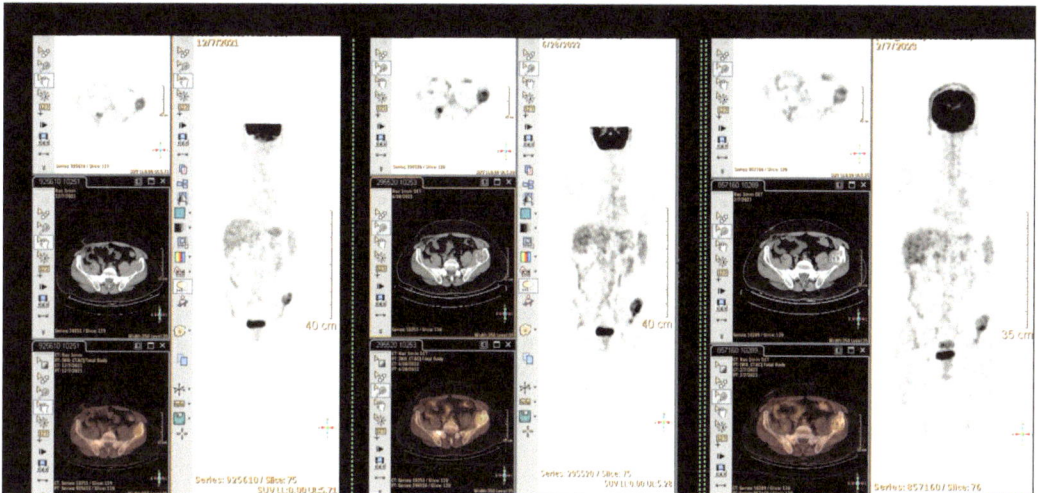

The figure below is of a 45 years old male with renal cell carcinoma treated with immunotherapy, pembrolizumab and axitinib after the first PET/CT. Inital follow-up PET/CT showed increase in uptake and size of the bone metas- tasis with subsequent decrease in uptake after 6 months with good response to treatment. We can also see a new increased uptake lesion in 2nd PET CT located in right sacumo, and other bone images

2.2.2 Hyperprogression

It is defined as an acceleration on tumor growth, there should be a duplication on tumor size in less than 2 months with clinical detrimental of the patients. The incidence is approximately in 15 % of the patients (5 % in patients with less than 65 years old and 20% in older patients). It is more common in patients over 65 treated with anti-PD1/PDL1 and in NSCLC, when this situation is suspected, the treatment should be immediately changed [5, 6].

Hyperprogression was observed in 29% of patients with head and neck cancer treated with antiPD-L1/PD-1 agents and correlated with a shorter PFS. It occurred in 39% of patients with at least a locoregional recurrence and 9% of patients with exclusively distant metastases [6].

Hyperprogressive disease in NSLC was significantly associated with more than 2 metastatic sites before PD-1/PD-L1 inhibitors compared with non-HPD (62.5% vs 42.6%) [7].

Some patients with MDM2 family amplification or EGFR aberrations had poor clinical outcome and significantly increased rate of tumor growth after single-agent checkpoint (PD-1/PD-L1) inhibitors [1].

The biological rationale may be related to that several primary and adaptive mechanisms of resistance to immunotherapy have been described. Response to immunotherapy seems to be conditioned by the infiltration of tumors by activated T-cells, other mechanism could be the absence of tumor recognition by T-cells, due to the lack of immunogenic tumor antigens, much more investigation should be done in this area.

	SUV Max 7/12/21	SUV Max 28/06/22	SUV Max 7/12 /22
sacrum	4,1	7,1	3,1
left iliac crest	4,9	7,1	4,2
9th dorsal vertebrae	4,6	6	4,5
8th rib	4,2	5	2,1
1st lumbar vertebrae	-	4,1	2,1
3rd lumbar vertebrae	-	3,4	3,1
10th dorsal vertebrae	-	4,9	4,5

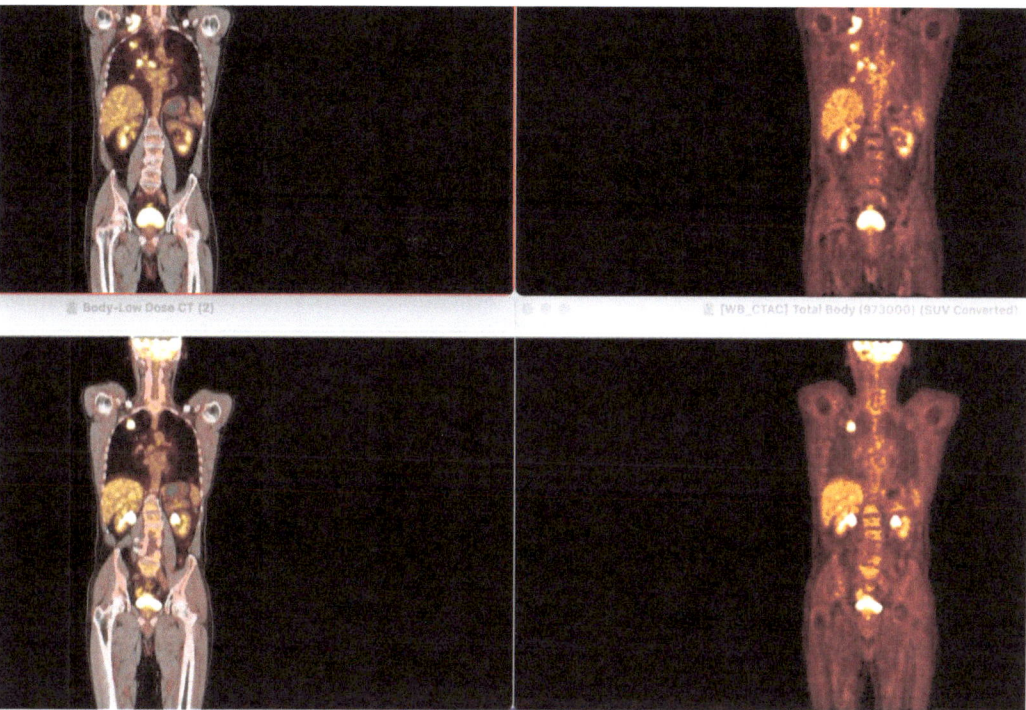

Male 61 years old. Lung carcinoma treated with nivolumab. In the upper image we can see definite progression in comparison with lower images

Even with increasing published data on hyperprogression, its definition is not consensual. Some authors used only radiological criteria, based on the variation of three-dimensional or unidimensional measurements of tumor burden over time to evaluate the rate of tumor growth before and after immunotherapy initiation. However, there is no definite evidence of hyperprogression regarding metabolic imaging, most of the reviewed bibliography is supported on CT findings. In this point PD (progressive disease) is the most practical approach and doubling size in CT, for suspecting hyperprogression on 18F PET CT.

Dissociated Response It is defined by a decrease or stabilization in some tumor sites with a concomitant increase in other sites.

Frequency: up to 10%.

It has better prognosis than homogeneous progression and these patients can benefit from adding other treatments like radiotherapy, surgery, or interventional radiology treatment.

It reflects the heterogeneity of tumors as well as their environment.

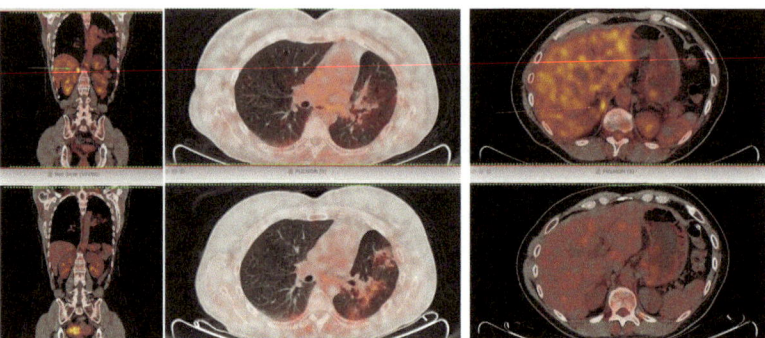

49 y Fem patient with relapsed Lung (NSCL) cancer treated with immunotherapy, after 6 months, we see good response in lung images, but there is a new increased uptake in right suprarenal gland, confirmed by surgery to be a small metastasis of 1.2 cm. Upper file: after 6 months treatment new PET CT

2.2.3 Durable Response

Female 60 y patient with melanoma resected and increased subcutaneous increased uptake (local persistent disease with increased uptake stable during 3 years.

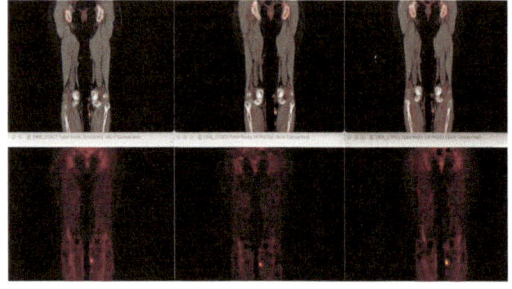

Immunorelated Adverse Effects (irAE) With these new drugs, more often with anti-PD1, there are adverse events related to immune activation, these effects are radically different from adverse effects related to cytotoxic drugs. Their presentation can range from mild and manageable, to severe and life threatening if not recognized early and treated with appropriate measures such as corticosteroids [8].The sensibility of PET CT for their diagnosis is much better than with others imaging modalities (CT), and the rapid identification and quick therapy, with immunosuppressive treatments, such as corticoids or TNFα antibody, improves patients evolution and allows to go on with the treatment [9]. Different irAE are more frequently seen with different drugs, e.g., ipilimumab, the first antibody approved by FDA, is seemingly more common with colitis and hypophysitis, while pneumonitis and thyroiditis are more common with nivolumab and pembrolizumab [10]. According to clinical reports, irAEs may occur at any time and cover multiple organs during the therapy (Fig. 2.2).

Fig. 2.2 irAEs can affect almost each organ system. Most of our organs may be affected with immune-related adverse events (irAEs), such as skin, liver, lung, pituitary, thyroid, gastrointestinal tract, and even the central nervous system. The severity of irAEs can range from mild and self-z. Available: Diagnosis and Management of Immune Related Adverse Events (irAEs) in Cancer Immunotherapy nYi-HeLiua1Xin. https://doi.org/10.1016/j.biopha.2019.109437

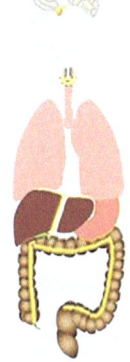

Neural:
- Serious Neurotoxicity (SNT)

Hepatotoxic:
- Hepatitis

Dermatological:
- Rash
- Pruritus

Endocrine:
- Hypophysitis
- Thyropathy

Respiratory:
- Pneumonitis

Gastrointestinal:
- Diarrhea
- Colitiss

Holistic:
- Cytokine release syndrome (CRS)

2.3   Mechanism

The involved mechanisms are suspected to be either a result of the induction of autoimmunity or a proinflammatory state [11]. Other situations related to the primary tumor are also supposed to be involved, like the tumor microenvironment (TME), immune infiltrate, adaptive immune response and neoantigen formation, so there are different incidences reported in different tumors.

Tumor-reactive T cells may modulate the production of antibodies by B cells and lead to antibody-mediated diseases.
Tumor-reactive T cells may modulate the production of antibodies by B cells and lead to antibody-mediated diseases.
Tumor-reactive T cells may modulate the production of antibodies by B cells and lead to antibody-mediated diseases.
Tumor-reactive T cells may modulate the production of antibodies by B cells and lead to antibody-mediated diseases.

Mechanisms underlying irAE

2.4   18FPET CT and irAE

The possibility of identifying inflammatory changes with F-18 FDG PET CT allows us to better diagnose this situation. There are different irAE, and the focus should be on the ones that can be life threatening: 34% of the patients according to Fujii et al. [12]. In "Incidence of immune-related adverse events and its association with treatment outcomes: the MD Anderson Cancer Center experience [11] experienced any grade of irAE, and 80% of them required systemic corticoids, and the most important conclusion related to this article is that this undesirable effects are associated to active immunostatus suggestive of potential clinical benefit for the patients. The incidence of these effects also is different according to the immune mechanism involved, and the frequency is with Anti CDLA 4: 54%; anti-PD1: 26%; anti PDL1: 13%. It is important for the imager to recognize the unique adverse events associated with immunotherapy to guide appropriate treatment and avoid potential imaging pitfalls that could be mistaken for metastatic progression of disease. The patterns that should be considered are:

• **Pneumonitis** is a very rare adverse effect. It is more frequent in the patients with the use of anti-PD-1 than anti-PD-L1 or anti-CTLA-4. But the compounding of PD-1 and CTLA-4 blockade was reported significantly higher frequency of the pulmonary toxicity than either single immune-check-point inhibitors, up to 5–10% at any grade and 2% at 3–4 grade. It involves death risk. There are four radiological CT patterns described for this complication [13]: (1) cryptogenic organizing pneumonia (COP) in 65% of patients. (2) Non-specific interstitial pneumonia in 15% of patients. (3) Hypersensitivity pneumonia in 10% and (4) Acute interstitial pneumonia (AIP)/acute respiratory distress syndrome (ARDS) in 10%. Regarding the **severity of the disease, there are 4 grades**:

– Grade 1 pneumonitis may be assessed by radiographic evidence and another CT may be repeated within 3–4 weeks to focus on the disease progression. Immunotherapy should be discontinued until improvement back to grade 1 or less, and administering prednisone under guidelines is essential for patients with grade 2 of pneumonitis. If pneumonitis is progressing to grade 3 or 4, it is suggested that immunotherapy should be ceased with the appropriate prescription of antibiotics and prednisolone. The median time to onset of pulmonary toxicity after initiation of immunotherapy is 2.3 months and tends to occur earlier in lung cancer (2.1 months) than in melanoma (5.2 months). Even after improvement of pneumonitis, occur with and without PD-1 antibody re-administration [14].

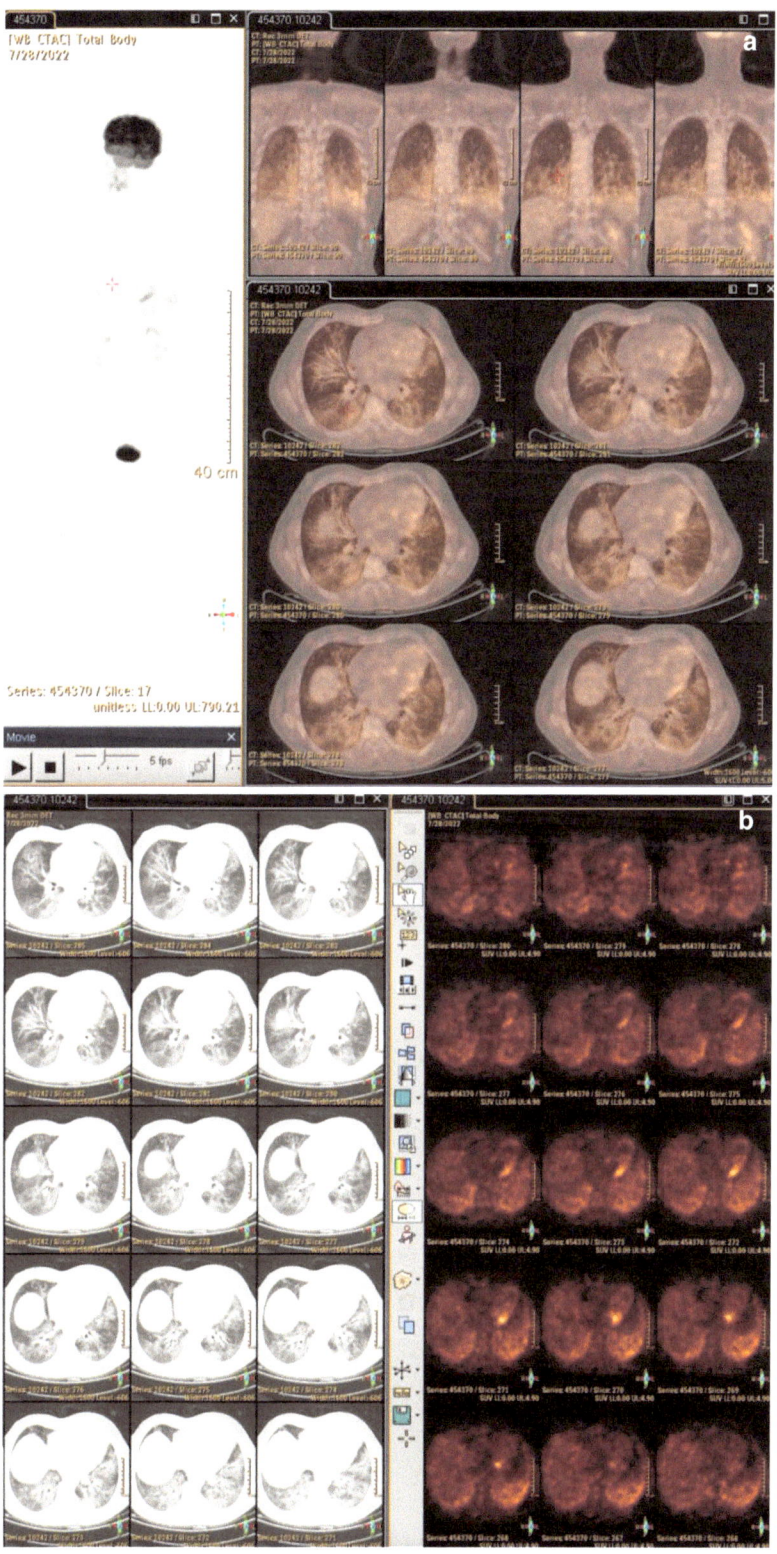

(**a, b**) Acute interstitial pneumonia in a patient treated with immunotherapy

Radiologic Patterns according to irAE	
Ct Patterns	CTFeatures
Acute Interstitial pneumonia /acute respiratory distress Syndrome	-Diffuse ground glass opacities (GGOs) -Consolidation -Lung volume loss
Nonspecific interstitiel Pneumonia	-Subtle GGOsand reticular opacities. -Peripheral and basilar distribution
Cryptogenic organizing pneumonia	-Multifocal consolidation and GGOs -Predominantly peripheral distribution
Hypersensitivity pneumonitis	-Diffuse GGOsand centrilobular nodules -Air trapping

- **Colitis** (more frequently within 6–7 weeks): It is associated to death risk when not treated as soon as diagnosed. Diarrhea and colitis are the main symptoms of gastrointestinal toxicities. In patients receiving ICPis, the incidence of all-grade diarrhea is reported to be higher with anti-CTLA-4 therapy, up to 30%. High grade diarrhea is also reported when nivolumab pluses ipilimumab, with the incidence up to 9%. There are two different patterns associated with Ipilimumab: **Diffuse Pancolitis**, that should be treated with corticoids, and during the diagnosis we should make the differential diagnosis with colitis related to oral hypoglycemics drug: many nuclear medicine departments stop metformin 24 h before 18FDG PET CT to avoid this situation. And **segmental colitis** which is associated with diverticulosis, restricted to a segment of colon and the treatment should include antibiotics [15]. In the CT we can see mesenteric vessel engorgement, bowel wall thickening (> 4mm irrespective of distension), or increased mucosal enhancement contrastct enhanced CT scan [16].

- Male 66 years old renal cancer with pulmonary secundarism. Treated at first with sunitinib no answer, he started therapy with Nivolumab 6 months ago. We can see segmental colitis confirmed with endoscopy. Images courtesy of Dr. Marcelo Claria, jefe de Diagnóstico por imagen Sanatorio Allende. Córdoba-Argentina.

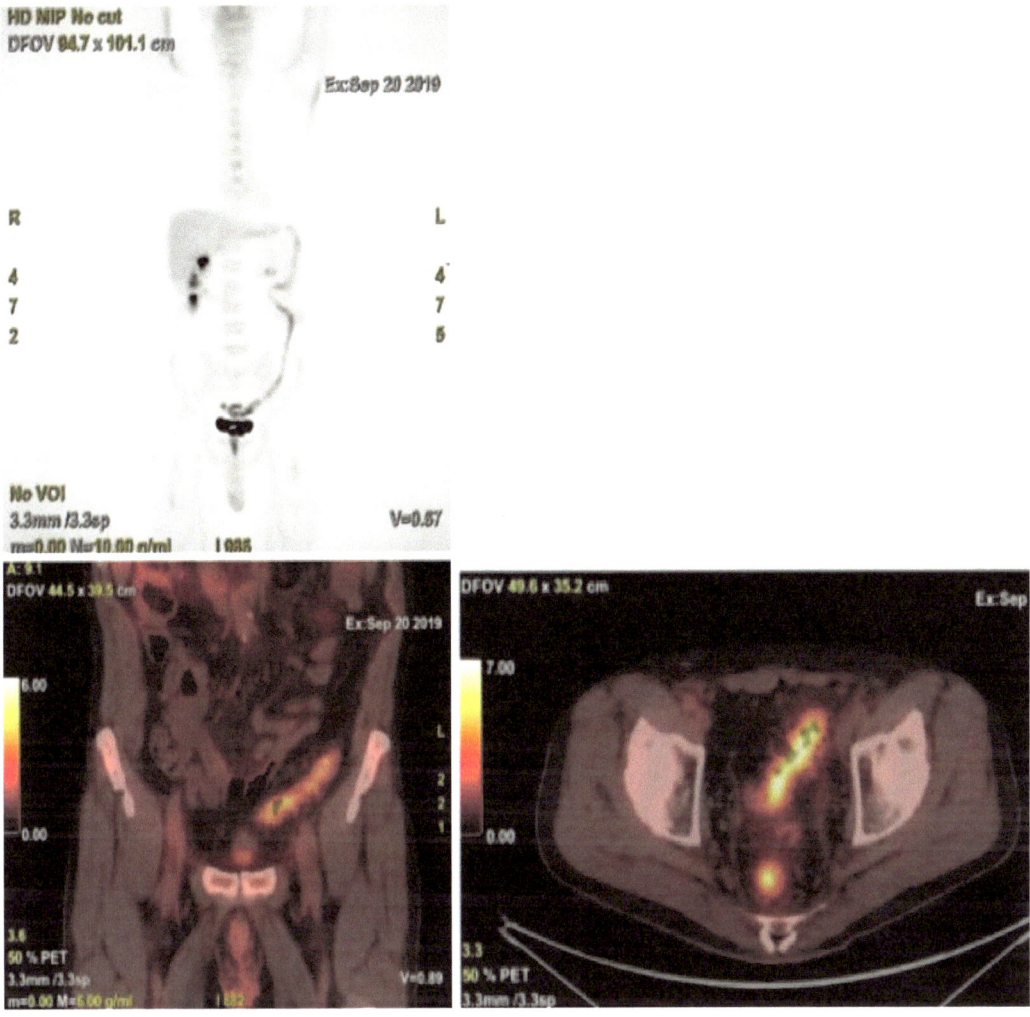

- **Pancolitis** after Pembrolizumab in a patient treated for melanoma. Images courtesy of Dr. Marcelo Claria, jefe de Diagnóstico por imagen Sanatorio Allende. Córdoba-Argentina

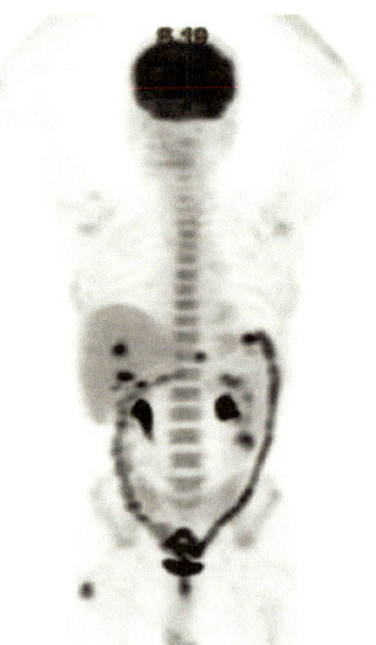 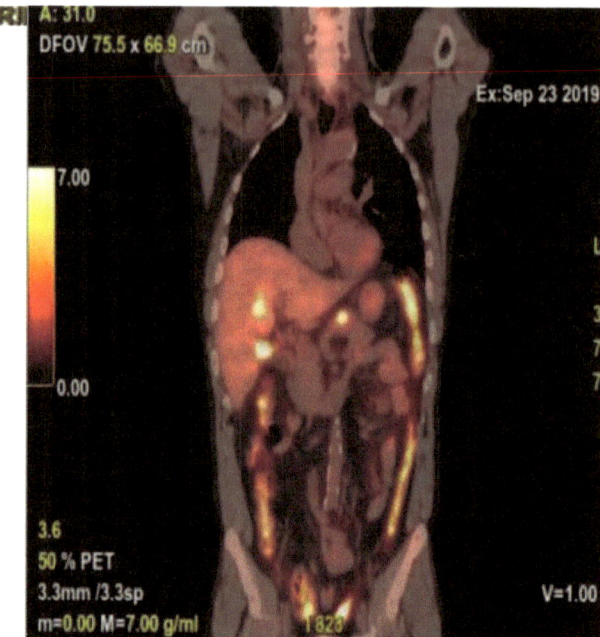

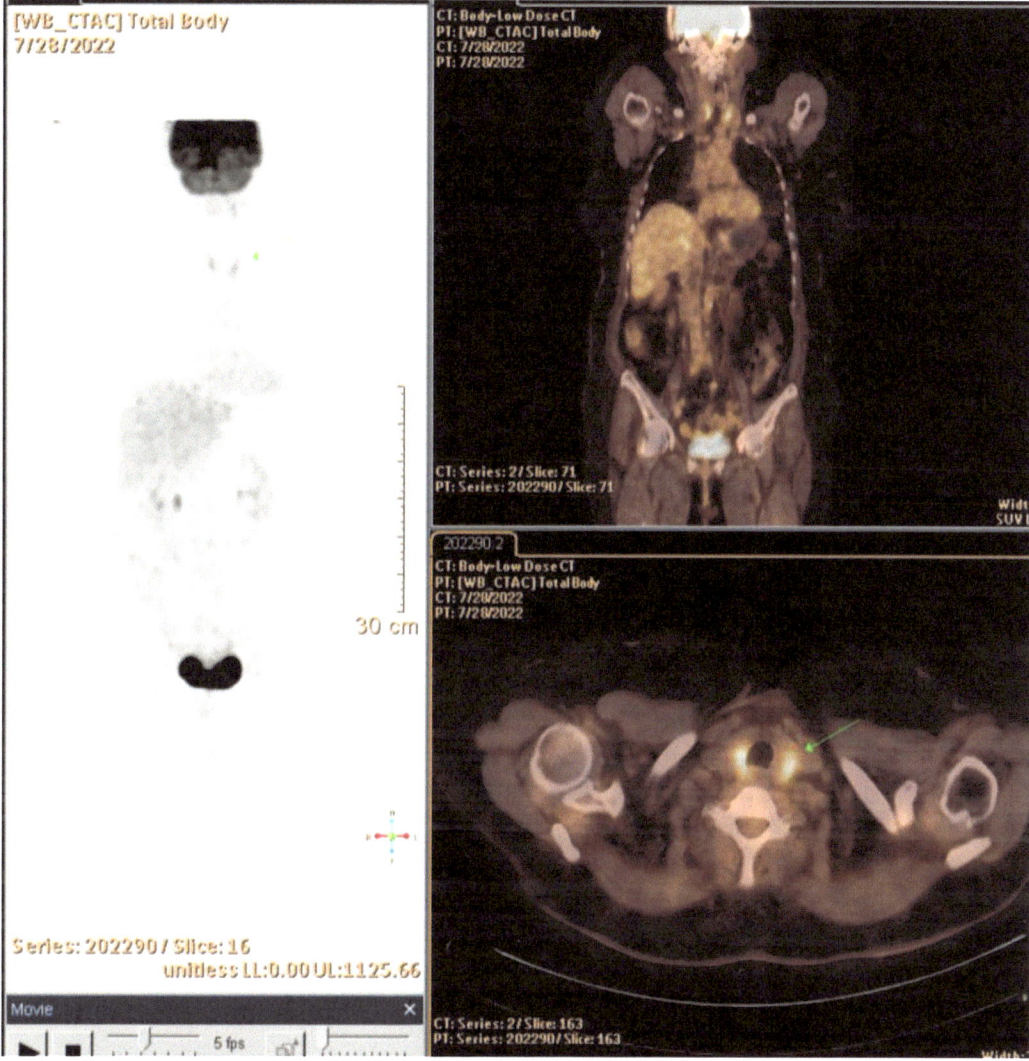

- **Hepatitis**: Starting at 3–9 weeks. The occurrence of hepatitis is less than 6% of patients receiving anti-PD-1 antibodies, about 7% of patients with CTLA-4 therapy and nearly 30% when CTLA-4 and PD-1/PD-L1 blockades are combined [17].
- **Adrenitis**
- **Pancreatitis** (−1%) in this case the typical pattern is increased diffuse uptake with the CT showing mildly enlarged pancreas with no peripancreatic inflammatory changes and rounded pancreatic contours that can be described as having the "sausage" appearance of autoimmune pancreatitis.
- **Hypophysitis** for Aide et al. [4], suggest the importance of starting the PET/CT by including the whole of skull in patients treated with immunotherapy. Also magnetic resonance imaging (MRI) of pituitary gland manifests specific imaging characteristics of enlarged pituitary glands and stalks.
- **Thyroiditis:** Thyropathy mainly includes primary hypothyroidism and hyperthyroidism, among which hypothyroidism is more common. Hypothyroidism generally develops at the 4th week with ipilimumab therapy and the 10th week in patients receiving nivolumab (more frequently between 7 and 20 weeks). It is very important to check that intense uptake deemed to be an immune-related sign was not present on the baseline scan, for example, diffuse thyroid uptake due to Hashimoto disease.

Moreover 18F-FDG PET/CT can predict the development of thyroiditis with subsequent hypothyroidism before laboratory testing after immunotherapy with nivolumab for lung cancer [28].

- Arthritis: shows diffuse periarticular FDG uptake in different joints like shoulders, elbow, wrists, hands, and hips.
- Gastritis
- Myocarditis

There are also other undesirable effects like dermatitis (such as rash, pruritus, and vitiligo but also may appear more serious effects like bullous pemphigoid, scleroderma-like skin changes, and severe cutaneous adverse reactions), fatigue, etc. not able to be recognized by 18FDG PET/CT.

It is also very important to compare previous studies, and to pay special attention to this irAE evolution in terms of metabolic behavior.

Incidence of irAEs with immunotherapeutic agents indicates an active immune status, suggestive of potential clinical benefit to the patient [12].

2.4.1 Therapy-Related Inflammation and Inverse Relation Liver SUV/Spleen SUV [18]

18F-FDG PET can help in the differentiation between progression and therapy-related inflammation, to define inflammatory changes it is important to consider particular patterns of tracer uptake [19]. Metabolic information provided by PET/CT is very important. And some items should be considered in lymph nodes and spleen. There are some important facts to consider regards lymph nodes:

Reactive nodes in the drainage basin of the primary tumor may be seen.

Reaction sarcoidosis like (5–7%) increased FDG uptake in mediastinal/hiliar nodes and may be in spleen. Symmetrical bilateral pattern of uptake in thorax, in enlarged hiliar/mediastinal lymph nodes suggesting sarcoidosis: lambda sign with or without portocaval nodes.

Preservation of fatty hilum.

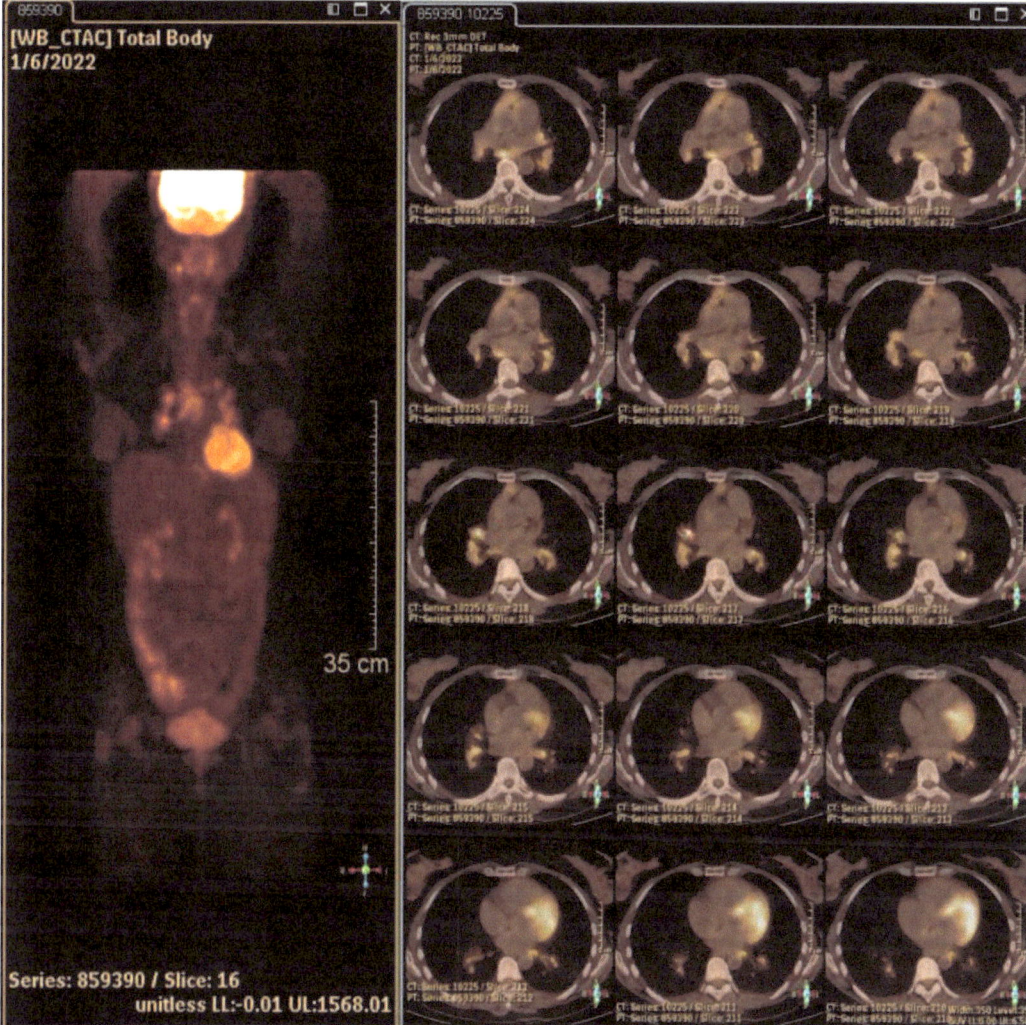

In patients with good evolution with the previous characteristics, FDG avidity can be a marker of immune activation rather than progressive disease [20]

2.5   Conclusion

There are four patterns when reporting 18FDG PET CT after immunotherapy that should be considered (a) pseudoprogression; (b) hyperprogression; (c) dissociated response; (d) durable response. Immune related adverse events should be considered and reported, as well as therapy-related inflammation like sarcoidosis like reaction are immunotherapy-related findings. It is necessary to write a practical guide for reporting these findings in order to harmonize our results.

References

1. Kato S, Goodman A, Walavalkar V, Barkauskas DA, Sharabi A, Kurzrock R. Hyperprogressors after immunotherapy: analysis of genomic alterations associated with accelerated growth rate. Clin Cancer Res. 2017;23(15):4242–50.
2. Hodi F, Ribas A, Daud A, et al. Evaluation of immune-related response criteria (irRC) in patients (pts) with advanced melanoma (MEL) treated with the anti-PD-1 monoclonal antibody MK-3475. J Clin Oncol. 2014;32(15):3006.

3. Kim HK, Baek S-W, Jeong Y, Yang Y, Kwon J, Han HS, An J-Y, Woo CG, Lee O-J, Lee TG, Lee KH. Pseudoprogression presenting as intestinal perforation in non-small cell lung cancer treated with anti-PD-1: a case report. Mol Clin Oncol. 2019;11(2):132–4.

4. Aide N, Hicks RJ, Le Tourneau C, Lheureux S, Fanti S, Lopci E. FDG PET/CT for assessing tumour response to immunotherapy: report on the EANM symposium on immune modulation and recent review of the literature. Eur J Nucl Med Mol Imaging. 2019;46(1):238–50.

5. Champiat S, Dercle L, Ammari S, Massard C, Hollebecque A, Postel-Vinay S, Chaput N, Eggermont A, Marabelle A, Soria J-C, Ferté C. Hyperprogressive disease is a new pattern of progression in cancer patients treated by anti-PD-1/PD-L1. Clin Cancer Res. 2017;23:8.

6. Saâda-Bouzid E, Defaucheux C, Karabajakian A, Coloma VP, Servois V, Paoletti X, Even C, Fayette J, Guigay J, Loirat D, Peyrade F, Alt M, Gal J, Le Tourneau C. Hyperprogression during anti-PD-1/PD-L1 therapy in patients with recurrent and/or metastatic head and neck squamous cell carcinoma. Ann Oncol. 2017;28:7.

7. Ferrara R, Caramella C, Texier M, Audigier Valette C, Tessonnier L, Mezquita L, Lahmar J, Mazieres J, Zalcman G, Brossea S, Westee V, Le Moulec S, Leroy L, Duchemann B, Veillon R, Planchard D, Boucher M, Koscielny S. Hyperprogressive disease in patients with advanced non-small cell lung cancer treated with PD-1/PD-L1 inhibitors or with single-agent. JAMA Oncol. 2018;4:1543–52.

8. Fujii T, Colen RR, Bilen MA, et al. Incidence of immune-related adverse events and its association with treatment outcomes: the MD Anderson Cancer Center experience. Investig New Drugs. 2018;36:638–46. https://doi.org/10.1007/s10637-017-0534-0.

9. Cousin S, Italiano A. Molecular pathways: immune checkpoint. Clin Cancer Res. 2016;22:4550–6.

10. Liu Y-H, Zang X-Y, Wang J-C, Huang S-S, Jiang X, Zhang P. Diagnosis and management of immune related adverse events (irAEs) in cancer immunotherapy. Biomed Pharmacother. 2019;120:109437. https://doi.org/10.1016/j.biopha.2019.109437.

11. Kaufman HL, Kirkwood JM, Hodi FS, Agarwala S, Amatruda T, Bines SD, Clark JI, Curti B, Ernstoff MS, Gajewski T, Gonzalez R, Hyde LJ, Lawson D, Lotze M, Lutzky J, Margolin K, McDermott DF, Morton D, Pavlick A, Richards JM, Sharfman W, Sondak VK, Sosman J. The Society for Immunotherapy of Cancer consensus statement on tumour immunotherapy for the treatment of cutaneous melanoma. Nat Rev Clin Oncol. 2013;10(10):588–9.

12. Fujii T; Colen RR; Bilen MA; Hess KR; Hajjar J; Suarez-Almazor ME; Alshawa A; Hong DS; Tsimberidou A; Janku F; Gong J; Stephen B; Subbiah V; Piha-Paul SA; Fu S; Sharma P; Mendoza T; Patel A; Thirumurthi S; Sheshadri A; Meric-Bernstam. Incidence of immune-related adverse events and its association with treatment outcomes: the MD Anderson Cancer Center experience. Invest New Drugs 2018; 36(4): 636-646. DOI: https://doi.org/10.1007/s10637-017-0534-0

13. Nishino M, Ramaiya NH, Awad MM, Sholl LM, Maattala JA, Taibi M, Hatabu H, Patrick A, Armand PF, Stephen F. PD-1 inhibitor-related pneumonitis in advanced cancer patients: radiographic patterns and clinical course, vol. 22. Clin Cancer Res; 2015. p. 24.

14. Koyauchi T, Inui N, Karayama M, et al. Clinical outcomes of anti-programmed death-1 antibody–related pneumonitis in patients with non-small cell lung cancer. SN Compr Clin Med. 2020;2:570–8. https://doi.org/10.1007/s42399-020-00259-3.

15. Kim KW, Ramaiya NH, Krajewski KM, Shinagare AB, Howard SA, Jagannathan JP, Ibrahim N. Ipilimumab-associated colitis: CT findings. Am J Roentgenol. 2013;200(5):468–74.

16. Tirumani SH, Ramaiya NH, Keraliya A, Bailey ND, Ott PA, Stephen Hodi F, Nishino M. Radiographic profiling of immune-related adverse events in advanced melanoma patients treated with ipilimumab. Cancer Immunol Res. 2015;3(10):1185–92. https://doi.org/10.1158/2326-6066.CIR-15-0102.

17. Reynolds K, Thomas M, Dougan M. Diagnosis and management of hepatitis in patients on checkpoint blockade. Oncologist. 2018;23(9):991–7. https://doi.org/10.1634/theoncologist.2018-0174. Epub 2018 May 31.

18. Anwar H, Sachpekidis C, Winkler J, et al. Absolute number of new lesions on 18F-FDG PET/CT is more predictive of clinical response than SUV changes in metastatic melanoma patients receiving ipilimumab. Eur J Nucl Med Mol Imaging. 2018;45:376–83. https://doi.org/10.1007/s00259-017-3870-6.

19. Sachpekidis C, Anwar H, Winkler J, et al. The role of interim 18F-FDG PET/CT in prediction of response to ipilimumab treatment in metastatic melanoma. Eur J Nucl Med Mol Imaging. 2018;45:1289–96. https://doi.org/10.1007/s00259-018-3972-9.

20. Tsai KK, Pampaloni MH, Hope C, et al. Increased FDG avidity in lymphoid tissue associated with response to combined immune checkpoint blockade. J Immunother Cancer. 2016;4:58. https://doi.org/10.1186/s40425-016-0162-9.

21. Seymour L, Bogaerts J, Perrone A, Ford R, Schwartz L, Mandrekar S. iRECIST: guidelines for response criteria for use in trials testing immunotherapeutics. Lancet Oncol. 2017;18:143–52.

22. Han B, Ryu J, Moon D, Shin M, Kim Y, L. HK. Bone SPECT imaging of vertebral hemangioma correlation with MR imaging and symptoms. Clin Nucl Med. 1995;20(10):916–21.

23. Beer L, Hochmair M, Prosch H. Pitfalls in the radiological response assessment of immunotherapy. Memory. 2018;11(2):138–43.

24. Wolchok JD, Hoos A, O'Day S, Weber JS, Hamid O, Lebbé C, Maio M, Binder M, Bohnsack O, Nichol G, Humphrey R, Hodi FS. Guidelines for the evaluation of immune therapy activity in solid tumors:

immune-related response criteria. Clin Cancer Res. 2009;15(23):7412–20.

25. Geukes Foppen MH, Rozeman EA, van Wilpe S, Postma C, Snaebjornsson P, van Thienen JV, et al. Immune checkpoint inhibition-related colitis: symptoms, endoscopic features, histology and response to management. ESMO Open. 2018;3:e000278.

26. Saada-Bouzid E, Defaucheux C, Karabajakian A, Coloma VP, Servois V, Paoletti X, et al. Hyperprogression during anti-PD-1/PD-L1 therapy in patients with recurrent and/or metastatic head and neck squamous cell carcinoma. Oxford Acad J. 2017;28:1605–11.

27. Anwar H, Sachpekidis C, Winkler J, Kopp-Schneider A, Haberkorn U, Hassel JC, et al. Absolute number of new lesions on (18)F-FDG PET/CT is more predictive of clinical response than SUV changes in metastatic melanoma patients receiving ipilimumab. Eur J Nucl Med Mol Imaging. 2018;45:376–83. https://doi.org/10.1007/s00259-017-3870-6.

28. Wong AN, McArthur GA, Hofman MS, Hicks RJ. The advantages and challenges of using FDG PET/CT for response assessment in melanoma in the era of targeted agents and immunotherapy. Eur J Nucl Med Mol Imaging. 2017;44(1):67–77. https://doi.org/10.1007/s00259-017-3691-7. Epub 2017 Apr 7.

29. Raad RA, Pavlick AC, Friedman K. Ipilimumab-induced hepatitis on 18F-FDG PET/CT in a patient with malignant melanoma. Clin Nucl Med. 2015;40(3):258–9. https://doi.org/10.1097/RLU.0000000000000606.

30. Eshghi N, Garland LL, Nia E, Betancourt R, Krupinski E, Kuo PH. 18F-FDG PET/CT can predict development of thyroiditis due to immunotherapy for lung cancer. J Nucl Med Technol. 2018;46(3):260–4.

31. Evangelista L. Molecular imaging and immunotherapy. Int J Biol Markers. 2020;35(1):37–41. https://doi.org/10.1177/1724600819899099.

32. Lopci E, Hicks RJ, Dimitrakopoulou-Strauss A, Dercle L, Iravani A, Seban RD, Sachpekidis C, Humbert O, Gheysens O, Glaudemans AWJM, Weber W, Wahl RL, Scott AM, Pandit-Taskar N, Aide N. Joint EANM/SNMMI/ANZSNM practice guidelines/procedure standards on recommended use of [18F]FDG PET/CT imaging during immunomodulatory treatments in patients with solid tumors version 1.0. Eur J Nucl Med Mol Imaging. 2022;49(7):2323–41. https://doi.org/10.1007/s00259-022-05780-2. Epub 2022 Apr 4. PMID: 35376991; PMCID: PMC9165250.

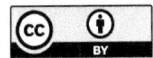

Surgery in Combination with Peptide Receptor Radionuclide Therapy: A Novel Approach for the Treatment of Advanced Neuroendocrine Tumours

Andrea Frilling and Ashley K. Clift

3.1 Introduction

Neuroendocrine tumours (NET)—recently reclassified under the auspices of 'neuroendocrine neoplasms' (NEN)—arise from widely distributed neuroendocrine cells and share the capacity to secrete hormones and vasoactive peptides. They encompass distinct tumour entities with variable clinical behaviour, ranging from indolent to highly aggressive. Most commonly they are seen in the gastro-entero-pancreatic (GEP) [1] and bronchopulmonary tracts [2]. The analysis of large registries demonstrates that NET are steadily increasing in incidence and prevalence, with approximately three- to sevenfold increases in the former over the past three decades, and an estimated prevalence of 35/100,000. In the gastrointestinal tract, NEN are the second most common malignancy after colon cancer [3].

The central management issue of NEN is that at initial diagnosis, lymph node metastases and distant metastases are frequently seen. In a substantial number of patients with initially localised disease, metastases occur later during their clinical course. Depending upon the primary tumour site, 65–95% of NET present with liver metastases [4, 5]. The incidence of hepatic metastases is highest in patients with small bowel NEN (SBNEN) (67–91%) and pancreatic NEN (PanNEN) (28.3–77%) [6, 7], in contrast to patients with well-differentiated appendiceal NEN who display hepatic involvement in under 1% of cases [8] and patients with type I gastric NET or those with small, mainly incidentally discovered rectal NET. In historical series with a very limited spectrum of treatment options, 5-year survival was 13–54% for NEN patients with liver metastases compared with 75–99% for those without hepatic involvement. Experience in Centres of Excellence indicates a 5-year overall survival of 56–83% for metastatic intestinal NEN and 40–60% for pancreatic NEN [9]. In patients with SBNEN, lymph node metastases, in addition to liver metastases, present a therapeutic challenge since they frequently compromise major mesenteric vascularity and encase the mesenteric root, inducing abdominal angina and intestinal ischemia.

A. Frilling (✉) · A. K. Clift
Department of Surgery and Cancer, Imperial College
London, London, UK
e-mail: a.frilling@imperial.ac.uk

© The Author(s) 2024
V. Prasad (ed.), *Beyond Becquerel and Biology to Precision Radiomolecular Oncology: Festschrift in Honor of Richard P. Baum*, https://doi.org/10.1007/978-3-031-33533-4_3

3.2 Molecular Imaging of Neuroendocrine Neoplasms

Molecular functional imaging has evolved into representing the cornerstone in diagnosis, staging, treatment selection, and follow-up of NEN. Scintigraphy with ^{111}In-pentetreotide has almost universally been replaced by hybrid positron emission tomography (PET)/computed tomography (CT) with ^{68}Ga-labeled somatostatin analogues (SSA) in the functional imaging of low-grade (G1) and intermediate-grade (G2) NEN [10–14]. Other PET agents utilised for diagnosis of neuroendocrine disease include ^{18}F-FDG (for G2 and high-grade NEN), ^{18}F-DOPA, ^{11}C-5-HTP, GLP1, ^{64}Cu-SSA and ^{68}Ga-labeled somatostatin receptor antagonists [15]. Hybrid PET/magnetic resonance imaging (MRI) appears to be superior to PET/CT in the staging of liver metastases, utilises the same anatomic imaging modality used as the gold standard for diagnosis and follow-up of neuroendocrine liver metastases [16]. Dual imaging with ^{68}Ga-DOTA and ^{18}F-FDG PET/CT is suggested to be performed in tandem in patients with higher-grade NEN to better capture the known heterogeneity of neuroendocrine disease, or if a clinical course indicates sudden change towards more aggressive tumour behaviour.

Meticulous staging of NEN before planned surgery is critical for optimal patient selection and accurate surgical strategy (Fig. 3.1). ^{68}Ga-DOTA-PET/CT has been shown to provide

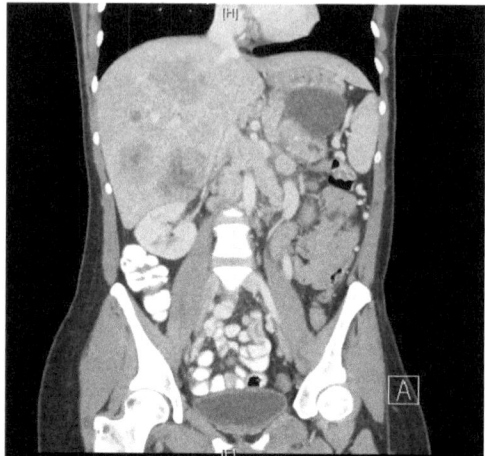
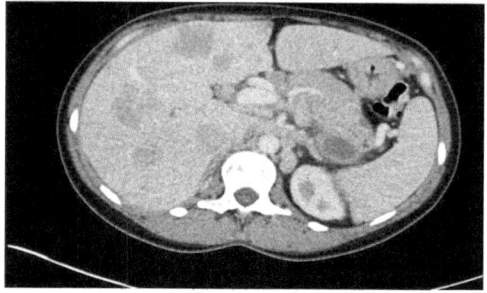

Fig. 3.1 Computed tomography of a patient with a distal pancreatic neuroendocrine neoplasm with liver metastases. This patient underwent distal pancreatectomy for treatment of the primary tumour, followed by peptide receptor radionuclide therapy to treat the liver metastases

additional information and predicate change in initial surgical planning either in terms of change in surgical strategy or switch to non-surgical treatment in up to one-third of patients [17, 18] (Figs. 3.2 and 3.3).

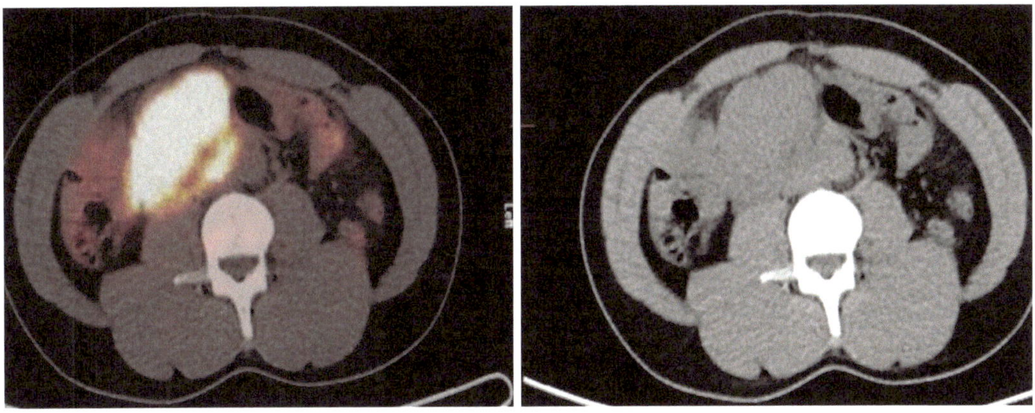

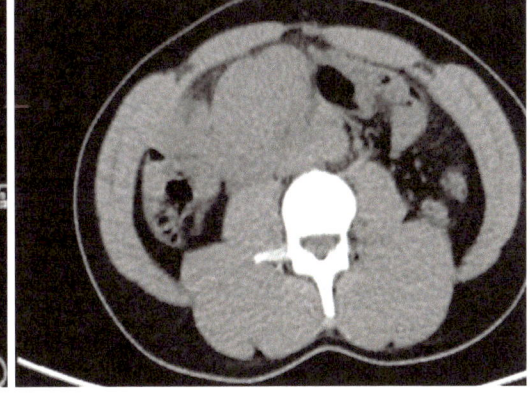

Fig. 3.2 Hybrid positron emission tomography (PET) using ^{68}Ga-DOTATATE with computed tomography (CT) demonstrating a patient with non-resectable, bulky mesenteric metastases from a small intestinal neuroendocrine tumour (well-differentiated, Ki67 1%)

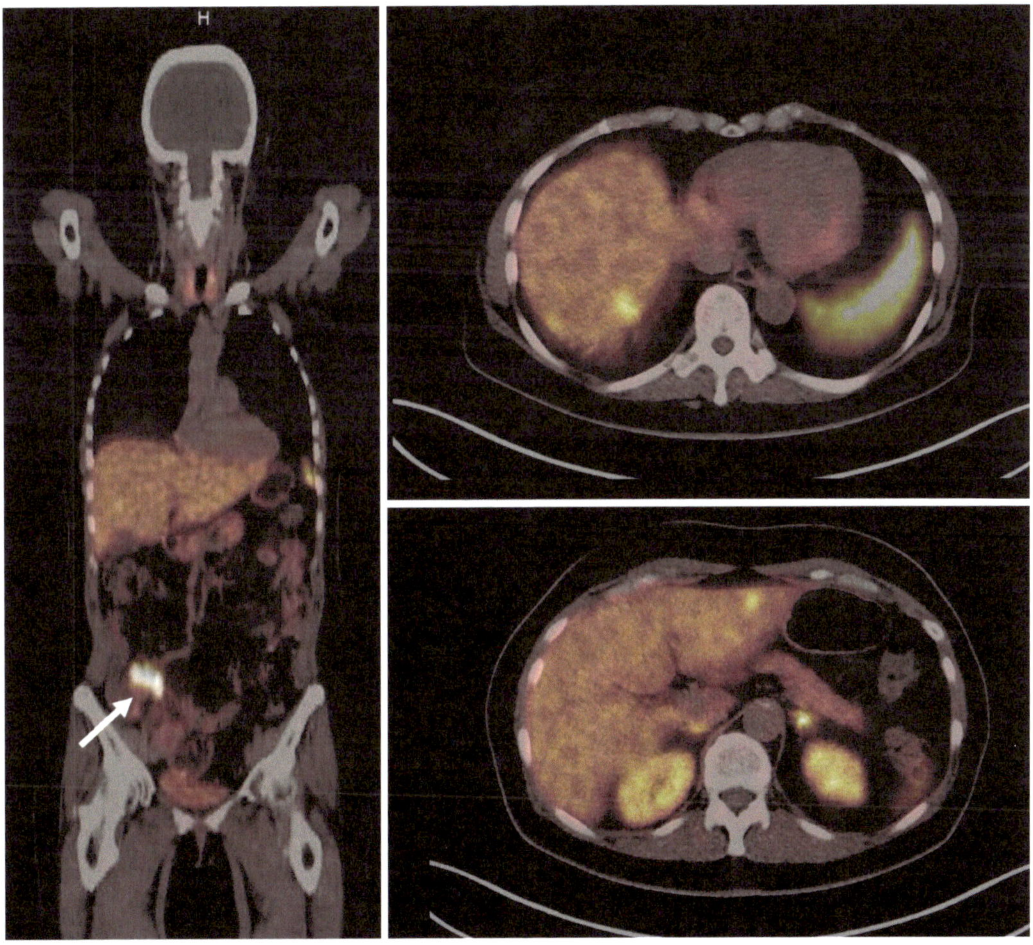

Fig. 3.3 Findings on ^{68}Ga-DOTATATE PET/CT for a patient with a metastatic small intestinal neuroendocrine neoplasm. This patient underwent resection of the primary tumour (arrow, left image), followed by debulking of liver metastases and then peptide receptor radionuclide therapy. Images provided courtesy of Professor Richard P. Baum and Dr D. Kaemmerer

3.3   Surgical Treatment

Radical surgery with an aim to eliminate the primary tumour including loco-regional lymph node metastases and distant metastases (particularly those in the liver) accounts for the first-line treatment of grade 1 and grade 2 NEN where possible. Surgery may also be a valid option for loco-regionally limited grade 3 NEN, especially in tumours with a Ki67 of ≤55% [19]. Although no randomised controlled trials exist comparing surgical versus non-surgical treatment, there is a large body of evidence generated in retrospective series showing that surgery provides the best long-term outcomes [20–22]. The proclivity of NEN to metastasize challenges the surgical approach since surgery as an isolated measure is frequently insufficient. Moreover, it requires embedding within multimodal treatment concepts and the cognisance of the surgeon in dealing with metastasised disease.

All patients with localised SBNET should be considered for curative resection [23, 24]. As up to 50% of SBNET are multifocal and most of them already metastatic to loco-regional lymph nodes at the time of diagnosis, meticulous exploration of the mesentery and palpation of the entire small bowel from Treitz's ligament to caecum is pivotal [25, 26]. A key issue in the resection of SBNEN is not necessarily the primary tumour per se, but the focus on preserving intestinal integrity whilst selectively resecting mesenteric lymph nodes. Extensive en bloc resections should be avoided as they may lead to short bowel syndrome. In case of multifocal focal tumour manifestation, multi-segmental resections might be required.

Patients with functioning PanNEN, irrespective of size, and those with primary tumours >2 cm are candidates for surgery encompassing typical resections including pancreaticoduodenectomy, distal pancreatectomy and total pancreatectomy, or atypical parenchyma-sparing resections [27]. Peripancreatic lymphadenectomy should be considered an integral part of a pancreatic resection with an exception of parenchyma-sparing procedures for benign insulinoma [28]. The indication for surgery and extent of surgery for multiple endocrine neoplasia (MEN)-1-associated PanNEN is a topic of controversial discussion, ranging from a rather conservative observational approach to extensive pancreatic resection [29, 30]. In general, nonfunctioning MEN-1-associated PanNEN smaller than 1 cm can be safely observed whilst tumours >2 cm should be resected. Indication for surgery is present in most of the patients with functioning MEN-1 PanNEN. Conflicting data exist also for small (≤2 cm) (nowadays frequently incidentally discovered) sporadic non-functioning PanNEN in asymptomatic patients. The threshold of ≤2 cm has been shown as a reliable selection criterion for surgical versus observational management in some series, whilst in others lymph node metastases and/or liver metastases were seen also in PanNEN less than 2 cm in size [31, 32]. Tumours causing ductal dilatation and G2/G3 PanNEN, even if below this threshold should be considered for resection [33]. In the future, biopsy-based genetic analysis of the primary tumour and novel preoperative risk scores may guide the decision to resect or to observe. Ki67 ≥3% and location of the tumour in the pancreatic head/uncinate process were shown to be associated with lymph node metastases in 21.4% of <2 cm in size PanNET, compared to 3.4% if Ki67 was <3% and the tumour located in the distal pancreas [34].

The role of resection of the primary tumour in presence of non-resectable LM in asymptomatic SBNEN or PanNEN patients is insufficiently defined. Randomised controlled trials comparing cohorts having primary tumour resection with those who were observed only and underwent surgery if symptoms occurred are lacking. Meta-analyses utilising data from retrospective series however indicate survival benefit for patients who had primary tumour resection in this setting [35]. Resecting an intestinal primary may avoid ileus, bowel obstruction, bleeding and desmoplastic reaction, and it may be associated with survival benefit [36]. For patients with asymptomatic PanNEN with non-resectable liver metastases, the recommendation for pancreatic resection is less convincing and burdened by selection bias. Surgery might be beneficial for younger patients free of comorbidities and tumour locations amenable to less extensive pancreatic resections [33].

The surgical treatment of neuroendocrine liver metastases (NE LM) involves resection with curative intention, cytoreductive surgery, or transplantation procedures [5, 37]. Patients with G1/G2 NEN with limited hepatic disease burden and highly selected patients with G3 tumours with Ki67 of ≤55% may be candidates for liver resection with curative intent. Only about 20% of all patients with NE LM are eligible for complete resection of liver deposits. Resection with curative intent is associated with the most favourable outcomes with a median 1-year, 3-year, 5-year, and 10-year overall survival (OS) rates of 94% (range 79–100%), 83% (range 63–100%), 70.5% (range 31–100%), and 42% (range 0–100%), respectively [38]. The wide range of reported overall survival reflects the importance of accurate patient selection. Whilst OS rates are overall favourable, early hepatic disease recurrence seen in approximately 80% of patients within the first three years following hepatectomy is a major clinical drawback [39]. This transforms liver resection with intended "curative" attempt to a de facto palliative treatment of NE LM, even if complete resection is achieved. Debulking surgery may be offered to patients with advanced G1/G2 NE LM unsuitable for radical hepatectomy, or to patients that are symptomatic either due to hepatic tumour bulk or hormone hypersecretion unresponsive to medical treatment [40]. Patients in whom at least 70% extirpation of tumour burden could be attained by parenchyma-sparing debulking procedures may benefit from surgery despite a rather short median liver progression-free survival of 11 months [41]. Liver transplantation is a generally accepted treatment option for highly selected patients with NE LM [42, 43]. Selection criteria for liver transplantation as defined by Mazzaferro et al. from Milan are: patients with low-grade NEN (with or without clinical symptoms), venous drainage of the primary tumour by the portal venous system, age ≤55 years, ≤50% liver involvement, complete resection of primary tumour and any extrahepatic disease prior to transplantation, and stable disease or disease response of at least 6 months before transplantation [44]. Under strict consideration of these selection criteria, 5-year and 10-year survival of 97.2% and 88.8%, respectively was reported [45]. Despite these impressive results and improvements of immunosuppressive protocols for patients transplanted for oncologic conditions, early disease recurrence remains a major clinical issue.

3.4 Surgery in Combination with Peptide Receptor Radionuclide Therapy

Peptide receptor radionuclide therapy (PRRT) with either ^{90}Y-octreotide or ^{177}Lu-DOTATATE or -DOTATOC was introduced into the treatment of metastasised NET in the early 1990s. Efficacy of PRRT in terms of favourable PFS and OS in NEN patients compared to historical controls has been shown in numerous phase I and II phase studies [46–49] and also prolonged PFS in the recent phase III NETTER-1 trial [50] (for more details please see contributions on peptide receptor radionuclide therapy in this Festschrift). The combination of surgical and medical-targeted therapeutic strategies within multimodal concepts offers an attractive possibility for long-term disease control by comprehensively eliminating macro- and microscopic neuroendocrine disease.

The combination of surgery and PRRT can be used in various clinical scenarios; (a) in neoadjuvant settings in patients with initially unresectable or borderline resectable NEN, (b) in adjuvant settings to minimise the risk of disease recurrence after radical surgery, (c) in palliative settings for treatment of remaining non-resectable disease after surgery, (d) as bridging prior to transplantation, or (e) as an upfront strategy to enhance the efficacy of PRRT by resecting the primary tumour. Such novel concepts have not yet been widely adopted and are mostly limited to single centres with interest and expertise in both advanced surgical procedures and theranostics.

In the first case reports, neoadjuvant Yttrium-90 (^{90}Y) DOTA-PRRT was shown to effectively down-stage initially unresectable NEN including those originating from midgut [51], pancreas [52], rectum [53] and stomach [54]. The concept of staged surgery with neoadjuvant ^{90}Y DOTA-PRRT has also been suggested for initially unresectable neuroendocrine liver metastases in case reports [55] and in small series [56]. In a Polish series of six patients with unresectable NEN, resection was achieved in two patients after tumour size reduction induced by PRRT [51]. In an Italian series comparing postoperative outcomes in patients with resectable/potentially resectable pancreatic NEN deemed at high risk of recurrence treated with or without neoadjuvant PRRT ($n = 23$ in each group), the incidence of nodal metastases was significantly lower in the PRRT group, and the PFS was significantly longer in the neoadjuvant group compared to the upfront surgery group [57]. Of interest, the risk of pancreatic fistula was lower in the neoadjuvant group compared to the group of patients who underwent upfront surgery. Most likely PRRT induces fibrosis which is known to reduce the risk of developing of pancreatic fistula [58]. A recent study comparing histopathological and immunophenotypic changes in pancreatic NEN after neoadjuvant PRRT revealed that neoadjuvant PRRT is associated with reduced tumour diameter, an increased percentage of stroma, preserved somatostatin receptor subtype 2A expression in most of the cases, and an increased CD163+ M2-polarised macrophage density [59]. Although the body of surgical data in NEN patients who underwent neoadjuvant PRRT is still scarce, postoperative complications do not occur more frequently than in not pre-treated patients. Peptide receptor radionuclide therapy has also a role as a bridging/downstaging procedure prior to liver or intestinal transplantation with an aim to stabilise macroscopical disease and target micrometastases [60]. To maximise the outcomes of neoadjuvant treatment for pancreatic neuroendocrine tumours, combined chemotherapy (Capecitabine/Temozolamide) and PRRT (chemo-PRRT) regimens have been brought into discussion [61].

Resection of the primary tumour in asymptomatic NET patients with unresectable distant metastases is a matter of ongoing debate [62–64]. In contrast, surgery for elimination of locoregional and/or debulking of distant disease followed by PRRT for remaining non-resectable distant metastases appears as a generally accepted approach in patients symptomatic due to local tumour effect [65]. Particularly those with small bowel NEN who are at risk of developing intestinal obstruction, bleeding, and desmoplastic mesenteric and patients with large pancreatic NEN at risk for significant local stomach and superior mesenteric vein compression [66] may benefit from this approach.

Recently, upfront locoregional primary tumour resection has been proposed in patients considered for peptide receptor radionuclide therapy. In a study reported by Bertani et al., patients who underwent upfront surgery showed higher stabilisation or objective response after PRRT and better median PFS (70 vs. 30 months) and OS (112 vs. 65 months) compared to patients who underwent solely PRRT [67]. Similar experience was reported by Kaemmerer et al. who demonstrated prolonged OS in patients who had primary tumour resected prior to PRRT [68].

3.5   Conclusions

Although surgery offers the best chance of disease cure, given the clinical challenges presented by the oft metastatic stage of NEN at initial diagnosis, this cannot be realised for many patients. Therefore, embedding surgery within a multimodal treatment concept alongside PRRT and driven by theranostic principles represents a novel approach that targets macro- and microdisease that may offer genuine advance in disease control. The combination of surgery and PRRT has only been reported in specialist centres with promising results from small series, but ideally a randomised controlled trial comparing neoadjuvant PRRT versus adjuvant PRRT versus PRRT alone is required to definitively assess this interesting therapeutic strategy. It is incumbent upon the NEN medical community to evaluate such novel treatment combinations to engender a divergence from a single modality focus that is often observed.

Conflict of Interest Both authors report that they have no conflicts to declare.

References

1. Clift AK, Kidd M, Bodei L, Toumpanakis C, Baum RP, Oberg K, et al. Neuroendocrine neoplasms of the small bowel and pancreas. Neuroendocrinology. 2019;110(6):444–76.
2. Fraenkel M, Faggiano A, Valk GD. Epidemiology of neuroendocrine tumors. Front Horm Res. 2015;44:1–23.
3. Dasari A, Shen C, Halperin D, Zhao B, Zhou S, Xu Y, et al. Trends in the incidence, prevalence, and survival outcomes in patients with neuroendocrine tumors in the United States. JAMA Oncol. 2017;3(10):1335–42.
4. Riihimäki M, Hemminki A, Sundquist K, Sundquist J, Hemminki K. The epidemiology of metastases in neuroendocrine tumors. Int J Cancer. 2016;139(12):2679–86.
5. Frilling A, Modlin IM, Kidd M, Russell C, Breitenstein S, Salem R, et al. Recommendations for management of patients with neuroendocrine liver metastases. Lancet Oncol. 2014;15(1):e8–21.
6. Panzuto F, Boninsegna L, Fazio N, Campana D, Pia Brizzi M, Capurso G, et al. Metastatic and locally advanced pancreatic endocrine carcinomas: analysis of factors associated with disease progression. J Clin Oncol. 2011;29(17):2372–7.
7. Miller HC, Drymousis P, Flora R, Goldin R, Spalding D, Frilling A. Role of Ki-67 proliferation index in the assessment of patients with neuroendocrine neoplasias regarding the stage of disease. World J Surg. 2014;38(6):1353–61.
8. Pawa N, Clift AK, Osmani H, Drymousis P, Cichock A, Flora R, et al. Surgical management of patients with neuroendocrine neoplasms of the appendix: appendectomy or more? Neuroendocrinology. 2017;106(3):242–51.
9. Pavel M, Baudin E, Couvelard A, Krenning E, Öberg K, Steinmüller T, et al. ENETS consensus guidelines for the management of patients with liver and other distant metastases from neuroendocrine neoplasms of foregut, midgut, hindgut, and unknown primary. Neuroendocrinology. 2012;95(2):157–76.
10. Sundin A, Arnold R, Baudin E, Cwikla JB, Eriksson B, Fanti S, et al. ENETS consensus guidelines for the standards of care in neuroendocrine tumors: radiological, nuclear medicine and hybrid imaging. Neuroendocrinology. 2017;105(3):212–44.
11. Deppen SA, Blume J, Bobbey AJ, Shah C, Graham MM, Lee P, et al. 68Ga-DOTATATE compared with 111In-DTPA-octreotide and conventional imaging for pulmonary and gastroenteropancreatic neuroendocrine tumors: a systematic review and meta-analysis. J Nucl Med. 2016;57(6):872–8.
12. Sadowski SM, Neychev V, Millo C, Shih J, Nilubol N, Herscovitch P, et al. Prospective study of 68Ga-DOTATATE positron emission tomography/computed tomography for detecting gastro-enteropancreatic neuroendocrine tumors and unknown primary sites. J Clin Oncol. 2016;34(6):588–97.
13. Hope TA, Bergsland EK, Bozkurt MF, Graham M, Heaney AP, Herrmann K, et al. Appropriate use criteria for somatostatin receptor PET imaging in neuroendocrine tumors. J Nucl Med. 2018;59(1):66–74.
14. Kulkarni HR, Baum RP. Theranostics with Ga-68 somatostatin receptor PET/CT: Monitoring response to peptide receptor radionuclide therapy. PET Clin. 2014;9(1):91–7.
15. Ito T, Jensen RT. Molecular imaging in neuroendocrine tumors: recent advances, controversies, unresolved issues, and roles in management. Curr Opin Endocrinol Diabetes Obes. 2017;24(1):15–24.
16. Hope TA, Pampaloni MH, Nakakura E, VanBrocklin H, Slater J, Jivan S, et al. Simultaneous (68) Ga-DOTA-TOC PET/MRI with gadoxetate disodium in patients with neuroendocrine tumor. Abdom Imaging. 2015;40(6):1432–40.
17. Ilhan H, Fendler WP, Cyran CC, Spitzweg C, Auernhammer CJ, Gildehaus FJ, et al. Impact of 68Ga-DOTATATE PET/CT on the surgical management of primary neuroendocrine tumors of the pancreas or ileum. Ann Surg Oncol. 2015;22(1):164–71.
18. Frilling A, Sotiropoulos GC, Radtke A, Malago M, Bockisch A, Kuehl H, et al. The impact of 68Ga-DOTATOC positron emission tomography/computed tomography on the multimodal management of patients with neuroendocrine tumors. Ann Surg. 2010;252(5):850–6.
19. Merola E, Rinke A, Partelli S, Gress TM, Andreasi V, Kollár A, et al. Surgery with radical intent: is there an indication for G3 neuroendocrine neoplasms? Ann Surg Oncol. 2020;27(5):1348–55.
20. Falconi M, Eriksson B, Kaltsas G, Bartsch DK, Capdevila J, Caplin M, et al. ENETS consensus guidelines update for the management of patients with functional pancreatic neuroendocrine tumors and non-functional pancreatic neuroendocrine tumors. Neuroendocrinology. 2016;103(2):153–71.
21. Niederle B, Pape UF, Costa F, Gross D, Kelestimur F, Knigge U, et al. ENETS consensus guidelines update for neuroendocrine neoplasms of the jejunum and ileum. Neuroendocrinology. 2016;103(2):125–38.
22. Fairweather M, Swanson R, Wang J, Brais LK, Dutton T, Kulke MH, et al. Management of neuroendocrine tumor liver metastases: long-term outcomes and prognostic factors from a large prospective database. Ann Surg Oncol. 2017;24(8):2319–25.

23. Larouche V, Akirov A, Alshehri S, Ezzat S. Management of small bowel neuroendocrine tumors. Cancer. 2019;11(9):1395.

24. Pasquer A, Walter T, Hervieu V, Forestier J, Scoazec J-Y, Lombard-Bohas C, et al. Surgical management of small bowel neuroendocrine tumors: specific requirements and their impact on staging and prognosis. Ann Surg Oncol. 2015;22(3):742–9.

25. Gangi A, Siegel E, Barmparas G, Lo S, Jamil LH, Hendifar A, et al. Multifocality in small bowel neuroendocrine tumors. J Gastrointest Surg. 2018;22(2):303–9.

26. Lardière-Deguelte S, de Mestier L, Appéré F, Vullierme M-P, Zappa M, Hoeffel C, et al. Toward a preoperative classification of lymph node metastases in patients with small intestinal neuroendocrine tumors in the era of intestinal-sparing surgery. Neuroendocrinology. 2016;103(5):552–9.

27. Maurizi A, Partelli S, Falconi M. Pancreatic surgery. Front Horm Res. 2015;44:139–48.

28. Lopez-Aguiar AG, Zaidi MY, Beal EW, Dillhoff M, Cannon JGD, Poultsides GA, et al. Defining the role of lymphadenectomy for pancreatic neuroendocrine tumors: an eight-institution study of 695 patients from the US Neuroendocrine Tumor Study Group. Ann Surg Oncol. 2019;26(8):2517–24.

29. Norton JA, Jensen RT. Resolved and unresolved controversies in the surgical management of patients with Zollinger-Ellison syndrome. Ann Surg. 2004;240(5):757–73.

30. Triponez F, Sadowski SM, Pattou F, Cardot-Bauters C, Mirallié E, Le Bras M, et al. Long-term follow-up of MEN1 patients who do not have initial surgery for small ≤2 cm nonfunctioning pancreatic neuroendocrine tumors, an AFCE and GTE study: Association Francophone de Chirurgie Endocrinienne & Groupe d'Etude des Tumeurs Endocrines. Ann Surg. 2018;268(1):158–64.

31. Chivukula SV, Tierney JF, Hertl M, Poirier J, Keutgen XM. Operative resection in early stage pancreatic neuroendocrine tumors in the United States: are we over- or undertreating patients? Surgery. 2020;167(1):180–6.

32. Finkelstein P, Sharma R, Picado O, Gadde R, Stuart H, Ripat C, et al. Pancreatic neuroendocrine tumors (panNETs): analysis of overall survival of nonsurgical management versus surgical resection. J Gastrointest Surg. 2017;21(5):855–66.

33. Sallinen VJ, Le Large TTY, Tieftrunk E, Galeev S, Kovalenko Z, Haugvik SP, et al. Prognosis of sporadic resected small (≤2 cm) nonfunctional pancreatic neuroendocrine tumors – a multi-institutional study. HPB. 2018;20(3):251–9.

34. Lopez-Aguiar AG, Ethun CG, Zaidi MY, Rocha FG, Poultsides GA, Dillhoff M, et al. The conundrum of < 2-cm pancreatic neuroendocrine tumors: a preoperative risk score to predict lymph node metastases and guide surgical management. Surgery. 2019;166(1):15–21.

35. Almond LM, Hodson J, Ford SJ, Gourevitch D, Roberts KJ, Shah T, et al. Role of palliative resection of the primary tumour in advanced pancreatic and small intestinal neuroendocrine tumours: a systematic review and meta-analysis. Eur J Surg Oncol. 2017;43(10):1808–15.

36. Capurso G, Rinzivillo M, Bettini R, Boninsegna L, Fave GD, Falconi M. Systematic review of resection of primary midgut carcinoid tumour in patients with unresectable liver metastases. Br J Surg. 2012;99(11):1480–6.

37. Frilling A, Clift AK. Surgical approaches to the management of neuroendocrine liver metastases. Endocr Metab Clin N Am. 2018;47(3):627–43.

38. Saxena A, Chua TC, Perera M, Chu F, Morris DL. Surgical resection of hepatic metastases from neuroendocrine neoplasms: a systematic review. Surg Oncol. 2012;21(3):e131–41.

39. Mayo SC, de Jong MC, Pulitano C, Clary BM, Reddy SK, Gamblin TC, et al. Surgical management of hepatic neuroendocrine tumor metastasis: results from an international multi-institutional analysis. Ann Surg Oncol. 2010;17(12):3129–36.

40. Osborne DA, Zervos EE, Strosberg J, Strosberg J, Boe BA, Malafa M, et al. Improved outcome with cytoreduction versus embolization for symptomatic hepatic metastases of carcinoid and neuroendocrine tumors. Ann Surg Oncol. 2006;13(4):572–81.

41. Morgan RE, Pommier SJ, Pommier RF. Expanded criteria for debulking of liver metastasis also apply to pancreatic neuroendocrine tumors. Surgery. 2018;163(1):218–25.

42. Fan ST, Le Treut YP, Mazzaferro V, Burroughs AK, Olausson M, Breitenstein S, et al. Liver transplantation for neuroendocrine tumour liver metastases. HPB. 2015;17(1):23–8.

43. Moris D, Tsilimigras DI, Ntanasis-Stathopoulos I, Beal EW, Felekouras E, Vernadakis S, et al. Liver transplantation in patients with liver metastases from neuroendocrine tumors: a systematic review. Surgery. 2017;162(3):525–36.

44. Mazzaferro V, Pulvirenti A, Coppa J. Neuroendocrine tumors metastatic to the liver: how to select patients for liver transplantation? J Hepatol. 2007;47(4):460–6.

45. Mazzaferro V, Sposito C, Coppa J, Miceli R, Bhoori S, Bongini M, et al. The long-term benefit of liver transplantation for hepatic metastases from neuroendocrine tumors. Am J Transplant. 2016;16(10):2892–902.

46. Bodei L, Kwekkeboom DJ, Kidd M, Modlin IM, Krenning EP. Radiolabeled somatostatin analogue therapy of gastroenteropancreatic cancer. Semin Nucl Med. 2016;46(3):225–38.

47. Brabander T, van der Zwan WA, Teunissen JJM, Kam BLR, Feelders RA, de Herder WW, et al. Long-term efficacy, survival, and safety of [177Lu-DOTA0,Tyr3] octreotate in patients with gastroenteropancreatic and bronchial neuroendocrine tumors. Clin Cancer Res. 2017;23(16):4617–24.

48. Baum RP, Kulkarni HR, Singh A, Kaemmerer D, Mueller D, Prasad V, et al. Results and adverse events of personalized peptide receptor radionuclide therapy with 90-Yttrium and 177-Lutetium in 1048 patients with neuroendocrine neoplasms. Oncotarget. 2018;9(24):16932–50.

49. Sabet A, Dautzenberg K, Haslerud T, Aouf A, Sabet A, Simon B, et al. Specific efficacy of peptide receptor radionuclide therapy with (177) Lu-octreotate in advanced neuroendocrine tumours of the small intestine. Eur J Nucl Med Mol Imaging. 2015;42(8):1238–46.

50. Strosberg J, El-Haddad G, Wolin E, Hendifar A, Yao J, Chasen B, et al. Phase 3 trial of 177Lu-dotatate for midgut neuroendocrine tumors. N Engl J Med. 2017;376(2):125–35.

51. Sowa-Staszczak A, Pach D, Chrzan R, Trofimiuk M, Stefańska A, Tomaszuk M, et al. Peptide receptor radionuclide therapy as a potential tool for neoadjuvant therapy in patients with inoperable neuroendocrine tumours (NETs). Eur J Nucl Med Mol Imaging. 2011;38(9):1669–74.

52. Kaemmerer D, Prasad V, Daffner W, Hörsch D, Klöppel G, Hommann M, et al. Neoadjuvant peptide receptor radionuclide therapy for an inoperable neuroendocrine pancreatic tumor. World J Gastroenterol. 2009;15(46):5867–70.

53. Ryan J, Akhurst T, Lynch AC, Michael M, Heriot AG. Neoadjuvant 90Yttrium peptide receptor radionuclide therapy for advanced rectal neuroendocrine tumour: a case report. ANZ J Surg. 2017;87(1–2):92–3.

54. Schmidt MC, Uhrhan K, Fischer T, Schmitz S, Markiefka B, Drzezga A, et al. Complete remission of metastatic neuroendocrine paragastric carcinoma after "neoadjuvant" peptide receptor radionuclide therapy and surgery. Clin Nucl Med. 2015;40(8):667–9.

55. Stoeltzing O, Loss M, Huber E, Gross V, Eilles C, Mueller-Brand J, et al. Staged surgery with neoadjuvant 90Y-DOTATOC therapy for down-sizing synchronous bilobular hepatic metastases from a neuroendocrine pancreatic tumor. Langenbeck's Arch Surg. 2010;395(2):185–92.

56. Chiapponi C, Lürssen N, Cremer B, Wahba R, Drebber U, Faust M, et al. Peptide receptor radionuclide therapy as a two-step strategy for initially unresectable liver disease from neuroendocrine tumors: a single-center experience. Endocrine. 2020;70(1):187–93. https://doi.org/10.1007/s12020-020-02341-1.

57. Partelli S, Bertani E, Bartolomei M, Perali C, Muffatti F, Grana CM, et al. Peptide receptor radionuclide therapy as neoadjuvant therapy for resectable or potentially resectable pancreatic neuroendocrine neoplasms. Surgery. 2017;163(4):761–7.

58. van Vliet EI, van Eijck CH, de Krijger RR, Nieveen van Dijkum EJ, Teunissen JJ, Kam BL, et al. Neoadjuvant treatment of nonfunctioning pancreatic neuroendocrine tumors with [177Lu-DOTA0,Tyr3] octreotate. J Nucl Med. 2015;56(11):1647–53.

59. Schiavo Lena M, Partelli S, Castelli P, Andreasi V, Smart CE, Pisa E, et al. Histopathological and immunophenotypic changes of pancreatic neuroendocrine tumors after neoadjuvant peptide receptor radionuclide therapy (PRRT). Endocr Pathol. 2020;31(2):119–31.

60. Frilling A, Giele H, Vrakas G, Reddy S, Macedo R, Al-Nahhas A, et al. Modified liver-free multivisceral transplantation for a metastatic small bowel neuroendocrine tumor: a case report. Transplant Proc. 2015;47(3):858–62.

61. Basu S, Parghane RV, Ostwal V, Shrikhande SV. Neoadjuvant strategies for advanced pancreatic neuroendocrine tumors: should combined chemotherapy and peptide receptor radionuclide therapy be the preferred regimen for maximizing outcome? Nucl Med Commun. 2018;39(1):94–5.

62. Lewis A, Raoof M, Ituarte PHG, Williams J, Melstrom L, Li D, et al. Resection of the primary gastrointestinal neuroendocrine tumor improves survival with or without liver treatment. Ann Surg. 2018;270(6):1131–7.

63. Citterio D, Pusceddu S, Facciorusso A, Coppa J, Milione M, Buzzoni R, et al. Primary tumour resection may improve survival in functional well-differentiated neuroendocrine tumours metastatic to the liver. Eur J Surg Oncol. 2017;43(2):380–7.

64. Daskalakis K, Karakatsanis A, Hessman O, Stuart HC, Welin S, Tiensuu Janson E, et al. Association of a prophylactic surgical approach to stage IV small intestinal neuroendocrine tumors with survival. JAMA Oncol. 2018;4(2):183–9.

65. Frilling A, Weber F, Saner F, Bockisch A, Hofmann M, Mueller-Brand J, et al. Treatment with (90)Y- and (177)Lu-DOTATOC in patients with metastatic neuroendocrine tumors. Surgery. 2006;140(6):968–76; discussion 976-7.

66. da Silva TN, van Velthuysen MLF, van Eijck CHJ, Teunissen JJ, Hofland J, de Herder WW. Successful neoadjuvant peptide receptor radionuclide therapy for an inoperable pancreatic neuroendocrine tumour. Endocrinol Diabetes Metab Case Rep. 2018;2018:18.

67. Bertani E, Fazio N, Radice D, Zardini C, Grana C, Bodei L, et al. Resection of the primary tumor followed by peptide receptor radionuclide therapy as upfront strategy for the treatment of G1–G2 pancreatic neuroendocrine tumors with unresectable liver metastases. Ann Surg Oncol. 2016;23:981–9.

68. Kaemmerer D, Twrznik M, Kulkarni HR, Hörsch D, Sehner S, Baum RP, et al. Prior resection of the primary tumor prolongs survival after peptide receptor radionuclide therapy of advanced neuroendocrine neoplasms. Ann Surg. 2019;274(1):e45–53. https://doi.org/10.1097/SLA.0000000000003237.

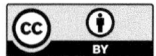

From Concept to Clinic and Commercialization: Cowboys Wanted

Christian P. Behrenbruch

The purpose of this chapter is threefold.

Firstly, it is an honor to be included in this *Festschrift,* a recognition and celebration of the enormous contribution Professor Richard Baum has made to the field of nuclear medicine. I would like to write a few words as to why Richard's contribution to nuclear medicine and theranostics has been so important from a commercial perspective, and why we need more innovators like him. Secondly, I want to review some of the reasons why, despite enormous potential, the field of nuclear medicine has not been as commercially successful as it could be, and the pitfalls we must address in order to deliver in the future. Finally, I'd like to highlight some of the areas that I am most excited about from a commercial perspective that will likely define the field over the next decade.

I've spent 20 years hunting money for imaging and nuclear medicine companies and over that time, through varying degrees of economic prosperity, I have received a great deal of candid feedback about how investors view the nuclear medicine industry. These perceptions offer provocative insights into our industry and I believe they are worth sharing, both for information and entertainment. Not all opinions will garner agreement.

4.1 Professor Richard Baum

Firstly, since this essay is delivered in honor and recognition of Richard, I would like to share a story about our esteemed colleague. In our field, there are few who have made such an immense contribution over such a long period of time, and even fewer who are such a force of nature. I first met Richard exactly ten years ago back in the early days of ImaginAb [1], where I was challenged by Richard to "get my act together" and do a first-in-human evaluation of an anti-PSMA antibody fragment (a minibody [2]) in an investigator-led study [3]. The truth is, I don't think Richard likes biologics much and were it not for the fact that the prostate PSMA[1] imaging

---

This opinion piece was written in mid-2020. The world of nuclear medicine (and the world more generally) has changed dramatically since then. We now have new approved prostate cancer imaging and therapy products from several vendors and there has been an almost Cambrian explosion of new radiopharma companies and venture capital interest. But just to illustrate that despite this step-change of excitement about nuclear medicine, many of the "gotcha's" still exist, I have left the content in place as a kind of personal "time capsule" and a test of whether I understand the future of this field or not.

Did my comments and predictions age well?

You decide.

C. P. Behrenbruch (✉)
Telix Pharmaceuticals Limited, Melbourne, VIC, Australia
e-mail: chris@telixpharma.com

---

[1] *PSMA* prostate-specific membrane antigen.

© The Author(s) 2024
V. Prasad (ed.), *Beyond Becquerel and Biology to Precision Radiomolecular Oncology: Festschrift in Honor of Richard P. Baum*, https://doi.org/10.1007/978-3-031-33533-4_4

field was so nascent, I very much doubt I would have piqued his interest. But I am grateful he was curious because, thanks to Richard, we got some preliminary data that enabled us to raise a "Series A" venture capital financing for the company. Without this, the company would have simply failed to launch. I will come back to this again at the end of this essay.

It was a delicate situation. We had manufactured a first batch of (approximately) clinical-grade material, we didn't have much of it to spare (and made at significant cost), but the company didn't have a lot of financial resources either. After several months of harassment from Richard (I admit) we sent him a summary of the manufacturing package, noting that we had only a very basic radiolabeling protocol. After a week of contemplation, I received an email from Richard indicating that he would be keen to do a straightforward biodistribution study in patients with advanced metastatic prostate cancer. We packaged up the precious vials of DOTA-conjugated fragment and sent them to him, with enough additional material for the highly talented radiochemistry team at ZentralKlinik Bad Berka to undertake some basic process development, validation runs and a first patient study. We were expecting to image 8 patients in total with SPECT, labeled with ^{111}In.

A few weeks went by, and we waited with great anticipation. Then one day a beautiful image appeared in my inbox. Then another. Then a more detailed biodistribution assessment and a rough dosimetry analysis. Then the 5th patient came. The images looked strange, a bit blurry (even by SPECT standards) and we were confused.

What had gone wrong?

Well, Richard had gone back to the first patient and substituted the indium for ^{177}Lu and, based on the dosimetry had given an approximately 45 mCi/m^2 dose of lutetium as a therapeutic dose. We were shocked, surprised, dumbfounded. It wasn't supposed to be a therapeutic agent, it was supposed to be an imaging agent! I traveled from Los Angeles to Levi, Finland[2] to have a meeting to discuss.

The meeting, which would forever change my view on the fundamental purpose of nuclear medicine, took place in a sauna at a resort a few hundred meters away from Santa's Arctic village. It was November, and there was already plenty of snow on the ground—a far cry from the gentle winter climate of Southern California. I was so irritated and jet lagged, I didn't really know what to say and I am sure my words blurted out in a jumbled mess. But Richard—as Richard often does—calibrated me on the facts of life.

He explained in his clear and typically direct manner, that his foremost mission is not to look at "interesting things" but to help his patients. He was encouraged (never went so far as to say "enthusiastic" I will note) by the imaging data and felt there was a chance to offer some benefit in the form of lutetium therapy. He explained that the patients had joined the study altruistically but that, in truth, there is little point in merely imaging disease. If patients are to benefit, then for a diagnostic there must be a corresponding therapeutic intervention, and without it—it is pointless. Pointless.

When you have spent a couple of years working on something with a pre-conceived idea of its value and purpose, to be re-calibrated in such a way is somewhat confronting. But what I observed in the years that followed is that I have met few clinician-scientists so committed and devoted to the patient. My personal lens of risk tolerance (or perhaps not) was simply an incomplete and perhaps even farcical viewpoint, and while it would clearly be unproductive for every investigator-led study to go off-piste, Richard *always* put the patient first.

The lesson I learned was simple—by all means do the experiment, but make sure that the purpose is maximized for the patient, not scientific curiosity. I wish I could say that this is an obvious and ingrained attribute of clinical research, but we all know that this is too often not the case, especially in nuclear medicine. It was a precious gift to me.

4.2   The Great Bexxar® Disaster

Moving on from sentimental rumination to business, the first reaction I typically get from investors in relation to anything nuclear medicine or radiopharmaceutical is a slight grimace and a slow exhalation of breath. A kinder investor audience will occasionally acknowledge that the technology is "nifty" but most just cut to the chase, namely that there are few good examples of high-quality nuclear medicine companies or commercially-successful products, even to this day. Investors prefer to see new ideas surrounded by relevant success stories and plenty of cash thrown at a given technology field. In investor parlance, they look for evidence that a company is "swimming where the water flows." Nuclear medicine is complex and hard to sell, both technically and in terms of historical performance.

In 2014 I met with New York investment bankers with the intention of taking ImaginAb public. At the time, the tally of nuclear medicine disasters was fairly substantial. Lantheus had just failed an IPO attempt [4], Immunomedics' share price was floundering about, Progenics wasn't impressing investors and the reputation of our industry was mostly one of mediocrity from past failures like Corixa to the distracted implosion of IBA's radiopharma business. While some of these companies have significantly reformed, even to the point of performing well, Bexxar and Zevalin® remain the epitome of our industry's remarkable ability to produce clinically outstanding products that failed miserably in the commercial world.

Most readers of this *festschrift* know the reason why Bexxar failed and I don't want this commentary to rehash old and mostly uninteresting history (although for those interested in an omprehensive written review, Luke Timmerman's analysis of Bexxar is excellent [5]). Fundamentally, taking revenue away from the oncologist was a recipe for commercial disaster and, at the time, there was more money in delivering chemotherapy than there was selling a "one-shot" wonder drug, irrespective of patient benefit [6]. However, to simplify the Bexxar failure to revenue conflict and patient ownership is to be analytically superficial. The fact remains that despite the impressive performance of Bexxar in follicular lymphoma (an astonishing 75% complete response) [7], the clinical trials that could have catapulted a radiopharmaceutical into the front-line of cancer care were not particularly comprehensive, were lethargically marketed, and arguably did not compel the field to change the standard of care at the time.

From the Bexxar experience we can ascertain two important lessons about how to commercialize novel nuclear medicine products. The first lesson is that to deliver a successful product, there needs to be a great clinical dataset. Fast-forwarding a decade from Bexxar, one only has to consider the relative commercial success of the Algeta/Xofigo® journey to appreciate the reward for doing things properly. The ALSYMPCA trial [8] was a robustly designed trial, intended to produce the necessary level of evidence, and it certainly delivered. For 3.6 months of median survival benefit [9], Algeta created almost $3B of value for shareholders between initial partnering funding and ultimate acquisition by Bayer [10]. I personally don't think anyone really believes that ^{223}Ra-dichloride is clinically any better than ^{153}Sm or ^{89}Sr (I certainly don't), but Algeta did the hard work and snagged a significant prize. More recently we had the NETTER trial [11] for Lutathera® (^{177}Lu-DOTATATE, AAA/Novartis) as another strong example of data-driven commercial outcomes for the field—and, of course, for patients. The point is, the growing call for robustly executed clinical trials is correct and necessary for the future of the field, for both clinical and commercial success.

4.3   "Us Versus Them"

The second insight from Bexxar relates to the turf battle between medical oncology and nuclear medicine. I have traveled extensively around the planet and observed the practice of nuclear medicine in many different clinical settings. Where there is a well-integrated team approach to treating cancer, experimental nuclear medicine (both diagnostic and therapeutic) thrives. But where there is an "us versus them" mentality, nuclear medicine remains relegated to the dungeon of the hospital and salvage patients waiting to exhale their last breath. It is a depressing and dreary place for otherwise outstanding science to exist.

This reality should encourage us to re-think the strategy for running clinical trials for nuclear medicine products, particularly therapeutic products. Does going head-head with standard care really sell the value proposition of nuclear medicine to an oncologist? Surely comparative trials that *integrate* standard care into the nuclear medicine treatment arm is a better way to go, especially given the therapeutic index typical of nuclear medicine approaches and the potential benefit in earlier stage patients? Considering some of the significant combination drug opportunities like androgen-deprivation therapy plus PSMA for prostate cancer [12], or combo radiation-checkpoint inhibitor studies [13], this would seem like a golden opportunity for our field. Especially since nuclear medicine therapies don't tend to have overlapping toxicities [14] and imaging (i.e., patient selection, treatment response assessment) is often "built-in" for free [15]. The question is, will nuclear medicine ever really "play nice" with medical oncology?

Of course, much has changed in the past 5 years and now we have some decent success stories to talk about, at least at face value. I could be unkind and note with disdain how long it took for radioactive somatostatin analogs to broadly impact patient care—or whine a bit and note that we probably could have had a highly effective PSMA therapy a decade before Endocyte and PSMA-617 [16, 17], but we are making progress. Like many, I playfully mocked Stefano Buono (with no small amount of envy mixed in, I fully admit) when he moved into the 69th floor of the Empire State Building in New York and re-invented AAA [18]. But what a magnificent success! The reward comes from being courageous enough to take light-touch manufacturing processes and patchy clinical data out of the realm of academia into the harsh glare of the real world. Did intellectual property underpin AAA's $4Bn valuation at the time it was acquired by Novartis? [19] Absolutely not—it was about doing the regulatory, manufacturing and clinical hard grind and finishing the job.

4.4 Intellectual Property: Who Cares?

Intellectual property (IP) is important but investors in our field probably worry too much about it. To be sure, we are probably going to see some interesting IP clashes in the near future, particularly around the PSMA small molecule programs [20]. There is also little doubt that IP infringement has hindered progress in the past. For example, we never had ^{18}F-choline imaging in the United States, largely because of the deterrent effect of IP ownership uncertainty. While many men in Europe genuinely benefitted from choline, Americans missed out. Of course, PSMA imaging mostly makes choline and fluciclovine (Axumin) [21] imaging mostly obsolete [22], but it's still disappointing to think of all the men that could have obtained some genuine benefit, not to mention the loss of a developmental incentive for the commercial ^{18}F networks that would have almost certainly paved the way for a more flexible and capable manufacturing capacity, especially in the United States.

Although IP doesn't particularly define our industry, especially given that it seems to take at least two decades for products to materialize (and thus composition of matter patents have expired anyhow), manufacturing and supply chain *does* define nuclear medicine, and this is where investors view our industry as especially challenging. There have been some interesting gambles—for example, when Bristol-Myers Squibb offloaded its imaging division to Avista Capital in 2008 [23], it was against the backdrop of a big pharma fear of the Cardiolite® patent cliff. Avista's bet was basically that patent expiration wouldn't particularly matter because supply chain and logistics trumped the importance of IP protection.

4.5 Imaging Is Not an Easy Business

It turned out that they were mostly right and although Lantheus is only now blossoming after its private equity hangover (with an incredibly low market capitalization relative to revenues, I might add), the Avista bet was a good one.

However, market conditions aside, it is somewhat sobering to compare Lantheus' failed 2014 IPO and slightly tepid (but ultimately successful) second-attempt in 2015 [24] with AAA's highly respectable 2015 public offering [25]. Both companies offer medical imaging products but AAA had a superior financial profile because their investment thesis was focused on therapeutic medicine, not diagnostic imaging. In reality, Richard's hot-tub pep talk is more than just about the patient, it also directly translates into value creation for shareholders.

Fundamentally, the commercial landscape of diagnostic nuclear medicine has undergone a dramatic shift. A decade or more ago, it was GE (via the Amersham acquisition), Siemens (PETNet), and IBA that were leading the charge in new nuclear medicine and PET tracers. Today none of those companies truly invest in new molecular imaging candidates and don't contribute much to the momentum of diagnostic nuclear medicine, let alone do anything earth shattering in radionuclide therapy. At one point, companies like GE and Siemens were interested in new tracers because they thought it would help them to sell capital equipment. As a case in point, PETNet was established by CTI (now Siemens), *precisely* to fuel demand for scanners, the metaphor being one of gas stations (cyclotron sites) and cars (PET scanners).

Although the roll-out strategy of cyclotron networks and the success of FDG PET is something that Henry Ford would have immediately recognized as akin to roads and gas stations, the price erosion and extreme commoditization of FDG has made it challenging for new high-value tracers to get to market. It's only recently with the advent of novel agents targeting PSMA (prostate) [26], CAIX (renal) [27], and immune cells (i.e., ^{18}F-AraG [28], anti-CD8 [29], and anti-PD1/L1 [30] constructs) that the potential patient benefit above that of FDG is sufficient to command a decent price tag. Blue Earth Diagnostics is a case in point and did a laudable job with fluciclovine (Axumin®), with a dose commanding $4000+ a pop in the United States, at least until the point where bundled reimbursement potentially crushes pricing [31].

There is also no doubt that the commercial failure of amyloid imaging, despite three FDA approvals representing a combined investment of well over a billion dollars from GE, Avid (Lilly), and Bayer (Piramal) [32], has fundamentally tainted investor appetite to invest in new imaging agents as a stand-alone value proposition. Alzheimer's imaging has clearly taught us that without a therapeutic intervention, an imaging agent is commercially useless [33]. With the possible dismissal of the "amyloid hypothesis" [34] likely follows the death of plaque imaging, despite arguable benefits to patient management [35]. Diagnostic nuclear medicine in cardiology and oncology plays a much more front-line role in guiding intervention, in the broadest sense, but the bar remains high for new stand-alone diagnostic products to truly show patient benefit. It is also at our peril that we ignore the various blood- and tissue-based diagnostic technologies that are making waves, and which certainly have the potential to compete in numerous applications [36].

4.6 Entrepreneurs Beware

What does this practically mean for the academic or entrepreneur (or, even better, academic-entrepreneur) who has a great idea for a new imaging tracer? Well, at a first pass, it probably means that there isn't a straightforward business case. I encounter a lot of small stand-alone diagnostic imaging tracer companies that struggle to obtain meaningful investment (to do the necessary trials). I personally wouldn't invest in a start-up that had an imaging tracer that wasn't directly tied to a therapeutic intervention, no matter how interesting the clinical application.

I also don't care much for made-up words like the term "theranostic" (and as an aside, I feel this term does our industry harm because it echos strongly of Theranos, the fraudulent blood diagnostics company [37] and we should endeavor to standardize a better term that investors reactively distrust less). However, I think that nothing in nuclear medicine is more important than the *concept* of theranostics. In fact, as we hurtle toward the era of personalized or "precision" medicine, it is truly our strategic advantage in comparison with other therapeutic modalities. It pains me to admit this because it means I personally wasted many years of my life trying to develop stand-alone diagnostic imaging products (in deference to Richard, I will admit my stupidity), but I firmly believe that in the long-term the strongest business model is where imaging is merely a cost of goods (COGS) of a therapy, and therefore should be as cheap and ubiquitous as possible.

Unfortunately, this isn't just history. New imaging tracers are still being developed to tackle a mostly theoretical unmet need. While I am as enamored as anyone with the beautiful images from FAPI [38], the world simply does not need another FDG and this new technology needs to developed to be more than "the next FDG". Indeed, one of the biggest business case impedi-ment to developing a new broad-use imaging agent is precisely the power and beauty of FDG. It's slightly unfortunate that our first great PET imaging may possibly be the best we'll ever have. FDG has big shoes to fill and unless the concordant therapeutic benefit of new strategies can be demonstrated, we will see plenty of new (however appealing) imaging agents fail to trans-form clinical care, and therefore add to the list of commercial failures by extension.

4.7   Build It and They Will Come

A "theranostic" strategy, the commitment to run-ning proper clinical trials and integrating with standard care could mean a very bright future for our field. Judging by the packed attendance at PSMA and NET conference presentations, it's clear we have plenty of attention from referral physicians. Richard has played a pivotal role in the creation of this incredible opportunity, includ-ing the momentum and enthusiasm we enjoy today. For the first time in a long time, it's exciting to be in nuclear medicine, but there are still plenty of ways to mess it up if we are not careful.

Aside from the marginally useful clinical studies we have a tendency to run, "big pharma" has traditionally shunned nuclear medicine

because of its manufacturing and supply chain complexity. Our products are complicated to make, are "melting ice cubes" and the just-in-time logistics of shipping a product anywhere in the world, every day, requires a heroic effort. Unfortunately, the supply chains that underpin our industry are not as strong as they need to be for future success.

The relentless commoditization of FDG means that our ^{18}F cyclotron networks are gener-ally in poor shape and need a significant level of investment to bring them up to the standard required to deliver multi-product capability, par-ticularly considering new manufacturing regula-tions in the United States and EU. This will be a significant investment headwind for new tracers, particularly ^{18}F-based PSMA tracers [39, 40] and notwithstanding the generally impressive com-mercial success of Axumin in the United States, roll-out was not particularly fast. For those with a penchant for ^{68}Ga, it's fair to say that most gen-erator vendors were caught short [41] and have unfortunately tarnished the reputation of gallium with investors.

4.8   A Fragile Supply Chain

On the therapeutic side, I believe we are on the verge of our first supply chain crunch for no car-rier added (NCA) ^{177}Lu. By the way, as an indus-try, we should *only* be using NCA lutetium if we are going to scale an industry based on responsi-ble waste management and a tenable environmen-tal profile. Although there is some optimization possible and there is talk of re-processing "raw" chemical-grade ^{177}Lu from various high-output reactor sources around the globe, scaling the sup-ply chain remains a non-trivial exercise. There are already some early signs of the "crunch", with vendors starting to sell preferential and guaran-teed access to production capacity [42], which I argue wouldn't happen if production was truly near-term scalable. Otherwise why diminish the value (and valuation) of the supply chain in such a simplistic way? Although there is seemingly a plethora of new NCA lutetium production proj-ects around the globe, only a small number are really serious and they are probably at risk of acquisition, possibly to the exclusion of the overall growth of the industry. If companies cannot access at least two or three credible, stable suppliers of isotope, then there will be insufficient resilience of supply to support product development and commercialization.

The issue goes considerably beyond lutetium. There are several promising ^{131}I products that are approved or close to market (Progenics [43], Y-mAbs [44]), but despite cheap and plentiful availability of iodine, manufacturing capacity for iodinated drug product remains extremely limited in virtually every territory. With a resurgence of interest in therapeutic nuclear medicine, driven by lutetium and the allure of alpha emitters, it's reasonable to assume that [131]I (and perhaps other useful flavors of iodine) [45] is going to see a renaissance too. Frankly, it's a very good isotope and worth a second life, even if success will mean investing in production and clinical infrastructure.

It almost doesn't matter what the therapeutic isotope is, the specialist manufacturing infrastructure is patchy. Capacity for clinical trials and even early commercialization of the odd orphan drug is available, but scale-up manufacturing essentially remains an unsolved problem in most parts of the world. I believe that the most powerful part of our ecosystem could end up becoming firms like Curium (the merger of IBA Molecular and Mallinckrodt's isotope business) [46] and Cardinal Health, and we are seeing considerable industry consolidation around manufacturing and production networks at present. There is a plausible scenario whereby a few dominant companies define the economics and market access reality of our industry. This in turn could have a suppressive effect on new product innovation as there would be little incentive to invest in early-stage clinical translation because it doesn't generate meaningful revenue and it's not evident that the larger supply chains are interested in investing in early-stage assets. New contract development and manufacturing organizations (CDMOs), like Evergreen Theragnostics [47], are badly needed to build this future capacity in a cost-effective way.

4.9 Future Frontiers

I am not particularly gifted at gazing into the crystal ball, I will save that task to Richard. Our field is still a moving target and we should persist in addressing the systemic risks of our industry. It would be hard to remain motivated and optimistic about new product development if there were not clear pathways forward to market. That said, there is always the temptation to skip past what we already have on our plate and play with the next shiny toy. Because our industry is so academically driven, we essentially have zero attention span and every time I attend the major scientific conferences I am reminded that part of the reason why we don't have great products impacting healthcare is because academics do the cool research, write the paper, run their clinical proof-of-concept (for another nice paper) and then move on. For the most part, new ideas don't end up in commercial ventures.

Although I am intrigued about the potential for alpha emitters (particularly [225]Ac, [211]At, and possibly [212]Pb) there is truthfully very little actual innovation going on here in my opinion. Putting a different isotope onto the same old targeting agents and declaring success isn't going to enable the field of alpha therapeutics [48]. We basically never did any meaningful prospective MTD/dose optimization studies with ^{177}Lu peptide therapies [49] and it doesn't look like anyone is really doing it with alpha emitters either, which is concerning for both the science and the patient. In the case of isotopes with complex decay chains like [225]Ac [50] or [227]Th (if one must) [51] there is so much more fundamental research and long-term follow-up to be done before we can robustly turn to our colleagues in mainstream oncology and say "we have something you should use." The fundamental radiobiology really isn't being done at all and it's going to hurt us at some point.

There is also a lot of mythology in our field. One of the great myths is that if we make our products more "drug-like" (i.e., use alphas) that mainstream pharma will finally buy into radiopharmaceuticals in a big way. Actually, there is no real basis for this assertion and Novartis' acquisition of AAA and Endocyte should be considered to be evidence of this misconception. What matters is cost-effective manufacturing and meaningful clinical data, not the seductive characteristics of a particular radionuclide. In my opinion, diversifying the manufacturing capability of our industry is vital, not just for therapeutics but for diagnostic imaging products too. The use of isotopes like ^{89}Zr and ^{64}Cu (to a limited extent) has the potential to alleviate the need to run large-scale networks of cyclotron production sites for imaging, which would have a big impact on production economics and patient access.

Finally, as I have already alluded, I think the most exciting future for the oncology-centric part of nuclear medicine, is immuno-oncology. On the imaging side, we have a growing number of PET tracers that provide an incredible window into the immune system and there is some evidence that mainstream pharma is paying attention [52]. On the therapeutic side, there is probably no therapeutic modality that is more synergistic with immuno-oncology drugs than targeted radiation, although the combination with external beam radiation is exciting too [53, 54]. If one considers the fundamental radiobiology, one could even argue that using targeted radiation to invoke an immune response in a highly complex and heterogeneous tumor micro-environment may be better accomplished with beta-rather than alpha-emitters (heresy, I know). We don't have to wait until tomorrow to explore this potential and I firmly believe it will become our industry's finest hour, providing that we can develop the analytical methods and clinical software applications to quantitate what is actually happening, and how to optimally cycle therapy for both toxicity and patient benefit.

4.10 Concluding Remarks

Buoyed by new optimism and the recognition that our industry has finally come of age, it's time to move out from our "spotty teenager" phase and into the relative grace of adulthood. With

industry and academia working together more effectively than ever, and academics increasingly demonstrating risk appetite for new commercial ventures, perhaps we will soon see a time where radiopharmaceuticals, and not CAR-Ts or gene editing tools, command the headline at mainstream biotech investor conferences.

As I have asserted, we need to work with mainstream oncology and integrate with standard care. We need to run scaled, prospective clinical studies that use meaningful comparators, not quasi-standards that don't reflect best practice [55]. Our manufacturing and supply chain needs to become more durable, flexible, and diversified.

However, my personal wish—offered with thanks and deference to our friend and colleague Richard—is that we also continue to take appropriate and patient-centric translational risks. Although the regulatory environment for nuclear medicine is not getting easier or less onerous, we still participate in a field that demands enormous cross-functional technical discipline to deliver. With this discipline and the elegance of what "theranostics" can achieve, we should be able to take measured risk, develop products in a more streamlined way, and deliver patient benefit faster than other fields of medicine. Commercial success, particularly for new startups, will utterly depend on this dynamic. Nuclear medicine has the potential to evolve from the "wild west" of the last couple of decades to a much more polished modality, but "cowboys" are still wanted, worthy of our finest - Richard Baum. Congratulations on your transformational and disruptive career!

Conflict of Interest Disclosure Founder and shareholder of Telix Pharmaceuticals Limited, ImaginAb Inc., Sofie Biosciences Inc., Mirada Medical Limited, Adaptix Limited.

References

1. ImaginAb, Inc. http://www.imaginab.com. Accessed 19 Jun 2020.

2. Wu AM, Senter BD. Arming antibodies: prospects and challenges for immunoconjugates. Nat Biotechnol. 2005;23(9):1137–46. https://doi.org/10.1038/nbt1141.

3. Kulkarni HR, Singh A, et al. PSMA-based radioligand therapy for metastatic castration-resistant prostate cancer: the bad Berka experience since 2013. J Nucl Med. 2016;57(3):97S–104S. https://doi.org/10.2967/jnumed.115.170167.

4. Perriello B. Report: Lantheus spikes IPO plans. Mass device. 2014. https://www.massdevice.com/report-lantheus-spikes-ipo-plans/. Accessed 19 Jun 2020.

5. Timmerman L. Why good drugs sometimes fail: the Bexxar Story. Xconomy. 2013. https://xconomy.com/national/2013/08/26/why-good-drugs-sometimes-fail-in-the-market-the-bexxar-story/. Accessed 19 Jun 2020.

6. Wilson WH. R-CHOP strikes again with survival benefit in follicular lymphoma. Blood. 2005;106(12):3678–9. https://doi.org/10.1182/blood-2005-09-3701.

7. Kaminsky MS, Tuck M, et al. 131I-tositumomab therapy as initial treatment for follicular lymphoma. N Engl J Med. 2005;352:441–9. https://doi.org/10.1056/NEJMoa041511.

8. Parker C, Nilsson S, et al. Alpha emitter radium-223 and survival in metastatic prostate cancer. N Engl J Med. 2013;369:213–23. https://doi.org/10.1056/NEJMoa1213755.

9. Heidegger I, Pichler R, et al. Radium-223 for metastatic castration-resistant prostate cancer: results and remaining open issues after the ALSYMPCA trial. Transl Androl Urol. 2018;7(Suppl 1):S132–4. https://doi.org/10.21037/tau.2017.10.06.

10. Genetic Engineering and Biotechnology News. Bayer clinches Algeta acquisition with $2.6B Bid. 2014. https://www.genengnews.com/news/bayer-clinches-algeta-acquisition-with-2-6b-bid/. Accessed 19 Jun 2020.

11. Strosberg J, El-Haddad G, et al. Phase 3 trial of 177Lu-dotatate for midgut neuroendocrine tumors. N Engl J Med. 2017;376:125–35. https://doi.org/10.1056/NEJMoa1607427.

12. Evans M, Smith-Jones PM, et al. Noninvasive measurement of androgen receptor signaling with a positron-emitting radiopharmaceutical that targets prostate-specific membrane antigen. Proc Natl Acad Sci. 2011;108(23):9578–82. https://doi.org/10.1073/pnas.1106383108.

13. Ko EC, Raben D, Formenti SC. The integration of radiotherapy with immunotherapy for the treatment of non-small cell lung cancer. Clin Cancer Res. 2018;24(23):5792–806. https://doi.org/10.1158/1078-0432.CCR-17-3620.

14. Wirsdorfer F, de Leve S, Jendrossek V. Combining radiotherapy and immunotherapy in lung cancer: can we expect limitations due to altered normal tissue toxicity? Int J Mol Sci. 2019;20(1):24. https://doi.org/10.3390/ijms20010024.

15. Divgi C. The current state of radiopharmaceutical therapy. J Nucl Med. 2018;59(11):1706–7. https://doi.org/10.2967/jnumed.118.214122.

16. Plieth J. From zero to hero, endocyte completes a remarkable transformation. Evaluate vantage. 2018. https://www.evaluate.com/vantage/articles/news/zero-hero-endocyte-completes-remarkable-transformation. Accessed 19 Jun 2020.

17. Bander NH, Milowsky MI, et al. Phase I trial of 177lutetium-labeled J591, a monoclonal antibody to prostate-specific membrane antigen, in patients with androgen-independent prostate cancer. J Clin Oncol. 2005;23(21):4591–601. https://doi.org/10.1200/JCO.2005.05.160.

18. Delaye F. Le spin-off du CERN qui vaut un milliard. Bilan. 2015. https://www.bilan.ch/techno/le_spin_off_du_cern_qui_vaut_un_milliard. Accessed 19 Jun 2020.

19. Genetic Engineering and Biotechnology News. Novartis to acquire advanced accelerator applications for $2.9B. 2015. https://www.genengnews.com/topics/drug-discovery/novartis-to-acquire-advanced-accelerator-applications-for-3-9b/. Accessed 19 Jun 2020.

20. Progenics Pharmaceuticals Inc. GlobeNewswire. 2019. https://www.globenewswire.com/news-release/2019/03/14/1753079/0/en/Progenics-Asserts-Ownership-of-PSMA-617-Intellectual-Property-Including-Composition-of-Matter-Patent.html. Accessed 19 Jun 2020.

21. BlueEarth Diagnostics Limited, A Bracco Company. https://www.blueearthdiagnostics.com/. Accessed 19 Jun 2020.

22. Calais J, Ceci F, et al. Prospective head-to-head comparison of 18F-fluciclovine and 68Ga-PSMA-11 PET/CT for localization of prostate cancer biochemical recurrence after primary prostatectomy. J Clin Oncol. 2019;37(7):15. https://doi.org/10.1200/JCO.2019.37.7_suppl.15.

23. Bristol-Myers Squibb Company. Avista Capital Partners completes acquisition of Bristol-Myers squibb medical imaging. 2008. https://news.bms.com/press-release/financial-news/avista-capital-partners-completes-acquisition-bristol-myers-squibb-medi. Accessed 19 Jun 2020.

24. NASDAQ Inc. Lantheus Holdings prices IPO at $6, below the range. 2015. https://www.nasdaq.com/articles/lantheus-holdings-prices-ipo-6-below-range-2015-06-24. Accessed 19 Jun 2020.

25. Advanced Accelerator Applications Inc. Advanced accelerator applications S.A. announces pricing of initial public offering. 2015. https://www.adacap.com/advanced-accelerator-applications-s-a-announces-pricing-of-initial-public-offering/. Accessed 19 Jun 2020.

26. Barakat A, Yacoub B, et al. Role of early PET/CT imaging with 68Ga-PSMA in staging and restaging of prostate cancer. Sci Rep. 2020;10:2705. https://doi.org/10.1038/s41598-020-59296-6.

27. Hekman M, Rijpkema M, et al. Positron emission tomography/computed tomography with ^{89}Zr-girentuximab can aid in diagnostic dilemmas of clear cell renal cell carcinoma suspicion. Eur Urol. 2018;74(3):257–60. https://doi.org/10.1016/j.eururo.2018.04.026.

28. Ronald JA, Kim B-S, et al. A PET imaging strategy to visualize activated T cells in acute graft-versus-host disease elicited by allogenic hematopoietic cell transplant. Cancer Res. 2017;77(11):2893–902. https://doi.org/10.1158/0008-5472.CAN-16-2953.

29. Pandit-Taskar N, Postow MA, et al. First-in-humans imaging with 89 Zr-Df-IAB22M2C anti-CD8 minibody in patients with solid malignancies: preliminary pharmacokinetics, biodistribution, and lesion targeting. J Nucl Med. 2020;61(4):512–9. https://doi.org/10.2967/jnumed.119.229781.

30. van de Donk PP, de Ruijter LK, et al. Molecular imaging biomarkers for immune checkpoint inhibitor therapy. Theranostics. 2020;10(4):1708–18. https://doi.org/10.7150/thno.38339.

31. Fischer JR. New bill calls for changing reimbursement for radiopharmaceuticals. DOTmed. 2019. https://www.dotmed.com/news/story/47993. Accessed 19 Jun 2020.

32. Jeffrey S. FDA approves third amyloid PET tracer for Alzheimer's. Medscape. 2014. https://www.medscape.com/viewarticle/822370. Accessed 19 Jun 2020.

33. Jack CR, Petersen RC. Amyloid PET and changes in clinical management for patients with cognitive impairment. JAMA. 2019;321(13):1258–60. https://doi.org/10.1001/jama.2019.1998.

34. Kametani F, Hasegawa M. Reconsideration of amyloid hypothesis and tau hypothesis in Alzheimer's disease. Front Neurosci. 2018;12:25. https://doi.org/10.3389/fnins.2018.00025.

35. Rabinovici GD, Gatsonis C, et al. Association of amyloid positron emission tomography with subsequent change in clinical management among medicare beneficiaries with mild cognitive impairment or dementia. JAMA. 2019;321(13):1286. https://doi.org/10.1001/jama.2019.2000.

36. Alix-Panabières C. The future of liquid biopsy (Outlook). Nature. 2020;579:S9. https://doi.org/10.1038/d41586-020-00844-5.

37. Carreyrou J. Bad blood: secrets and lies in a silicon valley startup. New York: Knopf; 2018.

38. Kratochwil C, Flechsig P, et al. 68Ga-FAPI PET/CT: tracer uptake in 28 different kinds of cancer. J Nucl Med. 2019;60(6):801–5. https://doi.org/10.2967/jnumed.119.227967.

39. Rowe SP, Macura KJ, et al. PSMA-based [^{18}F] DCFPyL PET/CT is superior to conventional imaging for lesion detection in patients with metastatic prostate cancer. Mol Imaging Biol. 2016;18(3):411–9. https://doi.org/10.1007/s11307-016-0957-6.

40. Giesel F, Knorr K, et al. Detection efficacy of 18F-PSMA-1007 PET/CT in 251 patients with biochemical recurrence of prostate cancer after radical prostatectomy. J Nucl Med. 2019;60(3):362–8. https://doi.org/10.2967/jnumed.118.212233.

41. Culter CS. Society of nuclear medicine and molecular imaging. Communication. 2018. https://s3.amazonaws.com/rdcms-snmmi/files/production/public/Ga68%20shortage%20letter.pdf. Accessed 19 Jun 2020.

42. ITM AG. ITM expands PSMA-617 supply agreement for no-carrier-added Lutetium-177. Bloomberg Business Wire. 2020. https://www.bloomberg.com/press-releases/2020-03-02/itm-expands-psma-617-supply-agreement-for-no-carrier-added-lutetium-177. Accessed 19 Jun 2020.

43. Progenics Pharmaceuticals Inc. AZEDRA® (iobenguane I 131) injection prescribing information. 2018. https://azedra.com/full-prescribing-information.pdf. Accessed 19 Jun 2020.

44. Kramer K, Pandit-Taskar N, et al. Intraventricular radioimmunotherapy targeting B7H3 for CNS malignancies. J Clin Oncol. 2019;37(15):e13592. https://doi.org/10.1200/JCO.2019.37.15_suppl.e13592.

45. Pirovano G, Jannetti SA, et al. Targeted brain tumor radiotherapy using an Auger emitter. Clin Cancer Res. 2020;26(12):2871–81. https://doi.org/10.1158/1078-0432.CCR-19-2440.

46. Curium Pharma. IBA molecular acquires Mallinckrodt nuclear imaging to create world-class radiopharmaceuticals Group. 2007. https://www.curiumpharma.com/2017/01/27/iba-molecular-acquires-mallinckrodt-nuclear-imaging-to-create-world-class-radiopharmaceuticals-group/. Accessed 19 Jun 2020.

47. Evergreen Theragnostics. Corporate web site. 2019. https://evergreentgn.com/. Accessed 19 Jun 2020.

48. Navalkissoor S, Grossman A. Targeted alpha particle therapy for neuroendocrine tumours: the next generation of peptide receptor radionuclide therapy. Neuroendocrinology. 2019;108:256–64. https://doi.org/10.1159/000494760.

49. Zhang J, Kulkarni H, et al. Long-term nephrotoxicity after peptide receptor radionuclide therapy (PRRT): myth or reality? J Nucl Med. 2019;60(1):567.

50. de Kruijff RM, Raavé R, et al. The in vivo fate of 225Ac daughter nuclides using polymersomes as a model carrier. Nat Sci Rep. 2019;9:11671. https://doi.org/10.1038/s41598-019-48298-8.

51. Hammer S, Hagemann UB, et al. Preclinical efficacy of a PSMA-targeted thorium-227 conjugate (PSMA-TTC), a targeted alpha therapy for prostate

cancer. Clin Cancer Res. 2019;12:2268. https://doi. org/10.1158/1078-0432.CCR-19-2268.

52. Niemeijer AN, Leung D, et al. Whole body PD-1 and PD-L1 positron emission tomography in patients with non-small-cell lung cancer. Nat Commun. 2018;9:4664. https://doi.org/10.1038/ s41467-018-07131-y.

53. Badiyan SN, Roach MC, et al. Combining immunotherapy with radiation therapy in thoracic oncology. J Thorac Dis. 2018;10(Suppl 21):S2492–507. https:// doi.org/10.21037/jtd.2018.05.73.

54. Pichler J, Wilson R. IPAX-1: phase I/II study of 131I-iodo-phenylalanine combined with external radi-

ation therapy as treatment for patients with glioblastoma multiforme. J Clin Oncol. 2020;38(15):2578. https://doi.org/10.1200/JCO.2020.38.15_suppl. TPS2578.

55. Hofman MS, Lawrentschuk N, et al. Prostate-specific membrane antigen PET-CT in patients with high-risk prostate cancer before curative-intent surgery or radiotherapy (proPSMA): a prospective, randomised, multicentre study. Lancet. 2020;395(10231):1208–16. https://doi.org/10.1016/S0140-6736(20)30314-7.

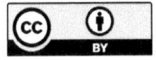

From Radiochemistry of the Lanthanides to [225]Ac and the Interference with Richard Baum

Gerd Juergen Beyer

5.1 Personal Introduction

In 1990, Heinz Schelbert, one of the pioneers of PET, has been asked during an invited lecture at the ZfK Rossendorf, why it happens that few newly created PET centers have significant success and others do not have at all. His answer was simple and clear: institutions where physicians accept scientists, for instance radio-chemists and physicists as equal partners and where they collaborate truly together, there the progress is programmed. In my scientific carrier, I have been privileged to have those fruitful collaborations, for instance with Prof. W. G. Franke, Clinic of Nuclear Medicine of the Medical Academy Dresden in the late 70-th–end 80-th and further at the end of my carrier with Richard Baum. He is one of those distinguished nuclear medical physicians, he is not only just collaborating with experts in different scientific disciplines (biochemistry, radiochemistry, physics, and others), he is promoting those close collaboration and has created a network around the world independent on political and economic situation in countries like Cuba, China, South Africa, and others. His strong engagement is motivating us in developing new techniques making new radionuclides available toward personalized nuclear medicine. In this contribution, I try to give a historical overview over the related research work that has been performed in Dresden, Dubna, and Geneva starting from the methodical developments for nuclear physics basic research in the late 60-th until the recent input especially with the Tb-isotopes to the Bad Berka activities guided by Richard Baum.

It was around 1954/1955: The International conference on peaceful use of nuclear technology in Geneva induced the foundation of national nuclear research centers all over the world, for instance CERN, JINR Dubna, KFK, Jülich, ZfK Rossendorf, etc. Nuclear technology became a fundamental part of the academic education programs. In the former GDR, the Faculty of Nuclear Technology at the Technical University Dresden was created including the chair "Radiochemistry". The new technology did fascinate me and with the age of 15 years, I decided that "Radiochemistry" should be the direction for my future professional carrier. The study in Radiochemistry at TU Dresden began in 1960 at TU Dresden. The Faculty of Nuclear Technology was closed down again in 1962, however direction Radiochemistry continued under the umbrella of inorganic chemistry. My first radioactive preparation I received in 1963 that was produced from Uranium-fission at the Rossendorf Research Reactor by Gerhard Wagner under the supervision of Prof. R. Muenze. G. Wagner finished his Radiochemistry study in Dresden 2

G. J. Beyer (✉)
Division of Nuclear Medicine, St. Louis, MO, USA
e-mail: gerd.beyer@cern.ch

© The Author(s) 2024
V. Prasad (ed.), *Beyond Becquerel and Biology to Precision Radiomolecular Oncology: Festschrift in Honor of Richard P. Baum*, https://doi.org/10.1007/978-3-031-33533-4_5

years earlier. Since that time, we kept close professional relations over a historical period of 55 years.

In this contribution, I try to give a historical overview of the developments of new radiochemical separation techniques which are relevant for making available special radionuclides for biomedical research and nuclear medical application and which have been performed in Dresden (Germany), Dubna (Russia), Geneva and CERN (Switzerland). It starts from the methodical developments for nuclear physics basic research in the late 60-th until the recent input especially with the Tb-isotopes to the Bad Berka activities guided by Richard Baum. Statements and conclusions are essentially strongly influenced by own experiences and a subjective point of view and should not be seen as a general scientific review.

A three-year research fellow ship position at the Joint Institute for nuclear research (JINR) Dubna was offered to me before finishing my diploma. Between the Radiochemistry at the TU Dresden and the Department of Nuclear Spectroscopy and Radiochemistry at the Laboratory of Nuclear Problems in Dubna very close relationships were already established. E. Herrmann (also absolvent of Radiochemistry, TU Dresden in 1963) was already delegated to Dubna and had introduced there a new extraction chromatographic process for separating short-lived light lanthanide isotopes from a very massive lanthanide target [1, 2] (see further below). This task is very similar to the task today: separating ^{177}Lu from massive Yb-targets. It was foreseen to replace E. Herrmann Dubna, since his three-year period was ending. After diploma 1965 and after about 1 year as scientific assistant position at the TU Dresden my scientific activity as radiochemist in Dubna started on 11 January 1967.

5.2 Situation of Nuclear Medicine in the 60-th

In the 60-th the Nuclear medicine was in the process switching from using rectilinear scanners to the planar scintillation camera. The number of available suitable isotopes was very limited. Intense R&D was going on to develop approaches

for using ^{99m}Tc as radiotracer for different imaging protocols. The breakthrough was found in 1969 with the introduction of Sn^{2+} as reducing agent for pertechnetate $[TcO_4^-]$ by R. Dreyer and R. Muenze. This invention opened the door to the cold KIT era [3, 4] and induced an enormous increase of the demand in ^{99}Mo/^{99m}Tc-generators.

In the beginning of the 60-th the atomic physicists were highly motivated to study short-lived nuclides far away from the line of beta-stability generally. In this concern, the region of lanthanides was of special interest because of a nuclear deformation in the lanthanide region. This nuclear deformation is also responsible for the alpha decay of several radionuclides in the middle of the lanthanide group (^{149}Tb!). Two international research projects were initiated at that time: ISOLDE at CERN (ISOLDE stays for Isotope Separation On Line Device) [5] and YASNAPP at the Joint Institute for Nuclear Research (JINR) Dubna (YASNAPP stays for **ya**dernaya **s**pectroscopia **na p**rotonom **p**utschke) [6]. The Idea for the ISOLDE Facility was born already in 1960 and the on-line separator went into operation in 1967 at CERN. After the shut-down of the synchrocyclotron (SC) at CERN in 1990 the new ISOLDE-2 facility was constructed and connected to the proton beam delivered from the CERN BOOSTER, the heart of the CERN accelerator cascade.

An off-line mass separator for the YASNAPP project in Dubna was proposed in 1967 and became operational in 1969. The semi-on-line system YASNAPP-1 went into full operation in 1971. It consisted of the isotope separator itself, a newly developed surface ionization ion source [7], a self-made fast rabbit system for transporting the irradiated targets to the separator, and a dedicated radiochemical laboratory nearby for fast separation of carrier-free nuclear reaction products from massive irradiated targets.

5.3 How to Make Sort-lived Nuclides Far from Beta Stability

High-energy proton-induced reaction (Spallation reaction) is an unspecific but very powerful and universal tool for producing radionuclides. The spallation process generates neutron-deficient nuclides of elements left from the target element; fragmentation gives n-rich nuclides of the light elements and fission generates neutron-rich nuclides of elements in the middle. As shown in Fig. 5.1 the higher the proton energy the higher

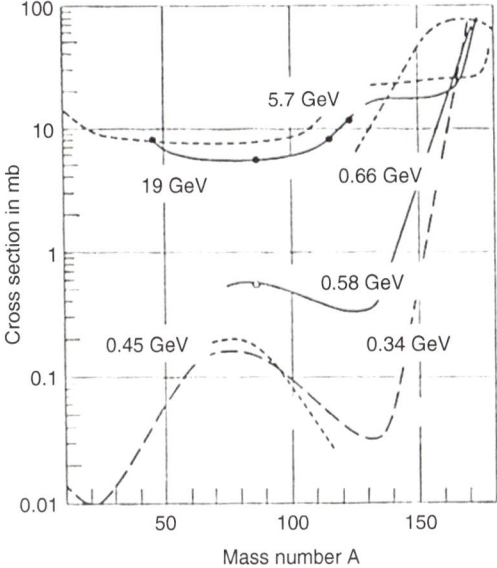

Fig. 5.1 Cross section for the formation of nuclides in interaction of high-energy protons with Ta-target (taken from [8])

the cross sections of the products far away from Z of the target element. With one heavy Z target element, we can produce practically all nuclides of the whole chart of nuclides. It was and is still a challenge for radiochemists and physicists to pick out one single nuclide from those very complex mixtures (Fig. 5.1).

Proton beams: The general difference between the two research projects highlighted in (Fig. 5.2) is the following: ISOLDE worked from the very beginning on-line, meaning an integrated unit of a target-ion source is directly connected to the analyzing magnet that separates the radioactive ion beams directly according to their atomic mass. A chemical separation one could make after mass separation, if required. The YASNAPP-1 project in Dubna started in reverse order: first, the radiochemical separation was done and thereafter the mass separation off-line.

In order to meet the physics interest to study the short-lived lanthanide isotopes new innovative separation techniques for lanthanides were developed in Dubna. In the following chapters, only few technologies for fast separations in the lanthanide region will be explained. A general overview one can find in [9].

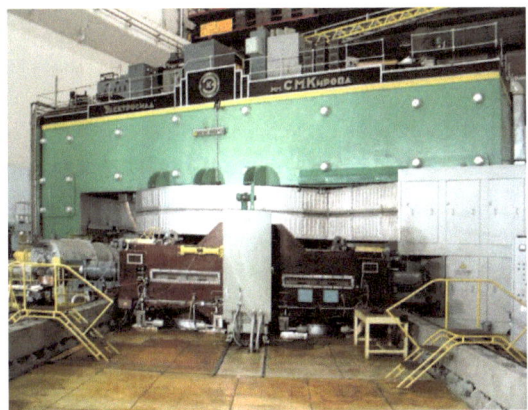
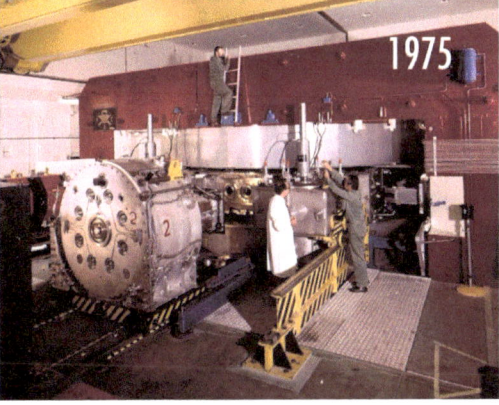

Fig. 5.2 (Left) Synchrocyclotron in Dubna (1984 reconstructed to a phasotron) providing a 660 MeV proton beam, this accelerator became operational in Dec 1949 and was the largest accelerator at that time. (Right) the synchrocyclotron at CERN, that delivered 600 MeV protons, operated from 1954 to 1990

5.4   Optimized Extraction Chromatography

From Fig. 5.1 we learned that when using 660 MeV protons as initial reacting particle interacting with a Ta-target the yield for nuclear reaction products (nuclides of the lanthanides) drops down relatively fast when we move away from Z of Ta. Consequently, there was the pressure to use massive lanthanides itself as target for producing strong sources of carrier-free short-lived radionuclides of the lanthanides. Figure 5.3 shows the radio-chromatogram for the separation of the carrier-free light lanthanides from a massive irradiated Er matrix. The point is that when loading the chromatographic column with macroscopic quantities of a lanthanide we find a very sharp front of the elution profile of the macroscopic component. This break-through point can be identified nicely and calibrated. In front of this break-through point the lighter lanthanides are eluted with high yield in carrier-free form, as long as the target material is not contaminated with lighter lanthanides. For cation exchange chromatography exist similar conditions, which can be used today for separating ^{177}Lu from massive Yb-targets for instance for shortening the separation time significantly.

The first ~150 ml eluate that contained the wanted short-lived carrier-free radionuclides of

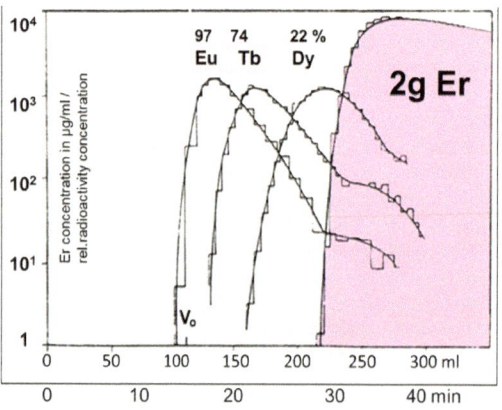

Fig. 5.3 Separation of lighter radio-lanthanides from massive Er-target by extraction chromatography: Column: 100 g silicagel, 26 × 410 mm (0.6 g HDEHP/1 g silicagel), elution with 2.68 M HCl, 7 ml/min at 40 °C (see [1, 2, 9])

the light lanthanides was evaporated and the products were thereafter separated into the different lanthanide fractions using a small separation column. The overall time for the isolation of a Tb-fraction from a 2 g Er target was about 45 min. In order to be faster one can make use of the mechanical recoil effect during the irradiation. G. Pfrepper proposed to irradiate suspension of very fine grain powders of insoluble materials (for instance phosphates of Lanthanides, Ta_2O_5, WO_3) as suspension in diluted mineral acid. After a simple filtration process, one can harvest up to 40% of the nuclear reaction products in the filtrate [10].

5.5   Separations Based on Szilard-Chalmers Effect

The 60-th was the high time of hot atom chemistry or recoil chemistry. My task for the research program in Dubna was to look after the potential using Szilard-Chalmers effects for preparative separations in the lanthanide region. The focus were complex compounds of the Lanthanides with complexions (polyamino-polycarboxylic acids) like EDTA or DTPA. First systematic isotope exchange studies were performed and the obtained results can be summarized as follows [11]:

The isotope exchange rate R in the system Ce^{3+}/[CeEDTA]$^-$ does not depend on the Ce^{3+} concentration.

The isotope exchange rate R depends linear on the H^+-concentration in the EDTA system (see Fig. 5.4 left).

The rate constant k_1 for the isotope exchange process is directly proportional to the stability constant β_{LnY} of the complex.

The exchange rate is generally low in neutral pH regions. This pH region is suitable to study the chemical effects of radioactive decay processes (see Fig. 5.4 right).

As a first conclusion of these results crystalline complex salts of the composition $(NH_4)_2$[Ln DTPA] x 2 H_2O were synthesized with a well-defined excess (0.1 Mol-%) of free Ln^{3+} (Ln = Er, Dy, Gd, Eu). About 1 g of those and material was

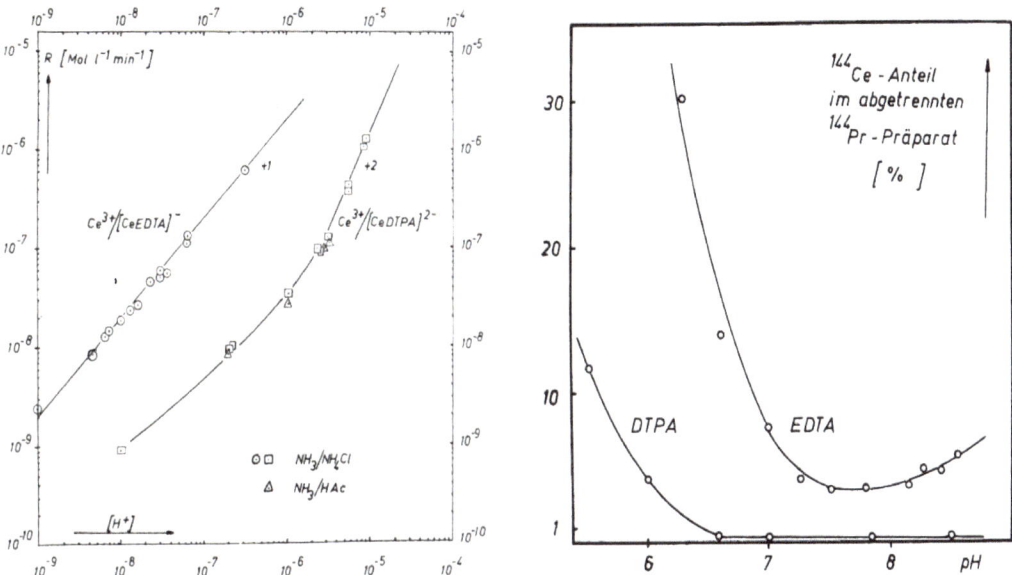

Fig. 5.4 Influence of the pH on the isotope exchange between Ce^{+3}-ions and complexed $[CeY]^{n+}$-ions, where Y is EDTA and DTPA. The isotope exchange is significantly smaller for the DTPA system ([11] for more details see text)

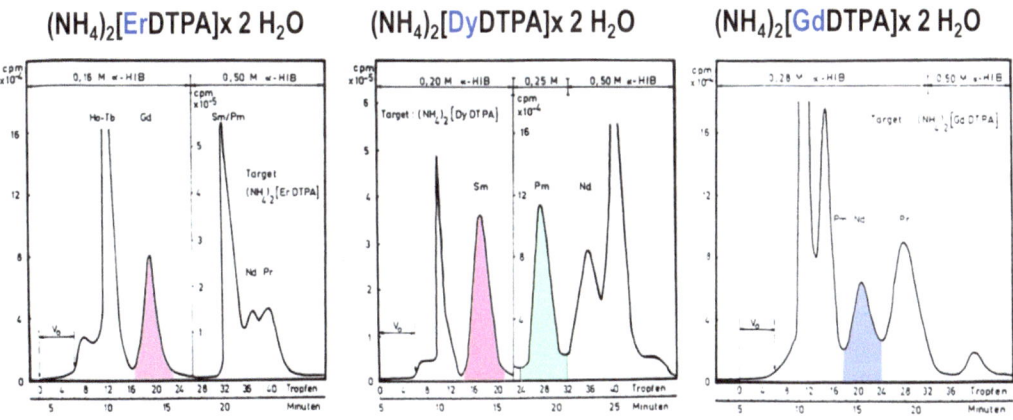

Column: 2.5 x 100 mm, Dowex 50 x8, 20 μm, NH_4^+-form; Elution: α-HIBA, pH=4.7, 0.15 ml/min

Fig. 5.5 Radio-chromatograms of preparative separation of short-lived radio lanthanides obtained in bombardment of different lanthanide DTPA complex compounds with 660 MeV protons

then irradiated with 660 MeV protons at the Dubna synchrocyclotron, thereafter dissolved in 5–8 ml H_2O that contained ~10 mg of a fine grain cation exchange resin (first we used "self-made" very fine resin, later on suitable resins became available on the market: Aminex A5). The nuclear reaction products stabilize as free ionic Ln^{3+}-ions. Because of the very low isotope exchange rate, we are able to collect the wanted short-lived

nuclides at the cation exchange resin within less than a minute and transfer this resin with the adsorbed products to a small cation exchange resin column for fast chromatographic separation [12]. Figure 5.5 shows those fast chromatographic separations for three different target complexes. The reader needs to consider that the radionuclides are short-lived and consequently during the separation process we generate daughter nuclides of neighboring elements. The fraction peaks look by far not that sharp as usual. The time needed for obtaining a clean fraction of a wanted lanthanide element took about 15 min; the total volume of one fraction was between 3–5 drops (~150 µl). The fastest separation was 8 minutes (for ^{144}Gd, half-life 4.5 min).

It was 1970 when P. Gregers Hansen, Prof. of Physics University of Aarhus (Denmark) and one of the Danish initiators of the ISOLDE program, visited the JINR Dubna. He was very much impressed by the obtained results of the fast radiochemical separation techniques for the Lanthanides and he invited me for a half-year fellowship position in his Institute of Physics in Aarhus (DK). His former radiochemist in that position (Helge Ravn) has been delegated to the ISOLDE project to CERN. I mention this because this was the real start of a close, continuous, and fruitful collaboration with CERN ISOLDE.

In Aarhus, I studied in detail the chemical effects of different radioactive decay processes. The Lanthanide group is indeed ideal for this kind of study; this group contains a complete range of radioisotopes having as complete a diversity of types of radiation and energy of radiation and half-life one would wish. Consequently, one could study the behavior of any decay mode without changing the basic chelating ligand. The different decay modes were: beta decay accompanied with gamma radiation with ignorable low (^{172}Er), medium (^{144}Ce) and high inner conversion rate (^{143}Ce), EC-decay mode (^{134}Ce, ^{135}Ce), isomeric decay with high inner conversion rate (^{137m}Ce). For producing the needed different radiotracers continuous access to the research reactor in Risö was assured (this research reactor has been shut down unfortunately since long time).

The result of this systematic studies can be summarized as follows [13]: The recoil energy of the beta decay is usually lower than the chemical binding energy, thus if we observe a bound brake this must be independent from the decay energy. Pure beta decay leads to 20 % bond brake due to

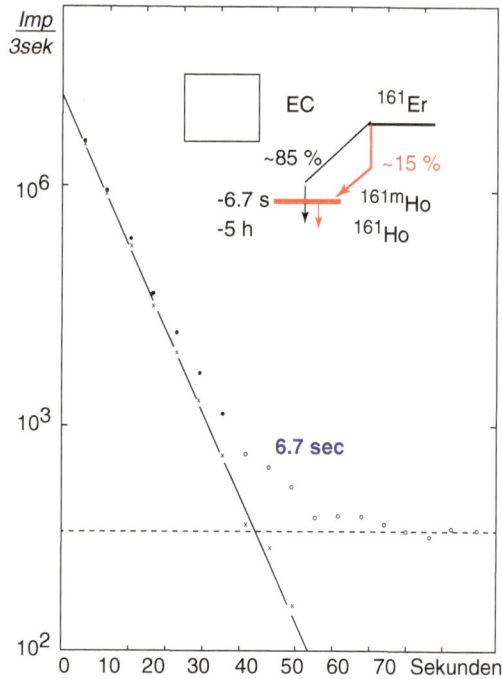

Fig. 5.6 New type of radionuclide generator based on chemical effects after radioactive decay. The mother nuclide ^{161}Er is been adsorbed as [^{161}Er DTPA]$^{2-}$-ion at a small anion-exchange column, the daughter products were eluted with a neutral 10^{-5}M Er^{3+}-solution [13, 14]

so-called electron shake-off effect. EC decay mode leads to 100% brake of any chemical binding due to Auger effect, independent on the decay energy. Same concerns all inner conversion processes. For alpha decay one has to consider very high recoil energies that cause in any case a complete destruction of the surrounding molecular environment.

These effects in combination with the knowledge of the isotope exchange kinetic allowed designing a completely new principle for radionuclide generators that are based on nuclear effects and not on chemical effects as usual. As an example in Fig. 5.6 the decay curve is shown for the 6.7 s half-life ^{161m}Ho. The mother nuclide ^{161}Er decays with ~15 % via EC to ^{161m}Ho and with ~85% the ground state of ^{161g}Ho. The ^{161}Er has been chelated with DTPA and fixed as [^{161}Er DTPA]$^{2-}$-ion at a small anion-exchange column, the daughter products were eluted with a neutral 10^{-5}M Er^{3+}-solution. F. Rösch [15] replaced the chelator DTPA later on by the macrocyclic chelator DOTA, which made the generator principle significantly more reliable.

1971 marked a significant milestone in the nuclear spectroscopy of short-lived lanthanide isotopes: the introduction of the surface ionization ion source developed in Dubna under the leadership of V. I. Raiko and H. Tyrroff [7]. With this new technique, we studied the ionization efficiencies for the different Lanthanides showing, that one can separate these isotopes with up to 80% efficiency within few minutes. The same research program we expanded to study the ionization efficiency for the Actinides. And 1991 is the time, when ^{225}Ac first time showed up in our research program. In [16] we describe a method to separate ^{225}Ac from irradiated Th-metal targets combining anion-exchange with the standard cation-exchange chromatography. In the same paper, we documented that the yield for the mass separation of Ac-radionuclides reached a value of 80%. This aspect since we will see later that one can use this technique to clean up ^{225}Ac from the unwonted side product ^{227}Ac. Similar separation yields we measured for some trans-Uranium elements, which we produced in heavy ion induced reaction at the heavy ion cyclotron U-300 of the Flerov Laboratory in Dubna.

A semi-on-line approach by inserting an unprocessed irradiated role of 15 mm × 2.5 mm × 100 μm Zr-Nb alloy foil target directly into the newly developed ion source was demonstrated first time for the identification of the ^{78}Rb [17]. We expected advantages for releasing the Rb from metal matrix because of the significant higher vapor pressure compared to that of the yttrium or lanthanides. This was the usually accepted hypothesis at that time. Later we will see that this hypothesis should be revised. However, with this Rb-experiment we initiated a serious program to study the transport of nuclear reaction products inside refractory metals with focus on the radio-lanthanides.

5.6 High-temperature Release Studies of Radio-lanthanides from Refractory Metals

For obtaining mono-isotope preparations directly from irradiated targets off-line or even on-line, the different radionuclides need to pass the following transport steps:

- Diffusion from the inner target matrix to the surface
- Desorption from the metal surface
- Effusion to the ionizer and finally
- Ionization

For the investigation of the transport processes a special experimental setup has been designed, which used the construction principles of the new Dubna surface ionization ion source. With this special furnace we were able to heat up small target samples within one minute from room temperature to ~3000 °C in vacuum (Fig. 5.7).

The temperature of the samples was controlled by two different techniques: first a W/W-Re thermocouple was inserted into a "black hole" in the bottom of each of the crucibles. Second, the vacuum furnace was tightened on top with a polished quartz plate that allowed measuring the temperature of the sample with a pyrometer. The temperature was adjusted by electron bombardment heating. The 1 mm thick W-winding is heated by few 100 A current to emit electrons, which are accelerated by an adjustable high-tension between 100 and 1000 V for bombarding the crucible. We could heat the small crucibles with up to 1 kW (1 A at 1000 V) power. Small samples of irradiated foils (660 MeV protons) of the following metals with different thicknesses were annealed at different temperatures for different periods: Ti, Zr, Nb, Hf, Ta, W, and Re. The results of these studies are published for each target element (e.g., Ta [18]) and summarized in [19]. Out of the large data set of our experimental results, only few aspects with relevance to the later bio-medical application are discussed later on.

Figure 5.8 illustrates that when heating the irradiated Zr-sample to only 1000 °C first the Y-nuclides are released from the sample and Sr

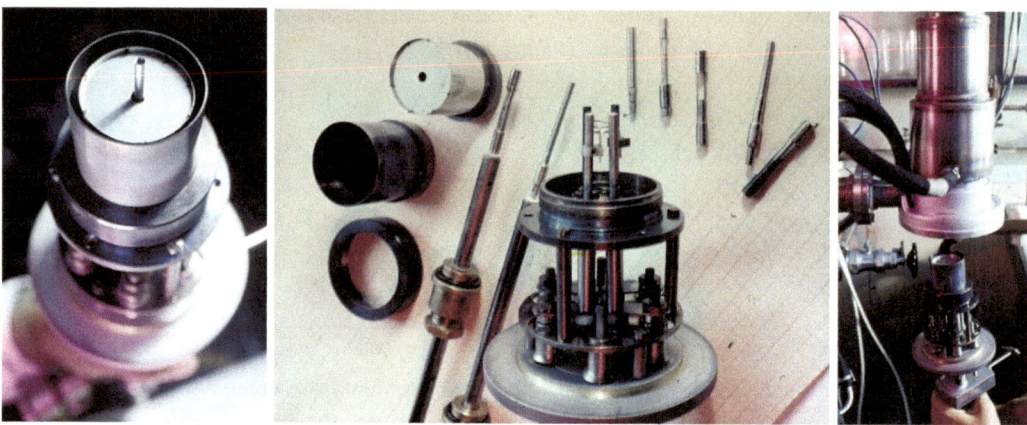

Fig. 5.7 Experimental vacuum-furnace for the study of high-temperature release of radio-lanthanides from irradiated refractory metal foils. Electron bombardment heating allowed heating up samples within one minute up to 3000 °C. **Left**: Insert with heat screens and an eight cm long conical Mo-crucible for thermo-chromatographic separation of radio-lanthanides. **Middle**: details of the furnace: heat screens, different configurations of crucibles and isolated holder for the crucibles. **Right**: Insertion of the furnace into the chilled vacuum stand

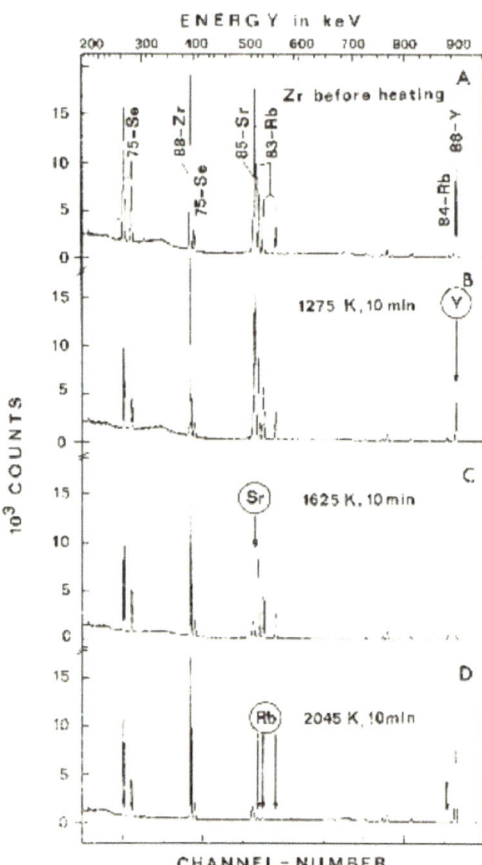

Fig. 5.8 Segments of gamma spectra of Zr-foil samples, irradiated with 660 MeV p (**a**) Zr-sample before heating, (**b**) same Zr-Sample after 10 min heating at 1000 °C, (**c**) after heating at 1340 °C, (**d**) after heating at 1760 °C

und Rb remain practically quantitatively inside the Zr sample. Sr is released only after heating to significant higher temperature (Fig. 5.8c) and Rb evaporates only closer to the melting point of Zr. Quantitatively we obtain a clear linear relationship between the radius of the diffusing specie and diffusion coefficient shown in Fig. 5.9 for two different metal target Zr and Ta.

Interesting is that we did not "lose" the Y (Fig. 5.8). The released Y-fraction was adsorbed quantitatively at the Ta-foil used as an envelope to protect the Zr-sample. The same effect was seen for the release of Sc from irradiated Ti and for the lanthanides released from Hf. We can expect to use this adsorption effect for a new separation technology for producing ^{225}Ac from irradiated Th. Furthermore, since the ^{225}Ra will remain in the Th-matrix we can use the thermic selective release of Ac as a kind of ^{225}Ra—^{225}Ac generator, providing "clean" ^{225}Ac (without ^{227}Ac—that is generated as contamination in the spallation process).

The adsorption enthalpies of the lanthanide nuclides at Ta-surface have been studied using the same vacuum furnace shown in Fig. 5.7 [20]. The adsorption enthalpies increase in the following order: Yb, Eu < Nd < Sc, Ce, Pm, La, Tm. < Gd < Lu, Y << Zr, Hf. The differences in the adsorption enthalpies can be used to separate the corresponding radio-lanthanides as shown in Fig. 5.10.

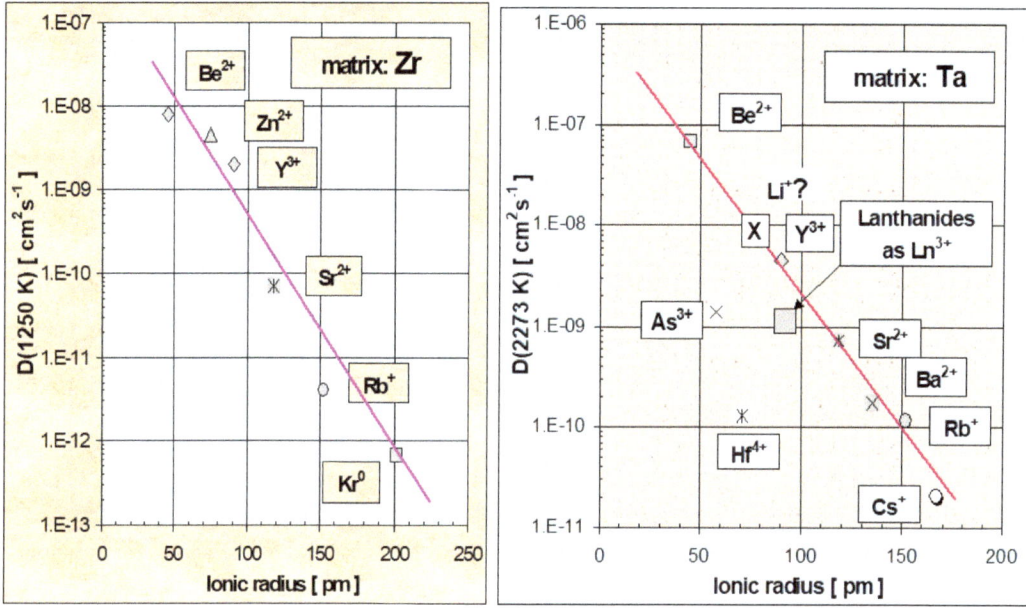

Fig. 5.9 Function of the diffusion coefficient of different nuclear reaction products in Zr (left) for 977 °C and Ta (right) for 2000 °C on the ionic radius of diffusing spe-cies. The samples were irradiated with 660 MeV protons at the Dubna synchrocyclotron

Fig. 5.10 Thermo-chromatographic separation of radio-lanthanides (details see text)

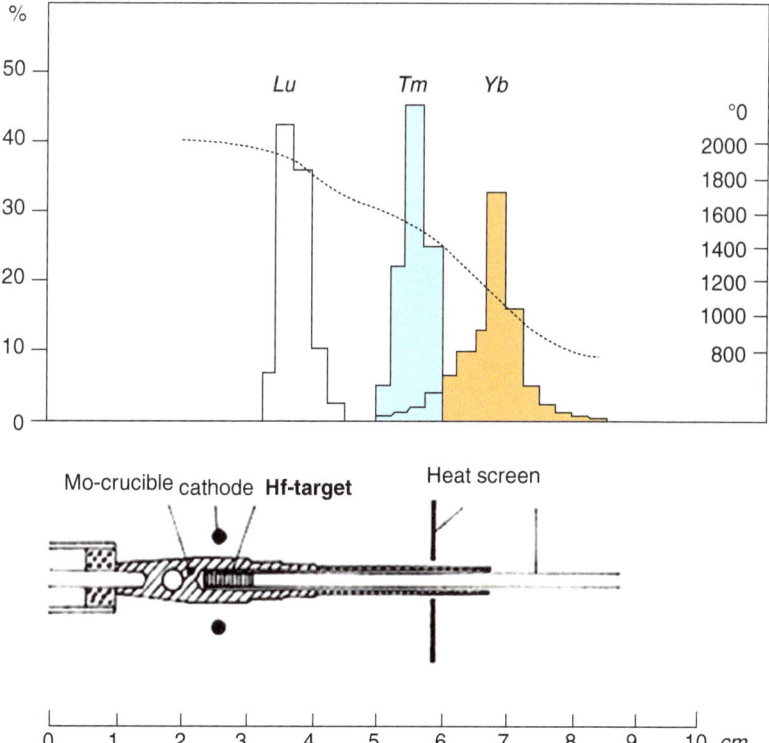

An irradiated Hf-foil target (660 MeV protons, Dubna Synchrocyclotron) has been inserted into the conical-shaped long Mo-crucible shown in Fig. 5.7. A Ta-tube has been inserted into that Mo-crucible as well. The conical shape of the Mo-crucible and the configuration of the heat screens allowed the formation of a temperature gradient along the crucible until the end of the Ta-tube from about ~2200 °C down to 600 °C. When heating the Hf-target by electron bombardment slightly above 2000 °C the lanthanide nuclides evaporate quantitatively from the Hf into the vacuum and then they are distributed along the Ta-tube according to their adsorption enthalpies, generating this nice vacuum-thermochromatogram. The same picture we obtained for Gd–Eu–Sm. The whole process took just 5 min.

5.7 ISOLDE and the On-line Production Lanthanide Nuclides

The above-discussed aspects of diffusion and adsorption of the spallation-produced radionuclides are finally implemented into the ISOLDE technology. Here we will concentrate only on the production of radionuclides of the lanthanides (Fig. 5.11).

By variation of the temperature-distribution in the target-ion source unit and variating the target configuration (foil thickness and grain size of powder), we can strongly influence the chemical selectivity of the extracted lanthanide element. This ISOL technique is a powerful tool to make also longer-lived radionuclides available for biomedical research and nuclear medical application.

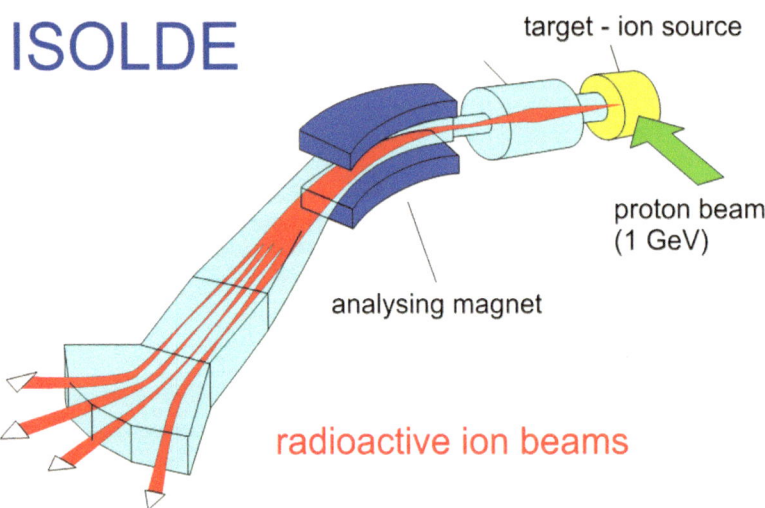

Fig. 5.11 ISOLDE principle: the high-energy proton beam hits a Ta-target, heated to ~2000 °C. The nuclear reaction products (mainly radio-lanthanides) releases from the target matrix by diffusion and desorption from the Ta-surface, effuse to the ionizing surface heated to about 2800 °C, they becomes ionized by surface ionization and the single charged ions are extracted from the target ion source system with 60 kV. The radioactive ion beam is passing the analyzing magnet where they are separated according to the atomic mass number A

5.8 Isotopes in Medicine: Situation in the 60-th

The early pioneering time of Nuclear Medicine was characterized by using "naked" radionuclides like ^{131}I or ^{89}Sr for nuclear medical application. With the introduction of the ^{99m}Tc-generator the radiochemists were occupied to search for useful reducing agents to bring the pertechnetate ion into an oxidation stage suitable for labelling of newly designed organic molecules. The general break through was reached 1969 with the introduction of Sn^{2+} as reducing agent by R. Dreyer and R. Münze [3], which marked the beginning of the cold KIT era around 1970 [4]. In that time, "new" isotopes were introduced into the nuclear medical practice: [67]Ga by C.L. Edwards in 1969 and 1973 the introduction of ^{123}I, ^{201}Tl, and [111]In. The first [^{18}F] FDG study was performed in around 1978. At this time of radio-isotope application in nuclear medicine (1975 I returned from Dubna to the ZfK Rossendorf and changed from the radiochemistry for nuclear physics basic research to the radiochemistry for medical isotope production. In a simple formless discussion in 1975 with Prof. R. Münze—in that time Head of the Radio-Isotope Department of the ZfK—he told me: "Look, there over we have this Russian cyclotron (U-120), they do something for nuclear medicine ([85]Sr). Look after, there shall outcome something more". In a second similar discussion, he said: "Here are some Japanese papers about lanthanide application in nuclear medicine, look what is behind". This was the stile in that time to transfer research tasks and induce initiative, essentially without further formalities, but also without providing additional resources. These little moments determined my later occupation and activities. It was a great pleasure supervising thereafter a small but powerful research group: F. Rösch, J. Steinbach, R. Bergmann, M. Kretzschmar, K. Schomäker, G. Kampf, G. Pimentel-Gonzales (Cuba) and others. Within a short time ^{67}Ga and ^{123}I were introduced into the nuclear medical practice of East Germany, [81]Rb/[81m]Kr-generators and ^{111}In followed. [211]At became the main subject with a strong internationally well-recognized

research group at the TU Dresden. Starting around 1980 the development for introduction of PET in the former GDR became the main research direction of our group. The second main research subject remained the radio-lanthanides for medicine. This was also the time for the interference with Richard Baum; our systematic studies of the bio-kinetic behavior of radio-lanthanides and actinium in tumor-bearing mice and rats and the developments to get access to longer-lived positron emitting metallic radionuclides together with F. Rösch played further on a dominant role in Richard Baum's carrier.

Initiated by the Japanese research on the bio-kinetic behavior of [169]Yb and [167]Tm (see for instance [21]) we confirmed in [22] that radio-lanthanides (e.g., [167]Tm) show the dramatic faster blood clearance compared to [67]Ga (Figs. 5.12 and 5.13).

The complete bio-kinetic study of [167]Tm was highlighted with the first planar scintigraphy patient study in 1978 in Dresden, Fig. 5.13 [22, 23].

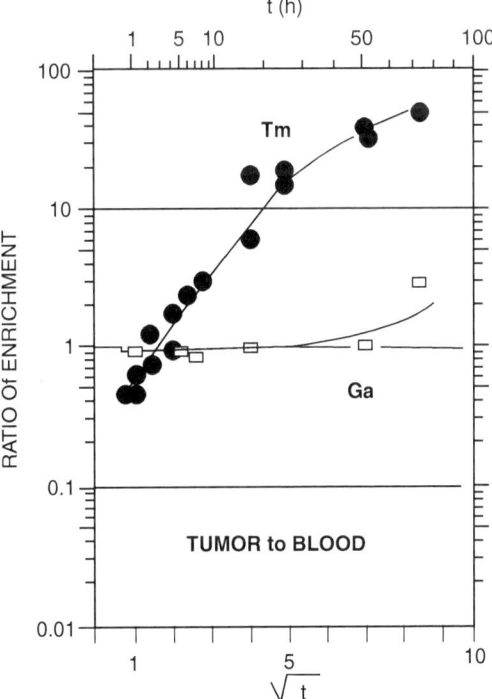

Fig. 5.12 Comparison of the blood clearance between [167]Tm and ^{67}Ga simultaneously injected as Citrate in tumor-bearing rats [22]

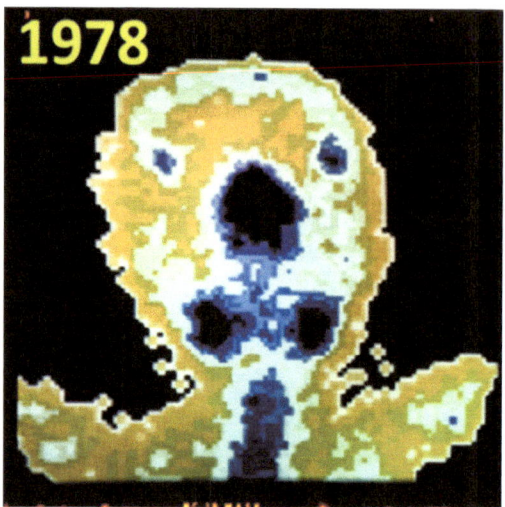

Fig. 5.13 First planar scintigraphy of a lymphoma patient 5 h p.i. 2 mCi [167]TmCit produced at CERN-ISOLDE

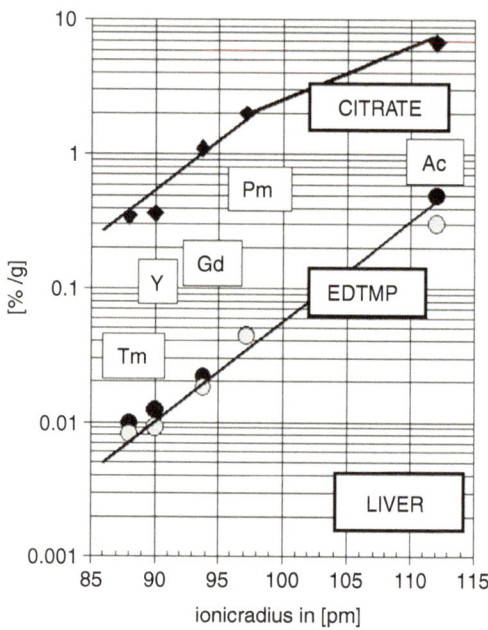

Fig. 5.14 Comparison of the bio-distribution of simultaneously injected radio-lanthanides and [225]Ac in Citrate and EDTMP solutions at 5 h p.i. in tumor-bearing rats [24, 26, 27]

In the following years, we collected bio-kinetic data for simultaneously injected cocktails of different radio-lanthanides, yttrium, and Ac in combination with different chelating ligands as citrate, EDTA, DTPA, NTA, and EDTMP. All radionuclide preparations were produced either in Dubna or at CERN ISOLDE as described above. From a stock of suitable long-lived radionuclides cocktails were mixed in a way that gamma spectroscopic technique allowed a clear data evaluation of the individual radio-tracer based on their characteristic gamma signals obtained from individual organ measurements. Few of the collected results will be presented here. For more details see [23–25].

Figure 5.14 illustrates two important results: The liver uptake of radio-lanthanides and Ac is strongly determined by the ionic radius of the Lanthanide nuclide. A liver uptake of ~0.01 %/g 2–5 h p.i. is accepted for nuclear medical in-vivo application. These low uptake values are obtained for the heavy Lanthanides and Y. For ^{67}Ga these values are reached only after ~48 h. The light lanthanides and Ac however show unacceptable high liver uptake because of the higher ionic radius. The second message is that when changing from Citrate to EDTMP ligand the liver uptake is reduced by a factor ~50. In further systematic experiments, we studied the influence of the EDTMP-ligand concentration (Fig. 5.15) [25].

In Fig. 5.15 we visualize clearly the competition between the two main excretion pathways: via kidney or liver: with increasing EDTMP concentration the excretion pathways for the individual lanthanides and Ac changes in favor of the urinary excretion. On the other hand, over a large range of EDTMP-concentration there is only little influence on the uptake in tumor and bone. Please note that the highest EDTMP-concentration used in this study was 30 mM, which is nearly three times the isotonicity. In this concern it should be mentioned, that there is no need to inject [153]SmEDTMP as such in palliative therapy of bone metastases. We have identical bio-distribution of the radio-lanthanides, if unlabeled EDTMP solution is injected first followed by the radio-tracer-injection thereafter independent on the chemical form: citrate complex or naked cation [28]. Due to these findings the author is convinced, that the main task of ETDMP in this kind of therapy is protecting the liver and not to link the radio-lanthanides into the bone

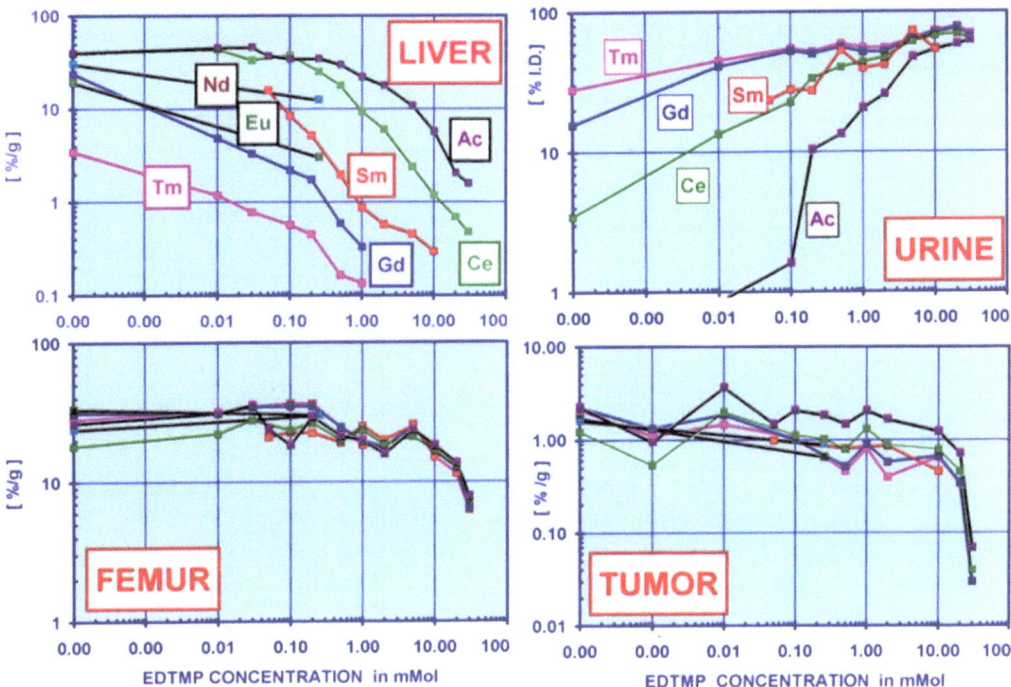

Fig. 5.15 Influence of the EDTMP concentration on the bio-kinetic behavior of radio-lanthanides and [225]Ac in tumor-bearing rats [25]

metastasis. The conclusion is, that we can practically use EDTMP as cold KIT in the same way as it is practiced for [99m]Tc.

In the 90-th we also started using chelated antibodies (DTPA-RITUXIMAB) and chelated peptides (Octreotide) (Fig. 5.16). In all cases, cocktails of radio-lanthanides and [225]Ac were used, meaning the radiotracers were injected simultaneously.

A combined summary of a large data matrix on our bio-kinetic studies performed over several years is presented in Fig. 5.16. For the citrate system, the T/L ratio is dramatically decreasing from about 1 for the heavy lanthanides down to 0.04 for Ac. The same tendency is seen for the EDTMP system (injected volume 0.5 ml per rat with a ligand concentration [EDTMP] = 2 mMol), however the T/L-ratios were about one order of magnitude better due to the reduced liver uptake in case of EDTMP compared to Citrate. In case of the DTPA-conjugated monoclonal antibodies no differences were observed for In and the heavy

lanthanides down to Pm. With higher ionic radius the T/L ratio decreases, reaching a value of 0.01 for Ac. The in-vivo stability is far below the requirement. Best values of the T/L ratio were obtained with Octreotides. The stability constant of the Pm-DTPA-mab complex ($pK_\beta \sim 22$) seems to be a threshold: for lower complex stability the in vivo stability of the metal-ligand complex becomes insufficient. Today we know that by changing the conjugated chelator DTPA by a macrocycle chelators like DOTA we increase the in vivo stability in a way, that there are no differences anymore between the different lanthanides. Even Ac can be used without changing of the tracer molecule. This was a great breakthrough into the direction of personalized nuclear medicine. Today we can use one basic bio-specific compound without any changes for any radionuclide of this group of elements independent on the decay mode and mode of application: for SPECT, PET, or therapy. A great step towards precision oncology.

Fig. 5.16 Comparison of the bio-distribution of different tumor seeking radio-tracers labeled with radio-lanthanides, [225]Ac and [111]In. The ratio of radioactivity uptake in tumor to liver tissue is plotted versus the ionic radius of the radio-metal [26, 27]. For more details see text

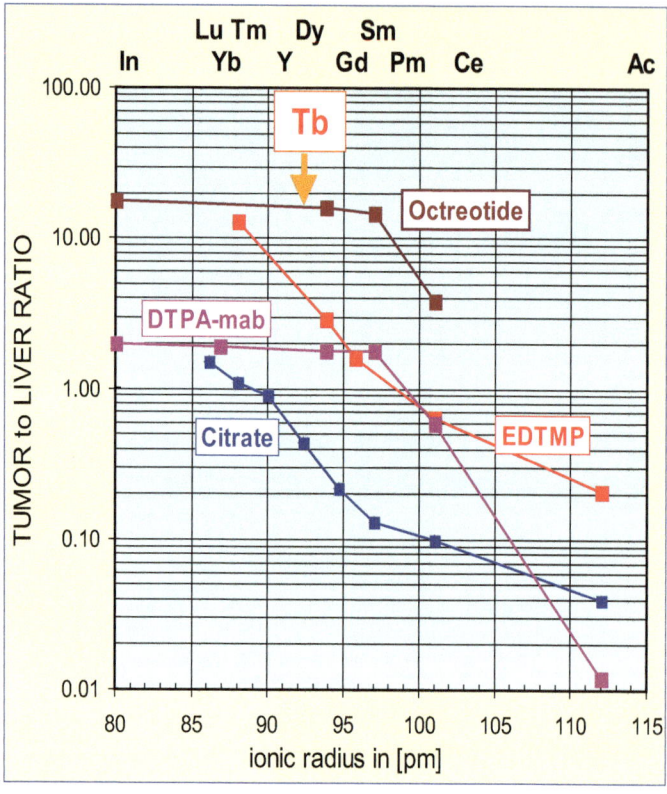

5.9   Metallic Positron Emitters

In the later 80-th we started in Rossendorf together with F. Rösch to think about metallic positron emitters for PET [29]. The list of potential candidates contained [44]Sc, ^{68}Ga, [86]Y, the positron emitters of the lanthanides, and others. This new direction became later on the dominant scientific field of F. Rösch with great impact in the activities of R. Baum especially when bringing the theranostic pair [68]Ga /^{177}Lu to the clinical routine. In the early 90-th we performed in Geneva several PET-phantom studies with the prototype of the rotating PET scanner (RPT 1), designed by David Townsend. This was the first PET scanner in Geneva. In Sept.1994 we performed a PET scan with a normal rabbit injecting the beautiful positron emitter [142]Sm (72 min), produced at ISOLDE [30], aiming to use this as tool **for individual in-vivo dosimetry** for the treatment with [153]SmEDTMP. The industrial producer of the [153]Sm EDTMP radiopharmaceutical for palliative treatment of bone metastases rejected the related proposal. Anyhow, this PET image of the rabbit done in 1994 was selected to beautify the cover page of the CERN Grey Book 1994 [31]. The time was simply not ready to understand the importance of the quantification, the terminus "Theranostica" was not yet born. PET scans with the mentioned RPT-1 scanner have been performed with other positron emitters of the lanthanides: [138]Nd/[138]Pr, [134]Ce/[134]La, [140]Nd/[140]Pr, and 1996 also with [152]Tb and [149]Tb. In Fig. 5.17 fragments of all those PET-scans are presented. With this only RPT-1 PET scanner, the images for [152]Tb were acceptable while for [149]Tb the quality was poor.

At the EANM congress 1998 in Berlin we presented a summary of the bio-kinetic studies with the focus on the alpha emitter [149]Tb asking the question: "Is [152]Tb suitable to monitor tissue doses in alpha therapy with [149]Tb using PET?" We also presented the table of the four interesting Tb-isotopes (Fig. 5.18) illustrating the unique

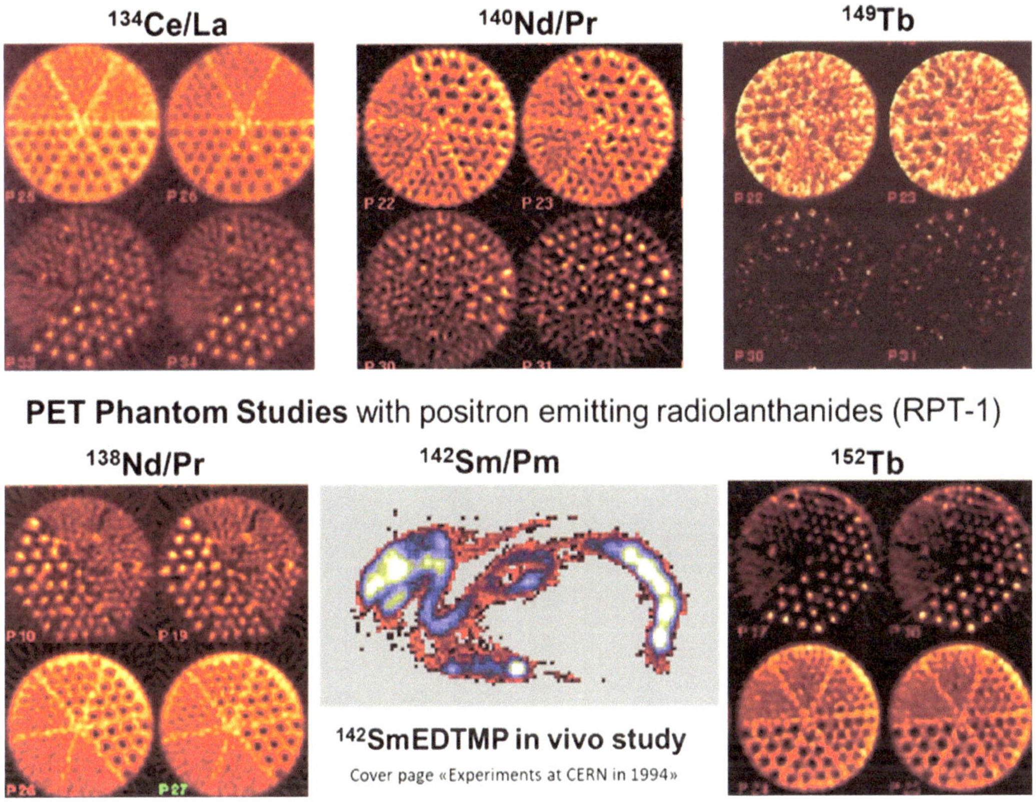

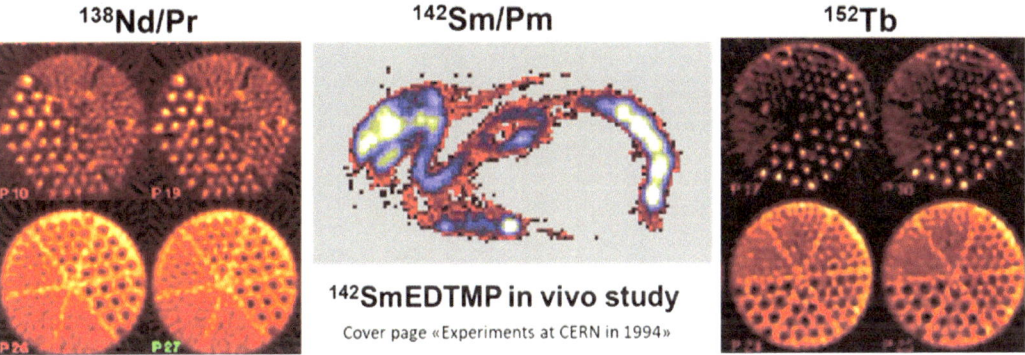

134Ce/La   **140Nd/Pr**   **149Tb**

PET Phantom Studies with positron emitting radiolanthanides (RPT-1)

138Nd/Pr   **142Sm/Pm**   **152Tb**

142SmEDTMP in vivo study
Cover page «Experiments at CERN in 1994»

Fig. 5.17 PET phantom studies with the Rotating Pet scanner at the University Hospital of Geneva using ISOLDE produced positron-emitting radionuclides of the lanthanides performed 1900–1995

Fig. 5.18 The four Tb isotopes with nuclear medical relevance for α- and β-therapy, PET, and SPECT [32, 33]

isotope $T_{1/2}$	decay mode	energy [keV]	branching [%]	production route
161Tb 6.9 d	ß⁻ max mean photons	590 195 48.9 74.6	100 14.8 9.8	^{160}Gd (n,γ) → ^{161}Gd → ß⁻ (3.6 min) ^{161}Tb
155Tb 5.32 d	EC photons	 86.2 105.3	100 31.8 24.9	Ta (p,spallation) ISOLDE diverse cyciotron reactions ^{155}Gd (p,n) ^{155}Tb
152Tb 17.5 h	ß⁺ max EC photons	2800	20 80 diverse	Ta (p,spallation) ISOLDE diverse cyciotron reactions
149Tb 4.1 h	α ß⁺ max EC photons	3970 1800	17 7 75 diverse	Ta (p,spallation) ISOLDE ^{142}Nd (^{12}C,4n) ^{149}Db ^{152}Gd (p,4n) ^{149}Tb other HI reactions

properties of terbium, combining all main decay modes suitable for specific nuclear medical applications: beta-therapy (^{161}Tb), SPECT imaging (^{155}Tb), PET-imaging (^{152}Tb), and finally alpha therapy (^{149}Tb) [32, 33]). Tb is the only element, which provides these unique universal possibili-

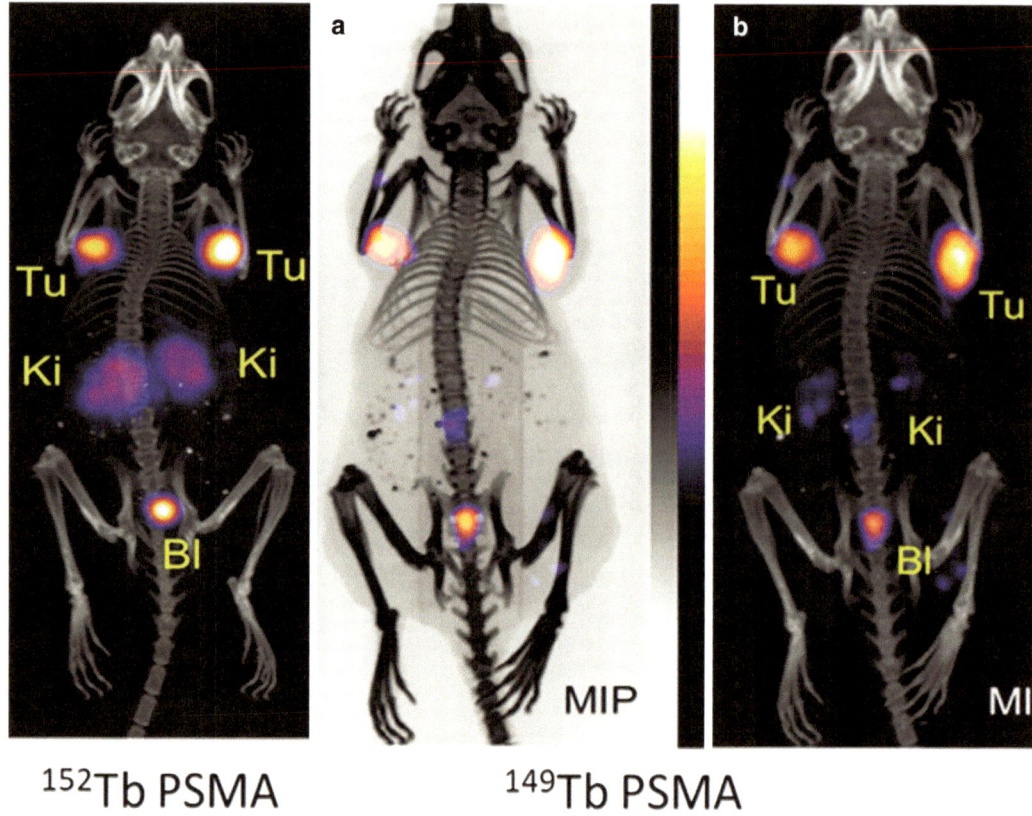

^{152}Tb PSMA ^{149}Tb PSMA

Fig. 5.19 PET/CT images of mice with ^{152}Tb PSMA (left) and ^{149}Tb PMSA (right) performed at PSI [25, 34]

ties. It is a great pleasure to see today, that great progress has been achieved due to the initiative of R. Baum together with his enthusiastic partners from PSI Ch. Mueller, Nick van der Meulen, and others [34, 35]. The latest highlight in this concern is the first PET/CT study of a patient using ^{152}Tb DOTATOC [36], where the ^{152}Tb was produced at CERN ISOLDE based on the technology described above (Fig. 5.19).

5.10 The Alpha Emitters ^{149}Tb and ^{225}Ac

In the Habil-Thesis 1978 (Beyer/Herrmann) [37] one can read at page 334, Vol 2, the following note: "...*Neben diesen für die nuklearmedizinische Diagnostik interessanten Nukliden sind mit den vorgestellten Targetvarianten auch weiche kurzlebige α-Strahler der Seltenen Erden zugänglich, die für die Therapie in der* Nuklearmedizin *Bedeutung erlangen könnten* (^{153}Dy, ^{151}Tb, ^{150}Tb *und* ***^{149}Tb***)".

Over nearly 20 years I had completely forgotten about ^{149}Tb, lost it out of my field of view. Mid 1990-th it was Barry Allen (Australia) who waked me up. He was in Geneva and we discussed the Targeted Alpha Therapy (TAT) with lanthanides—with ^{149}Tb! Next day we met in the hospital, I brought an old Dubna-prepring from 1971 with me about our spectroscopic studies of Tb-isomeres [38] showing that we had 1971 already serious activities of this interesting isotope ^{149}Tb in our hands. The ISOLDE schedule was changed immediately (fortunately ISOLDE had just the Ta-target in operation) and few days later we had a collection of mass number A = 149 in our lab in the hospital and made the chromatographic separation and we had around 400 MBq of ^{149}Tb in our hand. This was a real breakthrough: Barry Allen delegated one of his technicians to Geneva and we were starting to work on the Tb-isotopes, documented in several publications related to [152]Tb and [149]Tb see for example [39–41]. Since then the α-emitter [149]Tb became the focus of our lanthanide work. In [42] we described our very complex study about the evidence for single cell kill effect using [149]Tb RITUXIMAB. The conjugated antibody Rituximab we obtained from S. Larson (NY). The experiment with nude mice was designed by M.Miederer (Munich), the daudi cells came from Lausanne, cell cultivation and animal service was done in the Institute of Bio-Chemistry, Geneva University (Dir. Prof. R. Offord). The cell labeling was done by S. Vranješ from Belgrade, operation of the ISOLDE facility and the collection of A = 149 was done by J. Comor from Belgrade, the radiochemical purification of the [149]Tb, the labeling of the RITUXIMAB and QC as well as the gamma-spectroscopic data evaluation of the organ measurements of all animals was the job of

G. Beyer. It was a real surprise and great pleasure learning, that in three independent experimental runs 90 % of the animals that received the [149]Tb injection survived four months (until the moment when the financing was exhausted). We lost only one mice; G.Künzi said later on that he remembers, that the injection of the [149]Tb RITUXIMAB in one of the nude mice was not perfect (meaning not completely i.v.). Thus, terbium with his distinguished isotope [149]Tb and in his shadow the other three sisters ([152]Tb, [155]Tb, and [161]Tb) advanced to the most distinguished theranostic element. There is no other element in the periodic table, that combine all the four decay modes needed in nuclear medicine: β⁻ and β⁺, α and suitable photon radiation (note: [165]Er is the only pure Auger electron emitter in the lanthanide group). CERN-people named the [149]Tb later on the Swiss knife (Fig. 5.20).

Fig. 5.20 Surviving study with [149]Tb-RITUXIMAB in scid mice [42]

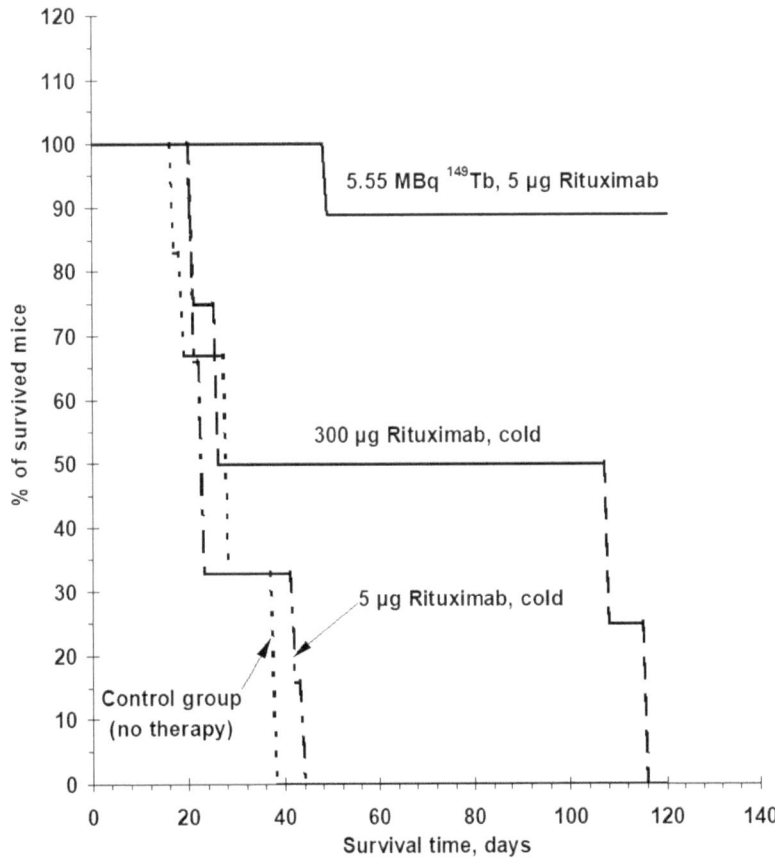

5.11 From "Radioactive Ion Beams for Bio-Medical Research" Until CERN Medicis: A New Facility

After the reunification of Germany (1991) I continued working directly at ISOLDE CERN (1991–1993) and thereafter until retirement in 2005 at the University Hospital of Geneva setting up the Geneva Cyclotron Unit for PET together with Ch. Morel. The main task at CERN was to study the potential of radioactive Ion beams for bio-medical research and nuclear medical application. Together with H. L. Ravn, U. Köster (both CERN at that time), and T. Ruth (Vancouver) we were fighting for acceptance of this technological approach (see for instance [43]). At that time our related proposal to CERN from 2005 [44, 45] did not yet find the required resonance by the CERN DG, because LHC had priority in all activities at CERN. A patent application has been formulated with the CERN Technology Transfer section [46]. Finally, with a delay of about 10 years the MEDICIS Project became a reality in 2014 [47] mainly based on the new initiative of Thierry Stora. A bright future can be expected for this pioneering system.

5.12 The ^{225}Ac Story

First time we made ^{225}Ac in 1971 by irradiating Th-metal with 660 MeV protons, separating the Ac by anion and cation exchange chromatography [16]. At that time we simply studied the ionization efficiency together with other actinide elements with our new surface ionization ion source. The Th-irradiation with protons was already a routine in Dubna especially for producing high purity ^{211}At from the decay of ^{211}Rn [48]. Our interest in ^{225}Ac appeared already in the 80-th when we studied the biokinetic behavior of the radio-lanthanides. The ^{225}Ac we produced ourselves either with the ISOLDE facility at CERN or by irradiating Th (or U) in Dubna. Our radiochemical separation schemes for separating ^{225}Ac from irradiated Th are described in [16] and for U_3O_8 in [49]: 27 g U_3O_8 were irradiated with

650 MeV protons at the Dubna phasotron. After three days of decay time the target was dissolved in 5M HNO_3. The U was separated by anion exchange chromatography using a Dowex 1×8 column. From the U-free solution the radio-lanthanides, Ac and Ra were coprecipitated with 100 mg Ba-carrier as $BaSO_4$ which was thereafter converted to $BaCO_3$. This sample containing the radio-lanthanides, Y, Ac, and Ra was shipped to Rossendorf for the final separation and purification [49].

For the first time, we used ^{225}Ac to label monoclonal antibodies in 1995 [50]. In that time the mab were still conjugated with DTPA, this conjugation one has to pay with one carboxylic group of the DTPA ending up with a chelator similar to EDTA only. The chelated mab labeled with ^{111}In and the heavy lanthanides showed practically identical and satisfactory biodistribution, however the complex stability for ^{225}Ac was significantly too low and consequently the in vivo stability was by far insufficient: Ac was trapped in the liver. After presenting those dates at a seminar at Sloan Kettering Hospital NY in 1995 Scheinberg asked, why you used ^{225}Ac and not ^{213}Bi. At Sloan Kettering Hospital they pioneered the TAT with ^{213}Bi which is obtained from an ^{225}Ac/^{213}Bi generator. The aim of our study was different, we simply wanted to compare the biokinetic behavior of Ac with the "golden" standard at that time (^{111}In) and with the lanthanides. But definitely this study initiated the motivation using the ^{225}Ac directly. The direct use of ^{225}Ac became possible in the moment when macrocycle chelators (like DOTA for example) replaced the former used DTPA and provided for Ac the same in vivo stability as for In or the lanthanides. H. Mäcke conjugated different peptides with different macrocycle chelators, which is the basis of the grandiose recent progress in radionuclide therapy. The beauty is that with this class of ligands we can use all the radionuclides of the group III of the periodic table (Ga and Sc, Y, lanthanides, and actinides) independent on their decay properties. This is a universal theranostic approach. Because of this development already at the beginning of the twenty-first century the quest for ^{225}Ac has grown significantly.

5.13   Where the ^{225}Ac Comes From

Until about 2003 the only source for ^{225}Ac in Germany or Europe was a nearly 1 kg stock of Th that is "contaminated" with about 1.5 GBq ^{229}Th and located at the Institut of Transuranium Elements (ITU Karlsruhe) and for the US about 5 GBq ^{229}Th stock at Oakridge (US). In Russia, a small fraction of the existing stock of ^{233}U has been processed making another source of ~0.5 GBq ^{225}Ac available [51]. Based on our Dubna experiences Shuikov initiated a program (around 2005) at the Troitzk LINAC for producing ^{225}Ac via the process Th(p;spall)^{225}Ac [52]. Since few years the US Department of isotopes is offering frequently ^{225}Ac products along this spallation process. The drawback of this process is that we have to consider a side production of ^{227}Ac that disturb the direct in-vivo application of the ^{225}Ac preparation.

In the scheme Fig. 5.21 the possible production routes for ^{225}Ac or ^{225}Ra are presented [53]. There are in principle three main strategies to access ^{225}Ac: the indirect production routes via ^{229}Th, the indirect production routes via ^{225}Ra and the direct production routes via spallation or ^{226}Ra (p,2n)^{225}Ac process. The problem with the process ^{226}Ra (p,2n)^{225}Ac is simply the fact that the normal reaction of protons with an energy higher than ~16 MeV is the fission process according to ^{226}Ra (p,f) FP. In order to avoid fission and for obtaining a relatively undisturbed ^{226}Ra(p,2n) ^{225}Ac process one needs to reduce the p-energy down to ~16 MeV. This means that one could run this process in principle with a classical PET cyclotron. However, we just scratch the excitation function and consequently the productivity is low. The licensing procedure and safety regulations related to alpha laboratories are other important issues. A small alpha workshop was

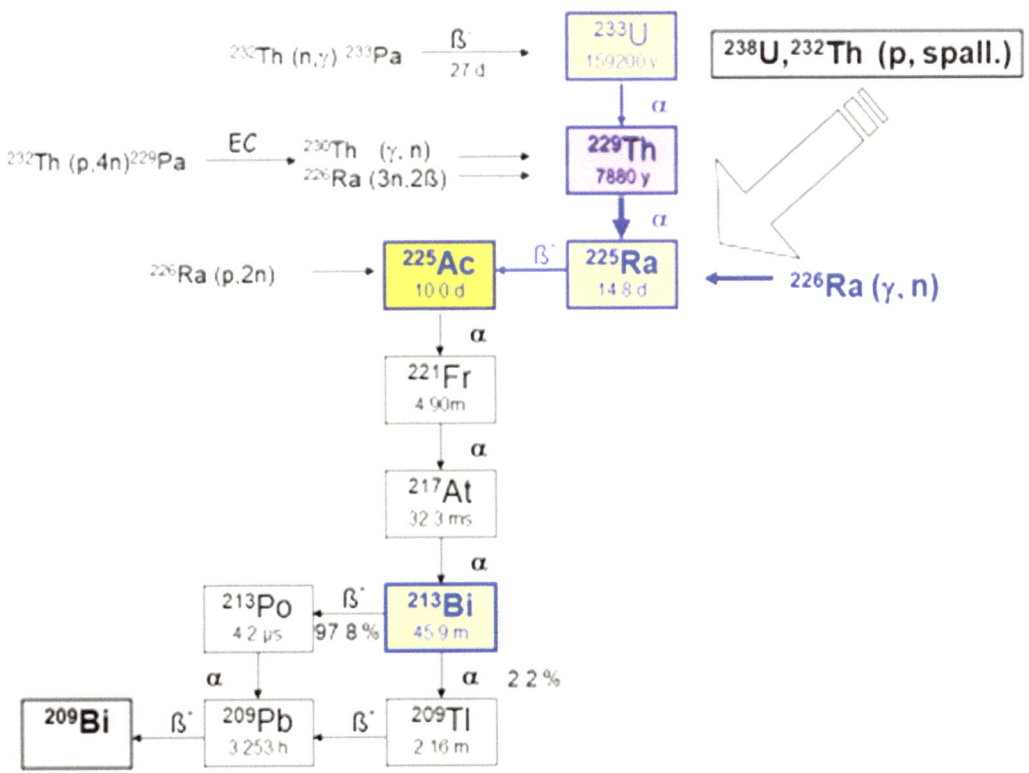

Fig. 5.21   The decay chain of ^{233}U and the potential production routes for ^{225}Ac [53]

organized in Dubna in 2003 with the participation of US representatives from the DOE, ROSATOM Authorities and mainly the Russian researchers. The interest of the US representatives was clearly to get access to the Russian resources for making ^{225}Ra and ^{225}Ac. With the Canadian firm Alpha IICH we started to organize a regular supply of small ^{225}Ac-preparations for R&D to the European market and succeeded to obtain four test samples of 18.5 MBq ^{225}Ac in 2004 from Russia (produced with the ^{229}Th/^{225}Ac generator principle described in [51]. The quality of these test samples was o.k. It took further about 15 years until a reliable supply of around 0.5 GBq ^{225}Ac from Russia is achieved now. By far the today's fast-growing demand in ^{225}Ac cannot be met with the existing resources. Today the discussion for project ideas for industrial scale ^{225}Ac production facilities continues at the platform of the regular TAT-workshops and conferences, last one being the TAT 11 Conference Ottawa (Canada) 2019 [54]. https://www.tat11.com/. Most promising seems to be the photonuclear process ^{226}Ra (γ, n) ^{225}Ra, a technology that has been proposed since long time. The needed high-power electron accelerators exists, the required quantities of ^{226}Ra are available. The bottleneck is that the investors are most likely not yet 100% convinced that the ^{225}Ac will play a serious role in future alpha therapy that justifies the high investment today. However, R. Baum's activities clearly demonstrated that ^{225}Ac will definitely play a dominant role in the future for treating cancer generally and effectively, within the International Centres for Precision Oncology ICPO. It is high time to establish a reliable industrial scale ^{225}Ac supply.

5.14 Summarizing

This contribution is a trial to draw the historical development of radiopharmaceuticals restricted to the radionuclides of the rare earth elements from the early beginning using them as naked metallic cation via chelates like Citrate or EDTMP and with labeled DTPA-conjugated mab's and -peptides until the modern radiopharmaceuticals based on peptides linked with macrocyclic chelators and further starting from simple scintigraphic imaging for diagnosis through quantitative PET imaging to the theranostic approaches of personalized nuclear medicine. The initial radiochemical and physicochemical developments in the field of rare earth elements definitely contributed to the progress in nuclear medicine, from diagnosis to precision oncology. R. Baum is one of the most distinguished medical specialists for precision oncology who understood the importance of scientific disciplines like radiochemistry, nuclear physics, or biochemistry as being unavoidable for success in the fight against cancer.

References

1. Herrmann E, Grosse-Ruyken H, Lebedev NA, Khalkin VA. Radiochimija. 1964;6:756.
2. Herrmann EJ. Chromatography. 1968;38:495.
3. Dreyer R, Muenze R. Markierung von Human Serum Albomin with 99m-Tc Wiss. Z K-Marx Uni Leipzig Nat Wiss R. 1969;18:629–33; Zur Tc-99m-Markierung von Serumalbumin; Isotopenpraxis 5 (1969) 296.
4. Eckelmann WC. J Am Coll Cardiol Img. 2009;2:364–8.
5. https://home.cern/news/series/meet-isolde/meet-isolde-where-did-it-all-begin.
6. Kalinnikov VG et al. D13-90-183 Dubna. 1990. https://inis.iaea.org/collection/NCLCollectionStore/_Public/23/049/23049399.pdf.
7. Beyer GJ, Herrmann E, Piotrovski A, Raiko VI, Tyrroff H. A new method for rare earth isotope separation. Nucl Instrum Methods. 1971;96(3):437.
8. Trabisch U, Bächmann K. Radiochim Acta. 1971;16:15.
9. Beyer GJ, Herrmann E, Tyrroff H. Gewinnung Trägerfreier Radionuklide der Lanthaniden. Isotopenpraxis. 1977;13(6):193–203.
10. Pfrepper G, Pfrepper R. Kernenergie. 1970;13:58.
11. Beyer GJ. Anwendung des Szilard-Chalmers Effekte zur schnellen Gewinnung trägerfreier Lanthanidaktivitäten aus Seltenerd-Komplexonaten für die Kernspektroskopie. PhD-Thesis, TU Dresden. 1969.
12. Beyer GJ, Große-Ruyken H, Khalkin VA, Pfrepper G. Complex compounds of the lanthanides with DTPA as target for irradiation with 660 MeV protons. J Inorg Nucl Chem. 1969;31:2135. https://www.sciencedirect.com/science/article/abs/pii/002219026990030X.
13. Beyer GJ, Grosse-Ruyken H, Khalkin VA. Eine Methode zur Trennung genetisch verknüpfter isobarer

und isomerer Nuklidpaare der Seltenen Erden. J Inorg Nucl Chem. 1969;31:1865. https://www.sciencedirect.com/science/article/abs/pii/0022190269804100?via%3Dihub.

14. Beyer GJ. Behaviour of rare earth daughter products in vivo after the radioactive decay of their parent nuclides chelated in bio-conjugates. INCFE5/COST D18, Geneva, 24-27 Aug 2003.

15. Zhernosekov KP, Filosofov DV, Qaim SM, Rösch F. A ^{140}Nd/^{140}Pr radionuclide generator based on physico-chemical transitions in ^{140}Pr complexes after electron capture decay of ^{140}Nd-DOTA. Radiochim Acta. 2007;95:319.

16. Beyer GJ, Herrmann E, Molnar F, Raiko VI, Tyrroff H. A highhly-efficient method for the separation of actinide isotopes. Radiochem Radioanal Lett. 1972;12(4-5):256–69.

17. Arlt R, Beyer GJ, Herrmann E, Habenicht W, Tyrroff H. On the identification of ^{78}Rb ($T_{1/2}$= 19 min). Radiochem Radioanal Lett. 1972;10(3):173.

18. Beyer GJ, Fromm WD, Novgorodov AF. Tracerdiffusion of different nuclear reaction product in polycristalline Ta. Nucl Instrum Methods. 1977;146:419.

19. Beyer GJ, Hagebo E, Novgorodov AF, Ravn HL. The role of diffusion in ISOL targets for the production of radioactive ion beams. NIM B. 2003;204:225–34. https://www.sciencedirect.com/science/article/abs/pii/S0168583X02019134.

20. Beyer GJ, Novgorodov AF, Khalkin VA. On the adsorption of ultra-small quantities of lanthanides, Sc, Y, Zr and Hf to polycrystalline Ta (in Russian). Radiokhimiya. 1978;96:589–97.

21. Ando A, Hisada K. Affinity of ^{167}Tm for malignant tumor and bone. Radioisotopes. 1975;24:41.

22. Beyer GJ, Franke WG, et al. Comparative kinetic study of simultaneously injected ^{167}Tm and ^{67}Ga-Citrate in normal and tumor bearing mice. Int J Appl Radiat Isot. 1978;29:673. https://www.sciencedirect.com/science/article/pii/0020708X78901059.

23. Beyer GJ, Muenze R, Fromm WD, Franke WG, Henke H, Khalkin VA, Lebedev NA. Spallation produced Thulium-167 for medical application. In: Medical radionuclide imaging 1980. Vienna: IAEA; 1981. https://inis.iaea.org/search/search.aspx?orig_q=RN:12641820.

24. Beyer GJ, Bergmann R, Schomäcker K, Rösch F, Schäfer G, Kulikov EV, Novgorodov AF. Comparison of the bio-distribution of ^{225}Ac and radio-lanthanides as citrate complexes. Isotopenpraxis. 1990;26(3):111–4.

25. Beyer GJ, Offord R, Künzi G, Aleksandrova Y, Ravn U, Jahn S, Backe J, Tengblad O, Lindroos M. The influence of EDTMP-concentration on the biodistribution of radio-lanthanides and 225-Ac in tumor bearing mice. Nucl Med Biol. 1997;24:367–72.

26. Beyer GJ. Radioactive ion beams for biomedical research and nuclear medical application. Hyperfine Interact. 2000;129:529. https://www.researchgate.net/publication/228797712_Radioactive_Ion_Beams_for_Bio-Medical_Research_and_Nuclear_Medical_Application.

27. Beyer GJ. Radioactive ion beams for bio-medical research and nuclear medical application. In: Advanced technology and particle physics (ICATPP-7). New York: World Scientific; 2002. p. 504–11.

28. Beyer GJ, Bergmann R, Kampf G, Mäding P, Rösch F. Simultaner Vergleich der Bioverteilung von ^{87}Y-CITRAT und ^{167}Tm-EDTMP an tumortragenden Ratten. Nucl Med. 1991;30:A21.

29. Rösch F, Beyer GJ. Studies on longer-living positron emitters under the aspect of radiopharmaceutica application. In: Bernhard G, editor. Annual report 1990. Rossendorf: Department of Radioactive Isotopes; 1991. p. 99–101. https://www.osti.gov/etdeweb/biblio/10121291.

30. Beyer GJ, Donath A, Morel C, Offord R, Künzi G, Ravn U, Aleksandrova Y, Jahn S, Lindroos M. 142-Samarium - a suitable positron emitter for uptake monitoring in 153-Sm EDTMP therapy. J Nucl Med. 1996;35(5):194.

31. Beyer GJ. Use of radioactive ion beams for biomedical research: 2. In-vivo dosimetry using positron emitting rare earth isotopes with the rotating prototype PET-scanner at the Geneva University Hospital (ISOLDE IS 331). CERN Greybook. 1994;1994:243–5.

32. Beyer GJ, Morel C, Slosman D, Sakar S, Allen BJ. Is ^{152}Tb suitable to monitor tissue dose in alpha therapy with 149Tb? (EANM 1998 Berlin). Eur J Nucl Med. 1998;25(8):1157.

33. Beyer G.J., and Roesch F. Radio-Lanthanides in nuclear medicine, 10th ICBIC, COST D-18 Florence, August 26-31, 2001.

34. Müller C, Vermeulen C, Köster U, Johnston K, Türler A, Schibli R. Alpha-PET with terbium-149: evidence and perspectives for radiotheranostics. EJNMMI Radiopharm Chem. 2016;1:5.

35. Müller C, Vermeulen C, Johnston K, Köster U, Schmid R, Türler A, et al. Preclinical in vivo application of ^{152}Tb-DOTANOC: a radio-lanthanide for PET imaging. EJNMMI Res. 2016;6:35. https://doi.org/10.1186/s13550-016-0189-4.

36. Baum R, Sing A, Benosova M, Vermeulen C, Gnesin S, Köster U, Johnston K, Müller SS, Kulkarni H, Türler A, Schibli R, Prior JO, van der Meulen NP, Müller C. Clinical evaluation of the radiolanthanide ^{152}Tb: first-in-human PET/CT with ^{152}Tb DOTATOC. Dalton Trans. 2017;46:14638–46.

37. Beyer GJ, Herrmann E. Zur Darstellung kurzlebiger radioactiver Nuklide für die Kernspektroskopie durch Spallation, habil-Schrift, TU Dresden, 26.10.1978, Vol 2, page 334.

38. Arlt R, Beyer GJ, Kuznetsov KV, Neubert W, Potempa AV, Hagemann U, Herrmann E. Untersuchung der kurzlebigen Isomere der isotope ^{148}Tb, ^{149}Tb, ^{150}Tb und ^{152}Tb Izv. An SSSR Ser Fiz. 1971;35:1612.

39. Allen BJ, Beyer GJ, Morel C, Offord R, Aleksandrova Y, Jahn S. Tb-149: a new radiolanthanide for targeted cancer therapy. 1996. https://www.osti.gov/etdeweb/biblio/20004328.

40. Allen BJ, Goozee G, Sarkar S, Beyer GJ, Morel C, Byrne AP. Production of [152]Tb by heavy ion reactions and proton induced spallation. Appl Radiat Isot. 2001;54(1):53–8.

41. Beyer GJ, Čomor JJ, Soloviev D, Hagebø E, Allen B, Dmitriev SN, Zaitzeva NG, Starodub GY, Molokanova LG, Vranješ S, Miederer M. Production routes of the alpha emitting [149]Tb for medical application. Radiochim Acta. 2002;90(5):247–52. https://www.researchgate.net/publication/236881833_Production_routes_of_the_alpha_emitting_149Tb_for_medical_application.

42. Beyer GJ, Miederer M, Vranješ-Durić S, Čomor JJ, Künzi G, Hartley O, Senekovitsch-Schmidtke R, Soloviev D, Buchegger F, ISOLDE Collaboration. Targeted alpha therapy in vivo: direct evidence for single cancer cell kill using [149]Tb-rituximab. EJNMMI. 2004;31(4):547–54. https://www.researchgate.net/publication/227074267_Targeted_alpha_therapy_in_vivo_Direct_evidence_for_single_cancer_cell_kill_using_149Tb-rituximab.

43. Beyer GJ, Ruth T. The role of electromagnetic separators in the production of radiotracers for bio-medical research and nuclear medical application. NIM B. 2003;204:694–700. https://www.sciencedirect.com/science/article/abs/pii/S0168583X03004890.

44. Drummond D, Susan A, Beyer GJ. Proposal to create a radiochemical laboratory at CERN for production of therapeutic alpha-emitting radionuclides using ISOLDE target techniques. Alpha IICH CERN Proposal March 2005 (unpublished).

45. Beyer GJ, Koester U, Ragnelli G, Ravn HL. High-tech radioisotope preparation at CERN-ISOLDE for life sciences research and medical application, Request to CERN, 10 March 2005.

46. Koester U, Beyer GJ, Ravn HL, Ragnelli G, Le Goff JM. Method for production of radioisotope preparations and their use in life science research, medical application and industry. CERN Patent application, C3019PCT, CERN TT Section, C30195PCT CERN, 2007.

47. dos Santos Augusto RM, Buehler L, Lawson Z, Marzari S, Stachura M, Stora T. CERN-MEDICIS (medical isotopes collected from ISOLDE): a new facility. Appl Sci. 2014;4:265–81. https://www.researchgate.net/publication/262495128_CERN-MEDICIS_medical_isotopes_collected_from_ISOLDE_A_new_facility.

48. Khalkin VA, Herrmann E, Norseev YV, Dreyer I. Chemiker-Zeitung. 1977;101:470–81.

49. Beyer GJ, Roesch F, Novgorodov AF, Kulikov EV. Preparation and chemical separation of [225]Ac. In: Muenze R, editor. Annual report 1990. Rossendorf: Department of Radioactive Isotopes; 1990. p. 17–20.

50. Beyer GJ, Offord RE, Künzi G, Jones RML, Ravn U, Aleksandrova Y, Werlin RC, Mäcke H, Jahn S, Tengblad. Biokinetic of monoclonal antibodies labelled with radio-lanthanides and [225]Ac in xeno-crafted nude mice. J Label Compd Radiopharm. 1995;37:529.

51. Tsoupko-Sitnikov V, Norseev Y, Khalkin VA. Generator of Actinium-225. J Radioanal Nucl Chem. 1996;205(1):75–83.

52. Zhuikov BL, Kalmykov SN, Ermolaev SV, Aliev RA, Kokhanyuk VM, Matushko VL, Tananaev IG, Myasoedov BF. Production of [225]Ac and [223]Ra by irradiation of Th with accelerated protons. Radiochemsitry. 2011;53:73–80.

53. Beyer GJ. Alpha emitting radionuclides – production and application. In: Baranova V, editor. Isotops I and II, properties, production and application, vol. 2. Moskva: FIZMATLIT; 2005. p. 372–89. https://www.researchgate.net/publication/257858681_Production_of_225Ac_and_223Ra_byirradiation_of_Th_with_accelerated_protons.

54. Zuckier LS. Proceedings from the TAT11. J Med Imaging Rad Sci. 2019;50:S115. https://www.tat11.com/.

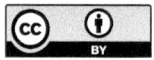

"How Do You Feel About Dosimetry?" The Gretchenfrage of Radionuclide Therapy

6

Matthias Blaickner

6.1 The Gretchenfrage

How is it now with thy religion, say?
I know thou art a dear good man,
But fear thy thoughts do not run much that way.
Faust; a Tragedy. Johann Wolfgang von Goethe

The lines above are uttered by Gretchen (diminutive of the given name Margarete) in Faust, Part one, the most known work of Johann Wolfgang von Goethe, who is considered by many the greatest German poet of all time. Gretchen's question (the "Gretchenfrage" in German) became a dictum for any issue which is both crucial as well as delicate. Gretchen, an innocent and faithful character asks Dr. Faust about his piety, with the respondent being secretly in league with the devil. Answering puts him in a dilemma. Honesty most probably would make his love interest leave and deceit always is the cornerstone of downfall and tragedy, so Faust evades the question. Ironically enough, he must have some kind of religious faith, since it would not make any sense for a categorical atheist to bond with a godlike, though sinister entity as Mephistopheles.

What does this have to do with dosimetry in Radionuclide Therapy, except the obvious geographical analogy, i.e., the cultural center Weimar as domain of Goethe and Schiller and the nearby Zentralklinik in Bad Berka as the scientific spearhead in the diagnosis and treatment with unsealed, radiolabeled compounds? Just like the Gretchenfrage, the question about the necessity, usefulness, and accuracy of dosimetry calculations in Radionuclide Therapy is both crucial as well as delicate. Crucial, because Radionuclide Therapy has proved its effectiveness in many studies and with regard to different nuclides [1–5]. Moreover, there is no doubt that the reduction of tumor mass stems from the effects of ionizing radiation on malignant cells rather than any other property of the radiolabeled compound.

And yet, in the field of Radionuclide Therapy, this radiobiological knowledge, developed and ensured by decades of radiation research, somehow cannot be transformed smoothly to an elegant correlation function with the calculated, absorbed radiation dose on one side, and the reduction of metastatic tissue on the other. This is the delicate aspect when it comes to dosimetry calculations in Radionuclide Therapy and not uncommonly physicians and medical physicists are tempted, just as Dr. Faust, to evade the question about its necessity, usefulness and accuracy, as well as the associated effort. An ongoing

M. Blaickner (✉)
Preclinical Molecular Imaging, AIT Austrian Institute of Technology GmbH, Seibersdorf, Austria

Department Computer Science, Competence Center Artificial Intelligence and Data Analytics, Fachhochschule Technikum Wien, University of Applied Sciences Technikum Wien, Wien, Austria
e-mail: matthias.blaickner@ait.ac.at;
matthias.blaickner@technikum-wien.at;
http://www.ait.ac.at; http://www.technikum-wien.at

© The Author(s) 2024
V. Prasad (ed.), *Beyond Becquerel and Biology to Precision Radiomolecular Oncology: Festschrift in Honor of Richard P. Baum*, https://doi.org/10.1007/978-3-031-33533-4_6

debate among scientists on the value of dosimetry beyond the preclinical phase of radiopharmaceutical development, such as the clinical implementation of personalized, image-based dosimetry, has been held in conferences and journals for years [6–9]. The purpose of this article is to give a structured and unbiased overview on the issue of dosimetry in Radionuclide Therapy, in the hope to spare the reader from Faust's lament:

And here, at last, I stand, poor fool!
As wise as when I entered school;

6.2 The Forms of Dosimetry in a Nutshell

The basis for all dosimetry in Nuclear Medicine is of course the MIRD (Medical Internal Radiation Dose) methodology. This article refrains from unrolling the mathematical and physical details, since there is plenty of excellent literature doing this, with [10] and [11] being just two examples.

Quantitative molecular imaging such as planar scintigraphy, SPECT/CT, and PET/CT is used to get hold of the tracer's bio-distribution within the patient whereas the radiation transport and the resulting dose deposition pattern solely depends on the radionuclide's emission spectrum and the geometry, i.e., the anatomy. The latter can be represented by phantoms, i.e., computational body models that have developed from being composed of simple geometric forms [12, 13] to the voxel-based ICRP (International Commission on Radiological Protection) reference phantoms [14]. Among the software packages that include these necessary data matrices were the original MIRDOSE [15] which then became OLINDA/EXM [16], as well as IDAC [17]. All the above offer so-called organ dosimetry, i.e., they calculate the mean absorbed radiation dose (AD) to an organ with both, the activity distribution in the source organ as well as the AD in the target organ being homogenously distributed over the organ's volume, with the option for adjustment to the weight of the patients' organs. In this simplified form of dosimetry, the AD to lesions can be approximated by the geometrical assumption of the lesion being a sphere (aka spherical model) [17].

Phantom-based organ dosimetry, as described in the last paragraph, is the most widely applied form of dosimetry. However, it is certainly not the most sophisticated form of personalized medicine. For this one needs to perform three-dimensional (3D), voxel-based dosimetry [18], where neither the source nor the target is represented by an a-priory phantom geometry, but by the patients' imaging data, i.e., PET/CT or SPECT/CT. There the heterogenous activity distribution is given by sequential, nuclear scans and the likewise heterogenous dose distribution is calculated on the voxel base (see Fig. 6.1) by means of Monte Carlo simulations [20] or some forms of convolutions with dose kernels [21–24]. Naturally this form of dosimetry is both, much more complex as well as prone to errors and only a few commercial software packages offer a workflow for it.

The expression theragnostics (also spelled theranostics) is a fusion of the word therapy and diagnosis. In nuclear medicine, this term describes the use of one or multiple tracers to either predict the absorbed dose in the course of treatment planning and with the help of a diagnostic scan, or to calculate dosimetry via accompanying imaging during therapy. Thereby, often pairs of radionuclides are used that either are isotopes of the same element or can be labeled to the same carrier molecule, thus assuming the biokinetics to be identical. Table 6.1 gives a short overview of the most common radionuclides used in theranostics. Both, phantom based as well as individual voxel-based dosimetry, can be used for thernostics and the following sections shall give you a review of the respective studies.

Absorbed dose images

Tumor 3   Tumor 11

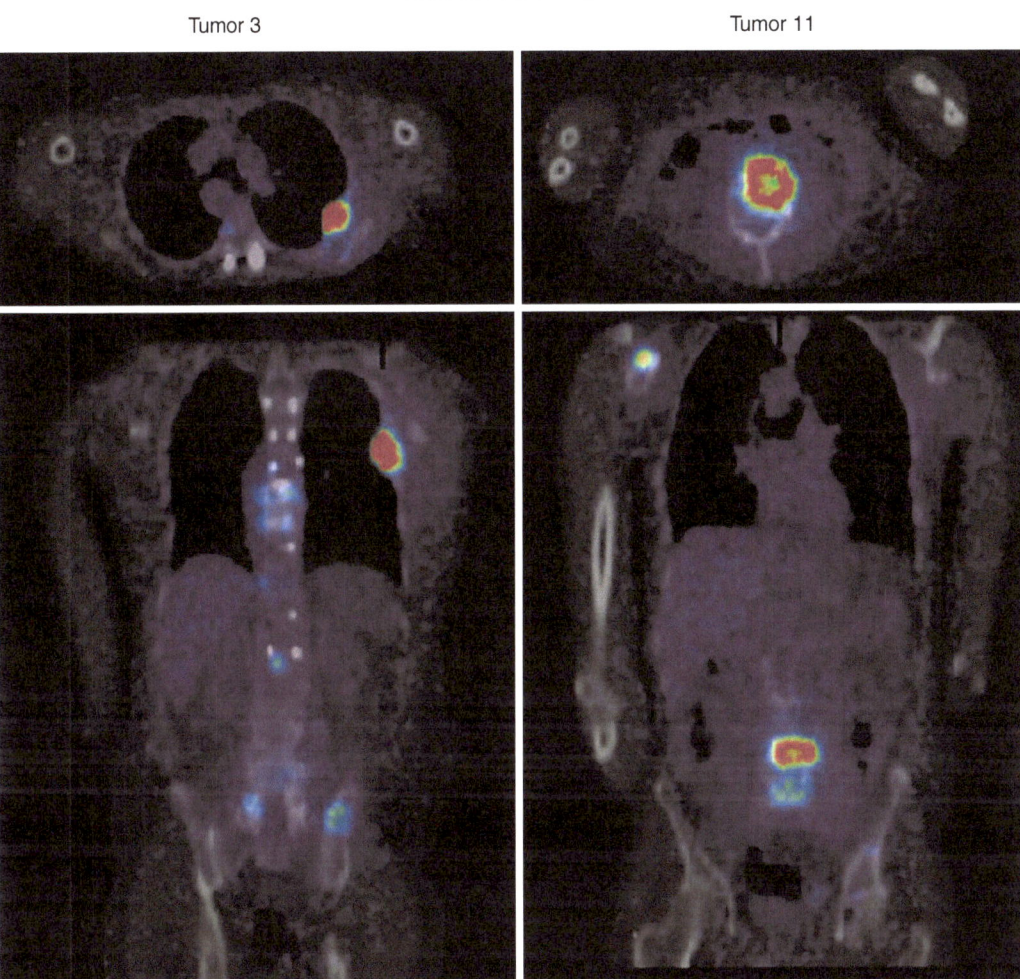

Fig. 6.1 Transverse and coronal cross sections depicting voxel-based absorbed dose images of two tumors (thyroid cancer). Adapted from [19]

Table 6.1 Combination of radionuclides used for theranostics in radionuclide therapy. Bold print indicates imaging data used for dosimetry

Diagnosis	Therapy	Indication	Remarks	References
[124]I-PET/CT	[131]I	Differentiated thyroid cancer	Gold standard for personalized dosimetry	[25–27]
^{123}I-SPECT/CT	[131]I	Differentiated thyroid cancer	Half-life too short for dosimetry	[26]
^{68}Ga-PET/CT	**[177]Lu SPECT/CT and/ or scintigraphy**	Metastatic/nonresectable neuroendocrine tumor, castration-resistant prostate cancer	Half-life of ^{68}Ga too short for dosimetry, ^{177}Lu-imaging during therapy is applied	[1, 28–30]

(continued)

Table 6.1 (continued)

Diagnosis	Therapy	Indication	Remarks	References
^{111}In-SPECT/CT and/or scintigraphy	[90]Y	Metastatic/nonresectable neuroendocrine tumors	–	[31, 32]
[86]Y-PET/CT	[90]Y	Metastatic/nonresectable neuroendocrine tumors	–	[33, 34]
–	^{90}Y-Bremsstrahlung SPECT-CT	Metastatic/nonresectable neuroendocrine tumors, hepatocellular carcinoma	At the experimental stage	[35, 36]
–	^{90}Y-PET/CT	Metastatic/nonresectable neuroendocrine tumors, hepatocellular carcinoma	At the experimental stage	[37–39]

6.3 Dose Quantities and Dose-Response in EBRT

In very general terms natural sciences is all about finding the right quantity to describe or model the phenomena observed. The basic quantity in radiation dosimetry is the mean absorbed dose (AD), which equals the energy deposited by ionizing radiation per unit mass of an anatomic structure (e.g., organ, tumor). This quantity is averaged for the mass and the irradiation time. In external beam radiotherapy (EBRT) multiple studies have demonstrated dose-response relationships between the lesions' AD and its response to the therapy, i.e., its shrinkage, often in the form of a sigmoidal dose-response curve [40, 41], as depicted in Fig. 6.2. When radiation oncologists perform treatment planning in EBRT they not only use the AD, but also other dosimetric concepts, such as dose volume histograms (DVH), the equivalent dose in 2 Gy fractions (EQD2) [43], or the biologic effective dose (BED). The latter takes into account the differences in dose rate, the repair half-time for sublethal tissue damage, the average doubling time for tumor clonogenic cells, as well as the assumed intrinsic radiosensitivity which is based on the linear-quadratic model [10, 44–46].

Just as for the AD, dose-response curves can be found in EBRT with respect to the BED [42].

When pondering about the dose-response relationship of tumor tissue, the unofficial supreme discipline of radiation oncology, one may not forget the dose-response relationships of healthy tissue, i.e., radiotoxicities, which is equally important for the patients' wellbeing. Here too, EBRT [47] as well as brachytherapy [43] have produced a remarkable evidence base.

Finally, the equivalent uniform (biological effective) dose (EUD) models the impact of the spatial dose distribution on the response [48]. The BED of each voxel is used to generate an EUD value for a specified volume (e.g., organ, tumor). Mathematically, in the case of dose non-uniformity the value of the EUD is always lower than the AD, which is why some studies suggested the EUD to be a better predictor of tumor response [19, 48–50]. Other quantities derived from voxel-based dosimetry include threshold approaches such as, e.g., D_{70} (the minimum dose to 70% of the voxels constituting the tumor volume) which in one study reliably predicted response or local failure in the treatment of hepatocellular carcinoma (HCC) with ^{90}Y resin microspheres [51]. Yet another study on this particular therapeutic field showed that the coverage of a lesion in terms of the DVH is much more predictive for progression-free survival (PFS) and overall survival (OS) than the mean absorbed dose [52].

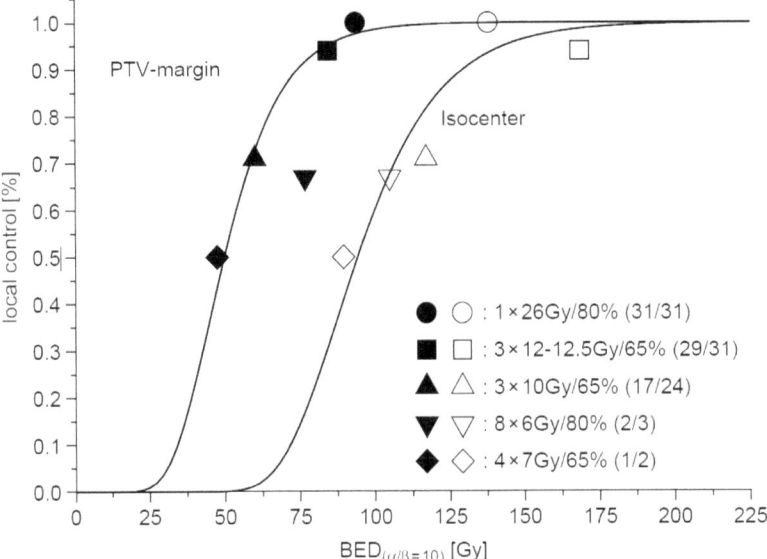

Fig. 6.2 The object of desire regarding the dosimetry of radionuclide therapy: a sigmoidal-shaped curve describing local tumor control dependent on BED (a/bZ10) of different EBRT irradiation regimes applied in Wuerzburg. The doses were calculated for the PTV-margin and the isocenter. The number of local failures compared to the total number of targets treated by the different fractionation regimes is shown in brackets. (From Wulf et al. [42])

6.4 Dose-Response I: Radiotoxicities in Radionuclide Therapy

The concept of BED was implemented in a multiregional kidney dosimetry model in MIRD Pamphlet No. 20 [46].

Bodei et al. [53] used this model and retrospective patient data to calculate a threshold for kidney toxicity at a BED of 40 Gy in patients without risk factors. Given the normally accepted tolerable dose for healthy kidneys of 23 Gy as known from EBRT [54], this value can now be exceeded since, e.g., the threshold BED of 40 Gy for ^{177}Lu-DOTATATE corresponds to an AD of 28 Gy. If fractionation is taken into account, i.e., multiple therapy cycles of radionuclide therapy, this value can even be increased to 35 Gy, thereby also increasing the potential dose to malignant tissue and demonstrating the practical value of dosimetry in radionuclide therapy, where the kidney is always the organ with the highest radiation burden.

Nevertheless, renal impairment is by far means not the only dose-effect of healthy tissue. For a comprehensive review it is referred to the formidable meta-analysis of Strigari and co-workers [55], who found 79 studies investigating dosimetry, of which 48 studies found an absorbed dose-effect correlation. Apart from renal toxicity, radiotoxicities due to radionuclide therapy mainly affect blood, marrow, and liver as listed in Table 6.2. A closer look reveals that liver toxicity only occurs in selective internal radionuclide therapy (SIRT), a treatment modality explicitly used to irradiate liver malignancies, thus explaining its high radiation burden. In researching the published literature on ^{177}Lu-PSMA therapy of metastatic castration-resistant prostate cancer, which became the rising star in radionuclide therapy within the last years, toxicities regarding kidney, blood and salivary gland were found to be minimal [3].

Altogether it can be said that dosimetry did a fine job in quantifying possible radiotoxicities, calculating threshold doses, and establishing

Table 6.2 Radiotoxicities reported in Radionuclide Therapy (except kidney which has a BED threshold dose of 40, see text above). NET stands for neuroendocrine tumors

Organ	Threshold dose (Gy)	Endpoint	Therapeutic Nuclide	Indication	Reference
Blood	2	High-grade bone marrow toxicity	[131]I	Differentiated thyroid carcinoma	[56]
Blood	1.7	High-grade bone marrow toxicity	[131]I	Differentiated thyroid carcinoma	[57]
Red marrow	2	Reduction in platelet counts	^{90}Y-DOTATOC	NET	[58]
Liver	50 (BED)	Liver normal tissue complication probability	[90]Y resin microspheres	Hepatocellular carcinoma	[59]
Liver	40	Radioembolization-induced liver disease	[90]Y resin microspheres	Hepatocellular carcinoma	[60]
Liver parenchyma	60	Liver decompensation	[90]Y glass microspheres	Hepatocellular carcinoma	[61]
Liver	60	G3 liver and blood toxicity	[166]Ho polylactic acid microspheres	Hepatocellular carcinoma	[62]
Lungs	50	Radiation pneumonitis	[90]Y Ivalon microspheres	Hepatocellular carcinoma	[63]

safety protocols, in some cases with the help of more sophisticated, radiobiological dose models as for the kidneys [46, 53], thereby making it possible to keep damage to healthy tissue in check and developing radionuclide therapy toward a cancer treatment modality with relatively mild side effects.

6.5 Dose-Response II: Tumor Response in Radionuclide Therapy

As alluded above, data from studies becomes sparse when the focus is on the dose-response of lesions, i.e., if one wants to correlate the tumor control with the radiation dose in the form of a dose-response curve as in Fig. 6.2. Table 6.2 gives an overview and concentrates on studies that actually reported dose-response curves, rather than mere threshold doses.

Pioneering work on this field includes the study of Koral and co-workers, who produced a sigmoidal curve relating AD and tumor volume for untreated patients suffering from low-grade follicular lymphoma and receiving ^{131}I-tositumomab [64]. Another work often cited is from Pauwels et al., who presented the first correlation between AD and tumor reduction for

gastroenteropancreatic neuroendocrine tumors (NET), treated with ^{90}Y-DOTATOC [32]. The most relevant study for peptide receptor radionuclide therapy (PRRT) however is a recent one by Ilan et al. [65] where the correlation between AD and tumor volume reduction of patients treated with ^{177}Lu-DOTATATE yielded Pearson coefficients R^2 never seen before, with 0.64 for tumors of diameter >2.2 cm and 0.91 (!) for tumors of diameter >4 cm (Fig. 6.3). Furthermore, Dewajara et al. [49] demonstrated a correlation between tumor reduction and EUD for refractory B-cell lymphoma treated with ^{131}I-tositumomab, albeit with rather low correlation coefficients (see Table 6.3).

When studying the results of Table 6.3 one should not forget all studies, that *didn't* report a dose-response relationship for lesions in radionuclide therapy. Substitutionally, two examples are given here: Jahn et al. [66] were unable to relate tumor shrinkage or biochemical response to the AD for small intestinal NET. Similarly, Barna et al. [67] looked into the dose-effect relationships in ^{177}Lu-PSMA I&T radionuclide therapy for metastatic castration-resistant prostate cancer by investigating 217 possible correlations between dosimetric quantities, biomarkers, and tumor shrinkage and only found 37 of them to be statically significant, none of them related to

Fig. 6.3 The scientific community would like to see more graphs like this: Tumor response in relation to tumor absorbed dose for all lesions evaluated with a diameter >2.2 cm (blue circles) and for lesions with a diameter >4.0 cm (red triangles). Taken from Cremonesi et al. [29], who adapted it from the original source, Ilan et al. [65]

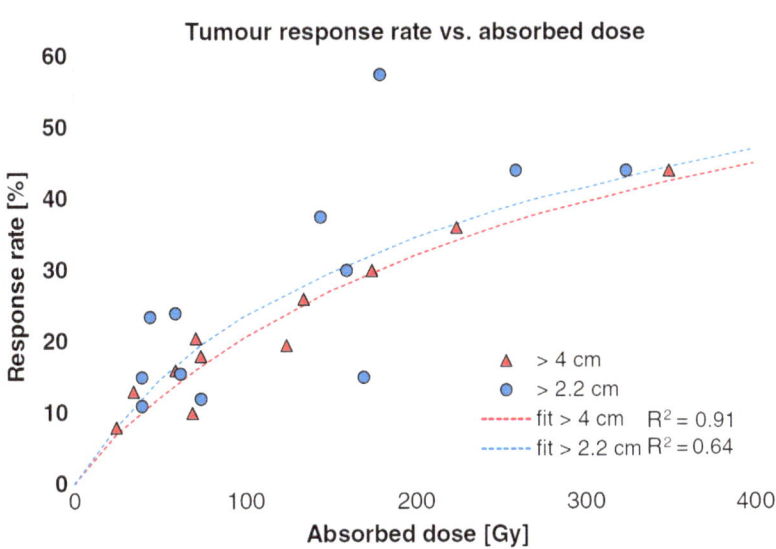

Table 6.3 Reported dose-response curves in radionuclide therapy

Study	Indication	Therapy	Imaging used for dosimetry	Form of dosimetry	Dose-response (R^2)
Pauwels et al. [32]	NET	^{90}Y-DOTATOC	^{86}Y-PET/CT	Phantom-based/ spherical model	Curve: AD vs. tumor reduction (0.5)
Ilan et al. [65]	Pancreatic NET	^{177}Lu-DOTATATE	^{177}Lu-SPECT/CT	Phantom-based/ spherical model	Curve: AD vs. tumor reduction (0.64, 0.91)[a]
Dewajara et al. [49]	Refractory B-cell lymphoma	^{131}I-tositumomab	^{131}I-SPECT/CT	Patient-specific/ voxel-based	Curve: AD (0.19) and EUD (0.36) vs. tumor reduction
Koral et al. [64]	Low-grade follicular lymphoma	^{131}I-tositumomab	^{131}I-SPECT	Phantom-based/ spherical model	Curve: AD vs. tumor reduction (0.44)

[a] See text for explanation

tumor reduction. For the sake of completeness, it has to be added that this study relied on planar scintigraphy rather than SPECT/CT.

In discussing the correlation between radiation dose and tumor reduction one should not forget the circumstances of radionuclide therapy, in particular the quantity and availability of data which of course has a huge impact on the likelihood to observe certain phenomena. Table 6.3 illustrates this issue by the fact that only one study actually performed voxel-based, patient-specific dosimetry [49] which inevitably is necessary for the calculation of a voxel-based quantity such as the EUD. This way the question remains whether the EUD is not reported more

frequently because (a) the associated prediction of tumor response is poor or (b) simply because of the lack of studies that take the trouble and effort to perform this more complex and laborious form of dose calculations.

Likewise, when comparing the number of cases in EBRT with the ones in Radionuclide Therapy, it is not realistic to expect the same degree of consolidation regarding dose-response relationships for tumor tissue. Moreover, patients undergoing radionuclide therapy almost always had several previous treatments, like hormonal therapy and/or chemotherapy, all of which affect the immune system as well as the individual state of health and subsequently also the tumor response. Certainly, the radio-oncologic lessons learned from EBRT cannot be extrapolated straightforward to Radionuclide Therapy, which in its application form rather resembles a systemic therapy than a local one.

6.6 The Answer to the Gretchenfrage

Facing the load of scientific studies cited above we return to the beginning, the Gretchenfrage:

How do we feel about dosimetry in Radionuclide Therapy?

In the scientific context one might reformulate it to:

What is the benefit of dosimetry in Radionuclide Therapy?

The term benefit in this discussion shall not only relate to scientific exploration, i.e., the investigation of dose-response relationships, but also to advantages for the individual patient and the clinical workflow. In EBRT the often-used keyword "Personalized Medicine" is realized by tailoring the spatial dose distribution to the individual case by means of several, adjustable parameters, such as angular distribution, frequency, and intensity modulation. Radionuclide Therapy is far away from this luxury and basically only has one adjusting screw, the administered activity. Here, personalized medicine implies the tailoring of the injected activity for the individual patient in a way, that malignant tissues receive the highest possible dose without the occurrence of radiotoxicities, thus avoiding under- as well as overtreatment.

Dosimetry calculations can do exactly that and in case of the combinations $^{124}I/^{131}I$ as well as $^{111}In/^{86}Y/^{90}Y$ enable an a-priory treatment planning. The diagnostic scan yields the tracer's biokinetics and uptake in lesions which are then used in the computation and prediction of the dose distribution of the therapeutic nuclide [19, 25–27, 31–34, 48]. In doing this, either phantom-based dose calculations including the spherical model for lesions or voxel-based dosimetry based

on patient-specific imaging data can be applied. Both procedures, in smaller or greater detail, provide the possibility of tailoring the administered activity for the sake of the best, individualized treatment. Reminding Table 6.3, voxel-based dosimetry does not necessarily produce a higher correlation coefficient. A voxel also constitutes a finite volume and there is no guarantee that it provides the absorbed dose at the biologically relevant scale, since dosimetry at a microscopic level remains inaccessible [9]. Nonetheless, it has to be kept in mind that the a-priory knowledge of the dose to malignant tissue in combination with published threshold doses for tumor response [55] and/or dose-response curves as in Table 6.3 enable the assessment of the expected course of the disease and therefore allow for prospective treatment planning.

This ideal scenario does of course not work for all forms of radionuclide therapy as outlined in Table 6.1. ^{68}Ga-PET/CT scans may be feasible for the correlation of lesions' SUV in PET with the absorbed dose from the later therapy or for the selection of appropriate candidates for PRRT (see [8] for a review), but cannot be used for a real dose calculation due to the short half-life of ^{68}Ga which is unable to produce the necessary biokinetics of the later phase. Still, dosimetry based on the accompanying ^{177}Lu scans is very useful, since the evaluation of the calculated organ and lesion doses of a cycle provides the necessary information to adjust the administered activity for all futures cycles and therewith enable a patient-specific optimization of radionuclide therapy. The incorporation of multiple cycles into the BED concept for kidney toxicity [53] is a good example for the value of optimization.

There is of course no guarantee that subsequent cycles will show the same relation between administered activity and absorbed dose, since uptake and biokinetics of irritated tissue, in particular lesions, will vary. Both, studies showing big differences [68] as well as minimal ones [69, 70], can be found in the literature. Another important result reported by Garkavij et al. [69] is that patients evaluated with planar-based dosimetry may have been undertreated compared to other methods. This is confirmed by Zechman et al.

[71] who showed in their review that the absorbed doses to the kidneys are systematically overestimated when using planar imaging.

Last but not least, in order to systematically *investigate* dosimetry in Radionuclide Therapy and dose-response effects, one has to *do* dosimetric studies. Solid and quantitative data which has way higher R^2 than in Table 6.3 are a prerequisite for personalized medicine and subsequently for the patient's welfare. Dosimetry might not be the *only* predictor for this, but certainly is an *essential* one. It's neither a magic flute nor will it generically explain all the effects in Radionuclide Therapy. But it can be used for personalized treatment planning as well as optimization, and it is getting better and more accurate with every new study performed.

Dr. Faust, in his despair to gain knowledge, even gives in to magic. Luckily as scientist we can rely on reason and evidence to face the same challenge:

> That I may know what the world contains
> In its innermost heart and finer veins.
> Faust; a Tragedy. Johann Wolfgang von Goethe

References

1. Kulkarni HR, Singh A, Schuchardt C, Niepsch K, Sayeg M, Leshch Y, et al. PSMA-based radioligand therapy for metastatic castration-resistant prostate cancer: the bad Berka experience since 2013. J Nucl Med. 2016;57(3):97S–104S. Available from http://www.ncbi.nlm.nih.gov/pubmed/27694180.
2. Baum RP, Kulkarni HR. Theranostics: from molecular imaging using Ga-68 labeled tracers and PET/CT to personalized radionuclide therapy - the bad Berka experience. Theranostics. 2012;2:437–47.
3. Baum RP, Kulkarni HR, Schuchardt C, Singh A, Wirtz M, Wiessalla S, et al. 177Lu-labeled prostate-specific membrane antigen radioligand therapy of metastatic castration-resistant prostate cancer: safety and efficacy. J Nucl Med. 2016;57(7):1006–13.
4. Riley AS, McKenzie GAG, Green V, Schettino G, England RJA, Greenman J. The effect of radioiodine treatment on the diseased thyroid gland. Int J Radiat Biol. 2019;95(12):1718–27.
5. Goldsmith SJ. Targeted radionuclide therapy: a historical and personal review. Semin Nucl Med. 2019;50(1):87–97.
6. Brans B, Bodei L, Giammarile F, Linden O, Luster M, Oyen WJG, et al. Clinical radionuclide therapy dosimetry: the quest for the "Holy Gray". Eur J Nucl Med Mol Imaging. 2007;34(5):772–86. Available from http://www.pubmedcentral.nih.gov/articlerender.fcgi?artid=1914264&tool=pmcentrez&rendertype=abstract.
7. Flux G, Bardies M, Chiesa C, Monsieurs M, Savolainen S, Strand S-E, et al. Clinical radionuclide therapy dosimetry: the quest for the "Holy Gray". Eur J Nucl Med Mol Imaging. 2007;34(10):1699–700. Available from http://www.ncbi.nlm.nih.gov/pubmed/17565497.
8. Blaickner M, Baum RP. Relevance of PET for pre-therapeutic prediction of doses in peptide receptor radionuclide therapy. PET Clin. 2014;9(1):99–112.
9. Chiesa C, Bardiès M, Zaidi H. Voxel-based dosimetry is superior to mean absorbed dose approach for establishing dose-effect relationship in targeted radionuclide therapy. Med Phys. 2019;46(12):5403–6.
10. Eberlein U, Cremonesi M, Lassmann M. Individualized dosimetry for theranostics: necessary, nice to have, or counterproductive? J Nucl Med. 2017;58(2):97S–103S.
11. Bolch WE, Eckerman KF, Sgouros G, Thomas SR. MIRD pamphlet No. 21: a generalized schema for radiopharmaceutical dosimetry–standardization of nomenclature. J Nucl Med. 2009;50(3):477–84. Available from http://www.ncbi.nlm.nih.gov/pubmed/19258258.
12. Snyder WS, Fisher HL, Ford MR, Warner GG. Estimates of absorbed fractions for monoenergetic photon sources uniformly distributed in various organs of a heterogeneous phantom. J Nucl Med. 1969;3:7–52.
13. Blaickner M, Kindl P. Diversification of existing reference phantoms in nuclear medicine: calculation of specific absorbed fractions for 21 mathematical phantoms and validation through dose estimates resulting from the administration of 18F-FDG. Cancer Biother Radiopharm. 2008;23(6):767–82.
14. Menzel H, Clement C, DeLuca PM. ICRP Publication 110. Realistic reference phantoms: an ICRP/ICRU joint effort. A report of adult reference computational phantoms. 2009.
15. Stabin MG. MIRDOSE: personal computer software for internal dose assessment in nuclear medicine. J Nucl Med. 1996;37(3):538–46.
16. Stabin MG, Sparks RB, Crowe E. OLINDA/EXM: the second-generation personal computer software for internal dose assessment in nuclear medicine. J Nucl Med. 2005;46(6):1023–7. Available from http://www.ncbi.nlm.nih.gov/pubmed/15937315.
17. Andersson M, Johansson L, Eckerman K, Mattsson S. IDAC-Dose 2.1, an internal dosimetry program for diagnostic nuclear medicine based on the ICRP adult reference voxel phantoms. EJNMMI Res. 2017;7(1):88. Available from http://www.ncbi.nlm.nih.gov/pubmed/29098485.
18. Flux G, Bardies M, Monsieurs M, Savolainen S, Strands S-E, Lassmann M. The impact of PET and SPECT on dosimetry for targeted radionuclide ther-

apy. Z Med Phys. 2006;16(1):47–59. Available from http://www.ncbi.nlm.nih.gov/pubmed/16696370.

19. Sgouros G, Hobbs RF, Atkins FB, Van Nostrand D, Ladenson PW, Wahl RL. Three-dimensional radiobiological dosimetry (3D-RD) with 124I PET for 131I therapy of thyroid cancer. Eur J Nucl Med Mol Imaging. 2011;38(1):41–7. Available from http://www.pubmedcentral.nih.gov/articlerender.fcgi?artid=3172686&tool=pmcentrez&rendertype=abstract.

20. Villoing D, Marcatili S, Garcia MP, Bardiès M. Internal dosimetry with the Monte Carlo code GATE: Validation using the ICRP/ICRU female reference computational model. Phys Med Biol. 2017;62(5):1885–904.

21. Reiner D, Blaickner M, Rattay F. Discrete beta dose kernel matrices for nuclides applied in targeted radionuclide therapy (TRT) calculated with MCNP5. Med Phys. 2009;36(11):4890–6.

22. Dieudonné A, Hobbs RF, Bolch WE, Sgouros G, Gardin I. Fine-resolution voxel S values for constructing absorbed dose distributions at variable voxel size. J Nucl Med. 2010;51(10):1600–7. Available from http://www.ncbi.nlm.nih.gov/pubmed/20847175.

23. Amato E, Minutoli F, Pacilio M, Campenni A, Baldari S. An analytical method for computing voxel S values for electrons and photons. Med Phys. 2012;39(11):6808–17. Available from http://www.ncbi.nlm.nih.gov/pubmed/23127074.

24. Lanconelli N, Pacilio M, Lo Meo S, Botta F, Di Dia A, Aroche AT, et al. A free database of radionuclide voxel S values for the dosimetry of nonuniform activity distributions. Phys Med Biol. 2012;57(2):517–33. Available from http://www.ncbi.nlm.nih.gov/pubmed/22217735.

25. Lassmann M, Reiners C, Luster M. Dosimetry and thyroid cancer: the individual dosage of radioiodine. Endocr Relat Cancer. 2010;17(3):161–72. Available from http://www.ncbi.nlm.nih.gov/pubmed/20448022.

26. Luster M, Clarke SE, Dietlein M, Lassmann M, Lind P, Oyen WJG, et al. Guidelines for radioiodine therapy of differentiated thyroid cancer. Eur J Nucl Med Mol Imaging. 2008;35:1941–59.

27. Sgouros G, Kolbert KS, Sheikh A, Pentlow KS, Mun EF, Barth A, et al. Patient-specific dosimetry for 131I thyroid cancer therapy using 124I PET and 3-dimensional-internal dosimetry (3D-ID) software. J Nucl Med. 2004;45(8):1366–72. Available from http://www.ncbi.nlm.nih.gov/pubmed/15299063.

28. Bodei L, Mueller-Brand J, Baum RP, Pavel ME, Hörsch D, O'Dorisio MS, et al. The joint IAEA, EANM, and SNMMI practical guidance on peptide receptor radionuclide therapy (PRRNT) in neuroendocrine tumours. Eur J Nucl Med Mol Imaging. 2013;40(5):800–16. https://doi.org/10.1007/s00259-012-2330-6.

29. Cremonesi M, Ferrari ME, Bodei L, Chiesa C, Sarnelli A, Garibaldi C, et al. Correlation of dose with toxicity and tumour response to 90 Y- and 177 Lu-PRRT provides the basis for optimization through individualized treatment planning. Eur J Nucl Med Mol Imaging. 2018;45(13):2426–41.

30. Okamoto S, Thieme A, Allmann J, D'Alessandria C, Maurer T, Retz M, et al. Radiation dosimetry for 177 Lu-PSMA I&T in metastatic castration-resistant prostate cancer: absorbed dose in normal organs and tumor lesions. J Nucl Med. 2017;58(3):445–50.

31. Cremonesi M, Botta F, Di Dia A, Ferrari M, Bodei L, De Cicco C, et al. Dosimetry for treatment with radiolabelled somatostatin analogues. A review. Q J Nucl Med Mol Imaging. 2010;54:37–51.

32. Pauwels S, Barone R, Walrand S, Borson-Chazot F, Valkema R, Kvols LK, et al. Practical dosimetry of peptide receptor radionuclide therapy with (90)Y-labeled somatostatin analogs. J Nucl Med. 2005;46(1):92–8. Available from http://www.ncbi.nlm.nih.gov/pubmed/15653657.

33. Helisch A, Förster GJ, Reber H, Buchholz H-G, Arnold R, Göke B, et al. Pre-therapeutic dosimetry and biodistribution of 86Y-DOTA-Phe1-Tyr3-octreotide versus 111In-pentetreotide in patients with advanced neuroendocrine tumours. Eur J Nucl Med Mol Imaging. 2004;31(10):1386–92. Available from http://www.ncbi.nlm.nih.gov/pubmed/15175836.

34. Förster GJ, Engelbach MJ, Brockmann JJ, Reber HJ, Buchholz HG, Mäcke HR, et al. Preliminary data on biodistribution and dosimetry for therapy planning of somatostatin receptor positive tumours: comparison of (86)Y-DOTATOC and (111)In-DTPA-octreotide. Eur J Nucl Med. 2001;28(12):1743–50. Available from http://www.ncbi.nlm.nih.gov/pubmed/11734910.

35. Fabbri C, Sarti G, Cremonesi M, Ferrari M, Di Dia A, Agostini M, et al. Quantitative analysis of 90Y Bremsstrahlung SPECT-CT images for application to 3D patient-specific dosimetry. Cancer Biother Radiopharm. 2009;24(1):145–54. Available from http://www.ncbi.nlm.nih.gov/pubmed/19243257.

36. Potrebko PS, Shridhar R, Biagioli MC, Sensakovic WF, Andl G, Poleszczuk J, et al. SPECT/CT image-based dosimetry for Yttrium-90 radionuclide therapy: application to treatment response. J Appl Clin Med Phys. 2018;19(5):435–43. https://doi.org/10.1002/acm2.12400.

37. Lhommel R, van Elmbt L, Goffette P, Van den Eynde M, Jamar F, Pauwels S, et al. Feasibility of 90Y TOF PET-based dosimetry in liver metastasis therapy using SIR-Spheres. Eur J Nucl Med Mol Imaging. 2010;37(9):1654–62. Available from http://www.ncbi.nlm.nih.gov/pubmed/20422185.

38. D'Arienzo M, Chiaramida P, Chiacchiararelli L, Coniglio A, Cianni R, Salvatori R, et al. 90Y PET-based dosimetry after selective internal radiotherapy treatments. Nucl Med Commun. 2012;33(6):633–40. Available from http://www.ncbi.nlm.nih.gov/pubmed/22407156.

39. Ho CL, Chen S, Cheung SK, Leung YL, Cheng KC, Wong KN, et al. Radioembolization with 90Y glass microspheres for hepatocellular carcinoma: significance of pretreatment 11C-acetate and 18F-FDG PET/

CT and posttreatment 90Y PET/CT in individualized dose prescription. Eur J Nucl Med Mol Imaging. 2018;45(12):2110–21. Available from http://www.ncbi.nlm.nih.gov/pubmed/29948107.

40. King CR. The dose–response of salvage radiotherapy following radical prostatectomy: a systematic review and meta-analysis. Radiother Oncol. 2016;121(2):199–203.

41. Kim HJ, Suh YG, Lee YC, Lee SK, Shin SK, Cho BC, et al. Dose-response relationship between radiation dose and loco-regional control in patients with stage II-III esophageal cancer treated with definitive chemoradiotherapy. Cancer Res Treat. 2017;49(3):669–77.

42. Wulf J, Baier K, Mueller G, Flentje MP. Doseresponse in stereotactic irradiation of lung tumors. Radiother Oncol. 2005;77(1):83–7. Available from http://www.ncbi.nlm.nih.gov/pubmed/16209896.

43. Georg P, Pötter R, Georg D, Lang S, Dimopoulos JCA, Sturdza AE, et al. Dose effect relationship for late side effects of the rectum and urinary bladder in magnetic resonance image-guided adaptive cervix cancer brachytherapy. Int J Radiat Oncol Biol Phys. 2012;82(2):653–7. Available from http://www.ncbi.nlm.nih.gov/pubmed/21345618.

44. Dale R, Carabe-Fernandez A. The radiobiology of conventional radiotherapy and its application to radionuclide therapy. Cancer Biother Radiopharm. 2005;20:47–51.

45. Baechler S, Hobbs RF, Prideaux AR, Wahl RL, Sgouros G. Extension of the biological effective dose to the MIRD schema and possible implications in radionuclide therapy dosimetry. Med Phys. 2008;35(3):1123–34. Available from http://www.pubmedcentral.nih.gov/articlerender.fcgi?artid=2974633&tool=pmcentrez&rendertype=abstract.

46. Wessels BW, Konijnenberg MW, Dale RG, Breitz HB, Cremonesi M, Meredith RF, et al. MIRD pamphlet No. 20: the effect of model assumptions on kidney dosimetry and response–implications for radionuclide therapy. J Nucl Med. 2008;49(11):1884–99. Available from http://www.ncbi.nlm.nih.gov/pubmed/18927342.

47. Dunavoelgyi R, Dieckmann K, Gleiss A, Sacu S, Kircher K, Georgopoulos M, et al. Radiogenic side effects after hypofractionated stereotactic photon radiotherapy of choroidal melanoma in 212 patients treated between 1997 and 2007. Int J Radiat Oncol Biol Phys. 2012;83(1):121–8. Available from http://www.ncbi.nlm.nih.gov/pubmed/21945109.

48. Prideaux AR, Song H, Hobbs RF, He B, Frey EC, Ladenson PW, et al. Three-dimensional radiobiologic dosimetry: application of radiobiologic modeling to patient-specific 3-dimensional imaging-based internal dosimetry. J Nucl Med. 2007;48(6):1008–16. Available from http://www.pubmedcentral.nih.gov/articlerender.fcgi?artid=2974276&tool=pmcentrez&rendertype=abstract.

49. Dewaraja YK, Schipper MJ, Roberson PL, Wilderman SJ, Amro H, Regan DD, et al. 131I-tositumomab radioimmunotherapy: initial tumor dose-response results using 3-dimensional dosimetry including radiobiologic modeling. J Nucl Med. 2010;51(7):1155–62. Available from http://www.ncbi.nlm.nih.gov/pubmed/20554734.

50. Chiesa C, Mira M, Maccauro M, Spreafico C, Romito R, Morosi C, et al. Radioembolization of hepatocarcinoma with 90Y glass microspheres: development of an individualized treatment planning strategy based on dosimetry and radiobiology. Eur J Nucl Med Mol Imaging. 2015;42(11):1718–38.

51. Kao YH, Steinberg JD, Tay YS, Lim GKY, Yan J, Townsend DW, et al. Post-radioembolization yttrium-90 PET/CT-part 2: dose-response and tumor predictive dosimetry for resin microspheres. EJNMMI Res. 2013;3(1):1–27.

52. Allimant C, Kafrouni M, Delicque J, Ilonca D, Cassinotto C, Assenat E, et al. Tumor targeting and three-dimensional voxel-based dosimetry to predict tumor response, toxicity, and survival after Yttrium-90 resin microsphere radioembolization in hepatocellular carcinoma. J Vasc Interv Radiol. 2018;29(12):1662–70. https://doi.org/10.1016/j.jvir.2018.07.006.

53. Bodei L, Cremonesi M, Ferrari M, Pacifici M, Grana CM, Bartolomei M, et al. Long-term evaluation of renal toxicity after peptide receptor radionuclide therapy with 90Y-DOTATOC and 177Lu-DOTATATE: the role of associated risk factors. Eur J Nucl Med Mol Imaging. 2008;35(10):1847–56.

54. Emami B, Lyman J, Brown A, Coia L, Goitein M, Munzenrider JE, et al. Tolerance of normal tissue to therapeutic irradiation. Int J Radiat Oncol Biol Phys. 1991;21(1):109–22. Available from http://www.ncbi.nlm.nih.gov/pubmed/2032882.

55. Strigari L, Konijnenberg M, Chiesa C, Bardies M, Du Y, Gleisner KS, et al. The evidence base for the use of internal dosimetry in the clinical practice of molecular radiotherapy, vol. 41. Berlin: Springer; 2014. p. 1976–88. Available from http://www.ncbi.nlm.nih.gov/pubmed/24915892.

56. Hartung-Knemeyer V, Nagarajah J, Jentzen W, Ruhlmann M, Freudenberg LS, Stahl AR, et al. Pretherapeutic blood dosimetry in patients with differentiated thyroid carcinoma using 124-iodine: predicted blood doses correlate with changes in blood cell counts after radioiodine therapy and depend on modes of TSH stimulation and number of preceding radioiodine therapies. Ann Nucl Med. 2012;26(9):723–9. Available from http://www.ncbi.nlm.nih.gov/pubmed/22802008.

57. Bianchi L, Baroli A, Lomuscio G, Pedrazzini L, Pepe A, Pozzi L, et al. Dosimetry in the therapy of metastatic differentiated thyroid cancer administering high 131I activity: the experience of Busto Arsizio Hospital (Italy). Q J Nucl Med Mol Imaging. 2012;56(6):515–21. Available from http://www.ncbi.nlm.nih.gov/pubmed/23358404.

58. Walrand S, Barone R, Pauwels S, Jamar F. Experimental facts supporting a red marrow uptake due to radiometal transchelation in 90Y-DOTATOC therapy and relationship to the decrease of

platelet counts. Eur J Nucl Med Mol Imaging. 2011;38(7):1270–80. Available from http://www. ncbi.nlm.nih.gov/pubmed/21318451.

59. Strigari L, Sciuto R, Rea S, Carpanese L, Pizzi G, Soriani A, et al. Efficacy and toxicity related to treatment of hepatocellular carcinoma with 90Y-SIR spheres: radiobiologic considerations. J Nucl Med. 2010;51(9):1377–85. Available from http://www. ncbi.nlm.nih.gov/pubmed/20720056.

60. Sangro B, Gil-Alzugaray B, Rodriguez J, Sola I, Martinez-Cuesta A, Viudez A, et al. Liver disease induced by radioembolization of liver tumors. Cancer. 2008;112(7):1538–46. https://doi.org/10.1002/cncr.23339.

61. Chiesa C, Mira M, Maccauro M, Romito R, Spreafico C, Sposito C, et al. A dosimetric treatment planning strategy in radioembolization of hepatocarcinoma with90Y glass microspheres. Q J Nucl Med Mol Imaging. 2012;56:503–8.

62. Smits MLJ, Nijsen JFW, van den Bosch MAAJ, Lam MGEH, Vente MAD, Mali WPTM, et al. Holmium-166 radioembolisation in patients with unresectable, chemorefractory liver metastases (HEPAR trial): a phase 1, dose-escalation study. Lancet Oncol. 2012;13(10):1025–34. Available from http://www.ncbi.nlm.nih.gov/pubmed/22920685.

63. Ho S, Lau WY, Leung TW, Chan M, Johnson PJ, Li AK. Clinical evaluation of the partition model for estimating radiation doses from yttrium-90 microspheres in the treatment of hepatic cancer. Eur J Nucl Med. 1997;24(3):293–8. Available from http://www.ncbi. nlm.nih.gov/pubmed/9143467.

64. Koral KF, Francis IR, Kroll S, Zasadny KR, Kaminski MS, Wahl RL. Volume reduction versus radiation dose for tumors in previously untreated lymphoma patients who received iodine-131 tositumomab therapy. Cancer. 2002;94(S4):1258–63.

65. Ilan E, Sandstrom M, Wassberg C, Sundin A, Garske-Roman U, Eriksson B, et al. Dose response of pancreatic neuroendocrine tumors treated with peptide receptor radionuclide therapy using 177Lu-DOTATATE. J Nucl Med. 2015;56(2):177–82.

66. Jahn U, Ilan E, Sandström M, Garske-Román U, Lubberink M, Sundin A. 177Lu-DOTATATE peptide receptor radionuclide therapy: dose response in small intestinal neuroendocrine tumors. Neuroendocrinology. 2019;110(7-8):662–70.

67. Barna S, Haug AR, Hartenbach M, Sazan R, Grubmüller B, Kramer G, et al. Dose calculations and dose-effect relationships in Lu-177-PSMA I&T radionuclide therapy for metastatic castration resistant prostate cancer. Clin Nucl Med. 2020;45(9):661–7.

68. Kairemo K, Kangasmäki A. 4D SPECT/CT acquisition for 3D dose calculation and dose planning in 177Lu-peptide receptor radionuclide therapy: applications for clinical routine. Recent Results Cancer Res. 2013;194:537–50. Available from http://www. ncbi.nlm.nih.gov/pubmed/22918781.

69. Garkavij M, Nickel M, Sjögreen-Gleisner K, Ljungberg M, Ohlsson T, Wingårdh K, et al. 177Lu-[DOTA0,Tyr3] octreotate therapy in patients with disseminated neuroendocrine tumors: analysis of dosimetry with impa1. Garkavij, M. et al. 177Lu-[DOTA0,Tyr3] octreotate therapy in patients with disseminated neuroendocrine tumors: analysis of dosimet. Cancer. 2010;116(4):1084–92.

70. Larsson M, Bernhardt P, Svensson JB, Wängberg B, Ahlman H, Forssell-Aronsson E. Estimation of absorbed dose to the kidneys in patients after treatment with 177Lu-octreotate: comparison between methods based on planar scintigraphy. EJNMMI Res. 2012;2(1):1–13.

71. Zechmann CM, Afshar-Oromieh A, Armor T, Stubbs JB, Mier W, Hadaschik B, et al. Radiation dosimetry and first therapy results with a 124I/131I-labeled small molecule (MIP-1095) targeting PSMA for prostate cancer therapy. Eur J Nucl Med Mol Imaging. 2014;41(7):1280–92. Available from http://www. ncbi.nlm.nih.gov/pubmed/24577951.

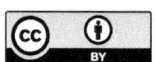

Lisa Bodei

It all began in Weimar, at the Goethe National Museum in Weimar, a magnificent and placid place. The place is redolent in history and culture, where Prof. Richard Baum organized the fourth Mitteldeutsches Neuroendokriner Tumor Symposium, in June 2013 (Fig. 7.1). Richard has always been a pioneer and the first to understand and disseminate the importance of many innovations, including the now popular theranostic concept. Unlike many conservative and "predictable" scientific gatherings, his meetings have always been *avant-garde* and pivotal in defining the trends for the future. To my delight and pleasure, I was invited to participate in what I knew would be a *tour de force* of the trailblazers of innovative nuclear medicine.

After more than 13 years of full immersion in peptide receptor radionuclide therapy (PRRT) of neuroendocrine tumors (NETs), I was in search of new inspirations to improve this excellent

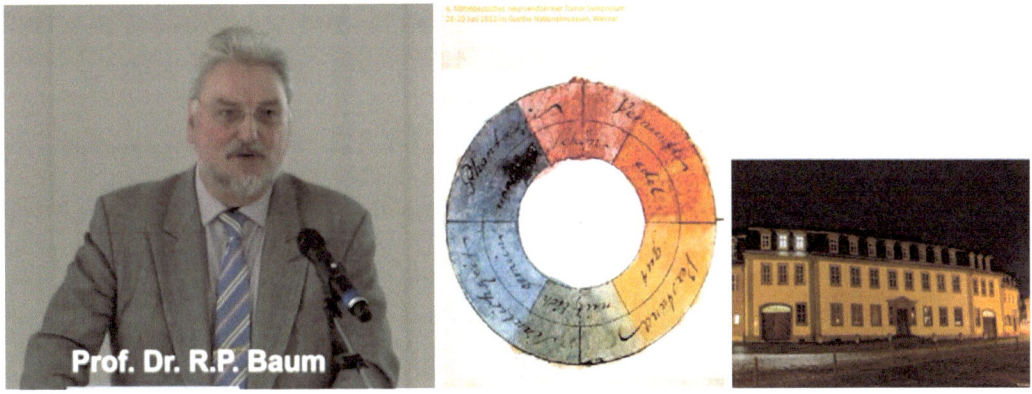

Fig. 7.1 It all started in Weimar. Prof. Richard P. Baum giving the introductory lecture at the fourth Mitteldeutsches neuroendokriner Tumor Symposium, in June 2013

L. Bodei (✉)
Molecular Imaging and Therapy Service, Department of Radiology, Memorial Sloan Kettering Cancer Center, New York, NY, USA
e-mail: bodeil@mskcc.org

© The Author(s) 2024
V. Prasad (ed.), *Beyond Becquerel and Biology to Precision Radiomolecular Oncology: Festschrift in Honor of Richard P. Baum*, https://doi.org/10.1007/978-3-031-33533-4_7

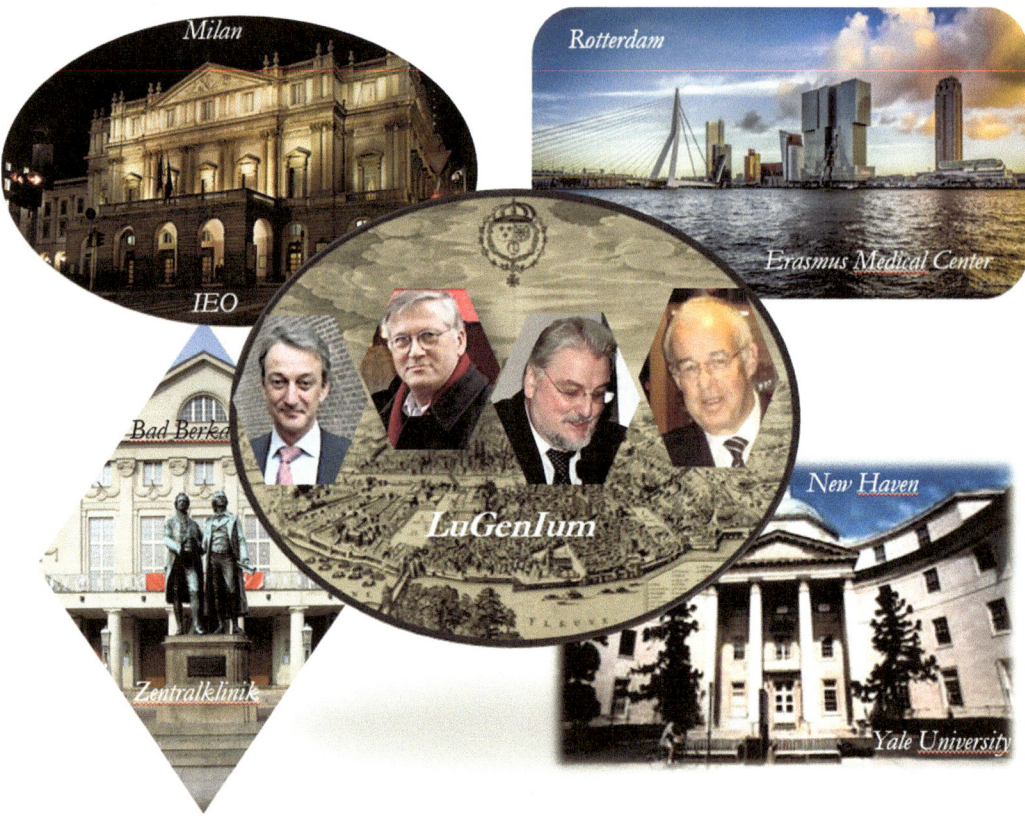

Fig. 7.2 The foundation of LuGenIum, with the contributions of Prof. Richard P. Baum (Bad Berka, GE), Prof. Irvin M. Modlin (Yale University, USA), Prof. Dik J. Kwekkeboom and Prof. Eric P. Krenning (Erasmus University, Rotterdam, NL)

treatment. I had been captured by the possibilities of accurate monitoring and prediction of therapy provided by blood transcriptome signatures for NETs, as proposed by the inventor of this field, Prof. Irvin M. Modlin of Yale University [1]. While walking through the rooms of Goethe's house, and inspired by the book and art collection that is so well-preserved there, I initiated a peripatetic discussion about the future of PRRT with Richard, Irvin, and Dik (the late and much beloved Prof. Dik J. Kwekkeboom from Erasmus University), who established ^{177}Lu-DOTATATE therapy. In the green study of the Master, I realized that three of the most important minds in the field of neuroendocrinology were there with me. "What if we could apply the sophisticated genomic techniques to PRRT?" I asked. The idea was met with considerable interest as well as skepticism. We then decided to meet in Lyon, during the EANM '13 annual meeting. There, among *pâté de foie gras* and a glass of *Côtes de Gascogne*, we decided to establish and fund a research group. In honor of the city of Lyon, whose old name was Lugdunum, we established *LuGenIum* (Fig. 7.2).

The scope of our innovative research venture was to understand the role of individual predisposition and specific tumor genomic profile in the response and toxicity to PRRT. Our specific aims were to, first, conduct a retrospective analysis of toxicity to PRRT (i.e., define the problem) in a large patient cohort, then to conduct two prospective studies (assess the efficacy of the ideas). Firstly, to identify NETs at a genomic level and assess the response to PRRT with a PCR-based blood analysis, and, secondly, to analyze markers of long-term toxicity in patients with NETs previously undergone to PRRT with a PCR-based blood analysis.

7.1 Retrospective Analysis of Toxicity

Given the increased use of PRRT in NETs and the numerous other therapies in patients undergoing PRRT, it is crucial to define the risk relationship between toxicity and therapy by identifying the risk factors. These factors are considered, by the clinicians, responsible of modulating the occurrence of adverse events after PRRT by altering the thresholds for toxicity to critical organs.

We assessed 807 subjects enrolled at my institution (at that time), the European Institute of Oncology (IEO) in Milan, who had received PRRT with ^{90}Y-, ^{177}Lu-, and ^{90}Y+^{177}Lu-somatostatin analog peptides. Our concept was to evaluate the renal and bone marrow toxicity, expressed by blood chemistry analysis, and the parameters then considered to modulate the tolerability, such as the risk factors, PRRT parameters, and clinical features [2]. To ensure a balanced assessment we utilized sophisticated statistical analysis with multiple regression, random forest feature selection, and recursive partitioning and regression trees.

We observed that severe nephrotoxicity was virtually absent after ^{177}Lu-peptides and was related to the administration of ^{90}Y-peptides. G1/G2 creatinine toxicity was present in 34.6% of all patients and G3/G4 toxicity in 1%. None of the patients treated with only ^{177}Lu-DOTATATE, however, developed severe toxicity. Bone marrow toxicity was low and comparable with other anti-neoplastic therapies. Myelodysplastic syndrome was observed in 2.35% of individuals, with a minority developing acute leukemias (1.1%). More interestingly, in our comparative analysis of nephrotoxicity, it was apparent that clinical factors, such as hypertension or prior nephrotoxic chemotherapy, as well as clinical features, such as anemia, failed to provide a basis for more than 34% of the cases of toxicity.

Similarly, in our comparative analysis of hematotoxicity, clinical factors, such as prior myelotoxic chemotherapies or bone marrow invasion, as well as clinical features, such as thrombocytopenia, could only be incriminated in ~30% of the cases of myeloproliferative disease. These data strongly suggest the existence of unidentified individual susceptibilities to radiation-associated disease, most likely of a genetic basis. Our inescapable conclusion was that personalized molecular approaches would be required to identify individual radiosensitivity.

7.2 Circulating NET Transcripts

The NETest is a gene expression assay that measures 51 NET marker transcripts in blood using real-time PCR [1, 3]. The 51 NETest genes are included in "14 omes". The assay utilizes multi-algorithmic analysis to quantify expression of gene clusters related to the tumor. NETest output is a score scaled 0–100 that represents the risk of NET disease. A normal score is ≤20, stable disease 21–40, progressive disease 41–100. The assay has demonstrated >90% accuracy, sensitivity and specificity for a NET diagnosis and residual/recurrent disease in numerous prospective studies and a recent meta-analysis [4–9].

7.3 Circulating NET Transcripts and SSR Imaging

The concept of adding an mRNA-based omic strategy to PRRT was based on our recognition of the need to improve the diagnostic and therapeutic approach to NETs. There was an obvious requirement to move from a mono-dimensional approach based on a single piece of information (i.e., somatostatin receptor expression) to a multidimensional one, based on the multiple simultaneous molecular measurements of the genes regulating tumor biology (behavior). We felt this was accomplishable if we could use the 51 "NET-defining" gene transcripts and their omic clusters to genomically characterize individual tumors.

Initially, we evaluated the relationship of the NETest with diagnostic imaging, namely Ga-68-based somatostatin analog PET (^{68}Ga-SSA-PET) [10]. Our hypothesis was that the integration of circulating molecular markers and a tissue index of proliferation with functional imagery would provide added functional information in respect of tumor biology and clinical behavior. We recruited two independent patient groups affected by gastroenteropancreatic (GEP) and bronchpulmonary (BP) NETs with positive ^{68}Ga-SSA-PET and evaluated all with NETest: 27 patients pre-PRRT as primary or salvage treatment from two Italian institutions, IEO, Milan and Istituto Tumori della Romagna (IRST), Meldola, and 22 patients referred for staging/restaging after various therapies at Charité University, Berlin. To understand the relationship between gene expression and imaging, we examined the maximum standardized uptake value (SUVmax) at PET and the circulating gene transcripts. Additional parameters included Ki-67 index, Chromogranin-A (CgA). Transcripts were measured by real-time quantitative reverse transcrip-

tion PCR (qRT-PCR) and multianalyte algorithmic analysis, CgA by enzyme-linked immunosorbent assay (ELISA). Statistical analysis to evaluate the strength of the relationships with the NETest included regression analyses, generalized linear modeling, and receiver-operating characteristic (ROC) curves.

Firstly, our regression model confirmed that the SUVmax measured in two centers were comparable. NETest was positive in 47 of 49 patients (96%), CgA was positive in 26 (54%) ($\chi^2 = 20.1$, $p < 2.5 \times 10^{-6}$, and 78% were G1-G2 according to WHO 2010 (Ki-67 < 20%). Gene transcript scores were predictive of imaging with >95% concordance and significantly correlated with SUVmax ($R^2 = 0.31$, root-mean-square error = 9.38). This meant that specific genes accurately predict the uptake: the genes MORF4L2 and HSF2, followed by somatostatin receptors SSTR1, 3, and 5 exhibited the highest correlation with SUVmax. Progressive disease was identified by elevated levels of a quotient of MORF4L2 expression and SUVmax [ROC-derived AUC (R^2 = 0.7, $p < 0.05$). As expected, no statistical rela-

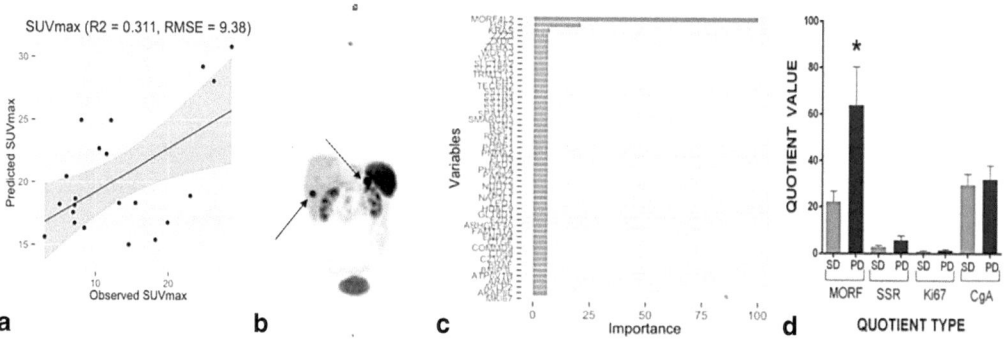

Fig. 7.3 Neuroendocrine specific multitranscriptomic analysis, NETest, predicts correlates with and predicts uptake at ^{68}Ga-labeled somatostatin analogue (SSA) PET with great concordance ((**a**) >95% concordance, R^2 = 0.31, root-mean-square error = 9.38). (**b**) Typical appearance of a ^{68}Ga-DOTATOC PET scan, maximum intensity projection (MIP) in a patient with elevated NETest, demonstrating an intensely avid pancreatic lesion (dotted arrow) as well as in intensely avid liver metastasis (solid arrow). (**c**) Histogram illustrating the genes contributing to predict the uptake at ^{68}Ga-SSA-PET: MORF4L2 and HSF2, are the most important. (**d**) Progressive disease was identified by elevated levels of a quotient of MORF4L2 expression and SUVmax [ROC-derived AUC (R^2 = 0.7, p < 0.05). A circulating gene-based quotient, therefore, has relevance for clinical management, because it adds functional biological multi-dimensionality to an image

tionship was identified between CgA and Ki-67 and imaging parameters (Fig. 7.3).

7.4 Circulating NET Transcripts and PRRT

We then moved on and tested the correlation of NETest and PRRT efficacy. Specifically, the aim of this segment of the research was to assess the accuracy of circulating NET transcripts as a measure of PRRT efficacy, and to identify prognostic gene clusters in baseline blood that could have relevance for PRRT efficacy [11]. Our hypothesis was that the measurement of circulating NET transcripts of patients undergoing PRRT would enable assessment of tumor response and provide biologically relevant information on an individual tumor. We prospectively enrolled 54 subjects with GEP and BP NETs. The majority (47/54) had low-grade NETs (G1/G2; BP typical/atypical), 31/49 were ^{18}FDG positive and 39/54 had progression at start. Disease status was assessed by RECIST1.1. Statistical analysis included chi-square, non-parametric measurements, multiple regression, receiver operating characteristic, and Kaplan-Meier survival curves. The disease control rate (stability, partial and complete responses) was 72% and median progression-free survival (PFS) was not reached (median follow-up: 16 months). Only grading (but not CgA, SSR expression, or FDG positivity) was associated with response ($p < 0.01$). At baseline, 94% of patients were NETest-positive, while CgA was elevated in 59%. NETest accurately (89%, $\chi^2 = 27.4$; $p = 1.2 \times 10^{-7}$) correlated with treatment response, while CgA was only 24% accurate. Additionally, we observed that pre-treatment expression of 8 genes representing clusters of genes regulating two components of tumor biology, namely growth-factor signaling (GFS) and metabolism (MTb), correlated with response. GFS and MTb omic clusters exhibited an AUC of 0.74 ± 0.08 (z-statistic = 2.92, $p < 0.004$) for response prediction (76% accuracy). Ki67 alone had no value as a predictor of treatment efficacy. To amplify the clinical utility using all modalities, we used a logistic regression model to integrate the GFS/

MTb parameter with grading. This provided a binary treatment prediction output: "predicted responder" (PPQ+); "predicted non-responder" (PPQ−) with an AUC of 0.90 ± 0.07, irrespective of tumor origin. The newly defined PRRT predicting quotient (PPQ) exhibited a 94% accurate correlation with PRRT responders (SD + PR + CR; 97%) vs. non-responders (91%).

7.5 Validation Study of PRRT Genomic Signature in Blood (PPQ) for the Prediction of ^{177}Lu-octreotate Efficacy

The characterization of the PPQ in the discovery cohort was the first demonstration of a pre-treatment parameter able to correlate with high accuracy with the response to PRRT. In so doing it accomplished longstanding unmet need in the radionuclide treatment of NETs, namely on a biological basis to accurately predict therapeutic efficacy. This parameter however needed validation in larger, independent cohorts to demonstrate that PPQ (an algorithm that integrates circulating NET-specific transcripts with tissue Ki67), would be able to differentiate PRRT-responders from PRRT-non-responders prior to the initiation of PRRT. In this respect, it was important to demonstrate that PPQ would behave as a predictive and not as a prognostic biomarker, by confirming that PPQ correlated only with PRRT response and not to other treatment strategies.

The study of PPQ as a predictive biomarker was undertaken in three independent ^{177}Lu-PRRT treated cohorts with a total of 158 subjects: the original developmental cohort, now enlarged to 72 subjects from IRST Meldola, Italy, and the two prospective validation cohorts from Zentralklinik Bad Berka, Germany ($n = 44$), and Erasmus Medical Center, Rotterdam, Netherlands ($n = 42$). Each cohort included predominantly well-differentiated, low-grade (G1–G2, 86–95%) GEP and BP NETs. To demonstrate the specificity of PPQ, we included two non-PRRT comparator cohorts: SSA-treated cohort I ($n = 28$; 100% G1–G2, 100% GEP) and II ($n = 51$; 98% low grade; 76% GEP-NET), and a watchful-waiting

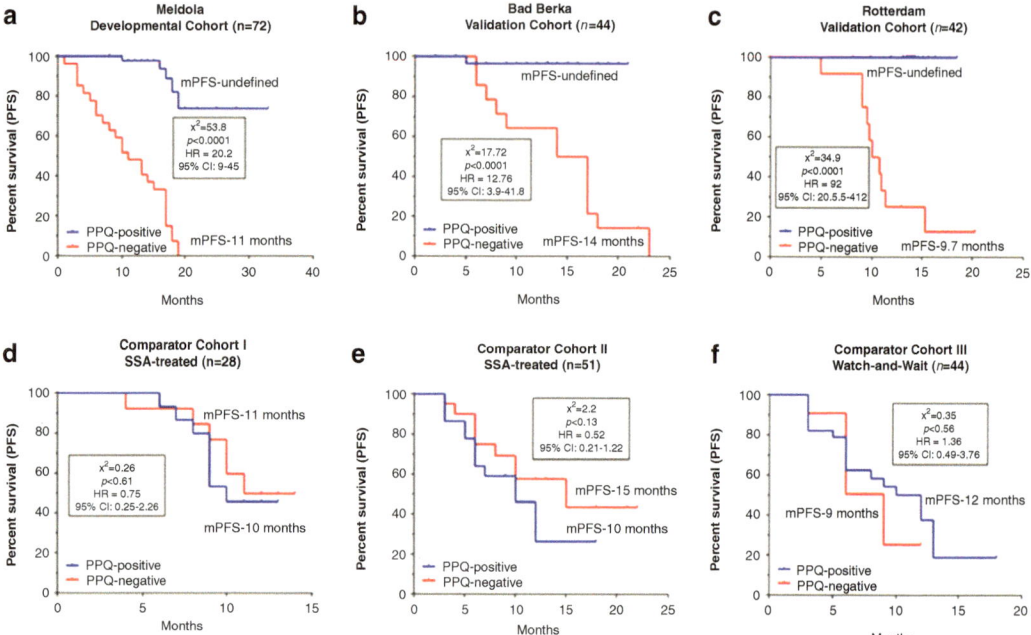

Fig. 7.4 PRRT Prediction Quotient for PFS prediction in PRRT-treated and non-treated cohorts. In the PRRT-treated cohorts (**a**–**c**) positive PPQ predicted a favorable PRRT outcome and was associated with undefined mPFS, while negative PPQ predicted a poor PRRT outcome and was associated with a mPFS of 11–14 months. In the comparator, non-PRRT treated cohorts (**d**–**f**), the prediction of PPQ did not make any difference in the outcome of therapy, resulting in similar mPFS for the PPQ positive and negative subjects. These results provide the demonstration that PPQ is a predictive biomarker and a measure of radiosensitivity

cohort ($n = 44$; 64% G1–G2; 91% GEP). Baseline parameters to be tested included PPQ, disease status, SSR, and CgA. Treatment response was evaluated using RECIST criteria [responder (stable, partial, and complete response) vs non-responder)]. Sample measurement and analyses were blinded to study outcomes. Statistical evaluation included Kaplan-Meier survival and standard test evaluation analyses.

In the developmental cohort, 56% responded to PRRT. The PPQ predicted 100% of responders and 84% of non-responders, with an accuracy of 93%. The two validation cohorts exhibited a response of 64 and 79%, respectively. In both, the PPQ was 95% accurate (Bad Berka: PPQ+ = 97%, PPQ− = 93%; Rotterdam: PPQ+ = 94%, PPQ− = 100%). Overall, the median PFS was not reached in PPQ+ vs PPQ− (10–14 months; HR: 18–77, $p < 0.0001$). In the two comparator cohorts, where SSA-treatment ($n = 79$) and watchful waiting ($n = 44$) were applied, the PRRT predictor (PPQ) had an accuracy of 47 and 50%,

respectively. Essentially, the predictive accuracy of flipping a coin! In addition, the PFS of the PPQ+ and PPQ− did not exhibit any significant differences in any of the two comparator cohorts. These data demonstrated that the PPQ measurement is an accurate predictor of radiosensitivity (Fig. 7.4).

7.6 Validation Study of Multigene NET-Specific Circulating Transcript Signature for the Monitoring of ^{177}Lu-octreotate Efficacy

Finally, we sought to validate the correlation of the multigene NET-specific circulating transcript signature with efficacy. Specifically, it was our intention to test the hypothesis that the NETest is able to over time monitor the response to PRRT and provide added value to the PPQ [12]. We prospectively evaluated whether the NETest was a

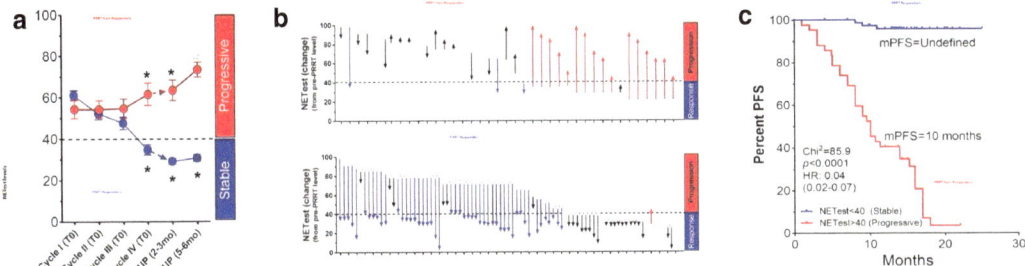

Fig. 7.5 NETest levels during PRRT. PRRT responders (blue, **a**, **b**) had significantly decreased NETest levels during and after PRRT. A decrease to NETest stable levels (NETest < 40) was significantly associated with a favorable outcome, represented by an undefined mPFS (blue, **c**). On the contrary, patients who did not respond to therapy (red, **a**, **b**) exhibited significantly increased NETest levels during and after PRRT. Increasing NETest levels to the progressive range (>40) were significantly associated with a poor outcome of PRRT, represented by a mPFS of 10 months (red, **c**). This is particularly valuable in light of the frequent pseudo-progression, related to the radiation inflammatory response, which limits the evaluation of PRRT outcome until after the end of PRRT

surrogate biomarker for RECIST in defining disease response and if NETest levels correlated with pretreatment PPQ prediction of efficacy. We included 122 prospectively enrolled patients with GEP and BP NETs undergoing PRRT with ^{177}Lu-peptides. These were divided into three cohorts (IRST, Meldola, Italy: $n = 72$; Zentralklinik Bad-Berka, Germany: $n = 44$; Erasmus University Rotterdam, Netherlands: $n = 41$). NETest was measured at baseline, at each PRRT cycle, and at follow-up (2–12 months). NETest is defined by a 1–100 score: stable disease is identified by a score <40, progression >40. CgA was used as a comparator. Samples were de-identified, and measurement and analyses were blinded. Kaplan-Meier survival and standard statistics were assessed. RECIST stabilization or response ("responder") occurred in 67%; 33% progressed. NETest significantly ($p <$ 0.0001) decreased in "responders" ($-47 \pm 3\%$); in "non-responders," NETst levels remained elevated ($+79 \pm 19\%$) ($p < 0.0005$). NETest monitoring accuracy was 98% (119/122). NETest levels >40 in the follow-up (indicating a progressive status) correlated with a shorter mPFS (10 months), as opposed to stable NETest levels (<40; not reached; HR 0.04 (95%CI, 0.02–0.07). PPQ was confirmed to predict response with high accuracy (118/122, 97%) with a 99% accurate positive and 93% accurate negative prediction. The combination of information deriving from the two genomic biomarkers demonstrated that NETest significantly ($p < 0.0001$) decreased in

PPQ-predicted responders ($-46 \pm 3\%$). Conversely, in PPQ-predicted non-responders the NETest remained elevated or increased ($+75 \pm 19\%$). Follow-up NETest values, stable vs progressive, reflected the PPQ prediction and the mPFS (not reached vs. 10 months; HR 0.06 (95%CI, 0.03–0.12). CgA was noncontributory: it decreased in 38% of PRRT responders and 56% of non-responders ($p = $ NS). In summary, these studies demonstrated two major outcomes. Firstly, the PPQ predicted PRRT response in 97%; secondly, the NETest accurately monitored PRRT response. Overall, it was evident that the PPQ is an effective predictive biomarker specific for PRRT and that the NETest provides an effective real-time surrogate marker of PRRT radiological response (Fig. 7.5). This is particularly valuable in light of the frequent pseudo-progression, related to the radiation inflammatory response, which limits the evaluation of PRRT outcome until after the end of PRRT [13]. It also provides evidence for further consideration in respect of health economic impact of repeated imaging as opposed to the use of a noninvasive biomarker assessment [14].

7.7 Future Developments

PRRT has demonstrated efficacy and tolerability in the treatment of well-differentiated neuroendocrine tumors. The work of the LuGenIum Consortium for Independent Research addressed some of the major challenges in its use, which are the prediction of efficacy and toxicity and the consequent patient stratification. Transcriptomic evaluations of blood and a combination of gene expression and specific SNPs, aided by machine learning algorithms, are worth consideration as key strategies to provide molecular tools that will enhance the efficacy and safety of PRRT [15].

Acknowledgments These results have been made possible by the support, knowledge, inspiration, and vision of Dik J. Kwekkeboom (of beloved memory), Eric P. Krenning, Irvin M. Modlin, and Richard P. Baum. I am also profoundly indebted to Irvin Modlin, Mark Kidd, and Ignat Drozdov who developed the NETest and whose felicitous intellectual support facilitated my work in the development of the PPQ. My gratitude also goes to my collaborators from Italy, particularly Giovanni Paganelli, Chiara M. Grana, and Stefano Severi; from Bad Berka, particularly Aviral Singh; and from Rotterdam, particularly, Wouter van de Zwan.

References

1. Modlin IM, Drozdov I, Kidd M. The identification of gut neuroendocrine tumor disease by multiple synchronous transcript analysis in blood. PLoS One. 2013;8:e63364.
2. Bodei L, Kidd M, Paganelli G, et al. Long-term tolerability of PRRT in 807 patients with neuroendocrine tumours: the value and limitations of clinical factors. Eur J Nucl Med Mol Imaging. 2015;42:5–19.
3. Modlin IM, Drozdov I, Alaimo D, et al. A multianalyte PCR blood test outperforms single analyte ELISAs (chromogranin A, pancreastatin, neurokinin A) for neuroendocrine tumor detection. Endocr Relat Cancer. 2014;21:615–28.
4. Oberg K, Modlin IM, De Herder W, et al. Consensus on biomarkers for neuroendocrine tumour disease. Lancet Oncol. 2015;16:435–46.
5. Pavel M, Jann H, Prasad V, Drozdov I, Modlin IM, Kidd M. NET blood transcript analysis defines the crossing of the clinical rubicon: when stable disease becomes progressive. Neuroendocrinology. 2017;104:170–82.
6. Modlin IM, Aslanian H, Bodei L, Drozdov I, Kidd M. A PCR blood test outperforms chromogranin A in carcinoid detection and is unaffected by proton pump inhibitors. Endocr Connect. 2014;3:215–23.
7. Pacak K, Kidd M, Meuter L, Modlin IM. A novel liquid biopsy (NETest) identifies paragangliomas and pheochromocytomas with high accuracy. Endocr Relat Cancer. 2021;28(11):731–44.
8. Modlin IM, Kidd M, Falconi M, et al. A multigenomic liquid biopsy biomarker for neuroendocrine tumor disease outperforms CgA and has surgical and clinical utility. Ann Oncol. 2021;32(11):1425–33.
9. Modlin IM, Kidd M, Frilling A, et al. Molecular genomic assessment using a blood-based MRNA signature (NETest) is cost-effective and predicts neuroendocrine tumor recurrence with 94% accuracy. Ann Surg. 2021;274:481–90.
10. Bodei L, Kidd M, Modlin IM, et al. Gene transcript analysis blood values correlate with ^{68}Ga-DOTA-somatostatin analog (SSA) PET/CT imaging in neuroendocrine tumors and can define disease status. Eur J Nucl Med Mol Imaging. 2015;42:1341–52.
11. Bodei L, Kidd M, Modlin IM, et al. Measurement of circulating transcripts and gene cluster analysis predicts and defines therapeutic efficacy of peptide receptor radionuclide therapy (PRRT) in neuroendocrine tumors. Eur J Nucl Med Mol Imaging. 2016;43:839–51.
12. Bodei L, Kidd MS, Singh A, et al. PRRT neuroendocrine tumor response monitored using circulating transcript analysis: the NETest. Eur J Nucl Med Mol Imaging. 2020;47:895–906.
13. Brabander T, van der Zwan WA, Teunissen JJM, et al. Pitfalls in the response evaluation after peptide receptor radionuclide therapy with [(177)Lu-DOTA(0),Tyr(3)]octreotate. Endocr Relat Cancer. 2017;24:243–51.
14. Liu E, Paulson S, Gulati A, et al. Assessment of NETest clinical utility in a U.S. Registry-based study. Oncologist. 2019;24:783–90.
15. Bodei L, Schöder H, Baum RP, et al. Molecular profiling of neuroendocrine tumours to predict response and toxicity to peptide receptor radionuclide therapy. Lancet Oncol. 2020;21:e431–43.

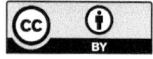

A Tree Can Be Recognized by Its Fruit

Marion de Jong

8.1 Introduction

A small German city named Bad Berka, which is situated in the south of the Weimar region, brought forth many famous people over time. These include both sons and daughters of Bad Berka and those strongly connected to the town (adapted from Wikipedia):

- Otto Fries (1849–1905), politician National Liberal Party (Germany), member of Reichstag
- Hugo Günther (1891–1954), party functionary (SPD/KPD/KPO/SED) and insurance director
- Hans Carl Nipperdey (1895–1968), law professor, first president of the Federal Labour Court
- Hartmut Griesmayr (born 1945), screenwriter and director
- Johann Wolfgang von Goethe (1749–1832), writer, stayed there often as a bathing guest
- Jakob Michael Reinhold Lenz (1751–1792), poet of Sturm und Drang
- Dietrich Georg von Kieser (1779–1862), medical doctor, worked as a physician in Berka
- Adolf Brütt (1855–1939), sculptor, worked in Bad Berka, since 1928 honorary citizen

- Martin Hellberg (1905–1999), author, actor and director
- Henry Augustus Siebrecht, florist, "Father of Fifth Avenue"
- Richard Baum, professor, physician, and scientist, Chef of the clinic for Molecular Radiotherapy at the Zentralklinik Bad Berka

The last person on this list, Prof. Richard Baum, is quite a special person. To describe him, I thought of a metaphor and expression taken from the bible (Luke 6:43-44): "An der Frucht erkennt man den Baum". That is because Richard Baum reminds me of a cherry tree; a firm tree, a highlight in the garden, solidly rooted in fertile ground, self-pollinating, but benefitting from other trees in the garden, and rich in delicious fruits that come in pairs. Paired fruits refer here to the field of theranostics (see below). For this contribution, I chose three themes:

- Fruits of Scientist Baum
- Fruits of Physician Baum
- Fruits of Friend Baum

8.2 Fruits of Scientist Baum

Radiolabeled somatostatin analogs were introduced more than 20 years ago for theranostics of patients with somatostatin receptor (especially subtype 2) expressing neuroendocrine tumors.

M. de Jong (✉)
Department of Radiology and Nuclear Medicine, Erasmus MC, Rotterdam, The Netherlands
e-mail: m.hendriks-dejong@erasmusmc.nl

© The Author(s) 2024
V. Prasad (ed.), *Beyond Becquerel and Biology to Precision Radiomolecular Oncology: Festschrift in Honor of Richard P. Baum*, https://doi.org/10.1007/978-3-031-33533-4_8

After injection into the body these small soma-tostatin peptide analogs can guide attached radio-activity to their target receptors overexpressed on tumor cells, enabling imaging or radionuclide therapy, dependent on the radionuclide of choice.

A few years later, the first clinical studies were carried out, also paving the way for the development of a variety of different radiolabeled peptide analogs for the diagnosis and treatment of tumors in many collaborative studies [1–10] (review: 11). Promising radiolabeled analogs used for positron emission tomography (PET) or peptide receptor radiotherapy (PRRT) include peptides targeting somatostatin receptors (SSTR), integrins, chemokine receptors, fibroblast activating protein (FAP), gastrin-releasing peptide receptor (GRPR), or the prostate-specific membrane antigen (PSMA) [11]. They are excellent examples of so-called theranostics, a combination of the terms therapeutics and diagnostics. It refers to the combination of a paired diagnostic/imaging tool or tracer used to identify a second tool (which may in fact be the same tracer now radiolabeled with a therapeutic radionuclide) for therapy, like the paired cherries in the cherry tree. Using this concept, "We can see what we treat and we can treat what we see". Theranostics comprise an interesting part of personalized or precision medicine: "The right treatment for the right patient at the right time and at the right dose".

Radiolabeled small peptides are an important class of radiopharmaceuticals applied for diagnosis and therapy of tumors. These small compounds possess beneficial properties as targeting probes in nuclear medicine: they are not immunogenic and show fast diffusion and target localization. Additionally, peptides can be easily modified, improving metabolic stability and adjusting favorable pharmacokinetics. In contrast to small molecular weight compounds, peptides are more tolerant of modifications. Because of the presence of endogenous enzymes (peptidases) for the degradation of peptides and proteins, the major disadvantage of peptides compared to small molecular mass probes could be the lower metabolic stability. A variety of strategies can overcome this problem, including

the introduction of unnatural amino acids, backbone cyclization, modifications, and the use of peptidase inhibitors [11, 12]. A relatively easy strategy for stability improvement toward peptidases is the application of d-amino acids or unnatural amino acids. In many cases, a combination of N/C-terminal modification with stabilization via d-amino acids or unnatural amino acids is used, as described for Tyr^3-octreotide or different RGD-derivatives. For a variety of tracers, backbone cyclization could be combined with the introduction of d-amino acids. However, not all amino acids in a sequence can be replaced either by the corresponding d-amino acid or by an unnatural amino acid without influencing the binding affinity. So, for another pathway to stabilize peptides, we hypothesized that the in vivo co-administration of specific enzyme inhibitors would improve peptide bioavailability and hence tumor uptake. Through single coinjection of the neutral endopeptidase inhibitor phosphoramidon (PA), we indeed were able to provoke remarkable rises in the percentages of circulating intact somatostatin, gastrin, and bombesin radiopeptides in mouse models, resulting in a clear increase in uptake in tumor xenografts in mice [12]. These approaches have also been applied in our collaborative research with Prof. Baum, resulting in the following fruits:

Gastrin-releasing peptide receptors (GRPR) represent attractive targets for tumor diagnosis and therapy because of their overexpression in major human cancers. Internalizing GRPR agonists were initially proposed for prolonged lesion retention, but a shift of paradigm to GRPR antagonists has been made, as radioantagonists, such as ^{99m}TcDB1 (^{99m}Tc-N4′-DPhe(6),Leu-NHEt(13)]BBN(6-13)), displayed better pharmacokinetics than radioagonists, in addition to their higher biosafety. We introduced ^{68}GaSB3, a ^{99m}Tc-DB1 mimic, carrying the chelator DOTA for labeling with the PET radiometal ^{68}Ga. SB3 and [(nat)Ga]SB3 bound to the human GRPR with high affinity, plus ^{67}GaSB3 displayed good in vivo stability. ^{67}GaSB3 showed high, GRPR-specific and prolonged retention in PC-3 xenografts in mice, but much faster clearance from the GRPR-rich pancreas. In patients in Bad Berka,

^{68}GaSB3 clearly visualized cancer lesions without adverse effects. Thus, 4 out of 8 breast cancer and 5 out of 9 prostate cancer patients showed pathological uptake on PET/CT. We concluded imaging with ^{68}GaSB3 to be promising in patients with primary breast or prostate cancer [13]. Afterward, we introduced, by replacement of the C-terminal Leu^{13}-Met^{14}-NH$_2$ dipeptide of SB3 by Sta^{13}-Leu^{14}-NH$_2$, the novel GRPR antagonist NeoBOMB1, labeled with different radiometals for theranostic use. NeoBOMB1 and ^{nat}Ga-, ^{nat}In-, and ^{nat}Lu-NeoBOMB1 bound again to GRPR with high affinity. They showed excellent metabolic stability in peripheral mouse blood. After injection in mice, all 3 tracers (^{67}Ga-, ^{111}In-, and ^{177}Lu-NeoBOMB1) showed comparably high and GRPR-specific uptake in the PC-3 xenografts. During a translational study in prostate cancer patients, ^{68}Ga-NeoBOMB1 rapidly localized in pathologic lesions, achieving high-contrast imaging, so the GRPR antagonist radioligands ^{67}Ga-, ^{111}In-, and ^{177}Lu-NeoBOMB1, independent of the radiometal applied, have shown comparable and most promising behavior in prostate cancer models and patients, in favor of future theranostic use in GRPR-positive cancer patients [14].

In another series of collaborative studies, we focused on the use of the potent alpha emitter bismuth-213 for radionuclide therapy [15–18]. So, we optimized the labeling conditions of ^{213}Bi-DOTATATE for preclinical applications of peptide receptor-targeted alpha therapy plus we evaluated whether ^{213}Bi-DOTATATE was suitable for the treatment of both larger neuroendocrine tumors overexpressing SSTR2 in comparison to its effectiveness in smaller tumors. Based on the results of the studies we concluded that ^{213}Bi-DOTATATE demonstrated a great therapeutic effect in both small and larger tumor lesions, whereas higher probability for stable disease was found in animals with small tumors.

In the text above, beautiful examples of translational research, from bench to bedside, have been shown. To further improve translational research, sophisticated cancer models are now available to address cancer-related research questions. Technological developments in probe synthesis and labeling have resulted in most promising imaging and therapeutic probes with the potential for basic research, as well as for translational and clinical applications. Moreover, translational collaborative studies as referred to above have shown that developments and improvements of multimodal imaging methods for use in animal research have substantially strengthened the field of preclinical theranostics. Improvements in all these research fields improved rapid translation of new therapies into the clinic [19].

We conclude that the future of radiopharmaceuticals for imaging and therapy is radiant. The field of theranostics will flourish even more when applying novel intra-arterial applications, targeting antagonists with better-targeting profiles, the application of novel radionuclides, including the powerful alpha emitters, and combination therapies.

8.3 Fruits of Doctor Baum

In Bad Berka, Prof. Baum and his team apply theranostics in cancer patients from all over the world with great success. Prof. Baum arrived in Bad Berka in 1997 to initiate a Nuclear Medicine department there; in the meantime, it became very well known for the application of theranostics. It has developed to an ENETS Center of Excellence where patients from many different parts of the world are being treated using PRRT with beta and alpha particle emitting radionuclides. PRRT is now approved by the European Medical Agency (EMA) and the Food and Drug Administration (FDA). In Bad Berka, around 1000 therapies are given each year in the large station with 22 beds. Not only patients with neuroendocrine tumors are being treated with PRRT, also patients suffering from other tumor types, like e.g. prostate cancer, can be treated now using novel theranostics, which is great news for all kinds of patients suffering from these cancers.

Prof. Baum is highly respected by his co-workers and patients, which is very understandable and well deserved, considering his enormous

different steps of the development and introduction of new theranostic radiopharmaceuticals.

Now it is time for a new adventure: Prof. Baum will start the Theranostics Center for Radiomolecular Precision Oncology in Wiesbaden: Richard, I wish you all the best and please continue the good work!

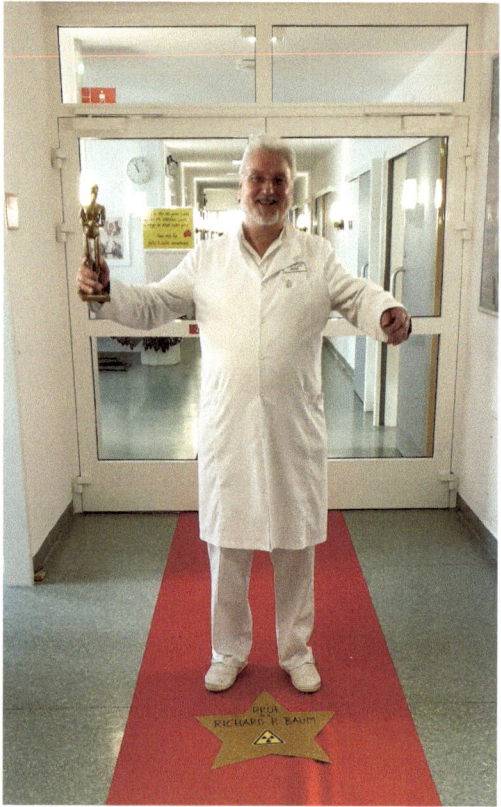

Fig. 8.1 Fruits of Doctor Baum

work load, enthusiasm, and drive to do the best possible for every patient. From the picture in Fig. 8.1 we can also clearly witness this. The successful theranostic work in Bad Berka is based on team work; like a cherry tree Prof. Baum can be self-pollinating, but he strongly benefits from fertile ground and the presence of other cherry trees around him.

8.3.1 Fruits of Our Friend Baum

Prof. Baum is a great colleague and friend, a treasure in our theranostic garden like a beautiful cherry tree: being considerate, very helpful, a source of inspiration, always in for a challenge, cheerful, and enthusiastic, albeit also demanding and ambitious. We both very much enjoyed the start of the theranostic adventure and I appreciate our collaborations, even though we worked in

References

1. Bodei L, Kidd M, Modlin IM, Prasad V, Severi S, Ambrosini V, et al. Gene transcript analysis blood values correlate with (6)(8)Ga-DOTA-somatostatin analog (SSA) PET/CT imaging in neuroendocrine tumors and can define disease status. Eur J Nucl Med Mol Imaging. 2015;42(9):1341–52.
2. Bodei L, Kidd M, Modlin IM, Severi S, Drozdov I, Nicolini S, et al. Measurement of circulating transcripts and gene cluster analysis predicts and defines therapeutic efficacy of peptide receptor radionuclide therapy (PRRT) in neuroendocrine tumors. Eur J Nucl Med Mol Imaging. 2016;43(5):839–51.
3. Bodei L, Kidd M, Paganelli G, Grana CM, Drozdov I, Cremonesi M, et al. Long-term tolerability of PRRT in 807 patients with neuroendocrine tumours: the value and limitations of clinical factors. Eur J Nucl Med Mol Imaging. 2015;42(1):5–19.
4. Bodei L, Kidd MS, Singh A, van der Zwan WA, Severi S, Drozdov IA, et al. PRRT genomic signature in blood for prediction of (177)Lu-octreotate efficacy. Eur J Nucl Med Mol Imaging. 2018;45(7):1155–69.
5. Bodei L, Kidd MS, Singh A, van der Zwan WA, Severi S, Drozdov IA, et al. PRRT neuroendocrine tumor response monitored using circulating transcript analysis: the NETest. Eur J Nucl Med Mol Imaging. 2020;47(4):895–906.
6. Caplin M, Sundin A, Nillson O, Baum RP, Klose KJ, Kelestimur F, et al. ENETS Consensus Guidelines for the management of patients with digestive neuroendocrine neoplasms: colorectal neuroendocrine neoplasms. Neuroendocrinology. 2012;95(2):88–97.
7. Oberg K, Krenning E, Sundin A, Bodei L, Kidd M, Tesselaar M, et al. A Delphic consensus assessment: imaging and biomarkers in gastroenteropancreatic neuroendocrine tumor disease management. Endocr Connect. 2016;5(5):174–87.
8. Strosberg J, El-Haddad G, Wolin E, Hendifar A, Yao J, Chasen B, et al. Phase 3 trial of (177)Lu-dotatate for midgut neuroendocrine tumors. N Engl J Med. 2017;376(2):125–35.
9. Strosberg J, Kunz PL, Hendifar A, Yao J, Bushnell D, Kulke MH, et al. Impact of liver tumour burden, alkaline phosphatase elevation, and target lesion size on treatment outcomes with (177)Lu-Dotatate: an analysis of the NETTER-1 study. Eur J Nucl Med Mol Imaging. 2020;47(10):2372–82.

10. Strosberg J, Wolin E, Chasen B, Kulke M, Bushnell D, Caplin M, et al. Health-related quality of life in patients with progressive midgut neuroendocrine tumors treated with (177)Lu-dotatate in the phase III NETTER-1 trial. J Clin Oncol. 2018;36(25):2578–84.

11. Rangger C, Haubner R. Radiolabelled peptides for positron emission tomography and endoradiotherapy in oncology. Pharmaceuticals. 2020;13(2):22.

12. Nock BA, Maina T, Krenning EP, de Jong M. "To serve and protect": enzyme inhibitors as radiopeptide escorts promote tumor targeting. J Nucl Med. 2014;55(1):121–7.

13. Maina T, Bergsma H, Kulkarni HR, Mueller D, Charalambidis D, Krenning EP, et al. Preclinical and first clinical experience with the gastrin-releasing peptide receptor-antagonist [(6)(8)Ga]SB3 and PET/CT. Eur J Nucl Med Mol Imaging. 2016;43(5):964–73.

14. Nock BA, Kaloudi A, Lymperis E, Giarika A, Kulkarni HR, Klette I, et al. Theranostic perspectives in prostate cancer with the gastrin-releasing peptide receptor antagonist NeoBOMB1: preclinical and first clinical results. J Nucl Med. 2017;58(1):75–80.

15. Chan HS, de Blois E, Konijnenberg MW, Morgenstern A, Bruchertseifer F, Norenberg JP, et al. Optimizing labelling conditions of (213)Bi-DOTATATE for preclinical applications of peptide receptor targeted alpha therapy. EJNMMI Radiopharm Chem. 2017;1(1):9.

16. Chan HS, de Blois E, Morgenstern A, Bruchertseifer F, de Jong M, Breeman W, et al. In vitro comparison of 213Bi- and 177Lu-radiation for peptide receptor radionuclide therapy. PLoS One. 2017;12(7):e0181473.

17. Chan HS, Konijnenberg MW, Daniels T, Nysus M, Makvandi M, de Blois E, et al. Improved safety and efficacy of (213)Bi-DOTATATE-targeted alpha therapy of somatostatin receptor-expressing neuroendocrine tumors in mice pre-treated with L-lysine. EJNMMI Res. 2016;6(1):83.

18. Chan HS, Konijnenberg MW, de Blois E, Koelewijn S, Baum RP, Morgenstern A, et al. Influence of tumour size on the efficacy of targeted alpha therapy with (213)Bi-[DOTA(0),Tyr(3)]-octreotate. EJNMMI Res. 2016;6(1):6.

19. de Jong M, Essers J, van Weerden WM. Imaging preclinical tumour models: improving translational power. Nat Rev Cancer. 2014;14(7):481–93.

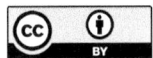

IAEA Strategy for Enhancing the Sustainability of Nuclear Medicine in Low- and Middle-Income Countries

9

Francesco Giammarile, Pilar Orellana, and Diana Paez

9.1 Introduction

The incidence and mortality associated with non-communicable diseases (NCDs) is on the rise globally. There has been a significant shift in the global disease burden in the past decades from communicable infectious diseases to non-communicable diseases, especially evident in low- and middle-income countries (LMICs). According to the World Health Organization (WHO), more than 38 million people die each year as a consequence of NCDs. It is expected that in the next 25 years the majority of new NCD cases and associated deaths will occur in LMICs. The increase in NCDs is related to several factors, including population growth, increased life expectancy and changes in lifestyle. The most frequent NCDs are cardiovascular diseases, cancer, chronic respiratory diseases and diabetes.

Medical imaging has revolutionized healthcare in the past decades as it has enabled the delivery of individual, patient-tailored disease management. Nuclear medicine (NM) techniques have become of paramount importance for the diagnosis and treatment of a wide range of health conditions, in particular NCDs.

For over 50 years, the International Atomic Energy Association (IAEA), an independent international organization related to the United Nations system, with a long history of promoting the safe, secure and peaceful uses of nuclear science and technology in its Member States (MS) provides assistance in building sustainable capacities in the use of medical use of radiation and radionuclides, including NM. The IAEA's Human Health program includes the Nuclear Medicine and Diagnostic Imaging (NMDI) sub-program which takes care of numerous initiatives aimed at fostering the integration of NM practice both in imaging and therapeutic applications into MS' healthcare systems.

On 25 September 2015, at the Summit on Sustainable Development, the 193 MS of the United Nations unanimously adopted the Sustainable Development Goals (SDGs), to improve the health status of vulnerable populations by ensuring universal and equitable access to quality healthcare, emphasizing their intention to significantly reduce the incidence of both communicable and non-communicable diseases. One target outlined in the agenda (target 3.4) aims "to reduce premature mortality from NCDs by one-third through prevention and treatment by 2030".

NM techniques can make significant contributions to the achievement of this SDG target. They evolved to allow for personalized healthcare, and they represent now an indispensable part of modern-day clinical practice. NM diagnostic and

F. Giammarile (✉) · P. Orellana · D. Paez
Nuclear Medicine and Diagnostic Imaging Section, Division of Human Health, IAEA, Vienna, Austria
e-mail: F.Giammarile@iaea.org

© The Author(s) 2024

V. Prasad (ed.), *Beyond Becquerel and Biology to Precision Radiomolecular Oncology: Festschrift in Honor of Richard P. Baum*, https://doi.org/10.1007/978-3-031-33533-4_9

therapeutic applications are very useful in addressing both NCDs and infectious diseases.

Despite the evident usefulness of NM techniques, in most MS, NM services are inadequate. The main factors affecting the expansion and sustainability of NM include high investment, operation and maintenance costs, inadequate qualified personnel and limited suppliers of radiopharmaceuticals [1–9].

9.2   Key Challenges

The routine use of NM might be impeded by significant obstacles. Limited infrastructure prevents countries from offering NM services to meet rising demand, especially for the management of cancer, CVDs and other NCDs [10–12]. The main constraints are:

Acquisition and Operation and Maintenance Costs The cost of establishing a nuclear medicine facility (including buildings and equipment) deters many MS. For countries with existing NM facilities, maintaining functional equipment is an issue. Countries who acquired their NM equipment through the IAEA technical cooperation programme, due to conflicting priorities (especially the need for response to communicable diseases) and limited financial resources, do not have adequate capacity for sustainable operation and maintenance, which include the cost of radiopharmaceuticals and equipment repairs. In addition, some countries are not able to replace the obsolete equipment without additional support from the IAEA.

Affordability NM is a relatively expensive tool. With limited or no health insurance, many patients cannot afford nuclear medicine procedures. The current global economic situation has kept health expenditure growth to almost zero in many low-income countries.

Awareness of the Role of Nuclear Medicine Although NM plays a key role in the current diagnostic imaging revolution, there is still a lack of knowledge among different stakeholders of the benefits and usefulness of the clinical applications of NM techniques. These need to be adequately explained. Most referring clinicians are not adequately informed about the NM discipline, as can be seen in inappropriate referrals. There is a stigma associated with the word 'nuclear' that may deter stakeholders from learning more about nuclear medicine, despite the high potential of radiolabelled molecules in diagnostic and therapeutic applications.

Human Resources To reach the full potential of nuclear medicine, there is a need to train the involved professionals throughout their careers. However, clinical and research personnel are scarce in all the disciplines involved in the practice of NM (i.e., chemists, radiopharmacists, physicians, physicists, clinician-scientists, technologists, etc.). This is, in many cases, due to a lack of specific training programmes that emphasize clinical applications, as well as a limited number of adequately equipped and well-staffed institutions capable of providing both academic and clinical trainings. Training in universities, medical institutions and industry has not been able to keep up with current demands. Furthermore, there is an impending leadership gap in the field. Nuclear medicine research requires a multidisciplinary team of individuals with extremely varied education and training. Only by training an adequate number of individuals in these various disciplines will nuclear medicine and molecular imaging reach its potential. Furthermore, there is a need to harmonize the training programs, in order to raise the level of knowledge and competencies of nuclear medicine specialists worldwide. Trainees come from diverse backgrounds and possess different knowledge and experience; hence, the training program requires an active and standardized approach to ensure compliance with at least the minimum standards needed to provide an optimal clinical nuclear medicine care.

Customs Practices Short half-lives radiopharmaceuticals need to be frequently imported. They must be cleared by customs upon arrival and delivered to the nuclear medicine centre immediately thereafter. However, in some countries, customs regulations are so cumbersome that clearing radiopharmaceuticals in time represents a real challenge.

Limited Suppliers of Radiopharmaceuticals Currently, the most important isotope used in nuclear medicine is metastable technetium-99 (Tc-99m). This radioisotope is produced from molybdenum-99 (Mo-99) in nuclear reactors that use highly enriched uranium (HEU) targets. There are only four producers of Tc-99m worldwide. Any interruption in production in one or more of these reactors results in a decrease of supply. This affects the accessibility of NM services and thus lifesaving treatment.

Inadequate Quality Assurance (QA) and Quality Control (QC) In LMIC, the limited availability of basic equipment used for QC, radiation protection and in medical physics research facilities, such as phantoms and certain radiation sources, poses another challenge to the practice of nuclear medicine.

Radiation Safety Radiation safety is a challenge for the practice of nuclear medicine. Each professional working with ionizing radiation should undergo compulsory monitoring for occupational radiation exposure. In countries, monitoring services for personnel are often provided by government agencies, such as radiation regulatory bodies. These services may also be provided by licensed, for-profit companies which charge more for the same services.

9.3 Interventions

The establishment, expansion and strengthening of NM services will contribute to reducing the incidence and impact of NCDs through early diagnosis, treatment and palliative care for the improved well-being of the population. The IAEA proposed several strategic interventions to be implemented concurrently for effective and sustainable NM services. The intention is to incorporate best practices for the establishment,

operation and maintenance of NM facilities and services, as well as for cost-recovery, expansion, human resource capacity building, and recruitment and retention of staff [10].

1. To increase the total number of NM centres
   (a) Prioritize NM in national health policy and budget through conducting national needs assessments and/or feasibility studies for nuclear medicine.
   (b) Establish domestic funding mechanisms, such as trust funds, for costly but essential medical services and facilities such as radiotherapy and nuclear medicine.
   (c) Formulate and implement national IAEA technical cooperation (TC) projects for the establishment of NM facilities.
   (d) Build and strengthen strategic partnerships.
2. To continuously educate the public and other stakeholders on the benefits and usefulness of the clinical applications of NM.
   (a) Publish and disseminate awareness-raising materials on the benefits of NM procedures and its critical diagnostic and therapeutic roles in a variety of clinical areas, including cardiology, oncology, paediatrics, neurology, endocrinology, infection, inflammation and pulmonology, to referring physicians and hospital managers.
   (b) Organizing NM events at national and regional levels.
   (c) Include introduction courses to NM in undergraduate medical degrees.
   (d) Educate customs officials and clearing and forwarding agents about the short half-life of radiopharmaceuticals and the need for urgent clearance.
3. To ensure that NM is recognized as a medical specialty in all MS.
   (a) Incorporate NM into national health policy frameworks, recognizing it as a medical speciality.
   (b) Strengthen the collaboration between existing NM professional societies and establish new ones, if absent, at national, regional, and international levels.

4. To have an adequate number of qualified NM professionals (including physicians, radiopharmacists, physicists, technologists and nurses) available in the NM centres.
    (a) Create a public structure and career ladder for NM.
    (b) Assess training needs, establish appropriate training curriculum and implement appropriate training programme, including continuous professional development programmes.
    (c) Recruit staff and create incentives for staff retention.
5. To establish appropriate cost recovery programmes to ensure a sustainable supply of radiopharmaceuticals, the operation and maintenance of equipment, and the replacement of ageing equipment.
    (a) Negotiate and conclude suitable contracts for the regular supply of radiopharmaceuticals with suppliers.
    (b) Negotiate and settle appropriate maintenance contracts for NM equipment that ensure that the warranty starts following proper installation and includes servicing and the replacement of parts.
    (c) Put in place long-term plans for the replacement of obsolete/ageing equipment as well as for the expansion and upgrading of NM services.
    (d) Produce locally radiopharmaceutical.
    (e) Provide financial autonomy or a dedicated operational budget for NM in order to maximize efficiency and flexibility.
6. To make NM more affordable.
    (a) Mobilize NGOs, local companies and philanthropists to support NM.
    (b) Establish schemes to help patients who cannot afford NM services.
    (c) Make NM consumables tax exempt since they are health related.
7. To increase the number of NM research studies, especially in the main clinical areas such as cardiology, oncology, paediatrics, neurology and endocrinology.
    (a) Mobilize resources to support the utilization of NM in clinical research.

    (b) Encourage NM professionals to actively participate in coordinated research activities in NM.
    (c) Promote the sharing and utilization of NM research findings with other stakeholders at national, regional, and international levels, and at NM conferences.
    (d) Collaborate with other national or international research institutes.
8. To enhance the safety of NM practice for both patients and physicians.
    (a) Establish and enforce safety regulations and guidelines.
    (b) Train qualified professionals in methods to enhance safety.
    (c) Promote quality assurance procedures.
    (d) Establish or strengthen occupational exposure control programmes.

While recognizing the need for continuity of support from the IAEA and other partners, the above-proposed interventions cannot be achieved without national ownership and leadership by individual governments. Each government is expected to provide equitable universal access to healthcare services, including NM.

9.4 Results

9.4.1 Technical Cooperation Programme

The technical cooperation (TC) programme is one of the mechanisms through which the IAEA directly helps its Member States to build, strengthen and maintain capacities for the safe, peaceful and secure use of nuclear technology in support of sustainable socioeconomic development. The TC programme addresses wide-ranging development objectives which include greater food productivity, better health and nutrition services, improved energy development, and sustainable energy production.

TC projects can be national, driven by the development priorities of a single Member State, or regional, when a group of Member States belonging to the same geographical area cooperate to create regional sustainability and self-reliance in the effective use of nuclear technologies. All Member States are eligible for support through TC projects, although in practice technical cooperation activities are focused on the needs and priorities of low-and-middle-income countries.

Through TC projects, the IAEA supports Member States by coordinating several activities aiming to build human resource capacity, and transfer know-how and technology. These activities include fellowships for individuals, scientific visit opportunities for more experienced professionals, training courses, meetings, missions of experts in the field, as well as procurement of technology and equipment.

TC projects related to nuclear medicine focus on the establishment of a nuclear medicine service (often the first in the country), the upgrade of existing departments with newer hybrid imaging modalities such as SPECT/CT or PET/CT, the enhancement of the clinical practice or the introduction of new diagnostic or therapeutic methodologies. Because of the multidisciplinarity of nuclear medicine, these projects usually include other components related to radiopharmacy, medical physics and safety.

Within a TC project fellowships are granted to health professionals to foster capacity building. These candidates are supported to spend an adequate period of time, in a well-established nuclear medicine service, for specialized and supervised hands-on training. The training programme is agreed with the hosting institute and is usually focused on a specific topic, for example, on the establishment and standardization of clinical protocols, the use of SPECT for cardiological and oncological studies, the therapeutic use of a certain radiopharmaceutical, the practical aspects of QA/QC of instrumentation and radioprotection, or the preparation of radiopharmaceuticals.

Education and training activities are a key component of TC projects and training courses are often included in the workplan to reach out to a larger number of health professionals. The use of international experts is another very effective

mean for the transfer of know-how. These experts are recruited by the IAEA and asked to support the project's counterparts on a specific aspect of the project. Being delivered locally, this kind of support is particularly important for solving specific issues and therefore for achieving the project's objectives. Finally, as one of the means for achieving their objectives, TC projects often include the procurement of important equipment or services based on the general aspects of sustainability and ownership [13].

9.4.2 Quality Assurance

In 2006, NMDI Section of the IAEA launched an initiative to design a program to help its constituency in MSs to self-assess the standard of their NM clinical practices and, if necessary, raise them up to accepted international standards. The output of that initiative has been a program called Quality Management Audits in Nuclear Medicine (QUANUM), based on comprehensive auditing missions of multidisciplinary teams.

The aim of the QUANUM program is threefold: in the first place to encourage the introduction of a routine process of conducting annual systematic audits in the clinical arena; secondly, to encourage the adoption of a culture of regular analyses and reviews of internal processes, both of them essential for positive growth in medical services and, third and even more important, to introduce the entire quality audit process, patient oriented, systematic and outcome based.

The QUANUM program proved to be applicable to a wide variety of institutions, from small practices to larger centres with PET/CT and cyclotrons. Clinical services rendered to patients showed a good compliance with international standards, while issues related to radiation protection of both staff and patients require a higher degree of attention. This should be considered as relevant feedback for the IAEA with regard to the effective translation of safety recommendations into routine practice. Training on drafting and application of Standard Operating Procedures (SOPs) should also be considered a priority [10–12].

9.4.3 Procurement

Over the years, NMDI Section of the IAEA has assisted over hundred low- and middle-income MS to acquire or strengthen their NM services. The Nuclear Medicine Resources Manual, for example, provides guidance to decision-makers on the different applications of nuclear medicine and on the prerequisites and resources needed to establish this service.

9.4.4 Education

Training in nuclear medicine is vital for the development of adequate capacities in MS. NMDI Section of the IAEA provided education and training opportunities to professionals throughout their careers, as part of a lifelong learning process.

As a promoter of optimal nuclear medicine practice, the IAEA published a *Training Curriculum for Nuclear Medicine Physicians*, which offers guidelines that are based on various publications, international recommendations as well as expert advice. The objective of this publication is to recommend a harmonized training programme for nuclear medicine physicians, allow trainees to develop the necessary knowledge, competencies and skills to practice this medical speciality and to ensure a safe and quality level of clinical nuclear medicine [7].

9.4.5 Coordinated Research Activities

The IAEA Coordinated Research Projects (CRPs) bring together research institutions throughout the world to collaborate on a well-defined research topic related to the acquisition and dissemination of new knowledge and technology in the various fields related to the peaceful use of atomic energy. Institutions and scientists from all around the world are selected to exchange information and work together on some relevant aspects related to the main topic,

thus creating international scientific networks and enhancing the capabilities of participating countries to be involved in state-of-the-art scientific research. The results are made freely available to the MS and the scientific community usually through IAEA publications, training material, or articles published in peer-reviewed journals [9].

9.5   Conclusion

The IAEA has a long tradition in assisting its Member States in the field of nuclear medicine. The main activities in this field are the production of guidance documents, the establishment of educational and training, the coordination of research activities and the support to Member States for establishing and safely operating nuclear medicine facilities through the technical cooperation programme. But enormous efforts are still needed, not only to ensure universal access to NM services, but also to make these services affordable and reliable.

References

1. International Atomic Energy Agency. Standard operating procedures for PET/CT: a practical approach for use in adult oncology. Vienna: International Atomic Energy Agency; 2013.
2. International Atomic Energy Agency. Clinical applications of SPECT/CT: new hybrid nuclear medicine imaging system. Vienna: International Atomic Energy Agency; 2008.
3. International Atomic Energy Agency. Appropriate use of FDG-PET for the management of cancer patients. Vienna: International Atomic Energy Agency; 2010.
4. International Atomic Energy Agency. Planning a clinical PET centre. Vienna: International Atomic Energy Agency; 2010.
5. International Atomic Energy Agency. Nuclear cardiology: its role in cost effective care. Vienna: International Atomic Energy Agency; 2012. Strategy for enhancing the sustainability of nuclear medicine in Africa, 2016. Vienna: International Atomic Energy Agency.
6. International Atomic Energy Agency. Nuclear cardiology: guidance on the implementation of SPECT myocardial perfusion imaging. Vienna: International Atomic Energy Agency; 2016.

7. International Atomic Energy Agency. Training curriculum for nuclear medicine physicians. Vienna: International Atomic Energy Agency; 2019.
8. International Atomic Energy Agency. Nuclear medicine resources manual ver 2.0 – a guide for decision makers. Vienna: International Atomic Energy Agency; 2020.
9. Coordinated research activities. 2019. Available from https://www.iaea.org/services/coordinated-research-activities.
10. Dondi M, Torres L, Marengo M, Massardo T, Mishani E, Van Zyl EA, Solanki K, Bischof Delaloye A, Lobato EE, Miller RN, Paez D, Pascual T. Comprehensive auditing in nuclear medicine through the IAEA QUANUM program. Part 1: the QUANUM program and methodology. Semin Nucl Med. 2017;47(6):680–6. https://doi.org/10.1053/j.semnuclmed.2017.07.003.
11. Dondi M, Torres L, Marengo M, Massardo T, Mishani E, Van Zyl EA, Solanki K, Bischof Delaloye A, Lobato EE, Miller RN, Ordonez FB, Paez D, Pascual T. Comprehensive auditing in nuclear medicine through the international atomic energy agency quality management audits in nuclear medicine program. Part 2: analysis of results. Semin Nucl Med. 2017;47(6):687–93. https://doi.org/10.1053/j.semnuclmed.2017.07.004.
12. Dondi M, Paez D, Torres L, Marengo M, Delaloye AB, Solanki K, Van Zyl EA, Lobato EE, Miller RN, Giammarile F, Pascual T. Implementation of quality systems in nuclear medicine: why it matters. An outcome analysis (quality management audits in nuclear medicine part III). Semin Nucl Med. 2018;48(3):299–306. https://doi.org/10.1053/j.semnuclmed.2017.12.001.
13. Casas-Zamora JA, Kashyap R. The IAEA technical cooperation programme and nuclear medicine in the developing world: objectives, trends, and contributions. Semin Nucl Med. 2013;43(3):172–80. https://doi.org/10.1053/j.semnuclmed.2012.11.007.

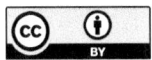

Majid Assadi, Reza Nemati, Hossein Shooli,
and Hojjat Ahmadzadehfar

10.1   Introduction

Malignant brain neoplasms are generally classified into primary neoplasms and metastatic
tumours. The former originate from the brain
parenchyma itself and the latter arise from body
systems other than the brain. Primary brain
tumours are typically sorted based on the WHO
classification (2016) into glioma tumours and
meningiomas as the most frequent tumours, and
other less frequent tumours [1]. Tumour recurrence is usually inevitable in about 90% of patients,
and then, regardless of frontline treatment strategies, the prognosis is less than 6 months.

Metastatic brain tumours usually originate
from lung, breast and skin (melanoma) tumours,
respectively. The overall survival duration for
patients with glioblastoma multiforme (GBM)
usually ranges between 14.6 and 16.8 months,
with a 24-month overall survival rate of 27–30%
[2–4].

Although the prevalence rate of brain tumours
is slightly increased, the disease prognosis is still
impoverished, particularly for high-grade
tumours [3, 5].

The optimal treatment for brain tumours
includes surgical resection and chemoradiotherapy in the routine clinical setting. However,
patients show variable responses to the currently
available treatments and many new therapeutics
fail to show effective therapeutic response in the
clinical trial phase; thus, prognosis still remains
poor and an effective treatment is lacking. The
causes underlying the different treatment
responses include the development of compensa-
tory resistance/escape pathways, pharmacodynamic failure (no therapeutic effect despite
sufficient drug activity on the target), pharmacokinetic failure (inadequate dose delivery to the
tumour), the barricading function of the blood-
brain barrier (BBB) and most importantly, the
inter- and intra-tumoral heterogeneity that both
allow the tumour cells to resist an across-the-
board treatment strategy. In addition, the infiltrative property of the tumours leads to recurrence at
or adjacent to the primary site of the tumour following each surgery, so that complete resection
of the tumour is impossible [6]. Thus, an across-
the-board treatment is ineffective in treating these
complex and heterogeneous tumours of the brain.

M. Assadi · H. Shooli
The Persian Gulf Nuclear Medicine Research Center,
Department of Nuclear Medicine, Molecular
Imaging, and Theranostics, Bushehr Medical
University Hospital, School of Medicine, Bushehr
University of Medical Sciences, Bushehr, Iran
e-mail: asadi@bpums.ac.ir

R. Nemati
Faculty of Medicine, Department of Neurology,
Bushehr Medical University Hospital, Bushehr
University of Medical Sciences, Bushehr, Iran

H. Ahmadzadehfar (✉)
Department of Nuclear Medicine, Klinikum
Westfalen, Dortmund, Germany
e-mail: Hojjat.ahmadzadehfar@klinikum-westfalen.de

© The Author(s) 2024
V. Prasad (ed.), *Beyond Becquerel and Biology to Precision Radiomolecular Oncology: Festschrift
in Honor of Richard P. Baum*, https://doi.org/10.1007/978-3-031-33533-4_10

The prerequisites for dealing with these tumours involve providing a tailored treatment by delivering the right drug to the right patient based on individual molecular and genetic characteristics; precision medicine seems to be a key solution. Precision medicine can provide a tailored treatment in order to meet the unsatisfied essentials for the treatment of brain tumours. In the context of neuro-oncologic care, the precision medicine concept is epitomized by target-based therapeutic approaches such as peptide receptor radionuclide therapy (PRRT) and radioimmunotherapy (RIT).

In detail, RIT involves the administration of a coupling of a radionuclide payload and a monoclonal antibody (mAb) that targets the cell-surface tumour-related antigens or the antigens within the tumour microenvironment [7]. This chapter aims to discuss the biologic targets used in the PRRT and RIT approach in brain tumours treatment and to highlight recent progress in radionuclide-based pharmaceutics and clinical trials. Finally, we provide perspectives and directions on the future PRRT and RIT in neuro-oncology cancer care. The substantial characteristics of ideal therapeutic radiopharmaceutical and available radiotracer for brain tumour imaging are shown in Tables 10.1 and 10.2, respectively.

10.1.1 Radionuclides Used in the Therapy

The therapeutic effect of radionuclide therapy depends on two radiobiologic properties: range and energy. Each of these parameters has a fundamental role in the processes inducing cell death. Two types of radionuclides are usually utilized: beta (^{131}I, ^{90}Y, ^{177}Lu) and alpha emitters (^{225}Ac, ^{213}Bi). The general properties of radionuclides for cancer therapy and the parameters affecting the uptake of radiopharmaceuticals in glioma tumours are summarized in Tables 10.3 and 10.4, respectively.

Table 10.1 Characteristics of ideal therapeutic radiopharmaceutical [8]

High specificity and affinity for the tumour cells
In vivo stability in human blood (not catabolized/metabolized)
$T_{1/2B}$ comparable with $T_{1/2P}$ of the radionuclide
Rapid targeting of tumour cells
Significant radioconjugate retention by the tumour cells for a period two- to three times longer than the $T_{1/2P}$ of the radionuclide
Absence of radioconjugate catabolism by the tumour cells
Absence or minimal uptake and retention by normal tissues/cells
Rapid elimination from the systemic circulation
Pharmacokinetics not tainted by repeated injection
Effective cell killing (high ionization particles to DNA)
Radionuclide distribution within the tumour cell clusters less
Heterogenous than the range of emitted particles
Delivering a therapeutic dose to all of the tumour cells
Irradiation cause only the cell death (no other radiation-related biological changes, for example, mutations and transformations into radio-resistant tumours)

Table 10.2 Currently available radiotracers for brain tumour imaging [9]

Biological measures	Radiotracer
Glucose transport across BBB and metabolism	2-Deoxy-2-[^{18}F] fluoro-d-glucose ([^{18}F] FDG)
Amino acid transport and protein synthesis	[^{11}C] methionine ^{18}F-fluoroethyltyrosine (^{18}F-FET)
Amino acid transport and dopamine metabolism	^{18}F-fluoro-L-3,4-dihydroxyphenylalanine (^{18}F-DOPA)
DNA replication	^{18}F-fluorothymidine (^{18}F-FLT)
Lipid metabolism	[^{11}C] choline/^{18}F-fluorocholine
Hypoxia	^{18}F-fluoromisonidazole (^{18}F-MISO) ^{18}F-azomycin arabinoside (^{18}F-FAZA) ^{64}Cu-methylthiosemicarbazone (^{64}Cu-ATSM)

Table 10.3 General properties of radionuclides for cancer therapy [8]

Decay type	Particles	NOP[a]	Range	LET	$E_{min} - E_{max}$
β^--particle	Energetic electrons	1	0.05–12 mm	~0.2 keV/μm	50–2300 keV[b]
α^{++}-particle	He nuclei	1	40–100 μm	~80 keV/μm	5–9 MeV[c]
EC/IC	Nonenergetic electrons	3–50	2–500 nm	~4–26 keV/μm	eV–keV[c]

EC electron capture, *IC* internal conversion, E_{max} maximum electron energy, E_{min} minimum electron energy, *LET* linear energy transfer
[a] Number of particles emitted per decaying atom
[b] Average (>1% intensity); continuous distribution of energy
[c] Monoenergetic

Table 10.4 Factors affecting uptake of radiopharmaceuticals in gliomas [9]

Tumour neovascularization and blood-brain barrier integrity
Histopathological grade
Rate of glucose metabolic
Rate of DNA proliferation
Synthesis of rate protein
Rate of Membrane (phospholipid) proliferation rate
Presence of membrane transporters on the tumour cells
Oxygenation status of tissue (hypoxia)
size of the lesion (partial volume effect)
Necrotic regions
Radiotherapy treatment

10.1.1.1 Alpha-Emitter Radionuclide

Alpha-emitting radionuclides have valuable advantages for use in targeted therapy. Alpha particles have a short range of <100 μm and a high level of linear energy transfer (LET ≈ 100 keV/μm) in human tissue. These features enable this radionuclide to deliver a critical cytotoxic dose to the targeted tumour cells while minimizing damage to the adjacent healthy tissues. Furthermore, cell death induced by alpha radiation is predominantly related to DNA double-strand breaks occurring along the trajectory of the profoundly ionizing particle and is mainly independent of both the phase of cell cycle and cellular oxygenation status [10, 11].

Moreover, it has been documented that alpha radiation is able to break the tumour's resistance to chemotherapeutics and irradiation (beta and gamma radiation) [12]; thus, targeted alpha therapy can provide an alternative option for the treatment of patients whose disease is refractory to standard therapies. It needs to be emphasized that the effect of radiation is not dependent on O [6]-methylguanine-DNA methyltransferase (MGMT) promoter methylation status, the most important predictive for the efficacy of treatment with temozolomide. Moreover, alpha-emitter particles perform better than temozolomide in vitro in treating multiple GBM cell lines as well as GBM stem cells (GSCs) [13].

^{225}Ac is an alpha emitter with a half-life of 9.9 days. The main decay path of ^{225}Ac comprises four net alpha-emitter particles with a high cumulative energy of 28 MeV and two beta-emitters of 1.6 and 0.6 MeV maximum energy. Gamma emissions are also produced in the ^{225}Ac decay path, allowing for limited in vivo imaging. Its relatively long half-life of 9.9 days and its multi-alpha particles emission in a rapid decay chain have made ^{225}Ac a critical cytotoxic radionuclide.

^{213}Bi is a hybrid alpha/beta emitter with a half-life of 46 minutes. It predominantly decays by beta emission to the very short-lived absolute alpha emitter ^{213}Po ($T1/2 = 4.2$ μs, $E = 8.4$ MeV) with a disintegration ratio of 97.8%. The residual 2.2% of ^{213}Bi decays into ^{209}Tl by emitting an alpha particle ($E = 5.5$ MeV, 0.16%, $E = 5.9$ MeV, 2.01%). The alpha particle emitted by ^{213}Po has an energy of 8.4 MeV and a path length of 85 μm in body tissues [14]. A summary of a-emitter particles used in the treatment of brain tumours is listed in Table 10.5.

10.1.1.2 Beta-Emitter Radionuclide

Currently, radionuclide therapy in human cancer therapy is mainly based on energetic β-emitting particles. These β-particles are negatively charged electrons emitted from the nucleus during the

Table 10.5 Physical properties of α-particle emitters [8]

Radionuclide	Half-life	Particle(s) emitted	E_{av} (MeV)[a]	R_{av} (μm)[b]
^{211}At	7.2 h	1α	6.79	60
^{213}Bi	46 min	1α, 2β	8.32	84
^{225}Ac	10 days	4α, 2β	6.83	61

[a] Mean energy of α-particles emitted per disintegration [15]

[b] Mean range for α-particles measured by second-order polynomial regression fit (data from [16]): $R = 3.87E + 0.75\ E^2 - 0.45$, where R represents the range (μm) in unit density matter and E represents the α-particle energy (MeV)

Table 10.6 Physical characteristics of β-Particle emitters [8]

Radionuclide	Half-life	$E^{\beta-}$ (max) (keV)[a]	$R^{\beta-}$ (max) (mm)[b]
^{177}Lu	6.7 days	497	1.8
^{131}I	8.0 days	606	2.3
^{188}Re	17.0 h	2120	10.4
^{90}Y	64.1 h	2284	11.3

[a] Maximum of energy of β particles emitted per disintegration

[b] Range (μm) for electrons by $E = 0.02 - 100$ keV calculated by Cole's equation [18]: $R = 0.043\ (E + 0.367)^{1.77} - 0.007$, whereas range (mm) for electrons with E (MeV) calculated using second order fits (data from [19]): $R\ (0.1 - 0.5$ MeV$) = 2.4E + 2.86E^2 - 0.14$, and $R\ (0.5 - 2.5$ MeV$) = 5.3E + 0.0034E^2 - 0.93$

decaying process of radioactive atoms and have different energies and a spectrum of ranges. After emission, as these β-particles pave their path, they lose their kinetic energies and finally take a contorted path and then stop. The recoil energy of the daughter nucleus is negligible due to its small mass [8]. The β-particle emission decayed by the beta-emitters has a maximum kinetic energy of 0.3–2.3 MeV and a penetration range of ~0.5–12 mm in soft tissue [17].

The β-particles range/cell diameter ratio enables β-particles to traverse the cells (10–1000). An important implication of the long range of the emitted electron is the cross-the-fire effect, a condition in which the radiation beam can irradiate the cells near the targeted cell without direct binding to those cells. A summary of beta-emitter particles used in the treatment of brain tumours is presented in Table 10.6.

10.1.2 Routes of Drug Administration

10.1.2.1 Systemic Administration of Radioconjugates

Typically, the systemic administration of therapeutics to treat various solid neoplasms ensures the delivery of a therapeutic dose to the tumour tissue; however, brain tumours represent an exception. Systemic drug application to brain tumours is restricted by several limitations, of which the most substantial is the intact BBB which prevents the distribution of drugs within the brain tissue. Nonetheless, the systemic administration of radiolabelled monoclonal antibodies (mAbs) via RIT approach for the treatment of brain tumours is possible in principle.

For instance, Emrich et al. attained an encouraging response following the intravenous (iv) administration of ^{125}I-labeled EGFR-mAb 425 for the treatment of patients with high-grade glioma tumours [20]. Another study compared the uptake of radioconjugates in tumours and demonstrated that, following the iv injection of radioconjugates, the levels of ^{131}I-labeled 81C6 (tumour-specific mAbs) were five times greater than those of co-injected ^{125}I-labeled 45.6 (tumour non-specific mAbs). These results were post-therapeutically controlled by a histological examination of tissue biopsies. Furthermore, Zalutsky et al. concluded that the level of ^{131}I-labelled 81C6 was up to 200 times greater than that in normal brain tissue based on the biopsies [21]. Remarkably, they studied the tumour dose delivery of the mAbs to the glioma tumours after iv and intra-carotid administration of a radiolabelled-mAb. They found that there is no significant difference in drug delivery between iv and intra-carotid application of the radiolabelled-mAb, but that the intra-carotid injection may be associated with carotid cannulation-related complications.

10.1.2.2 Locoregional Application of Radioconjugates

The locoregional application of the therapeutic is defined as the direct injection of a radiolabelled-mAb either in the tumoral tissue, a tumour cyst or a surgically created resection cavity (SCRC). This method is the best of choice for drug delivery to brain tumours, mainly because it can circumvent the BBB, the most important physical barrier impeding drug penetration into the brain tissue. Other benefits of locoregional application include its capacity to deliver a high dose of radiation to the tumour while minimizing systemic toxicity and interference with potential human antibodies against mouse antigen (HAMA). Locoregional administration of the therapeutic is done either via convection-enhanced delivery (CED) or Ommaya reservoir [22].

The CED method involves the implantation of a catheter through which therapeutic products can be applied using constant, low, positive pressure bulk flow. Pre-clinical and clinical investigations have revealed that CED can provide effective therapeutic delivery to substantial volumes of the brain and brain tumour. However, catheter technology has several shortcomings that impede the technique from being reliable and reproducible as will be discussed below. Furthermore, the only completed phase III study of GBM did not demonstrate a survival advantage for patients treated with a trial therapeutic administered via CED. Although many ongoing efforts have been made to implement innovative catheter designs and imaging approaches, there is still a long way to go to introduce an effective locoregional drug delivery system [23].

10.2 Peptide Receptor Radionuclide Therapy

10.2.1 Biologic Targets for PRRT

10.2.1.1 Neurokinin Type 1 Receptor

Neurokinin type 1 (NK-1R) is one of three different types of mammalian tachykinin receptors that belong to the seven transmembrane G-protein-coupled receptor family. NK-1R applies its effect by activating phospholipase C, then producing inositol triphosphate [24]. The ligand for NK-1R is substance-P (SP) [25]. Furthermore, the over-expression of NK1-R in glioma tumours has provided a basis for NK-1R-targeted therapy for the treatment of brain tumours. So far, the administration of ^{225}Ac-DOTA-substance-P has shown promising results in pre-clinical studies [13]. Also, Królicki et al. reported promising results for using ^{213}Bi-DOTA-substance P in recurrent GBM [26].

10.2.1.2 Glioma Chloride Channels

A chloride ion channel was found to be ubiquitously expressed in glioma tumours while lacking in normal brain tissue [27]. Also, the expression level of glioma chloride channel (GCC) is related to the tumour grade, such that 90% or more of high-grade gliomas and all GBMs express GCC [27]. Therefore, GCC can be used either as a diagnostic biomarker or as a target for therapy. Chlorotoxin (CTX) is a 36-amino acid protein that is isolated from the venom of the giant yellow Israeli scorpion (*Leiurus quinquestriatus*); it effectively inhibits the molecular currents passing through the GCC with approximately 80% effectiveness [27].

TM-601 is an artificial form of CTX and is a lyophilized, sterile and pyrogen-free compound. ^{131}I-TM-601 comprises TM-601 as a targeting component coupled with ^{131}I as a radionuclide payload [28]. This radiolabelled therapeutic is approved for phase I of clinical trials and the results are promising to start phase II.

10.2.1.3 Somatostatin Receptor

The peptide somatostatin is excreted by the endocrine, neural and immune systems and is ubiquitously expressed by several tissues of the body. Its functions include neuroregulation (motor, sensory and cognition) and cellular growth blockage by paracrine and autocrine routes [29, 30]. Somatostatin function is induced through transmembrane G protein-coupled receptors; the molecule enters the cell after binding to the ligand [31]. To date, six subclasses of somatostatin receptors (SSTRs) have been found: SSTR 1, 2A, 2B, 3, 4 and 5.

Many brain tumours express different subclasses of SSTR on their cell surface; these include primary brain neoplasms such as glioma tumours, meningioma neoplasms, paediatric tumours of the brain (medulloblastomas), pituitary adenomas and supratentorial primitive neuroendocrine tumours (PNETs) [32–35]. Dutour et al. [36] revealed that glioma and meningioma tumours express at least one, and sometimes different multiple subclasses of SSTR. They provided the proofs on identifying SSTRs in tumours and the surrounding tissues, predominantly in the blood vessels related to tumour neovascularization.

So far, three ^{68}Ga-DOTA peptides have been produced for clinical imaging; these include ^{68}Ga-DOTA-TOC, ^{68}Ga-DOTA-NOC and ^{68}Ga-DOTA-TATE. The ability to bind to SSTR2 is the common characteristic of ^{68}Ga-DOTA peptides, but they differ in terms of their SSTR subtype affinity profile [37].

A summary of the ideal characteristics of the biologic target for targeted cancer therapy is listed in Table 10.7.

Table 10.7 Ideal target for target-based radionuclide therapy

Ubiquitous and homogeneous expression on the tumour cells
Absence or minimal expression on the normal cells
Intrinsic tumoricidal property
Ability to pass through the BBB
Sufficient and homogeneous distribution in the tumour tissue
High target affinity and Stable ligand binding in the low nanomolar range
Rapid elimination from systemic circulation
Absence or trivial side effect profile

10.2.2 Clinical Studies

As mentioned earlier, the treatment-challenging properties of high-grade brain tumours and the failure of an across-the-board treatment to improve overall survival (OS) indicate an urgent need to develop an effective therapeutic. In this regard, precision medicine can provide a tailored treatment based on the individual biologic targets expressed by the tumours. PRRT is an initiative approach to more accurately treat these tumours.

The first PRRT study was conducted by Merlo et al. [38]. They treated 11 patients (seven low-grade and four anaplastic glioma patients) by locoregional administration of ^{111}In-DOTA0D-Phe1Tyr3]-octreotide (^{111}In-DOTATOC) and ^{90}Y-labeled DOTATOC. In this proof-of-concept study, patients were treated with intra-tumoral injection of radioconjugate via a port-a-cath-like device. Furthermore, they showed a homogeneous distribution and stable peptide-to-receptor binding of ^{111}In-DOTATOC on the tumour cells surface. The administered dose was one-to-four fractions based on the tumour volume; 1110 MBq of ^{90}Y-labeled DOTATOC was the maximum dose per each injection. Six stable diseases and the shrinking of a cystic low-grade astrocytoma tumour were achieved. The toxicity profile included secondary perifocal oedema. The authors claimed that the activity/dose ratio (MBq/Gy) may serve as a potential prognostic factor for the clinical course of the disease.

Recently, we assessed the treatment efficacy of intravenous ^{177}Lu-DOTATATE in patients with high-grade astrocytoma; the results were promising (Fig. 10.1).

However, further well-designed studies to determine absorbed dose; more precise protocols based on tumour invasiveness, aggressiveness, malignant transformation and histological classification; as well as long-term outcome and the effect of this therapeutic on laboratory parameters are highly warranted. A list of selected clinical studies is presented in Table 10.8.

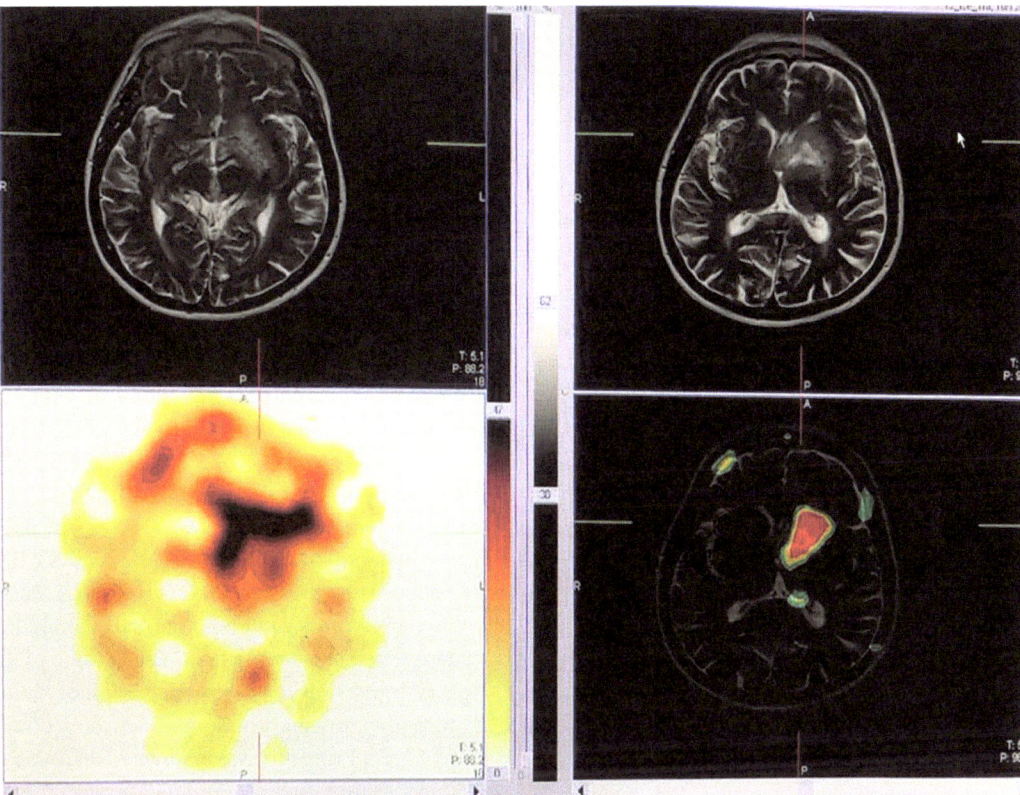

Fig. 10.1 Peptide receptor radionuclide therapy for 63-year-old women with glioblastoma multiforme in left striatum. There is remarkable uptake in the tumour on post-therapy images using 177Lu-DOTATATE (3.7 GBq). The patient had received three cycles of 177Lu-DOTATATE and achieved a stable course since starting therapy. This figure also depicts the ubiquitous and homogeneous distribution of the radioconjugate throughout the tumour tissue following iv injection

Table 10.8 Selected PRRT in the brain tumours

Drug	Phase	Target/vector	Results	Toxicity profile	Notes
PRRT in newly diagnosed disease					
^{90}Y-labeled DOTATOC [38]	Pilot study	Radiolabelled-peptide against SSTR administered locoregionally	Six disease stabilization Shrinkage of one low-grade astrocytoma	Only perifocal oedema	Sufficient drug distribution Stable peptide to ligand binding
^{90}Y-labeled DOTATOC [39]	Pilot study	Radiolabelled-peptide against SSTR administered locoregionally	13–45 months of steroid-free in progressive gliomas		
^{177}Lu-DOTATATE [40]	Pilot study	Radiolabelled-peptide against SSTR administered intravenously	One complete remission Three partial remission One stable disease	No major side effect was reported	They included 10 patients and 50% were responsive to treatment
^{90}Y-DOTATAGA-SP [25]		Radiolabelled-peptide against SSTR administered locoregionally	Disease stabilization and clinical status improvement were observed	Radionecrosis and transient treatment-associated brain oedema	This study provided the evidence for specificity of the drug for gliomas

(continued)

Table 10.8 (continued)

Drug	Phase	Target/vector	Results	Toxicity profile	Notes
PRRT in recurrent disease					
^{90}Y-labeled DOTATOC [41]	Pilot study	Radiolabelled-peptide against SSTR administered locoregionally by Rickham reservoir	One complete remission Two partial remission	Minor side effect reported	Three patients were included and all were responsive to treatment

10.3 Immune-Based Radionuclide Therapy

10.3.1 Biologic Targets for RIT

10.3.1.1 Tenascin-C

Tenascin-C (TN-C) is a hexa-brachion polymorphic glycoprotein of the extracellular matrix (ECM) expressed in both normal conditions and disorders. TN-C is expressed far and wide in pathologic conditions such as wound healing, inflammatory processes and tumorigenesis; it also has a short-term physiological expression during embryogenesis and organogenesis [42]. Regarding tumorigenesis, the key function of TN-C is to ease the migration of tumour cells from the ECM to other body parts [43]. Approximately 90% of glioma tumour cells show extensive expression of TN-C, particularly glioblastomas, contrary to normal cells which express it to a minor extent [42, 44, 45]. TN-C was shown to have immunoreactivity in the tumoral vessels and the tumour networks of high-grade astrocytoma tumours [46]. Furthermore, TN-C is expressed in the tumoral vessels in higher levels in high-grade compared to low-grade astrocytoma tumours [46]. TN-C expression is associated with proliferative rate, angiogenesis and progressive growing pattern [46]. Regarding the overexpression of TN-C in gliomas and its crucial role in tumour proliferation, migration, progression and angiogenesis, it seems that targeting TN-C can serve as a targeted therapy approach based on tumour biology in selected patients [46–48]. So far, several antibodies have been designed to target TN-C; these are classified as murine monoclonal antibodies (mmAbs) and chimeric antibodies (cAbs). mmAbs against TN-C include BC-2, BC-4, 81C6, ST2146, ST2485, F16 and P12; cAbs consist of ch81C6 [49–51]. These antibodies have been studied in the preclinical setting; if they show promise, they are eligible for translation into clinical trials [52, 53].

10.3.1.2 Epidermal Growth Factor Receptor

Epidermal growth factor receptor (EGFR) is a transmembrane protein that functions as a receptor for a protein ligand belonging to the epidermal growth factor family [54]. The binding of the ligand to the EGFR causes the phosphorylation of receptor tyrosine kinase and activates downstream signal transduction pathways involved in cellular proliferation rate regulation, differentiation and survival [54]. Moreover, EGFR overexpression is associated with some cancers such as brain neoplasms [55]. It has been detected in about 57% of GBM tumours [55]. EGFR has an important role in tumour cell proliferation and survival; therefore, EGFR blockage can interrupt intracellular signalling. Thus, it has gained meaningful attention as a biological target for RIT in brain tumours. Thus far, two types of therapeutics have been made to inhibit EGFR activity: mAbs that target EGFR and tyrosine kinase inhibitors (TKIs) that prohibit EGFR-related signalling pathways. These mAbs include nimotuzumab, cetuximab and monoclonal antibody-425, while the TKIs consist of erlotinib and gefitinib. Both of these drug types have been investigated in preclinical and clinical trials [56–65].

10.3.1.3 Neural Cell Adhesion Molecule

Neural cell adhesion molecule (NCAM) is a glycoprotein on the cell surface that has Ig-like and fibronectin type III (FnIII) domains in its structure and is classified in the immunoglobulin (Ig) superfamily. Within the central nervous system (CNS), these molecules contribute to cell group formation, NCAM-related neurite outgrowth and synaptic plasticity [66, 67]. Because NCAM has been found ubiquitously in some cancers such as brain neoplasms, NCAM-targeted therapy for these tumours has received significant attention. Several mAbs have been created against NCAM including ^{131}I-UJ13A, ^{131}I-ERIC-1 and ^{90}Y-ERIC1; they have been tested in pre-clinical and clinical studies of RIT for brain neoplasms [68–71].

10.3.1.4 Histone H1

Tumour necrosis therapy (TNT) is an innovative strategy in the targeted therapy of cancers; it uses mAbs or fragments of such to aim at an intracellular antigen of the necrotic debris of the tumour [72]. Tumours of the brain contain areas of necrosis in which the cells have higher cell membrane permeability; thus, several immunoglobulins are able to enter the cells [72]. Furthermore, histone H1 is a linker histone; it is found in the nucleus and is involved with nucleosomal arrays for increased compacting of the nucleosomes in order to form a higher-level chromatin structure [73]. There is a widespread expression of the molecule in the necrotic areas of brain tumours. Therefore, it can be targeted using a mAb equipped with a radionuclide payload [72]. ChTNT-1/B mAb is a genetically engineered chimeric mAb capable of specifically binding to the DNA-bound histone H1 in order to form an insoluble and non-diffusible anchor for the bounded mAb [72]. Recently, it has been attached to ^{131}I and has been applied in the treatment of GBM tumours [72, 74].

10.3.2 Future Novel Targets

10.3.2.1 Fibulin-3

Fibulin-3 is a glycoprotein of the extracellular matrix (ECM) typically detected in healthy connective tissues. The molecule is absent in normal brain tissue; however, it is expressed by GBM cells and is found in the ECM of tumour tissue [75–77]. Moreover, fibulin-3 can initiate Notch and NF-κB signalling pathways by autocrine and paracrine paths that have not been described in healthy tissues [75, 77, 78]. Fibulin-3 intensifies the capacity for invasion, neovascularization and survival in the tumour-initiating cell population of GBM; it is related with poor prognosis and represents a biomarker of active progression [79, 80]. Hence, the pivotal role of fibulin-3 in the biology of GBM and the significant tumour-to-background ratio potentially make it an appealing molecular target for cancer therapy. Nandhu et al. introduced a function-inhibitor antibody that targets fibulin-3, named mAb428.2, that was designed to treat GBM tumours in a mouse model [81]. They treated mice carrying xenograft subcutaneous or intracranial GBM by administration of mAb428.2 via either iv or intra-tumoral injection. The results show promise; mAb428.2 successfully bound to the target and inhibited the fibulin-3 from starting ADAM17, Notch and NF-κB signalling in the cells of GBM and finally reduced tumour growth, invasion and neovascularization, and improved the survival of the mice.

Another study reported that anti-fibulin-3-targeted therapy for GBM can strengthen anti-tumour inflammatory response [82]. Taking the available evidence together, fibulin-3 represents a promising biological target for the treatment of these tumours, particularly for RIT where it is joined with a radionuclide payload. Also, fibulin-3-based RIT may provide promising therapeutics due to a high tumour-to-background ratio that enables it to reach the tumour tissue while minimizing damage to the nearby non-tumoral tissues.

10.3.3 Clinical Studies

The clinical studies of the application of RIT in brain tumours are summarized in Tables 10.9 and 10.10.

Table 10.9 Selected therapeutic design for RIT in the brain tumours

Therapeutic design	Drug	Study data	Results	Notes
Newly diagnosed disease				
mAb	Nimotuzumab	Randomized phase III of chemoradiation+nimotuzumab versus chemoradiation alone [56]	mOS: 22.3 months vs.19.6 months PFS (12-month): 25.6% vs. 20.3%	In subset analyses of patients with EGFR amplification, PFS was 31.8% in experimental arm versus 23% in the chemoradiation arm ($P = 0.88$)
TKI	Erlotinib	Single-arm phase II combined with chemoradiation [57]	mOS: 15.3 months PFS (6-month): NA	NA
TKI		Single-arm phase II combined with chemoradiation [58]	mOS: 19.3 months PFS (6-month): 12%	EGFR overexpression did not affect outcomes
TKI	Gefitinib	Single-arm phase II combined with radiotherapy [59]	mOS: 11.5 months PFS (6-month): 40%	EGFR overexpression did not affect outcomes
		Single-arm phase II after radiotherapy [60]	mOS: 12 months PFS (12-month): 17%	*EGFR* overexpression and/or amplification and/or presence of EGFRvIII did not affect outcomes
Recurrent disease				
TKI	Erlotinib	Randomized phase II of erlotinib versus temozolomide or carmustine [83]	ORR: 3.7% vs. 9.6% mOS: 7.7 months vs. 7.3 months PFS (6-month): 11.4% vs. 24%	• Outcomes favoured patients in the control arm; EGFR amplification did not affect outcomes • EGFRvIII associated with poor survival outcomes
		Single arm phase II study of erlotinib [61]	ORR: 0% mOS: 6 months PFS (6-month): 3%	NA
		Single arm phase II study of erlotinib [62]	ORR: 6% mOS: 10 months PFS (6-month) PFS: 20%	EGFR (assessed by FISH or IHC), EGFRvIII and PTEN (both assessed by IHC) status did not affect outcomes
TKI	Gefitinib	Single-arm phase II study [61]	ORR: 5% mOS: 6 months PFS (6-month): 14%	EGFR amplification and/or overexpression did not affect outcomes
		Single-arm phase II study [64]	ORR: 0% mOS: 10 months PFS (6-month): 13%	EGFR amplification and/or mutation did not affect outcomes
mAb	Cetuximab	Stratified phase II with patients with EGFR amplification [65]	ORR: 7.1% mOS: 5 months PFS (6-month): 7%	EGFR amplification (without mutation) was associated with marginal improvement in PFS (3 months versus 1.6 month; $P = 0.006$) but not OS (5.6 months versus 4 months; $P = 0.12$) in subset analysis of patients from whom tissue was available (35 of 55)[131]
		Stratified phase II study with patients without EGFR amplification [65]	ORR: 5.5% mOS: 4.8 months PFS (6-month): 11%	

FISH fluorescent in situ hybridization, *IHC* immunohistochemistry, *mAb* monoclonal antibody, *NA* not available, *ORR* overall response rate, *OS* overall survival, *PFS* progression-free survival, *TKI* tyrosine kinase inhibitor

Table 10.10   Selected ADC therapy studies for high-grade gliomas

Drug	Phase	Target/vector	Results	Toxicity profile	Notes
Radioimmunotherapy in recurrent disease					
[188]Re-nimotuzumab [84]	I	Radiolabelled-ant EGFR antibody administered by Ommaya reservoir	ORR: NA mOS: 19 months 6-month PFS: NA	Liver-function test abnormalities, neurological deterioration, radionecrosis	MTD = 3 mg for 10 mCi [188]Re-labelled-antibody
[211]At-ch81C6 [85]	I	Radiolabelled-chimeric anti-tenascin antibody administered by Rickham reservoir	ORR: NA mOS: 14.3 months 6-month PFS: NA	Visual deficit, nausea, fatigue, infections, HAMA, seizures, headaches, aphasia, numbness	
^{131}I-BC2/BC-4 [53]	I/II	Radiolabelled-anti tenascin antibody	ORR: 22% mOS: 21 months 6-month PFS: NA	Headaches, HAMA	
Cotara(^{131}I-chTNT--1/B) [74]	II	Radiolabelled-anti histone-H1 antibody applied by CED	ORR: 18% mOS: 9.5 months 6-month PFS: NA	Memory impairment, reduced consciousness, fatigue, abdominal pain, catheter complications, headaches, hemiparesis, seizures, cerebral oedema, confusion, agitation	Efficacy data are available only for patients with recurrent disease receiving 1.25 mCi/cm^3 and 2.5 mCi/cm^3
Radioimmunotherapy in newly diagnosed disease					
[125]I-mAb 425 [86]	II	Intravenous delivery of radiolabelled mouse anti-EGFR antibody (with radiotherapy + temozolomide)	ORR: NA mOS: 20.4 months 6-month PFS: NA	Flushing, hypotension, occasional nausea, skin irritation, HAMA	Median OS was 10.2 months for a cohort of patients receiving radiotherapy alone
[131]I-81C6 [87]	Pilot study	Locoregional delivery of radiolabelled mouse anti-tenascin antibody (with radiotherapy + chemotherapy)	ORR: NA mOS: 22.6 months 6-month PFS: NA	Seizures, hematologic, neurological, infective, thrombotic complications	NA
^{131}I-BC2/BC4 [53]	I/II	Locoregional delivery of radiolabelled mouse anti-tenascin antibody (with conventional surgery and post-operative radiotherapy ± chemotherapy)	ORR: NA mOS: 19 months 6-month PFS: NA	Headaches, HAMA	• Data shown are only for patients with glioblastoma • mOS: 25 months for patients with small-volume (<2 cm^3) disease

CED convection-enhanced delivery, *HAMA* human anti-mouse antibody, *MTD* maximum tolerated dose, *NA* not available, *mOS* median of overall survival, *PFS* progression-free survival, *RCC* renal-cell carcinoma, *ORR* overall response rate

10.3.4 Challenges and Future Directions

10.3.4.1 Challenges

Brain tumours present as aggressive tumours with very poor prognosis despite optimal available treatment. Of those several reasons for therapeutic failure mentioned above, two represent the crucial parameters contributing to clinical trial failure; thus, should be considered as among important factors for treatment planning. The first is the physical barricading function of the BBB and the latter is inter- and intra-tumoral heterogeneity.

10.3.4.2 The Blood-Brain Barrier (BBB)

Given the biologic properties of the intact BBB, many drugs are prohibited from passing through it to reach the brain parenchyma; an interrupted BBB allows the selective passage of larger substances (antibodies or larger peptides). However, all the parts of brain tumours are not covered by the interrupted BBB and some parts are not accessible due to shielding behind an intact BBB.

The locoregional administration of therapeutics (chemotherapeutic or radiolabelled payloads) is designed to circumvent this obstacle in the treatment strategy. However, this method has faced some challenging issues including significant local toxicity profile, lack of anti-tumour efficacy (pharmacodynamic failure) and local complications such as radioconjugate leaking, local pain, local bleeding and local infection/inflammation.

Another approach is the application of drugs that are small enough to pass through the intact BBB. However, an effective drug of sufficiently small molecular size has yet to be developed.

Before the introduction of tumour-selective therapeutics, cancers were treated by nonspecific cytotoxic drugs that harm many parts in the body with early/late and transient/permanent complications. Given the low therapeutic effect, high cytotoxic profile of the drugs and their significant side effects, survival remained impoverished. Therefore, the precision medicine concept aimed to introduce targeted therapy to selectively target tumour cells while minimizing damage to other parts of the body. Notable progress has been made, but several challenges still remain.

10.3.4.3 Tumoral Heterogeneity

Another important factor in treatment failure is tumour heterogeneity. Tumour heterogeneity may be classified as inter- and intra-tumoral heterogeneity depending upon the different genetic characteristics and molecular profile not only between patients but also within each subject. It is well-known that high-grade brain tumours are composed of multiple tumour cell colonies with different genetic properties and molecular profiles. Interestingly, the precision medicine concept, which involves giving the right drug to the right patient, can provide a personalized solution to circumvent inter- and intra-tumoral heterogeneity.

There is an unmet need in regard to the lack of classification of patients in clinical trials based on the molecular and genetic profile of their tumours; the intertumoral heterogeneity in brain tumours usually results in an inhomogeneous patient group that shows variable therapeutic responses to the same treatment. Therefore, these heterogeneities necessitate the sorting of patients with high-grade tumours according to genetic characteristics, molecular profile and constitutional tumoral cell colonies. This approach can optimize the precision medicine concept to circumvent inter-tumoral heterogeneity by aiming to deliver the right drug to the right patients in order to provide the optimal therapeutic benefits (Fig. 10.2).

So far, few clinical trials have incorporated molecular and genetic properties into their study design and patients are simply divided into a new case group and a recurrent disease group. However, these patient groups are highly inhomogeneous due to vast tumoral heterogeneity and overly simple classification strategies. Moreover, an assessment of treatment efficacy in an inhomogeneous patient group will probably lead to inconclusive results and misinterpretation of the true therapeutic benefits, and may mask the responding patient population.

Regardless of the many possible reasons for the failure of a clinical trial, inhomogeneous

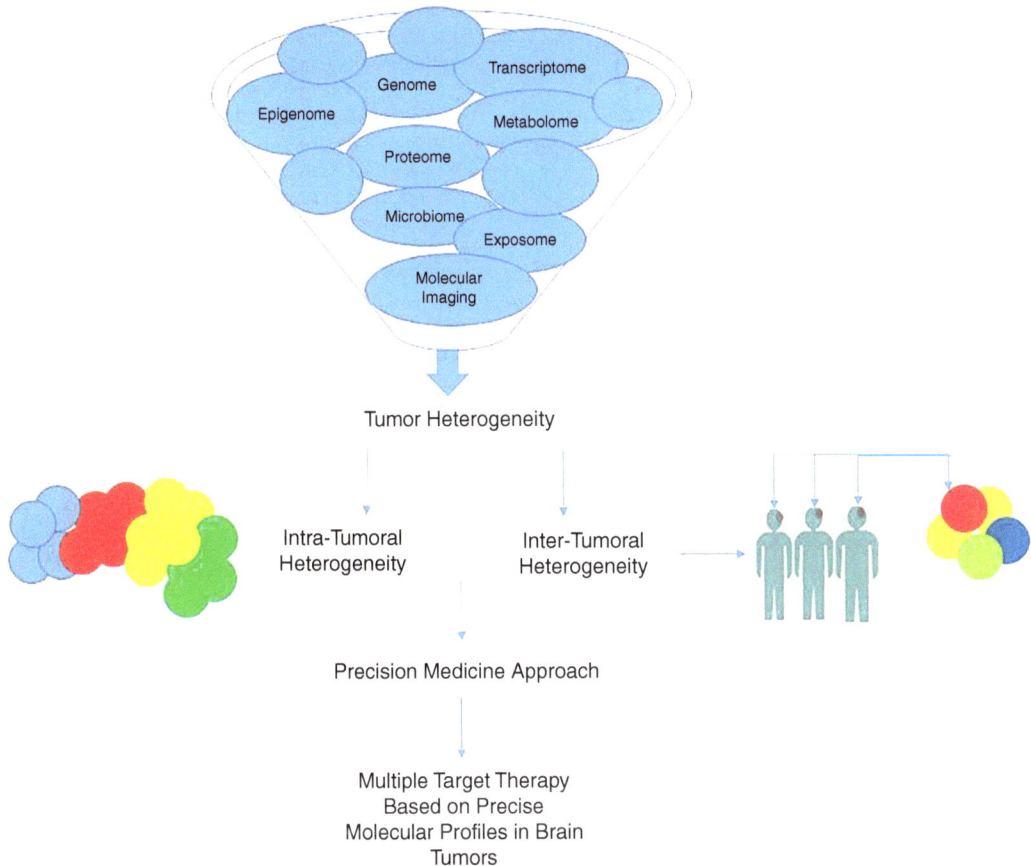

Fig. 10.2 Precision medicine approach in brain tumours

patient population and intertumoral heterogeneity are major issues that challenge the merits of an effective clinical trial and have yet to be addressed. This obstacle can be tackled by incorporating individual biologic data into patient classification, such as molecular profile, genetic characteristics and the immunologic properties of the tumour cell colonies.

Unfortunately, the molecular, genetic and immunologic characteristics of high-grade glioma tumours have not been fully discovered to date. Therefore, an alternative strategy is to identify and separate patients who respond to a given drug in a routine clinical trial, and to explore the biologic properties contributing to the therapeutic response. This alternative strategy can grant us a better insight into the biologic principles of tumorigenesis and help to identify biomarkers for patient classification and disease prognostication.

Following biology-based classification of the patients, another issue that needs to be addressed is that of intratumoral heterogeneity, which can be eluded by targeting multiple biologic targets in order to target all of the constitutional tumoral colonies. The best solution is the coupling of a radionuclide payload and an mAb with an intrinsic tumoricidal property that allows us to fight cancer cells more efficiently.

10.3.5 Conclusion

Early and effective intervention is mandatory in the early stages of high-grade gliomas due to the extensive and irreversible destruction of healthy neural tissues by the tumour. It is time to reconsider recommending an across-the board treatment without patient classification based on individual biologic profile. Biology-based patient classification and individual-based multiple-targeted therapy are essential prerequisites of a tailored personalized management that would pave the way toward an effective treatment for brain tumours.

References

1. Louis DN, Perry A, Reifenberger G, von Deimling A, Figarella-Branger D, Cavenee WK, et al. The 2016 World Health Organization classification of tumors of the central nervous system: a summary. Acta Neuropathol. 2016;131(6):803–20.
2. Stupp R, Mason WP, Van Den Bent MJ, Weller M, Fisher B, Taphoorn MJ, et al. Radiotherapy plus concomitant and adjuvant temozolomide for glioblastoma. N Engl J Med. 2005;352(10):987–96.
3. Stupp R, Hegi ME, Mason WP, Van Den Bent MJ, Taphoorn MJ, Janzer RC, et al. Effects of radiotherapy with concomitant and adjuvant temozolomide versus radiotherapy alone on survival in glioblastoma in a randomised phase III study: 5-year analysis of the EORTC-NCIC trial. Lancet Oncol. 2009;10(5):459–66.
4. Chinot OL, Wick W, Mason W, Henriksson R, Saran F, Nishikawa R, et al. Bevacizumab plus radiotherapy–temozolomide for newly diagnosed glioblastoma. N Engl J Med. 2014;370(8):709–22.
5. Stummer W, Pichlmeier U, Meinel T, Wiestler OD, Zanella F, Reulen HJ. Fluorescence-guided surgery with 5-aminolevulinic acid for resection of malignant glioma: a randomised controlled multicentre phase III trial. Lancet Oncol. 2006;7(5):392–401.
6. Gaspar LE, Fisher BJ, Macdonald DR, Leber DV, Halperin EC, Schold SC Jr, et al. Supratentorial malignant glioma: patterns of recurrence and implications for external beam local treatment. Int J Rad Oncol. 1992;24(1):55–7.
7. Pouget J-P, Navarro-Teulon I, Bardiès M, Chouin N, Cartron G, Pèlegrin A, et al. Clinical radioimmunotherapy—the role of radiobiology. Nat Rev Clin Oncol. 2011;8(12):720.
8. Kassis AI. Radiotargeting agents for cancer therapy. Expert Opin Drug Deliv. 2005;2(6):981–91.
9. Volterrani D, Erba PA, Carrió I, Strauss HW, Mariani G. Nuclear medicine textbook: methodology and clinical applications. Cham: Springer; 2019.
10. Wulbrand C, Seidl C, Gaertner FC, Bruchertseifer F, Morgenstern A, Essler M, et al. Alpha-particle emitting 213Bi-anti-EGFR immunoconjugates eradicate tumor cells independent of oxygenation. PLoS One. 2013;8(5):64730.
11. Barendsen G, Koot C, Van Kersen G, Bewley D, Field S, Parnell C. The effect of oxygen on impairment of the proliferative capacity of human cells in culture by ionizing radiations of different LET. Int J Radiat Biol Relat Stud Phys Chem Med. 1966;10(4):317–27.
12. Friesen C, Glatting G, Koop B, Schwarz K, Morgenstern A, Apostolidis C, et al. Breaking chemoresistance and radioresistance with [213Bi] anti-CD45 antibodies in leukemia cells. Cancer Res. 2007;67(5):1950–8.
13. Majkowska-Pilip A, Rius M, Bruchertseifer F, Apostolidis C, Weis M, Bonelli M, et al. In vitro evaluation of 225Ac-DOTA-substance P for targeted alpha therapy of glioblastoma multiforme. Chem Biol Drug Des. 2018;92(1):1344–56.
14. Sgouros G, Roeske JC, McDevitt MR, Palm S, Allen BJ, Fisher DR, et al. MIRD Pamphlet No. 22 (abridged): radiobiology and dosimetry of alpha-particle emitters for targeted radionuclide therapy. J Nucl Med. 2010;51(2):311–28.
15. Jain RK. Physiological barriers to delivery of monoclonal antibodies and other macromolecules in tumors. Cancer Res. 1990;50(3):814–9.
16. Netti PA, Hamberg LM, Babich JW, Kierstead D, Graham W, Hunter GJ, et al. Enhancement of fluid filtration across tumor vessels: implication for delivery of macromolecules. Proc Natl Acad Sci. 1999;96(6):3137–42.
17. Knapp FF, Dash A. Radiopharmaceuticals for therapy. Cham: Springer; 2016.
18. Wright H, Hamm R, Turner J, Howell R, Rao D, Sastry K. Calculations of physical and chemical reactions with DNA in aqueous solution from Auger cascades. Oak Ridge: Oak Ridge National Lab; 1989.
19. Esteban JM, Schlom J, Mornex F, Colcher D. Radioimmunotherapy of athymic mice bearing human colon carcinomas with monoclonal antibody B72.3: histological and autoradiographic study of effects on tumors and normal organs. Eur J Cancer Clin Oncol. 1987;23(6):643–55.
20. Emrich JG, Brady LW, Quang TS, Class R, Miyamoto C, Black P, et al. Radioiodinated (I-125) monoclonal antibody 425 in the treatment of high grade glioma patients: ten-year synopsis of a novel treatment. Am J Clin Oncol. 2002;25(6):541–6.
21. Zalutsky MR, Moseley RP, Coakham HB, Coleman RE, Bigner DD. Pharmacokinetics and tumor localization of 131I-labeled anti-tenascin monoclonal antibody 81C6 in patients with gliomas and other intracranial malignancies. Cancer Res. 1989;49(10):2807–13.
22. Gholamrezanezhad A, Shooli H, Jokar N, Nemati R, Assadi M. Radioimmunotherapy (RIT) in brain tumors. Nucl Med Mol Imaging. 2019;2019:1–8.
23. Vogelbaum MA, Aghi MK. Convection-enhanced delivery for the treatment of glioblastoma. Neuro-Oncology. 2015;17(2):ii3–8.
24. Maggi CA. The mammalian tachykinin receptors. Gen Pharmacol Vasc S. 1995;26(5):911–44.

25. Kneifel S, Cordier D, Good S, Ionescu MC, Ghaffari A, Hofer S, et al. Local targeting of malignant gliomas by the diffusible peptidic vector 1,4,7,10-tetraaz acyclododecane-1-glutaric acid-4,7,10-triacetic acid-substance p. Clin Cancer Res. 2006;12(12):3843–50.

26. Królicki L, Bruchertseifer F, Kunikowska J, Koziara H, Królicki B, Jakuciński M, et al. Safety and efficacy of targeted alpha therapy with 213 Bi-DOTA-substance P in recurrent glioblastoma. Eur J Nucl Med Mol Imaging. 2019;46(3):614–22.

27. Ullrich N, Gillespie GY, Sontheimer H. Human astrocytoma cells express a unique chloride current. Neuroreport. 1996;7(5):1020–4.

28. Mamelak AN, Rosenfeld S, Bucholz R, Raubitschek A, Nabors LB, Fiveash JB, et al. Phase I single-dose study of intracavitary-administered iodine-131-TM-601 in adults with recurrent high-grade glioma. J Clin Oncol. 2006;24(22):3644–50.

29. Reichlin S. Somatostatin. N Engl J Med. 1983;309(24):1495–501.

30. Patel YC. Molecular pharmacology of somatostatin receptor subtypes. J Endocrinol Investig. 1997;20(6):348–67.

31. Cescato R, Schulz S, Waser B, Eltschinger V, Rivier JE, Wester HJ, et al. Internalization of sst2, sst3, and sst5 receptors: effects of somatostatin agonists and antagonists. J Nucl Med. 2006;47(3):502–11.

32. Ramirez C, Cheng S, Vargas G, Asa SL, Ezzat S, Gonzalez B, et al. Expression of Ki-67, PTTG1, FGFR4, and SSTR 2, 3, and 5 in nonfunctioning pituitary adenomas: a high throughput TMA, immunohistochemical study. J Clin Endocrinol Metab. 2012;97(5):1745–51.

33. Fruhwald MC, O'Dorisio MS, Pietsch T, Reubi JC. High expression of somatostatin receptor subtype 2 (sst2) in medulloblastoma: implications for diagnosis and therapy. Pediatr Res. 1999;45(5):697–708.

34. Fruhwald MC, Rickert CH, O'Dorisio MS, Madsen M, Warmuth-Metz M, Khanna G, et al. Somatostatin receptor subtype 2 is expressed by supratentorial primitive neuroectodermal tumors of childhood and can be targeted for somatostatin receptor imaging. Clin Cancer Res. 2004;10(9):2997–3006.

35. Sharma P, Mukherjee A, Bal C, Malhotra A, Kumar R. Somatostatin receptor-based PET/CT of intracranial tumors: a potential area of application for 68 Ga-DOTA peptides? AJR Am J Roentgenol. 2013;201(6):1340–7.

36. Dutour A, Kumar U, Panetta R, Ouafik L, Fina F, Sasi R, et al. Expression of somatostatin receptor subtypes in human brain tumors. Int J Cancer. 1998;76(5):620–7.

37. Shooli H, Dadgar H, Wang YJ, Vafaee MS, Kashuk SR, Nemati R, et al. An update on PET-based molecular imaging in neuro-oncology: challenges and implementation for a precision medicine approach in cancer care. Quant Imaging Med Surg. 2019;9(9):1597–610.

38. Merlo A, Hausmann O, Wasner M, Steiner P, Otte A, Jermann E, et al. Locoregional regulatory peptide receptor targeting with the diffusible somatostatin analogue 90Y-labeled DOTA0-D-Phe1-Tyr3-octreotide (DOTATOC): a pilot study in human gliomas. Clin Cancer Res. 1999;5(5):1025–33.

39. Schumacher T, Hofer S, Eichhorn K, Wasner M, Zimmerer S, Freitag P, et al. Local injection of the 90Y-labelled peptidic vector DOTATOC to control gliomas of WHO grades II and III: an extended pilot study. Eur J Nucl Med Mol Imaging. 2002;29(4):486–93.

40. Assadi M, Nemati R, Shooli H, Rekabpour J, Amini A, Ravanbod M, et al., editors. Peptide receptor radionuclide therapy for high-grade glioma brain tumors: variable clinical response in a pilot study. Barcelona: EANM; 2019.

41. Heute D, Kostron H, von Guggenberg E, Ingorokva S, Gabriel M, Dobrozemsky G, et al. Response of recurrent high-grade glioma to treatment with (90) Y-DOTATOC. J Nucl Med. 2010;51(3):397–400.

42. Herold-Mende C, Mueller MM, Bonsanto MM, Schmitt HP, Kunze S, Steiner HH. Clinical impact and functional aspects of tenascin-C expression during glioma progression. Int J Cancer. 2002;98(3):362–9.

43. Martin D, Brown-Luedi M, Chiquet-Ehrismann R. Tenascin-C signaling through induction of 14-3-3 tau. J Cell Biol. 2003;160(2):171–5.

44. Leins A, Riva P, Lindstedt R, Davidoff MS, Mehraein P, Weis S. Expression of tenascin-C in various human brain tumors and its relevance for survival in patients with astrocytoma. Cancer. 2003;98(11):2430–9.

45. Ventimiglia JB, Wikstrand CJ, Ostrowski LE, Bourdon MA, Lightner VA, Bigner DD. Tenascin expression in human glioma cell lines and normal tissues. J Neuroimmunol. 1992;36(1):41–55.

46. Kim CH, Bak KH, Kim YS, Kim JM, Ko Y, Oh SJ, et al. Expression of tenascin-C in astrocytic tumors: its relevance to proliferation and angiogenesis. Surg Neurol. 2000;54(3):235–40.

47. Brack SS, Silacci M, Birchler M, Neri D. Tumor-targeting properties of novel antibodies specific to the large isoform of tenascin-C. Clin Cancer Res. 2006;12(10):3200–8.

48. De Santis R, Albertoni C, Petronzelli F, Campo S, D'Alessio V, Rosi A, et al. Low and high tenascin-expressing tumors are efficiently targeted by ST2146 monoclonal antibody. Clin Cancer Res. 2006;12(7):2191–6.

49. Reardon DA, Akabani G, Edward Coleman R, Friedman AH, Friedman HS, Herndon JE, et al. Phase II trial of murine 131I-labeled antitenascin monoclonal antibody 81C6 administered into surgically created resection cavities of patients with newly diagnosed malignant gliomas. J Clin Oncol. 2002;20(5):1389–97.

50. Reardon DA, Zalutsky MR, Bigner DD. Antitenascin-C monoclonal antibody radioimmunotherapy for malignant glioma patients. Expert Rev Anticancer Ther. 2007;7(5):675–87.

51. Riva P, Franceschi G, Riva N, Casi M, Santimaria M, Adamo M. Role of nuclear medicine in the treatment

of malignant gliomas: the locoregional radioimmunotherapy approach. Eur J Nucl Med. 2000;27(5):601–9.

52. Riva P, Franceschi G, Frattarelli M, Lazzari S, Riva N, Giuliani G, et al. Loco-regional radioimmunotherapy of high-grade malignant gliomas using specific monoclonal antibodies labeled with 90Y: a phase I study. Clin Cancer Res. 1999;5(10):3275–80.

53. Riva P, Franceschi G, Frattarelli M, Riva N, Guiducci G, Cremonini AM, et al. 131I radioconjugated antibodies for the locoregional radioimmunotherapy of high-grade malignant glioma: phase I and II study. Acta Oncol. 1999;38(3):351–9.

54. Herbst RS. Review of epidermal growth factor receptor biology. Int J Rad Oncol. 2004;59(2):21–6.

55. Brennan CW, Verhaak RG, McKenna A, Campos B, Noushmehr H, Salama SR, et al. The somatic genomic landscape of glioblastoma. Cell. 2014;157(3):753.

56. Westphal M, Heese O, Steinbach JP, Schnell O, Schackert G, Mehdorn M, et al. A randomised, open label phase III trial with nimotuzumab, an anti-epidermal growth factor receptor monoclonal antibody in the treatment of newly diagnosed adult glioblastoma. Eur J Cancer. 2015;51(4):522–32.

57. Brown PD, Krishnan S, Sarkaria JN, Wu W, Jaeckle KA, Uhm JH, et al. Phase I/II trial of erlotinib and temozolomide with radiation therapy in the treatment of newly diagnosed glioblastoma multiforme: North Central Cancer Treatment Group Study N0177. J Clin Oncol. 2008;26(34):5603–9.

58. Prados MD, Chang SM, Butowski N, DeBoer R, Parvataneni R, Carliner H, et al. Phase II study of erlotinib plus temozolomide during and after radiation therapy in patients with newly diagnosed glioblastoma multiforme or gliosarcoma. J Clin Oncol. 2009;27(4):579–84.

59. Chakravarti A, Wang M, Robins HI, Lautenschlaeger T, Curran WJ, Brachman DG, et al. RTOG 0211: a phase 1/2 study of radiation therapy with concurrent gefitinib for newly diagnosed glioblastoma patients. Int J Radiat Oncol Biol Phys. 2013;85(5):1206–11.

60. Uhm JH, Ballman KV, Wu W, Giannini C, Krauss J, Buckner JC, et al. Phase II evaluation of gefitinib in patients with newly diagnosed grade 4 astrocytoma: Mayo/North Central Cancer Treatment Group Study N0074. Int J Rad Oncol. 2011;80(2):347–53.

61. Raizer JJ, Abrey LE, Lassman AB, Chang SM, Lamborn KR, Kuhn JG, et al. A phase II trial of erlotinib in patients with recurrent malignant gliomas and nonprogressive glioblastoma multiforme postradiation therapy. Neuro-Oncology. 2010;12(1):95–103.

62. Yung W, Vredenburgh J, Cloughesy T, Nghiemphu P, Klencke B, Gilbert M, et al. Safety and efficacy of erlotinib in first-relapse glioblastoma: a phase II open-label study. Neuro-Oncology. 2010;12:1061–70.

63. Franceschi E, Cavallo G, Lonardi S, Magrini E, Tosoni A, Grosso D, et al. Gefitinib in patients with progressive high-grade gliomas: a multicentre phase II study by Gruppo Italiano Cooperativo di Neuro-Oncologia (GICNO). Br J Cancer. 2007;96(7):1047–51.

64. Rich JN, Reardon DA, Peery T, Dowell JM, Quinn JA, Penne KL, et al. Phase II trial of gefitinib in recurrent glioblastoma. J Clin Oncol. 2004;22(1):133–42.

65. Neyns B, Sadones J, Joosens E, Bouttens F, Verbeke L, Baurain J-F, et al. Stratified phase II trial of cetuximab in patients with recurrent high-grade glioma. Ann Oncol. 2009;20(9):1596–603.

66. Leshchyns'ka I, Sytnyk V, Morrow JS, Schachner M. Neural cell adhesion molecule (NCAM) association with PKCβ2 via βI spectrin is implicated in NCAM-mediated neurite outgrowth. J Cell Biol. 2003;161(3):625–39.

67. Sytnyk V, Leshchyns'ka I, Schachner M. Neural cell adhesion molecules of the immunoglobulin superfamily regulate synapse formation, maintenance, and function. Trends Neurosci. 2017;40(5):295–308.

68. Hopkins K, Chandler C, Bullimore J, Sandeman D, Coakham H, Kemshead J. A pilot study of the treatment of patients with recurrent malignant gliomas with intratumoral yttrium-90 radioimmunoconjugates. Radiother Oncol. 1995;34(2):121–31.

69. Papanastassiou V, Pizer B, Coakham H, Bullimore J, Zananiri T, Kemshead J. Treatment of recurrent and cystic malignant gliomas by a single intracavity injection of 131I monoclonal antibody: feasibility, pharmacokinetics and dosimetry. Br J Cancer. 1993;67(1):144.

70. Jones D, Lashford L, Dicks-Mireaux C, Kemshead J. Comparison of pharmacokinetics of radiolabeled monoclonal antibody UJ13A in patients and animal models. NCI Monogr. 1987;3:125–30.

71. Path F, Kemshead JT, Path F. Direct injection of 90Y MoAbs into glioma tumor resection cavities leads to limited diffusion of the radioimmunoconjugates into normal brain parenchyma: a model to estimate absorbed radiation dose. Int J Rad Oncol. 1998;40(4):835–44.

72. Shapiro WR, Carpenter SP, Roberts K, Shan JS. 131I-chTNT-1/B mAb: tumour necrosis therapy for malignant astrocytic glioma. Expert Opin Biol Ther. 2006;6(5):539–45.

73. Shahbazian MD, Grunstein M. Functions of site-specific histone acetylation and deacetylation. Annu Rev Biochem. 2007;76:75–100.

74. Patel SJ, Shapiro WR, Laske DW, Jensen RL, Asher AL, Wessels BW, et al. Safety and feasibility of convection-enhanced delivery of Cotara for the treatment of malignant glioma: initial experience in 51 patients. Neurosurgery. 2005;56(6):1243–52; discussion 52-3.

75. Kobayashi N, Kostka G, Garbe JH, Keene DR, Bachinger HP, Hanisch FG, et al. A comparative analysis of the fibulin protein family. Biochemical characterization, binding interactions, and tissue localization. J Biol Chem. 2007;282(16):11805–16.

76. Giltay R, Timpl R, Kostka G. Sequence, recombinant expression and tissue localization of two novel extracellular matrix proteins, fibulin-3 and fibulin-4. Matrix Biol. 1999;18(5):469–80.

77. Hu B, Thirtamara-Rajamani KK, Sim H, Viapiano MS. Fibulin-3 is uniquely upregulated in malignant gliomas and promotes tumor cell motility and invasion. Mol Cancer Res. 2009;7(11):1756–70.

78. Hiddingh L, Tannous BA, Teng J, Tops B, Jeuken J, Hulleman E, et al. EFEMP1 induces γ-secretase/Notch-mediated temozolomide resistance in glioblastoma. Oncotarget. 2014;5(2):363.

79. Nandhu MS, Kwiatkowska A, Bhaskaran V, Hayes J, Hu B, Viapiano MS. Tumor-derived fibulin-3 activates pro-invasive NF-κB signaling in glioblastoma cells and their microenvironment. Oncogene. 2017;36(34):4875–86.

80. Nandhu MS, Hu B, Cole SE, Erdreich-Epstein A, Rodriguez-Gil DJ, Viapiano MS. Novel paracrine modulation of Notch–DLL4 signaling by fibulin-3 promotes angiogenesis in high-grade gliomas. Cancer Res. 2014;74(19):5435–48.

81. Nandhu MS, Behera P, Bhaskaran V, Longo SL, Barrera-Arenas LM, Sengupta S, et al. Development of a function-blocking antibody against fibulin-3 as a targeted reagent for glioblastoma. Clin Cancer Res. 2018;24(4):821–33.

82. Longo SL, Behera P, Viapiano MS, Nandhu MS. Inhibition of fibulin-3 reverses macrophage polarization in glioblastoma and increases antitumor inflammatory responses. Cancer Res. 2018;78(13):1706.

83. van den Bent MJ, Brandes AA, Rampling R, Kouwenhoven MC, Kros JM, Carpentier AF, et al. Randomized phase II trial of erlotinib versus temozolomide or carmustine in recurrent glioblastoma: EORTC brain tumor group study 26034. J Clin Oncol. 2009;27(8):1268–74.

84. Casaco A, Lopez G, Garcia I, Rodriguez JA, Fernandez R, Figueredo J, et al. Phase I single-dose study of intracavitary-administered Nimotuzumab labeled with 188 Re in adult recurrent high-grade glioma. Cancer Biol Ther. 2008;7(3):333–9.

85. Zalutsky MR, Reardon DA, Akabani G, Coleman RE, Friedman AH, Friedman HS, et al. Clinical experience with α-particle–emitting 211At: treatment of recurrent brain tumor patients with 211At-labeled chimeric antitenascin monoclonal antibody 81C6. J Nucl Med. 2008;49(1):30–8.

86. Li L, Quang TS, Gracely EJ, Kim JH, Emrich JG, Yaeger TE, et al. A phase II study of anti-epidermal growth factor receptor radioimmunotherapy in the treatment of glioblastoma multiforme. J Neurosurg. 2010;113(2):192–8.

87. Reardon DA, Zalutsky MR, Akabani G, Coleman RE, Friedman AH, Herndon JE, et al. A pilot study: 131I-antitenascin monoclonal antibody 81c6 to deliver a 44-Gy resection cavity boost. Neuro-Oncology. 2008;10(2):182–9.

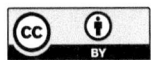

Modern Diagnostic and Therapeutic Approaches in Thyroid Diseases: Theranostics and the Changing Role of Radioactive Isotopes

11

Frank Grünwald, Amir Sabet,
Christina L. Q. Nguyen Ngoc, W. Tilman Kranert,
and Daniel C. L. Gröner

It is a great honor and a great pleasure to contribute to a Festschrift for Professor Richard Baum, a very good friend, a brilliant scientist, and one of the leading clinically active physicians in the field of coupling diagnostic and therapeutic approaches using radioactive isotopes—the so-called "theranostics".

Outside nuclear medicine, theranostic represents the tight connection of diagnostic procedures and therapeutic regimens, resulting in personalized medicine. Diagnostic tools on a molecular level are gaining more and more importance with the upcoming development of highly specific drugs such as kinase inhibitors and immunotherapeutic substances. Due to dramatic progresses in radiochemistry and radiopharmacy, molecular imaging with radioactive isotopes coupled with specific treatment options becomes a central issue with respect to the meaning of radioactive isotopes in modern medicine, focused on multimodal treatment regimens. It is not so easy to give an exact definition for the use of isotopes in theranostics: it is related to a substance, that "finds its way" to target tissue (by specific molecular mechanisms) which might be—benign or malignant—the pathologic tissue, e.g., a neuroendocrine tumor, or a (healthy) target for pathological processes like the thyroid gland in Graves' disease for autoantibodies.

Radioactive iodine was the first isotope in history engaged in a theranostic approach, initially used to treat thyroid diseases. The first radioiodine treatments were done in the early 1940s and published in 1946 [1]. The first therapy in Europe was performed by Cuno Winkler in 1948 [2]. Based on the high effectivity of the sodium iodine transporter, highly specific uptake and striking effects could be achieved with radioiodine therapy. I-131 was discovered by Glenn Seaborg and John Livingood at the University of California. Initially, I-128 was used in animal studies, it was substituted by I-130 and finally I-131 with respect to superior physical and logistic characteristics. Iodine-123 for scintigraphic and SPECT imaging and I-124 for PET imaging followed. Like in all other theranostic applications, radioactive iodine isotopes can be used to perform dosimetry with respect to target organs as well as to critical organs to minimize side effects.

It took several decades and overwhelming successes in radiochemistry to copy the observed convincing effects of radioiodine treatment in the

F. Grünwald (✉) · A. Sabet · C. L. Q. Nguyen Ngoc
W. T. Kranert · D. C. L. Gröner
Department of Nuclear Medicine, Hospital of the Johann Wolfgang Goethe University Frankfurt/Main, Frankfurt/Main, Germany
e-mail: gruenwald@em.uni-frankfurt.de

V. Prasad (ed.), *Beyond Becquerel and Biology to Precision Radiomolecular Oncology: Festschrift in Honor of Richard P. Baum*, https://doi.org/10.1007/978-3-031-33533-4_11

therapy of other diseases, particularly in cancer. The classic theranostic feature of I-131 with beta- and gamma-radiation can still be addressed as a blueprint for modern treatment regimens with radioactive isotopes. Nevertheless, compared to the time before 2000, the "classic" indications for radioiodine treatments are decreasing worldwide. Several reasons for this issue have to be discussed:

Mazzaferri and his group [3, 4] proved dramatic advantages of therapy regimens to treat differentiated thyroid cancer including radioiodine therapy not only in metastatic disease to destroy

radioiodine-positive metastases (Fig. 11.1), but also to ablate remnant tissue in cases without visible remnant or metastatic malignant tissue. Outcome of patients treated with radioiodine improved markedly [3, 4] with respect to progression-free survival as well as overall survival. The reasons for the superiority of remnant ablation are obvious: besides the possible destruction of intrathyroidal micrometastases in tissue remnants, the conditions for an optimal follow-up are based on the absence of scintigraphically detectable (also benign) thyroid tissue and negative serum thyroglobulin as the most important tumor

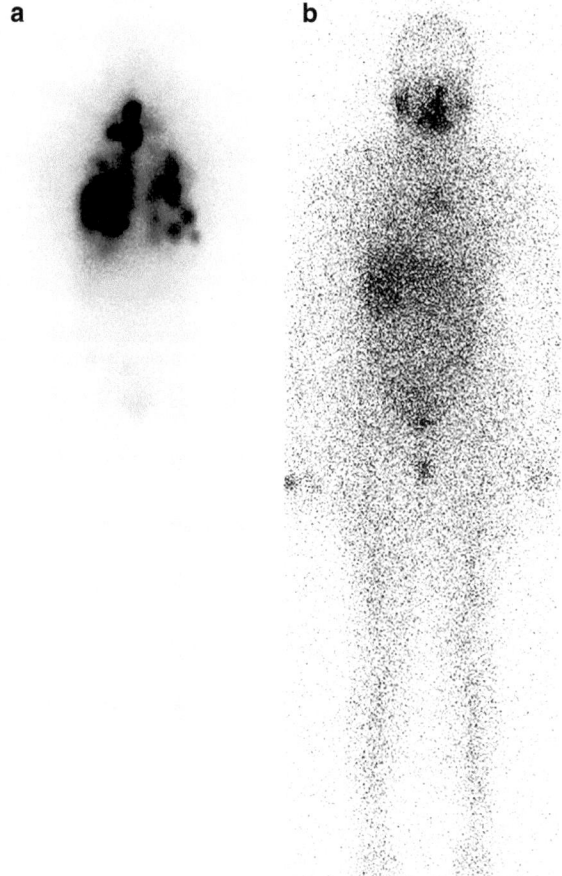

Fig. 11.1 59-year-old female patient after thyroidectomy and central lymph node dissection because of papillary thyroid cancer (pT2m, pN1a (9/42)). (**a**) Whole-body scan after first radioiodine application: multiple radioiodine-positive lung metastases (thyroglobulin: 113 ng/mL). (**b**) Whole-body scan after second radioiodine application, showing the treatment success of the first radioiodine

therapy: only faint residual thoracic radioiodine uptake (thyroglobulin: 0.1 ng/mL). (**c**) CT scan before radioiodine treatment: multiple small lung metastases. (**d**) CT scan 6 months after high dose radioiodine treatment: remission of the lung metastases. (**e**) CT scan 1 year after high dose radioiodine treatment: further regression of the lung metastases

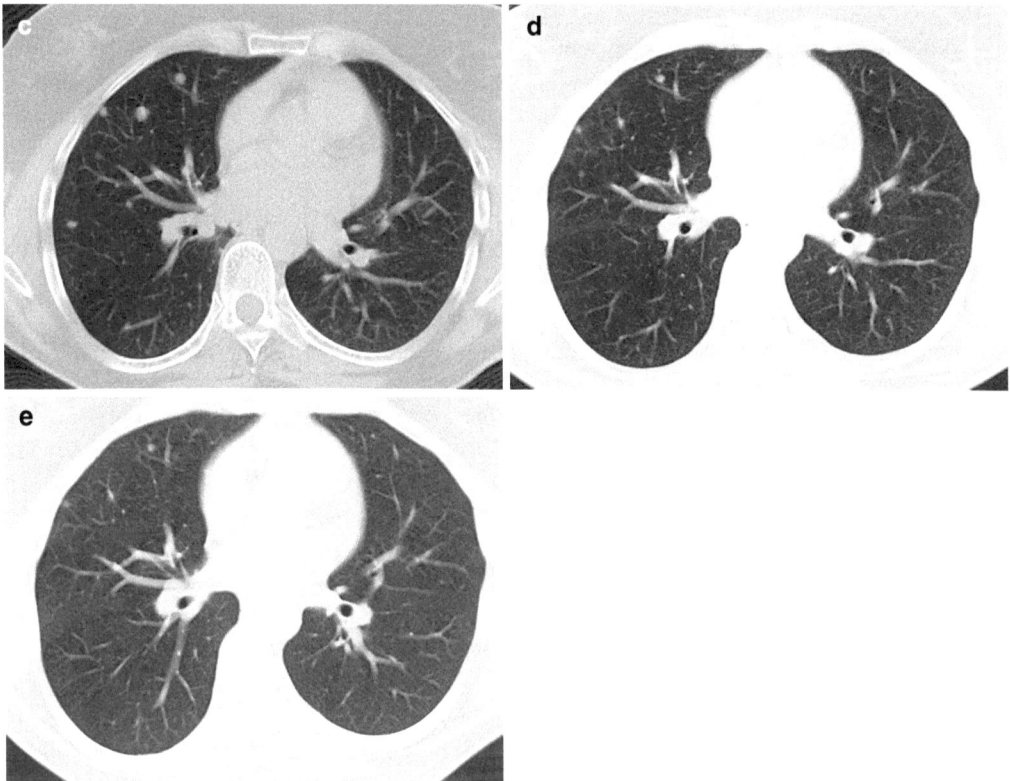

Fig. 11.1 (continued)

marker in differentiated thyroid cancer. Nevertheless, in some guidelines, written during the last years, e.g., published by the American Thyroid Association (ATA) [5] recently, besides restrictions concerning scintigraphy (recommended only, if TSH is suppressed) radioiodine treatment is considered less important and recommended only in higher tumor stages of differentiated thyroid cancer. Moreover, in papillary microcarcinoma, active surveillance is discussed instead of surgery (and ablation radioiodine therapy) [6, 7].

The reasons for these recommendations remain somewhat unclear. Partly, they are based on a number of publications dealing with possible secondary malignancy after radioiodine therapy in thyroid cancer, e.g., by Iyer et al. and other groups [8–11]. Several drawbacks of these papers make it difficult to follow the arguments against the use of treatment regimens, proven to be effective for several decades. Especially the effect of intensified surveillance (subsequently to radioiodine therapy) and resulting changes in early diagnosis in various cancers (addressed as secondary malignancies) were not taken into account. Moreover, cancers diagnosed as early as 6 months after radioiodine application were counted as secondary malignomas, contradicting radiation biology experiences, that it takes several years or even decades to develop stochastic radiation burdens, as described in these papers. In addition, a dose-effect relationship which should be expected in diseases, caused by a distinct factor, was not observed in most of these studies. A well-written paper dealing with some weak arguments concerning secondary malignancies (referring to a paper published by Molenaar et al. [12]) was published by Tulchinsky et al. [13]. A partial harmonization of ATA guidelines with especially European understandings [14] of optimal treatment regimens could be achieved in the "Martinique process" [15] by specialists from several continents. A second reason for the decreasing number of radioiodine treatment in thyroid cancer worldwide might be the emerging importance of screening programs, including thyroid ultrasound [16]. On one hand, subsequently, thyroid cancers are detected at lower tumor stages with less nodal or distant metastatic involvement [17] and therefore decreased need for ablative radioiodine therapy (besides changes in the guidelines recommendations). On the other hand, higher detection rates could cause more radioiodine treatments (only those cases, in which the tumor would otherwise not be clinically obvious during lifetime). Surgical techniques have been improved, causing lower volumes of remnant tissue after thyroidectomy, resulting in lower numbers of radioiodine treatment cycles and lower amounts of radioiodine needed for complete remnant tissue ablation. Radioiodine uptake and thyroglobulin-guided radioiodine ablation was proven to be superior to fixed doses with respect to efficacy as well as side effects [18]. Risk-adapted treatment schedules are important also in metastatic disease with respect to the known outcome difference between synchronous and metachronous manifestation of distant metastases [19]. Whereas initial data did not show inferiority of low-dose (1.1 GB) radioiodine ablation in low-risk patients [20], in subsequently published papers it was proven that low-risk patients as well as high-risk patients benefit from higher activities [21]. Using I-124, Jentzen et al. [22] reported high success rates in dosimetry-guided therapeutic regimens.

Also in benign thyroid diseases, especially in Plummer's disease, we observe a decreasing number of radioiodine treatments (and also amounts of radioiodine needed), due to earlier detection of subclinical hyperthyreosis by screening programs and TSH measurements in standard clinical work-up. In addition, in former iodine deficiency areas, prevalence of functional autonomy is decreasing with the improvement of nutritional iodine supply [23, 24].

In diagnostic approaches, the use of radioisotopes decreases with respect to thyroid diseases as well since several guidelines recommend scintigraphy only in case of TSH suppression (see above). It is difficult to follow this argumentation since papers dealing with the prevalence of functional autonomy prove the necessity of scintigraphy also in cases with known thyroid nodules and normal TSH, because autonomic foci can be detected in many patients suffering from nodular goiter and presenting with normal TSH [25, 26]. Not only the need for treating functional autonomy, e.g., by radioiodine, can be derived from scan results, but also, with respect to deciding on the malignancy risk of suspicious nodules, it is important to avoid biopsy of hot nodules since these often show up as follicular neoplasia, which in general has to be addressed as an indication for surgery with histological work-up of the lesion, if the nodule is cold but is misleading in case of hot nodules. Other techniques, like elastography or power Doppler, might give some additional information on the tissue characteristics of thyroid nodules but are not able to replace scintigraphy [27, 28]. In addition, the thyroid scan is important to differentiate between thyroiditis with thyroid hormone releasing from destructed follicles and Graves' disease with hyperthyreosis [29].

New fields for the use of radioactive isotopes in malignant thyroid diseases were established within the last two decades and particularly the last few years—especially with respect to interdisciplinary settings. The loss of radioiodine uptake, due to the loss of sodium iodine symporter (or its embedding in the cell membrane) markedly decreases prognosis [30]. In addition to morphological imaging with ultrasound, CT, and MRI, various functional imaging techniques were established to detect malignant tissue within the thyroid gland as well as radioiodine-negative tumor sites after thyroidectomy and ablative therapy.

Besides "functional scintigraphy" with Tc-99 m-pertechnetate or I-123, "metabolic imaging "with Tc-99 m-Hexakis-(2-methoxy-2-methylpropylisonitrile) (MIBI), and—if available—FDG-PET scan have proven to contribute significantly to the characterization of suspicious thyroid nodules [31, 32]. The very high negative predictive value of MIBI scintigraphy (>90%) has brought this technique to clinical routine in the work-up of thyroid nodules. FDG-

PET has its major role in the detection of radioiodine-negative lesions in differentiated thyroid cancer [33, 34] and medullary thyroid cancer [35] and is superior to morphological imaging with CT and MRI. MIBI scintigraphy can be useful during follow-up and recurrence detection when FDG-PET/CT is not available [36, 37]. Radioiodine refractory condition is—according to paper published by Cabanillas et al. [38]—defined as

– Lack of radioiodine uptake on posttherapy scan (>1.1 GB).
– Lack of radioiodine uptake on whole body scan in known structural disease.
– Lack of demonstratable ability of the tumor to concentrate sufficient radioiodine for a tumoricidal effect (<80 Gy in metastatic foci),
– Structural progression 6–12 months after radioiodine therapy.
– Rising Tg levels 6–12 months after radioiodine therapy.
– Continued progression despite cumulative activities of >20 GBq.

In these situations, other treatment options have to be discussed. Conventional chemotherapy (e.g., with doxorubicin or cisplatin) did not show positive effects in most cases and was used in some patients suffering from anaplastic or poorly differentiated thyroid carcinomas [39]. Recently, particularly multikinase inhibitors emerged as promising treatment options. They showed positive effects as to tumor shrinkage and progression-free survival [38]. Sorafenib was approved on the basis of the DECISION trial, which showed a prolonged progression-free survival from 5.8 to 10.8 months [40] with no significant effect on the overall survival. Lenvatinib was approved by the FDA on the basis of the SELECT trial [41]. Progression-free survival was 18.3 months in the verum group and 3.6 months in the placebo group [41]. The response rate was as high as 65%, including 4 complete remissions. Therefore, lenvatinib seems to be the most promising kinase inhibitor (without considering possible effects on radioiodine uptake of other drugs) hitherto.

Former approaches to reinduce radioiodine uptake and therefore engage the radioisotope theranostic principle were done with retinoic acid [42, 43] and rosiglitazine [44]. In about 30% of all cases, radioiodine uptake in initially radioiodine-negative tumor lesions could be achieved by retinoic acid. Nevertheless, there are only few cases with reported clinical success for this kind of redifferentiation therapy.

According to a number of recently published results, molecular profiling could be extremely helpful in radioiodine refractory cancer [45–51] with respect to evaluating individual outcome prognosis as well as choosing optimal targeted therapy [52]. Immune checkpoint inhibitors proved to be effective in various cancer types and can be expected to be helpful also in some patients suffering from thyroid cancer. A new approach was the use of selumetinib [53]. It was effective to increase radioiodine uptake and shrink tumor mass, especially in RAS-mutated tumors. In 12 out of 20 patients, radioiodine uptake was increased significantly, causing partial remission in 5 cases [53]. Recently, dabrafenib was shown to be able to reinduce striking radioiodine uptake in BRAF-positive cases [54]. All these data are leading back to the above-mentioned personalized treatment (also called theranostic), coupled with genetic tumor characterization. Larger series are necessary to evaluate the success rate, the intensity of iodine uptake, and the therapeutical effects of dabrafenib in initially radioiodine-refractory cancer.

In general, increasing importance of mutation analyses can be expected in the near future, e.g., for larotrectinib, a highly selective inhibitor of the three tropomyosin receptor kinase proteins TRKA, TRKB, and TRKC. Larotrectinib is a tissue unspecific kinase inhibitor ("tissue agnostic") and is approved for all cancer types with NTRK fusion. Only around 1% of all malignant tumors are NTRK-positive, but (besides salivary gland cancer and sarcomas) papillary thyroid cancers have the highest likelihood to be NTRK-positive. Only a few cases were reported [55], but this substance might become more important in the therapy of radioiodine-negative/refractory papillary thyroid cancer in the future.

Since all these drugs have remarkable side effects (hypertension, diarrhea, fatigue, weight loss, hand-foot skin reaction), which are in part severe and can be life-threatening, their toxicity has to be kept in mind when weighing advantages against disadvantages of starting kinase inhibitor treatments. Especially in slow-growing thyroid cancers, it is really difficult to find the right time point to start with the treatment when symptoms become more evident and/or progression of the disease accelerates. According to the ATA guidelines, multi-kinase inhibitors should be engaged in case of a diameter increase of more than 20% within 6 months [5]. Other groups [56] recommended to start with kinase inhibitors, when the tumor diameter is >1 cm and progression occurred within less than 12 to 14 months.

But also "classic" isotope theranostics (besides iodine isotopes) which were developed for other cancer types, e.g., somatostatin receptor positive neuroendocrine tumors, proved to be helpful in some cases of differentiated thyroid cancer (Fig. 11.2). Somatostatin receptor overexpression has been demonstrated in normal thyroid as well as thyroid cancer cells [57–62]. A series of 16 patients had been treated with PRRT by the group of Richard Baum. Stable disease was observed in 36%, and partial response in 18% [63]. Since PSMA-positivity could be demonstrated not only in prostate cancer but also in several other tumor types, PSMA-specific ligands were used for diagnosis and therapy in various cancers. PSMA ligand uptake was also seen in differentiated thyroid cancer (by incident as well as in specific work-up of cases with suspected recurrence [64, 65]) and Lu-177 ligands have been used to treat radioiodine-refractory differentiated thyroid cancer [66].

Fibroblast activation protein inhibitor (FAPI) is overexpressed in cancer-associated fibroblasts in many tumors and Ga-68-PET/CT was proven to be a suitable diagnostic tool in various cancers, including differentiated thyroid cancer [67]. Perhaps FAPI can be used as a theranostic substance in the future—labeling with Actinum-225 and Yttrium-90 has been described [68, 69]. Nevertheless, Ga-68-FAPI uptake in poorly differentiated thyroid cancer was rather low [70].

C-X-C chemokine receptor type 4 (CXCR-4)-mediated uptake of radioactive ligands has been used for diagnostic (with Ga-68-Pentixafor) [71] as well as therapeutic (with Lu-177-Pentixather) [72–74] approaches. The chemokine receptor CXCR-4 is overexpressed in various tumors (including solid tumor tissue such as breast cancer, pancreatic adenocarcinoma, hepatocellular carcinoma, lung and colorectal cancer) and is linked to tumor invasiveness and resulting poorer outcome [71]. In addition, CXCR-4 is positive in inflammatory diseases [74]. A meta-analysis, dealing with CXCR-4 expression in thyroid tissue, showed a distinct overexpression in papillary cancer (OR 67!) and a weak overexpression also in thyroiditis (OR 1.7) [75]. Therefore, due to very high overexpression in papillary cancer, this theranostic substance might be a promising solution for iodine refractory cases in the future.

Also in benign thyroid diseases new fields for the use of radioisotopes can be defined: Around 15 years ago, thermal ablation procedures were introduced successfully to clinical routine in the treatment of thyroid nodules [76–79]. Initially addressed as an alternative to radioiodine treatment and therefore a competing technique, it could be proven that it is possible to combine both techniques for optimal treatment of nodular goiter, especially with hot and cold nodules present in one thyroid gland [80]. In Graves' disease, total thyroid ablation (TTA) was proven to be superior to surgery alone with respect to improvement of endocrine orbitopathy. In patients treated by TTA, endocrine orbitopathy could be reduced significantly [81].

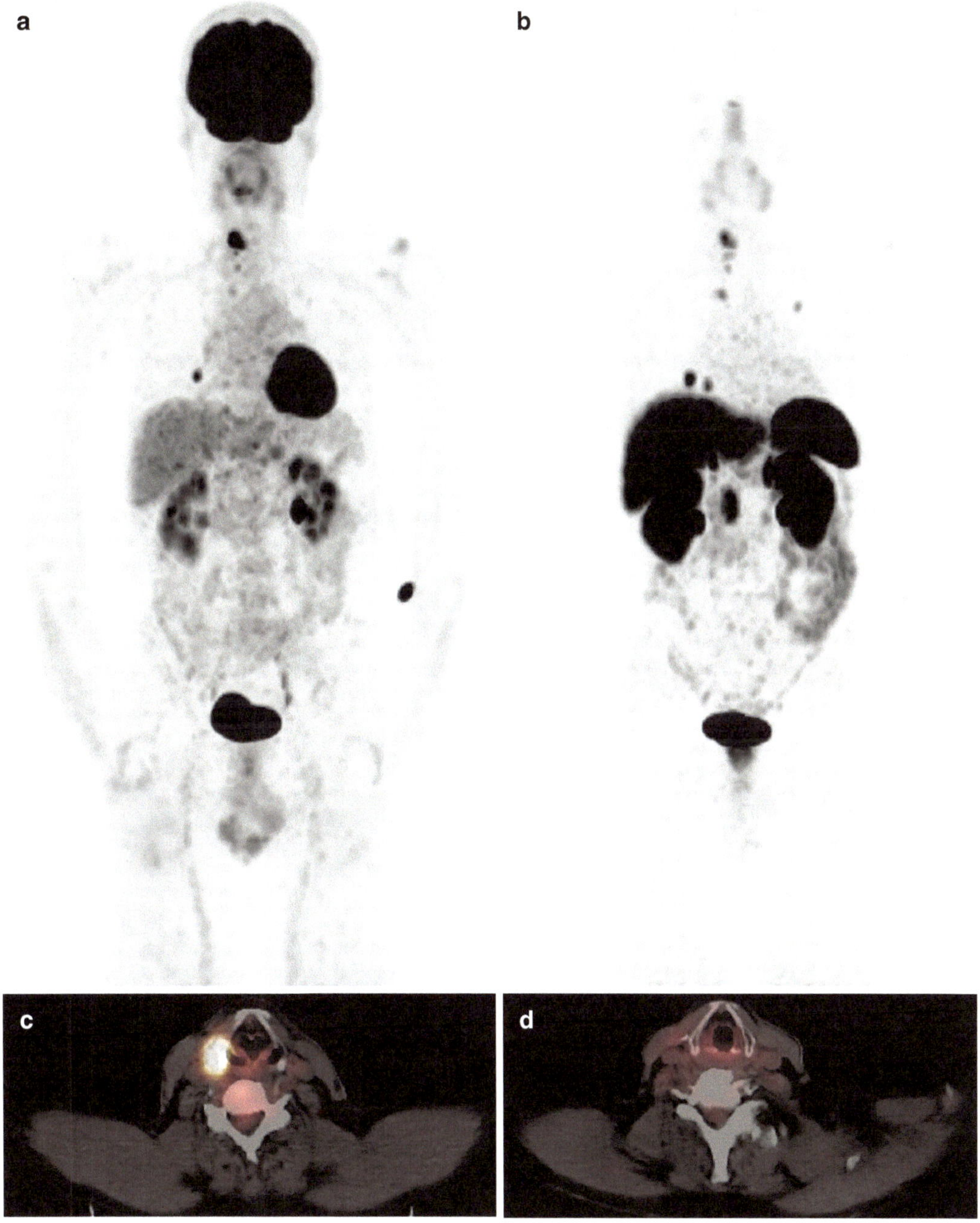

Fig. 11.2 60-year-old male patient after thyroidectomy, several subsequent operations, several radioiodine treatments (including one therapy after retinoic acid pretreatment) because of follicular Hürthle cell carcinoma (pT3m cN1) without significant radioiodine uptake. (**a**) FDG-PET/CT (MIP) showing local recurrence and lung metastases. (**b**) Ga-68-DOTATATE-PET/CT (MIP) showing somatostatin receptor positivity in tumor lesions. (**c**) FDG-PET/CT (transversal slice) before treatment with Lu-177-DOTATATE showing high glucose metabolism in local recurrence (including lymph nodes). (**d**) FDG-PET/CT (transversal slice) after treatment with Lu-177-DOTATATE showing therapeutic success (decreased glucose metabolism)

11.1   Conclusion

Thyroid scintigraphy has to face competition with several other diagnostic procedures, but it has still an undoubtable major role in the functional characterization of thyroid nodules. Although treatment of other diseases, particularly systemic malignant diseases, is more vigorously attracting the nuclear medicine scientific community, the use of radioisotopes in thyroid diseases offers important fields for new developments and optimization besides the classic and well-established techniques of thyroid theranostic, radioiodine, which is the historical origin of all theranostic principles, based on molecular mechanisms in the thyroid gland.

References

 1. Hertz S, Roberts A. Radioactive iodine in the study of thyroid physiology; the use of radioactive iodine therapy in hyperthyroidism. JAMA. 1946;131:81–6.
 2. Biersack HJ, Grünwald F. Thyroid cancer. Berlin, Heidelberg: Springer-Verlag; 2005.
 3. Mazzaferri EL, Jhiang SM. Long-term impact of initial surgery and medical therapy on papillary and follicular thyroid cancer. Am J Med. 1994;97:418–28.
 4. Mazzaferri EL. Radioiodine and other treatments and outcomes. In: Braverman LE, Utiger RD, editors. The thyroid. Philadelphia: Lippincott-Raven. p. 922–45.
 5. Haugen BR, Alexander EK, Bible KC, Doherty GM, Mandel SJ, Nikiforov YE, et al. 2015 American thyroid association management guidelines for adult patients with thyroid nodules and differentiated thyroid cancer. Thyroid. 2016;26:1–133.
 6. Leboulleux S, Tuttle RM, Pacini F, et al. Papillary thyroid microcarcinoma: time to shift from surgery to active surveillance? Lancet Diabetes Endocrinol. 2016;4:933–42.
 7. Griffin A, Brito JP, Bahl M, Hoang JK. Applying criteria of active surveillance to low-risk papillary thyroid cancer over a decade: how many surgeries and complications can be avoided? Thyroid. 2017;27:518–23.
 8. Iyer NG, Morris LG, Tuttle RM, Shaha AR, Ganly I. Rising incidence of second cancers in patients with low-risk (T1N0) thyroid cancer who receive radioactive iodine therapy. Cancer. 2011;117:4439–46.
 9. Marti JL, Jain KS, Morris LGT. Increased risk of secondary malignancy in pediatric and young adult patients treated with radioactive iodine for differentiated thyroid cancer. Thyroid. 2015;25:681–7.
10. Lang BH, Wong IO, Wong KP, Cowling BJ, Wan KY. Risk of second primary malignancy in differentiated thyroid carcinoma treated with radioactive iodine therapy. Surgery. 2012;151:844–50.
11. Silva-Vieira M, Carrilho Vaz S, Esteves S, Ferreira TC, Limbert E, Salgado L, Leite V. Second primary cancer in patients with differentiated thyroid cancer: does radioiodine play a role? Thyroid. 2017;27:1068–76.
12. Molenaar RJ, Sidana S, Radivoyevitch T, Advani AS, Gerds AT, Carraway HE, Angelini D, Kalaycio M, Nazha A, Adelstein DJ, Nasr C, Maciejewski JP, Majhail NS, Sekeres MA, Mukherjee S. 10a Risk of hematologic malignancies after radioiodine treatment of well-differentiated thyroid cancer. J Clin Oncol. 2018;36:1831–9.
13. Tulchinsky M, Binse I, Campennì A, Dizdarevic S, Giovanella L, Jong I, Kairemo K, Kim CK. Radioactive iodine therapy for differentiated thyroid cancer: lessons from confronting controversial literature on risks for secondary malignancy. J Nucl Med. 2018;59:723–5.
14. Luster M, Aktolun C, Amendoeira I, Barczynski M, Bible KC, Duntas LH, et al. European perspective on 2015 American Thyroid Association management guidelines for adult patients with thyroid nodules and differentiated thyroid cancer: preceedings of an Interactive International Symposium. Thyroid. 2019;29:7–26.
15. Tuttle RM, Ahuja S, Avram AM, Bernet VJ, Bourguet P, Daniels GH, et al. Controversies, consensus, and collaboration in the use of ^{131}I therapy in differentiated thyroid cancer: a joint statement from the American Thyroid Association, the European Association of Nuclear Medicine, the Society of Nuclear Medicine and Molecular Imaging, and the European thyroid association. Thyroid. 2019;29:461–70.
16. Ahn HS, Welch HG. South Korea's thyroid-cancer "Epidemic"—Turning the Tide. N Engl J Med. 2015;373:2389–90.
17. Farahati J, Mäder U, Gilman E, Görges R, Maric I, Binse I, Hänscheid H, Herrmann K, Buck A, Bockisch A. Changing trends of incidence and prognosis of thyroid carcinoma. Nuklearmedizin. 2019;58:86–92.
18. Jin Y, Ruan M, Cheng L, Fu H, Liu M, Sheng S, Chen L. Radioiodine uptake and thyroglobulin-guided radioiodine remnant ablation in patients with differentiated thyroid cancer: a prospective, randomized, open-label, controlled trial. Thyroid. 2019;29:101–10.
19. Sabet A, Binse I, Dogan S, Koch A, Rosenbaum-Krumme SJ, Biersack HJ, Biermann K, Ezziddin S. Distinguishing synchronous from metachronous manifestation of distant metastases: a prognostic feature in differentiated thyroid carcinoma. Eur J Nucl Med Mol Imaging. 2017;44:190–5.
20. Schlumberger M, Catargi B, Borget I, Deandreis D, Zerdoud S, Bridji B, Bardet S, Leenhardt L, Bastie D, Schvartz C, Vera P, Morel O, Benisvy D, Bournaud C, Bonichon F, Dejax C, Toubert ME, Leboulleux S, Ricard M, Benhamou E, Tumeurs de la Thyroïde Refractaires Network for the Essai Stimulation Ablation Equivalence Trial. Strategies of radioiodine ablation in patients with low-risk thyroid cancer. N Engl J Med. 2012;366:1663–73.
21. Verburg FA, Mäder U, Reiners C, Hänscheid H. Long-term survival in differentiated thyroid cancer is worse

after low-activity initial post-surgical 131I therapy in both high- and low-risk patients. J Clin Endocrinol Metab. 2014;99:4487–96.

22. Jentzen W, Hoppenbrouwers J, van Leeuwen P, van der Velden D, van de Kolk R, Poeppel TD, Nagarajah J, Brandau W, Bockisch A, Rosenbaum-Krumme S. Assessment of lesion response in the initial radioiodine treatment of differentiated thyroid cancer using 124I PET imaging. J Nucl Med. 2014;55:1759–65.

23. Happel C, Kranert WT, Bockisch B, Korkusuz H, Grünwald F. I-131and Tc-99m-Uptake in focal thyroid autonomies. Development in Germany since the 1980s. Nuklearmedizin. 2016;55:236–41.

24. Manz F, Böhmer T, Gärtner R, Grossklaus R, Klett M, Schneider R. Quantification of iodine supply: representative data on intake and urinary excretion of iodine from the German population in 1996. Ann Nutr Metab. 2002;46:128–38.

25. Graf D, Helmich-Kapp B, Graf S, Veit F, Lehmann N, Mann K. Functional activity of autonomous adenoma in Germany. Dtsch Med Wochenschr. 2012;137:2089–92.

26. Görges R, Kandror T, Kuschnerus S, Zimny M, Pink R, Palmedo H, et al. Scintigraphically "hot" thyroid nodules mainly go hand in hand with a normal TSH. Nuklearmedizin. 2011;50:179–88.

27. Happel C, Truong PN, Bockisch B, Zaplatnikov K, Kranert WT, Korkusuz H, Ackermann H, Grünwald F. Colour-coded duplex-sonography versus scintigraphy. Can scintigraphy be replaced by sonography for diagnosis of functional thyroid autonomy? Nuklearmedizin. 2013;52:186–91.

28. Etzel M, Happel C, von Müller F, Ackermann H, Bojunga J, Grünwald F. Palpation and elastography of thyroid nodules in comparison. Nuklearmedizin. 2013;52:97–100.

29. Dietlein M, Dressler J, Eschner W, Leisner B, Reiners C, Schicha H. Procedure guideline for thyroid scintigraphy (version 3). Deutsche Gesellschaft für Nuklearmedizin; Deutsche Gesellschaft für Medizinische Physik. Nuklearmedizin. 2007;46:203–5.

30. Spitzweg C, Bible KC, Hofbauer LC, et al. Advanced radioiodine-refractory differentiated thyroid cancer: the sodium iodide symporter and other emerging therapeutic targets. Lancet Diabetes Endocrinol. 2014;2:830–42.

31. Schmidt M, Schenke S. Update 2019 for MIBI scintigraphy in cold thyroid nodules. Der Nuklearmediziner. 2019;07:174–82.

32. Schenke S, Zimny M, Rink T, et al. Tc-99m-MIBI scintigraphy of hypofunctional thyroid nodules. Comparison of planar and SPECT imaging. Nucl Med. 2014;53:105–10.

33. Grünwald F, Kälicke T, Feine U, Lietzenmayer R, Scheidhauer K, Dietlein M, et al. Fluorine-18 fluorodeoxyglucose positron emission tomography in thyroid cancer: results of a multicentre study. Eur J Nucl Med. 1999;26:1547–52.

34. Feine U, Lietzenmayer R, Hanke JP, Held J, Wöhrle H, Müller-Schauenburg W. Fluorine-18-FDG and iodine-131-iodide uptake in thyroid cancer. J Nucl Med. 1996;37:1468–72.

35. Diehl M, Risse JH, Brandt-Mainz K, Dietlein M, Bohuslavizki KH, Matheja P, et al. Fluorine-18 fluorodeoxyglucose positron emission tomography in medullary thyroid cancer: results of a multicenter study. Eur J Nucl Med. 2001;28:1671–6.

36. Grünwald F, Briele B, Biersack HJ. Non-131I-scintigraphy in the treatment and follow-up of thyroid cancer. Single-photon-emitters or FDG-PET? Q J Nucl Med. 1999;43:195–206.

37. Grünwald F, Menzel C, Bender H, Palmedo H, Willkomm P, Ruhlmann J, Franckson T, Biersack HJ. Comparison of 18FDG-PET with 131iodine and 99mTc-sestamibi scintigraphy in differentiated thyroid cancer. Thyroid. 1997;7:327–35.

38. Cabanillas ME, Terris DJ, Sabra MM. Information for clinicians: approach to the patient with progressive radioiodine-refractory thyroid cancer-when to use systemic therapy. Thyroid. 2017;27:987–93.

39. Saller B. Treatment with cytotoxic drugs. In: Biersack HJ, Grünwald F, editors. Thyroid Cancer. Heidelberg, Berlin: Springer-Verlag; 2005. p. 171–86.

40. Brose MS, Nutting CM, Jarzab B, Elisei R, Siena S, Bastholt L, et al. Sorafenib in radioactive iodine-refractory, locally advanced or metastatic differentiated thyroid cancer: a randomized, double-blind phase 3 trial. Lancet. 2014;384:319–28.

41. Schlumberger M, Tahara M, Wirth LJ, Robinson B, Brose MS, Elisei R, et al. Lenvatinib versus placebo in radioiodine-refractory thyroid cancer. N Engl J Med. 2015;372:621–30.

42. Grünwald F, Menzel C, Bender H, Palmedo H, Otte R, Fimmers R, et al. Redifferentiation therapy-induced radioiodine uptake in thyroid cancer. J Nucl Med. 1998;39:1903–6.

43. Simon D, Körber C, Krausch M, Segering J, Groth P, Görges R, Grünwald F, et al. Clinical impact of retinoids in redifferentiation therapy of advanced thyroid cancer: final results of a pilot study. Eur J Nucl Med Mol Imaging. 2002;29:775–82.

44. Elola M, Yoldi A, Emparanza JI, Matteucci T, Bilbao I, Goena M. Redifferentiation therapy with rosiglitazone in a case of differentiated thyroid cancer with pulmonary metastases and absence of radioiodine uptake. Rev Esp Med Nucl. 2011;30:241.

45. Landa I, Ibrahimpasic T, Boucai L, Sinha R, Knauf JA, Shah RH, et al. Genomic and transcriptomic hallmarks of poorly differentiated and anaplastic thyroid cancers. J Clin Invest. 2016;126:1052–66.

46. Liu T, Wang N, Cao J, Sofiadis A, Dinets A, Zedenius J, et al. The age- and shorter telomere-dependent TERT promotor mutation in follicular thyroid cell-derived carcinomas. Oncogene. 2014;33:4978–84.

47. Xing M, Liu R, Liu X, Murugan AK, Zhu G, Zeiger MA, et al. BRAF V6000E and TERT promotor mutations cooperatively identify the most aggressive pap-

illary thyroid cancer with highest recurrence. J Clin Oncol. 2014;32:2718–26.

48. Kunstman JW, Juhlin CC, Goh G, Brown TC, Stenman A, Healy JM, et al. Characterization of the mutational landscape of anaplastic thyroid cancer via whole-exome sequencing. Hum Mol Genet. 2015;24:2318–2.

49. Latteyer S, Tiedje V, König K, Ting S, Heukamp LC, Meder L, et al. Targeted next-generation sequencing for TP53, RAS, BRAF, ALK and NF1 mutations in anaplastic thyroid cancer. Endocrine. 2016;54:733–41.

50. Melo M, da Rocha AG, Vinagre J, Batista R, Peixoto J, Tavares C, et al. TERT promotor mutations are a major indicator of poor outcome in differentiated thyroid carcinoma. J Clin Endocrinol Metab. 2014;99:E754–65.

51. Shi X, Liu R, Qu S, Zhu G, Bishop J, Liu X, et al. Association of TERT promotor mutation 1,295,228CT with BRAF V600E mutation, older patient age, and distant metastasis in anaplastic thyroid cancer. J Clin Endocrinol Metab. 2015;100: E:632–7.

52. Cabanillas ME, Ryder M, Jimenez C. Targeted therapy for advanced thyroid cancer: kinase inhibitors and beyond. Endocr Rev. 2019;40:1573–604.

53. Ho AL, Grewal RK, Leboeuf R, Sherman EJ, Pfister DG, Deandreis D, et al. Selumetinib-enhanced radioiodine uptake in advanced thyroid cancer. N Engl J Med. 2013;368:623–32.

54. Rothenberg SM, McFadden DG, Palmer E, Daniels GH, Wirth LJ. Redifferentiation of radioiodine-refractory BRAF V600E-mutant thyroid carcinoma with dabrafenib. Clin Cancer Res. 2015;21:1028–35.

55. Hong DS, DuBois SG, Kummar S, Farago AF, Albert CM, Rohrberg K, et al. Larotrectinib in patients with TRK fusion-positive solid tumours: a pooled analysis of three phase 1/2 clinical trials. Lancet Oncol. 2020;21:531. https://doi.org/10.1016/S1470-2045(19)30856-3.

56. Tuttle RM, Brose MS, Grande E, Kim SW, Tahara M, Sabra MM. Novel concepts for initiating multi-targeted kinase inhibitors in radioactive iodine refractory differentiated thyroid cancer. Best Pract Res Clin Endocrinol Metab. 2017;31:295–305.

57. Chodhury PS, Gupta M. Differenteiated thyroid cancer theranostics: radioiodine and beyond. Br J Radiol. 2018;91:20180136. https://doi.org/10.1259/bjr.20180136.

58. Ain KB, Taylor KD, Tofiq S, Venkataraman G. Somatostatin receptor subtype expression in human thyroid and thyroid carcinoma cell lines. J Clin Endocrinol Metab. 1997;82:1857–62.

59. Lincke T, Singer J, Kluge R, Sabri O, Paschke R. Relative quantification of indium-111 pentetreotide and gallium-68 DOTATOC uptake in the thyroid gland and association with thyroid pathologies. Thyroid. 2009;19:381–9.

60. Zatelli MC, Tagliati F, Taylor JE, Rossi R, Culler MD, Uberti EC. Somatostatin receptor subtypes 2 and 5 differentially affect proliferation in vitro of the human medullary thyroid carcinoma cell line. J Clin Endocrinol Metab. 2001;86:2161–9.

61. Forssell-Aronsson EB, Nilsson O, Bejegard SA, Kölby L, Bernhardt P, Mölne J, et al. In-111-DTPA-D-Phe1--octreotide binding and somatostatin receptor subtypes in thyroid tumors. J Nucl Med. 2000;41:636–42.

62. Middendorp M, Selkinski I, Happel C, Kranert WT, Grünwald F. Comparison of positron emission tomography with [(18)F]FDG and [(68)Ga]DOTATOC in recurrent differentiated thyroid cancer: preliminary data. Q J Nucl Med Mol Imaging. 2010;54:76–83.

63. Budiawan H, Salavati A, Kulkarni HR, Baum RP. Peptide receptor radionuclide therapy of treatment-refractory metastatic thyroid cancer using Yttrium-90 and Lutetium-177 labeled somatostatin analogs; toxicity, response and survival analysis. Am J Nucl Med Mol Imaging. 2014;4:39–52.

64. Lengana T, Lawal IO, Mokoala K, Vorster M, Sathekge MM. 68Ga-PSMA: a one-stop shop in radioactive iodine refractory thyroid cancer? Nucl Med Mol Imaging. 2019;53:442–5.

65. Ngoc CN, Happel C, Sabet A, Bechstein WO, Grünwald F. Iodine avid papillary thyroid cancer showing PSMA-expression in 68Ga-PSMA ligand PET/CT. Nuklearmedizin. 2019;58:50–1.

66. Assadi M, Ahmadzadehfar H. 177Lu-DOTATATE and 177Lu-prostate-specific membrane antigen therapy in a patient with advanced metastatic radioiodine-refractory differentiated thyroid cancer after failure of tyrosine kinase inhibitors treatment. World J Nucl Med. 2019;18:406–8.

67. Kratochwil C, Flechsig P, Lindner T, Abderrahim L, Altmann A, Mier W, Adeberg S, Rathke H, Röhrich M, Winter H, Plinkert PK, Marme F, Lang M, Kauczor HU, Jäger D, Debus J, Haberkorn U, Giesel FL. Ga-68-FAPI PET/CT: tracer uptake in 28 different kinds of cancer. J Nucl Med. 2019;60:801–5.

68. Langbein T, Weber WA, Eiber M. Future of theranostics: an outlook on precision oncology in nuclear medicine. J Nucl Med. 2019;60(Suppl 2):13S–9S.

69. Watabe T, Liu Y, Kaneda-Nakashima K, Shirakami Y, Lindner T, Ooe K, Toyoshima A, Nagata K, Shimosegawa E, Haberkorn U, Kratochwil C, Shinohara A, Giesel F, Hatazawa J. Theranostics targeting fibroblast activation protein in the tumor stroma: Cu-64 and Ac-225 labelled FAPI-04 in pancreatic cancer xenograft mouse models. J Nucl Med. 2019;61:563. https://doi.org/10.2967/jnumed.119.233122.

70. Giesel FL, Kratochwil C, Lindner T, Marschalek MM, Loktev A, Lehnert W, Debus J, Jäger D, Flechsig P, Altmann A, Mier W, Haberkorn U. Ga-FAPI PET/CT: biodistribution and preliminary dosimetry estimate of 2 DOTA-containing FAP-targeting agents in patients with various cancers. J Nucl Med. 2019;60:386–92.

71. Werner RA, Kircher S, Higuchi T, Kircher M, Schirbel A, Wester HJ, Buck AK, Pomper MG, Rowe SP, Lapa C. CXCR4-directed imaging in solid tumors. Front Oncol. 2019;14:770. https://doi.org/10.3389/fonc.2019.00770.

72. Herrmann K, Schottelius M, Lapa C, Osl T, Poschenrieder A, Hanscheid H, et al. First-in-human experience of CXCR4-directed endoradiotherapy with 177Lu- and 90Y-labeled pentixather in advanced-stage multiple myeloma with extensive intra- and extramedullary disease. J Nucl Med. 2016;57:248–51.
73. Lapa C, Herrmann K, Schirbel A, Hanscheid H, Luckerath K, Schottelius M, et al. CXCR4-directed endoradiotherapy induces high response rates in extra-medullary relapsed multiple myeloma. Theranostics. 2017;7:1589–97.
74. Kircher M, Herhaus P, Schottelius M, Buck AK, Werner RA, Wester HJ, Keller U, Lapa C. CXCR4-directed theranostics in oncology and inflammation. Ann Nucl Med. 2018;32:503–11.
75. Wu Z, Cao Y, Jiang X, Li M, Wang G, Yang Y, Lu K. Clinicopathological significance of chemokine receptor CXCR4 expression in papillary thyroid carcinoma: a meta-analysis. Minerva Endocrinol. 2020;45:43. https://doi.org/10.23736/S0391-1977.
76. Yue W, Wang S, Wang B, Xu Q, Yu S, Yonglin Z, et al. Ultrasound guided percutaneous microwave ablation of benign thyroid nodules: safety and imaging follow-up in 222 patients. Eur J Radiol. 2013;82:e11–6.
77. Sung JY, Baek JH, Jung SL, Kim JH, Kim KS, Lee D, Kim WB, Na DG. Radiofrequency ablation for auton-omously functioning thyroid nodules: a multicenter study. Thyroid. 2015;25:112–7.
78. Baek JH, Kim YS, Lee D, Huh JY, Lee JH. Benign predominantly solid thyroid nodules: prospective study of efficacy of sonographically guided radiofre-quency ablation versus control condition. AJR Am J Roentgenol. 2010;194:1137–42.
79. Grünwald F. Alternative techniques in benign diseases. In: Goretzki P, editor. Thyroid. Berlin: Lehmanns Media; 2017. p. 87–105.
80. Happel C, Korkusuz H, Koch DA, Grünwald F, Kranert WT. Combination of ultrasound guided per-cutaneous microwave ablation and radioiodine ther-apy in benign thyroid diseases. A suitable method to reduce the 131I activity and hospitalization time? Nuklearmedizin. 2015;54:118–24.
81. Li HX, Xiang N, Hu WK, Jiao XL. Relation between therapy options for Graves' disease and the course of Graves' ophthalmopathy: a systematic review and meta-analysis. J Endocrinol Invest. 2016;39:1225–33.

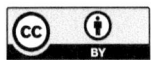

Cardiotoxicity of Targeted Therapies: Imaging of Heart Does Matter

Raffaella Calabretta and Marcus Hacker

12.1 Cancer Targeted Therapies

Molecular targeted therapies are characterized by blocking essential biochemical pathways or mutant proteins that are required for cancer cell growth and survival [1]. The *National Cancer Institute* defines a target therapy as "type of treatment that uses drugs or other substances to identify and attack specific types of cancer cells with less harm to normal cells. Some targeted therapies block the action of certain enzymes, proteins, or other molecules involved in the growth and spread of cancer cells. Other types of targeted therapies help the immune system kill cancer cells or deliver toxic substances directly to cancer cells and kill them. Targeted therapy may have fewer side effects than other types of cancer treatment. Most targeted therapies are either small molecule drugs or monoclonal antibodies" [2]. Targets selected for molecular targeted therapy include growth factors, signalling molecules, cell-cycle proteins, modulators of apoptosis and molecules that promote angiogenesis, among many others ([3], Fig. 12.1). Targets that are commonly used for imaging and therapy in nuclear medicine practice are radiolabelled peptides. Peptides are important regulators of growth, cellular function and intercellular communication and they act as neurotransmitters, regulating immune response and information transduction. Peptide ligands are neurotransmitters, hormones, chemokines, cytokines and growth factors. Receptors targeted with radiolabelled peptides have become an important topic, particularly in nuclear oncology [4].

Targeted cancer therapeutics are amongst the major treatment options for cancer today, together with cytotoxic chemotherapies. These treatments are more selective for cancer cells and improve the quality of life for cancer patients undergoing therapy [5]. However, these molecular targets are expressed also in normal cells, which explains the different grades of toxicity, resulting from the disruption of normal cellular function. Along with the benefits of disease stabilization different adverse events are reported [6, 7]. The radiopeptide treatments improve survival in cancer patients without significant evidence of cardiac function impairment.

R. Calabretta · M. Hacker (✉)
Division of Nuclear Medicine, Department of Biomedical Imaging and Image-guided Therapy, Medical University of Vienna, Vienna, Austria
e-mail: marcus.hacker@meduniwien.ac.at

© The Author(s) 2024
V. Prasad (ed.), *Beyond Becquerel and Biology to Precision Radiomolecular Oncology: Festschrift in Honor of Richard P. Baum*, https://doi.org/10.1007/978-3-031-33533-4_12

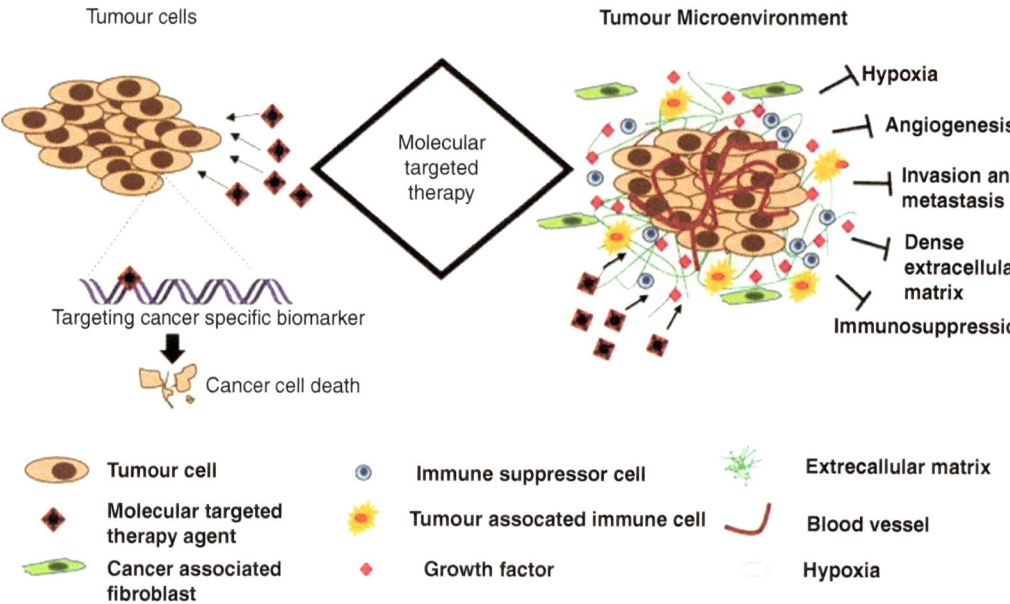

Tumour cells

Tumour Microenvironment

Molecular targeted therapy

Hypoxia
Angiogenesis
Invasion and metastasis
Dense extracellular matrix
Immunosuppression

Targeting cancer specific biomarker

Cancer cell death

	Tumour cell		Immune suppressor cell		Extrecallular matrix
	Molecular targeted therapy agent		Tumour assocaled immune cell		Blood vessel
	Cancer associated fibroblast		Growth factor		Hypoxia

Fig. 12.1 Summary of molecular targeted therapy mechanisms. Molecular targeted therapy on cancer focuses on targeting specific cancer-associated molecules that are highly expressed in cancer cells or by modulating the tumour microenvironment related to tumour vasculature, metastasis or hypoxia. (*Y.T. Lee et al.* [3])

12.2 Cardiotoxicity of Cancer Targeted Therapy

One frequent side effect in targeted therapies is cardiotoxicity. Cardiotoxicity related to cancer therapy is a broad term and includes any functional or structural heart injury related to cancer treatment. Cardiotoxicity is well known to occur secondary to cancer chemo and radiotherapy and may lead to premature morbidity and death among cancer survivors because of the direct effects of the cancer treatment on heart function and structure. Cardiotoxic effects have also been observed in novel targeted therapies. In the context of underlying cardiovascular diseases (CVD), which are the leading cause of death in the Western world, it may accelerate the development of CVD, especially in the presence of traditional cardiovascular risk factors [7–10]. To identify patients at risk for cardiotoxicity from cancer therapy, it is crucial to detect previous subclinical cardiac abnormalities and to perform an early detection of possible cardiovascular complications during treatment by increasing, for example, the surveillance frequency [10, 11].

Myocardial dysfunction and heart failure (HF), frequently described as *cardiotoxicity*, are the most concerning cardiovascular complications of cancer therapies and cause an increase in morbidity and mortality [10]. Cardiotoxicity is grouped into two categories, based on different pathological changes and clinical characteristics:

– Type I: traditional, related to traditional chemotherapy.
– Type II: targeted, related to novel targeted therapeutic agents.

Anthracyclines are the prototype of type I agents and are associated with a significant risk of left ventricular dysfunction (LVD) or HF, compared with non-anthracycline therapies [12]. The pathophysiological mechanisms differ by drug and include accelerated atherosclerosis, coronary spasm, vascular endothelial damage and arterial thrombotic events [13]. In addition to cardiac dysfunction, which is typical for anthracycline-based chemotherapies, targeted cancer therapy-induced cardiotoxicities may manifest also as elevated blood pressure, atherosclerosis, thromboembolism, pericardial thickening and arrhythmia [12]. Unfortunately, the understanding of the underlying pathophysiology and natural history of cardiotoxicity remains limited. Therefore, it is critical to perform an early patient risk stratification [13].

12.3 Diagnostic Tools to Detect Myocardial Toxicity

12.3.1 Anamnesis and Risk Stratification

The first step to identify patients at increased risk for cardiotoxicity consists of a careful baseline anamnesis. Demographic (age, family history of CVD), lifestyle (smoking, obesity, high alcohol intake, sedentary habit) and other cardiovascular risk factors (i.e. arterial hypertension, diabetes mellitus, hypercholesterolemia) should be collected to perform a patient risk stratification before cancer therapy. Previous cancer treatments should be also recorded.

12.3.2 Electrocardiography

Electrocardiography (ECG) is recommended in all patients before and during the cancer treatments. It is useful to detect any ECG signs of cardiac toxicity, either transitory or chronic, including ST-T wave changes, conduction disturbances, arrhythmias, and others [10, 13].

12.3.3 Cardiac Biomarkers

The use of cardiac biomarkers during cardiotoxic chemotherapy may be considered in order to detect early cardiac injury. They are accurate, reproducible, widely available, and high-sensitive Troponin I, high-sensitivity Troponin I, B-type natriuretic Peptide (BNP) and NT-proBNP are generally recorded. However, there is currently no clear evidence about the role of cardiac biomarkers to detect cardiotoxicity due to both targeted molecular therapies as well as traditional chemotherapy [10].

12.3.4 Imaging Modalities for Cardiotoxicity Screening

Cardiac imaging modalities include echocardiography, cardiac magnetic resonance imaging, positron emission tomography, conventional nuclear imaging techniques, cardiac computer tomography and coronary computer tomography angiography. Functional testing with exercise or stress agents is also routinely used to diagnose either LV myocardial ischaemia or other LV perfusion abnormalities [10, 13, 14].

12.3.4.1 Echocardiography

Cancer patients treated with potentially cardiotoxic therapy are at high risk of developing myocardial dysfunction and congestive HF. LV ejection fraction (LVEF) as a global marker of LV systolic function is currently used and several strategies have been applied over the past decades to detect it. Cardiac dysfunction resulting from exposure to cancer treatments was first recognized in the 1960s, with the widespread introduction of anthracyclines into the oncologic therapeutic setting. Different definitions of cancer therapeutics–related cardiac dysfunction (CTRCD) have been historically used [15]. A joint committee of the American Society of Echocardiography and the European Association of Cardiovascular Imaging defined the CTRCD as a decrease in the LVEF of >10% points, to a value <53% (normal reference value for two-dimensional (2D) echocardiography). The decrease should be confirmed by repeated cardiac imaging. The repeat study should be performed 2–3 weeks after the baseline diagnostic study showing the possible initial decrease in LVEF. That should be further categorized as symptomatic or asymptomatic, or with regard to reversibility [16].

2D-echocardiography is the method of choice to detect the LVEF before, periodically during and after potential cardiotoxic cancer therapy. This is because of its wide availability, reproducibility, versatility, lack of radiation exposure and also safety in patients with concomitant renal disease. The modified 2D-biplane Simpson method is recommended for estimation of LVEF and LV volumes. Echocardiography allows the evaluation of left and right ventricular dimensions, volumes, and function as well as valvular, and pericardial pathology. [10, 13, 16] Despite some limitations, the incorporation of modern techniques such as myocardial contrast echocardiography, three-dimensional (3D) echocardiography, Doppler tissue imaging and speckle-tracking echocardiography offer a prudent compromise between cost-effectiveness and clinical predictive value [14].

12.3.4.2 Cardiac Magnetic Resonance

Cardiac magnetic resonance (CMR) is a helpful tool for the evaluation of cardiac structures, myocardial function as well as pericardium. Late gadolinium enhancement (LGE) imaging may be useful to detect scarring or fibrosis and can sensitively detect a myocardial infarction. The quantitative myocardial perfusion mapping allows to quantify the regional myocardial perfusion reserve. CMR is an excellent test for the comprehensive evaluation of cardiac masses and infiltrative conditions. Accuracy and reproducibility are characteristics of CMR, despite its limited availability [10, 12].

12.3.4.3 Nuclear Positron Emission Tomography

Positron emission tomography (PET) is the gold standard technique to assess myocardial perfusion and metabolism in nuclear medicine practice, due to its high spatial and temporal resolution and high diagnostic sensitivity and accuracy. Hybrid systems with either computer tomography (CT) or magnetic resonance imaging (MRI) have been used.

The use of cardiac PET, and in particular of quantitative myocardial perfusion PET, has been growing during the last decade. [^{13}N]-labelled ammonia, [^{15}O]-labelled water and ^{82}Rubidium have been employed as effective myocardial perfusion tracers. The acquisition protocols using dynamic acquisitions allow the absolute quantification of LV myocardial blood flow (MBF) at rest and after stress as well as the derivation of LV coronary flow reserve (CFR). Gating, that is an ECG synchronized registration, provides functional information such as LVEF, left ventricular volumes, wall motion and wall thicken-

ing. Moreover, quantitative PET makes possible to assess the presence of LV microvascular dysfunction, which is involved in various cardiac diseases, including the early stages of coronary artery atherosclerosis, hypertrophic and dilated cardiomyopathy, and hypertensive heart disease. Nevertheless, the acquisition and analysis of quantitative PET requires a high level of expertise [17, 18]. PET is also the gold standard technique to analyse myocardial metabolism or to assess myocardial viability using 2-[^{18}F]fluorodeoxyglucose (FDG). Clinical studies applying cardiac PET to monitor for cardiotoxicity related to cancer target therapies are limited. Recent publications report accurate estimation of left and right functional parameters also from routine dynamic whole-body FDG PET scans for oncological purposes, which could open a new perspective for further clinical applications of the PET examinations [19].

Targeted cancer therapy-induced cardiotoxicities may manifest also as a development or a progression of atherosclerosis. During the past decade, studies suggested that PET/CT with FDG is a valid tool to assess and to reliably quantify atherosclerotic inflammatory activity by evaluating the glucose metabolism of corresponding immune cells and to predict severe cardio- and cerebrovascular events in oncological patients [20, 21]. Recently, it was reported a significant increase of arterial inflammation in large arteries in patients suffering from melanoma treated with immune checkpoint inhibitor therapy, using FDG PET/CT imaging [22].

Patients with haematological malignancies could rarely develop light chain amyloidosis, which may present with cardiac amyloidosis, an infiltrative cardiomyopathy, often presenting as heart failure with preserved LVEF. Echocardiography and CMR imaging are useful for the diagnosis of cardiac amyloidosis but they cannot reliably distinguish it from other infiltrative heart diseases. PET/CT with radiopharmaceuticals that were originally developed for the detection of cerebral amyloid deposits and diagnosis of Alzheimer's disease, like ^{18}F-florbetair or ^{11}C-PIB have recently shown promising results for the detection of cardiac and extra-cardiac amyloidosis [23].

12.3.4.4 Conventional Nuclear Imaging

The American Society of Clinical Oncology guidelines 2016 recommend the use of multiple gated acquisition (MUGA) with technetium-99m [^{99m}Tc] labelled red blood cells to assess LVEF, if such a measurement is not feasible by echocardiography and CMR. Limitations include a radiation exposure and its inability to assess additional information on cardiac structure [10, 16].

An increasing number of Nuclear Medicine sites are routinely using single photon emission computer tomography (SPECT) systems to diagnose coronary artery disease or to detect myocardial ischemia. ECG-gated cardiac SPECT allows for reliable estimating myocardial perfusion as well as functional parameters (LVEF, LV volumes), LV wall motion and LV wall thickening with high accuracy [24].

12.3.4.5 Cardiac Computed Tomography, Angio-Coronary Computer Tomography

Whilst cardiotoxicity related to cancer therapy generally focuses on LV impairment, cancer treatments can cause other clinical cardiac syndromes including coronary events, pericardial disease, valvular heart diseases, pulmonary hypertension and right ventricular dysfunction. CT coronary angiography provides a non-invasive anatomical assessment of coronary artery disease. Among the immune and targeted therapeutics, those inhibiting the vascular endothelial growth factor (VEGF) signalling pathway have an increased risk for coronary thrombosis, which can be detected non-invasively by this technique [10, 12, 13].

12.4 Summary

Molecular targeted therapies are characterized by blocking essential biochemical pathways or mutant proteins that are required for cancer cell growth and survival. Targeted cancer therapeutics are amongst the major treatment options for cancer today. These treatments are more selective for cancer cells and improve the quality of life for cancer patients undergoing therapy. Nevertheless, one frequent side effect in targeted therapies is cardiotoxicity, frequently described as myocardial dysfunction and HF. Cardiotoxicity includes also any subsequent functional or structural heart injury, with a possible accelerated development of CVD. The early identification of patients at risk for cardiotoxicity from cancer target therapies and the early diagnosis of CV complications related to cancer treatments are crucial. Anamnesis and risk stratification are the first steps of the diagnostic process to detect myocardial toxicity. ECG detects cardiac electrical changes, cardiac biomarkers may be considered to detect early cardiac injury. Imaging modalities for cardiotoxicity screening include echocardiography, the method of choice to detect the LVEF, and CMR imaging, to evaluate cardiac structures, myocardial function and infiltrative conditions. Nuclear PET is the gold standard technique to assess LV myocardial perfusion and metabolism, to detect the development or a progression of acoronary artery therosclerosis and to identify cardiac and extra-cardiac amyloidosis. Conventional imaging in nuclear medicine practice includes MUGA and cardiac SPECT. Cardiac CT is a valid tool to detect morphological pathologies of heart, pericardial disease, valvular heart diseases, pulmonary hypertension, or right ventricular dysfunction. CT coronary angiography provides a non-invasive anatomical assessment of coronary artery disease.

References

1. Vanneman M, Dranoff G. Combining immunotherapy and targeted therapies in cancer treatment. Nat Rev Cancer. 2012;12(4):237–51.
2. https://www.cancer.gov/publications/dictionaries/cancer-terms/def/targeted-therapy.
3. Lee YT, Tan YJ, Oon CE. Molecular targeted therapy: treating cancer with specificity. Eur J Pharmacol. 2018;834:188–96.
4. Ambrosini V, Fani M, Fanti S, Forrer F, Maecke HR. Radiopeptide imaging and therapy in Europe. J Nucl Med. 2011;52(Suppl 2):42S–55S.
5. Miller MJ, Foy KC, Kaumaya PT. Cancer immunotherapy: present status, future perspective, and a new paradigm of peptide immunotherapeutics. Discov Med. 2013;15(82):166–76.
6. Widakowich C, De Castro G Jr, De Azambija E, Dihn P, Awada A. Review: side effects of approved molecu-

lar targeted therapies in solid cancers. Oncologist. 2007;12:1443.

7. Zuppinger C, Suter TM. Cancer therapy-associated cardiotoxicity and signaling in the myocardium. J Cardiovasc Pharmacol. 2010;56(2):141–6.

8. WHO. Cardiovascular diseases (CVDs). Fact sheet no. 317. Geneva: World Health Organization; 2015. http://www.who.int/mediacentre/factsheets/fs317/en/.

9. 2016 ESC/EAS guidelines for the management of dyslipidaemias. Eur Heart J. 2016;37:2999–3058.

10. Zamorano JL, Lancellotti P, Rodriguez Muñoz D, Aboyans V, Asteggiano R, Galderisi M, Habib G, Lenihan DJ, Lip GYH, Lyon AR, Lopez Fernandez T, Mohty D, Piepoli MF, Tamargo J, Torbicki A, Suter TM, ESC Scientific Document Group. 2016 ESC Position Paper on cancer treatments and cardiovascular toxicity developed under the auspices of the ESC Committee for Practice Guidelines: The Task Force for cancer treatments and cardiovascular toxicity of the European Society of Cardiology (ESC). Eur Heart J. 2016;37(36):2768–801.

11. Poulin F, Thavendiranathan P. Cardiotoxicity due to chemotherapy: role of cardiac imaging. Curr Cardiol Rep. 2015;17(3):564.

12. Chen Z, Ai D. Cardiotoxicity associated with targeted cancer therapies. Mol Clin Oncol. 2016;4(5):675–81.

13. Seraphim A, Westwood M, Bhuva AN, Crake T, Moon JC, Menezes LJ, Lloyd G, Ghosh AK, Slater S, Oakervee H, Manisty CH. Advanced imaging modalities to monitor for cardiotoxicity. Curr Treat Options Oncol. 2019;20(9):73.

14. Plana JC, Galderisi M, Barac A, Ewer MS, Ky B, Scherrer-Crosbie M, Ganame J, Sebag IA, Agler DA, Badano LP, Banchs J, Cardinale D, Carver J, Cerqueira M, DeCara JM, Edvardsen T, Flamm SD, Force T, Griffin BP, Jerusalem G, Liu JE, Magalhães A, Marwick T, Sanchez LY, Sicari R, Villarraga HR, Lancellotti P. Expert consensus for multimodality imaging evaluation of adult patients during and after cancer therapy: a report from the American Society of Echocardiography and the European Association of Cardiovascular Imaging. J Am Soc Echocardiogr. 2014;27(9):911–39.

15. Khouri MG, Douglas PS, Mackey JR, Martin M, Scott JM, Scherrer-Crosbie M, Jones LW. Cancer therapy-induced cardiac toxicity in early breast cancer: addressing the unresolved issues. Circulation. 2012;126(23):2749–63.

16. Awadalla M, Hassan MZO, Alvi RM, Neilan TG. Advanced imaging modalities to detect cardiotoxicity. Curr Probl Cancer. 2018;42(4):386–96.

17. Sciagrà R, Lubberink M, Hyafil F, Saraste A, Slart RHJA, Agostini D, Nappi C, Georgoulias P, Bucerius J, Rischpler C, Verberne HJ, Cardiovascular Committee of the European Association of Nuclear Medicine (EANM). EANM procedural guidelines for PET/CT quantitative myocardial perfusion imaging. Eur J Nucl Med Mol Imaging. 2021;48:1040–69.

18. Sciagrà R. Quantitative cardiac positron emission tomography: the time is coming! Scientifica (Cairo). 2012;2012:948653.

19. Rasul S, Beitzke D, Wollenweber T, et al. Assessment of left and right ventricular functional parameters using dynamic dual-tracer [13N]NH3 and [18F]FDG PET/MRI. J Nucl Cardiol. 2020;29:1003.

20. Bucerius J, Hyafil F, Verberne HJ, Slart RH, Lindner O, Sciagra R, Agostini D, Übleis C, Gimelli A, Hacker M, Cardiovascular Committee of the European Association of Nuclear Medicine (EANM). Position paper of the Cardiovascular Committee of the European Association of Nuclear Medicine (EANM) on PET imaging of atherosclerosis. Eur J Nucl Med Mol Imaging. 2016;43(4):780–92.

21. Rominger A, Saam T, Wolpers S, Cyran CC, Schmidt M, Foerster S, Nikolaou K, Reiser MF, Bartenstein P, Hacker M. 18F-FDG PET/CT identifies patients at risk for future vascular events in an otherwise asymptomatic cohort with neoplastic disease. J Nucl Med. 2009;50(10):1611–20.

22. Calabretta R, Hoeller C, Pichler V, Mitterhauser M, Karanikas G, Haug A, Li X, Hacker M. Immune checkpoint inhibitor therapy induces inflammatory activity in large arteries. Circulation. 2020;142:2396.

23. García-González P, Cozar-Santiago MDP, Maceira AM. Cardiac amyloidosis detected using 18F-florbetapir PET/CT. Rev Esp Cardiol (Engl Ed). 2016;69(12):1215.

24. Verberne HJ, Acampa W, Anagnostopoulos C, Ballinger J, Bengel F, De Bondt P, Buechel RR, Cuocolo A, van Eck-Smit BL, Flotats A, Hacker M, Hindorf C, Kaufmann PA, Lindner O, Ljungberg M, Lonsdale M, Manrique A, Minarik D, Scholte AJ, Slart RH, Trägårdh E, de Wit TC, Hesse B, European Association of Nuclear Medicine (EANM). EANM procedural guidelines for radionuclide myocardial perfusion imaging with SPECT and SPECT/CT: 2015 revision. Eur J Nucl Med Mol Imaging. 2015;42(12):1929–40.

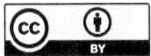

The Evolution of n.c.a. ^{177}Lu to n.c.a. ^{177}Lu-Edotreotide for the Treatment of Neuroendocrine Tumours. Sixteen Years of Collaboration Between Zentralklinik Bad Berka and ITM

13

P. Harris, R. Henkelmann, S. Marx, and K. Zhernosekov

13.1 Introduction

Diagnostic and therapeutic radionuclides offer an excellent platform for the development of innovative drugs, which enable non-invasive visualization of diseases and complementary targeted treatments. The concept of personalized medicine is realized! This innovation in nuclear medicine together with an increasing demand for high-quality radionuclides and radiopharmaceuticals has triggered the expansion of nuclear medicine as a hospital speciality, together with the development of a new radiotheranostics industry.

This chapter describes the successful development of no-carrier-added (n.c.a.) Lutetium-177 and of n.c.a. ^{177}Lu-edotreotide as examples of the successful collaboration between an academic nuclear medicine institution and industry.

13.2 No-Carrier-Added Lutetium-177: The Gold Standard for Radionuclide Treatment

After the introduction of suitable macrocyclic chelators into the targeting molecules, trivalent radiometals such as Yttrium-90 (pure high energy β^--emitter) gained importance for the targeted therapeutic treatment of serious oncological disease [1]. Lutetium-177 in particular, has demonstrated excellent physical properties to enable the precise delivery of cytotoxic dose of beta irradiation to small and large malignant lesions. Furthermore, by emitting soft beta radiation (E_β 133.6 keV) Lutetium-177 radiolabelled compounds have a favourable safety profile particularly in terms of nephrotoxicity. Small components of photons (112.9 keV, 6% and 208.4 kEv, 10%) enable the visualization and quantitative estimation (dosimetry) of biodistribution by means of SPECT, without having a negative impact on safety (Table 13.1). Starting with Lutetium-177-based treatments of somatostatin receptor-positive tumours in the late 1990s, the use of radionuclide has dramatically increased. A number of novel therapies are being developed for the treatment of serious oncologi-

P. Harris · R. Henkelmann (✉) · S. Marx
K. Zhernosekov
ITM Isotopen Technologien Muenchen AG,
Munich, Germany
e-mail: Richard.Henkelmann@itm.ag

© The Author(s) 2024
V. Prasad (ed.), *Beyond Becquerel and Biology to Precision Radiomolecular Oncology: Festschrift in Honor of Richard P. Baum*, https://doi.org/10.1007/978-3-031-33533-4_13

Table 13.1 Characteristics of industrially available therapeutic β⁻-emitters [2]

Nuclide	$T_{1/2}$	$E_{β^-,av}$ [MeV]	$E_γ$ [keV] ($I_γ$ [%])	Mean Tissue range [mm]	Imaging / Dosimetry	Specific activity/ Radionuclidic purity	Energy deposition
⁹⁰Y*	64.053 h	0.934	-	3.9	no	no-carrier-added/ high purity	hard betas for large and heterogeneous tumors (min 5 mm lesions)
¹⁷⁷Lu**	6.647 d	0.134	112.9 (6) 208.4 (10)	0.67	yes excellent	1) carrier-added/ low purity 2) no-carrier-added/ high purity	soft betas for small tumors (min 0.5 mm lesions)
¹³¹I	8.0252 d	0.182	284.3 (6) 364.5 (82) 636.9 (7)	0.91	yes low resolution	no-carrier-added/ high purity	Large gamma-component might result in hematox

* two in EU registered precursors (EZAG; IBA)

** two in EU registered precursors (carrier-added Lumark (IDB / AAA); no-carrier-added EndolucinBeta (ITG))

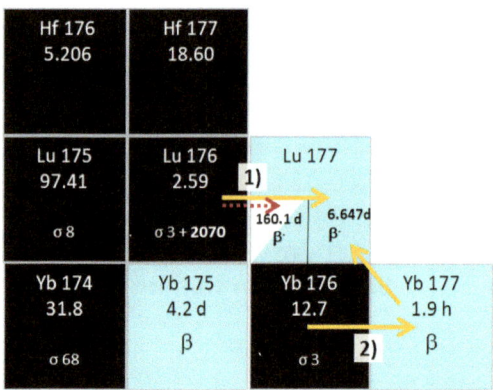

1) ^{176}Lu(n,γ)^{177}Lu

2) ^{176}Yb(n,γ)^{177}Yb → ^{177}Lu

Fig. 13.1 Excerpt of the Karlsruhe nuclide chart

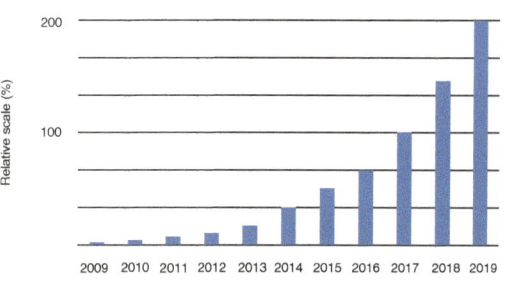

Fig. 13.2 Relative amount of no-carrier-added Lutetium-177 commercialized by ITM AG reflecting the dramatic year-on-year increase of Lutetium-177-based therapies in cancer

cal diseases using tumour receptor targeting, including PSMA and FAP [3, 4].

An important aspect of the successful development of Lutetium-177-based therapies is the availability of a radionuclide with specific activity suitable for the radiolabelling of targeting molecules. The first carrier-added preparations of Lutetium-177 for radiolabelling became commercially available from the early 2000s. Lutetium-177 can be easily produced in a nuclear reactor by the irradiation of the highly enriched stable isotope Lutetium-176 (Fig. 13.1). A high cross-section for the neutron capture reaction enables a reasonable specific activity to be achieved, although the final preparation still consists of a mixture of the stable and radioactive isotopes Lu-176 and Lu-177, respectively. The

main drawback of this manufacturing pathway is the co-accumulation of long-lived metastable Lutetium-177 m (half-life 160.44 days). Depending on the irradiation parameters, the fraction of this long-lived radionuclidic impurity varies from 0.2 to 0.7%. The disposal of solid and especially liquid wastes, contaminated with the long-lived impurity, is costly and laborious.

A significant enhancement for the future development of targeted radionuclide therapies was the implementation of no-carrier-added Lutetium-177. If the neutron capture reaction leads to an intermediate β⁻-unstable nuclide, then a secondary formed radioisotope is an isoton to the target nucleus. In this case the radionuclide can be isolated from the target material chemically in a no-carrier-added form. Thus the irradiation of highly-enriched Ytterbium-176 with neutrons results in short-lived Yb-177, which decays to desired Lu-177 (Fig. 13.2). Furthermore, only the ground state (i.e., Lu-177 g) is generated, providing the highest radionuclidic purity of the preparation free from Lu-177 m contamination.

A challenge in the manufacturing of no-carrier-added Lutetium-177 is the chemical purification of the radioisotope from the massive Ytterbium-176 targets. Two adjacent members of the lanthanide series Yb(III) and Lu(III) are chemically very similar and their chemical separation becomes a difficult scientific task. For production of industrial quantities of no-carrier-added Lutetium-177, gram amounts of Ytterbium-176 must be utilized. In contrast, the accumulated radionuclide corresponds to several micrograms of Lutetium mass.

ITM AG (through its affiliate ITG GmbH) has developed and implemented a unique automated process for the chemical processing of massive irradiated Ytterbium-176 targets and the fast isolation of no-carrier-added Lutetium-177 isotope. In 2007, ITG commenced the first irradiations of enriched Ytterbium-176 for the industrial production of no-carrier-added Lutetium-177 at the Munich research reactor FRMII. Due to the limited operation cycles of research nuclear reactors and in order to secure the weekly production and supply of Lu-177, it was necessary to build up a reactor network with a large number of medium- and high-flux reactors worldwide. Currently, ITM closely cooperates with research reactors in Belgium, France, Netherlands, Poland, South Africa and the USA.

An important characteristic of the no-carrier-added form is the fact that the quality doesn't depend on the performance among different nuclear reactors, with the highest level of specific activity being ensured for all radionuclide preparations. Furthermore, the specific activity of no-carrier-added Lutetium-177 remains high over the shelf-life of the product. Currently, ITM supplies its European registered product (EndolucinBeta™) worldwide to nuclear medicine departments and to industrial partners for the radiolabelling of tumour-targeting molecules (Fig. 13.2).

13.3 No-Carrier-Added Lutetium-177-Edotreotide for Treatment of Neuroendocrine Tumours

Originally developed in Basel, Switzerland, the synthetic somatostatin analogue edotreotide (or DOTATOC) has been evaluated and clinically used in combination with Yttrium-90 for the therapy of somatostatin receptor-positive tumours. Currently, Ga-68-edotreotide PET imaging agents are approved in Europe and in the USA for visualisation of neuroendocrine tumours (NETs). Excellent pharmacokinetic properties of this peptide combined with the outstanding characteristics of Lutetium-177 make it even more attractive for therapeutic use.

Favourable pharmacokinetics properties of edotreotide were initially reported by comparing the behaviour of ^{111}In-labelled edotreotide with ^{111}In-labelled DOTATATE in the same patients [5]. Particular emphasis was given to kidney uptake and to the tumour-to-kidney ratio. Whereas the mean absorbed dose to the red marrow was similar, ^{111}In-edotreotide demonstrated a comparably higher tumour-to-kidney absorbed dose ratio. Interestedly, the urinary excretion rate of radiolabelled edotreotide was significantly higher than for DOTATATE, whereas the tumour doses were within the same range. This initial study was performed without a reno-protective amino acid infusion.

Later on, the Bad Berka group investigated the in vivo behaviour of the ^{177}Lu-labeled peptides DOTATATE, DOTANOC, and DOTATOC. The aim of the study was to compare the pharmacokinetics and dosimetry of these three different peptides, considering inter- and intra-patient variability in a large cohort of patients with GEP NETs [6]. This study confirmed the favourable pharmacokinetic properties of radiolabelled edotreotide previously demonstrated by Forrer and colleagues. Edotreotide has a more rapid clearance from healthy organs compared to DOTATATE and DOTANOC providing a high tumour to background ratio and hence a high targeted dose of radiation to the tumour. The authors concluded that of the three peptides, ^{177}Lu-edotreotide results in the highest tumour-to-kidney ratio, indicating that it is and is a very appropriate choice for the therapy of GEP NETs.

The first systematic evaluation of treatment data with no-carrier-added ^{177}Lu-edotreotide in patients with GEP NETs was performed by Professor R. P. Baum at the Zentralklinik Bad Berka, Germany [7]. In this retrospective study, the efficacy and safety of treatment with ^{177}Lu-edotreotide were evaluated in 56 subjects with metastasised, progressive NET (50% gastroenteric, 27% pancreatic, 23% other primaries) who had not received previous PRRT treatment prior to a new diagnosis of progression. Subjects received on average 2.1 (range 1–4) cycles of ^{177}Lu-edotreotide as the sole treatment, administered in median doses of 7.0 GBq, at approximately three-monthly treatment intervals. Forty-three percent (24/56) of the study population underwent only a single ^{177}Lu-edotreotide cycle. Of these, 15 died from progressive disease prior to further PRRT. In total, 26 patients (46%) had died at data-base lock. When stratified for the number of ^{177}Lu-edotreotide cycles received (1 vs. ≥2), subjects treated only once were found to have a significantly lower Karnofsky performance status (KPS) at baseline (70.4 vs. 89.4, $p < 0.001$), indicating more advanced disease stage. In the total population (A), median progression-free (PFS) and overall survival (OS) were 17.4 and 34.2 months, respectively (Figs. 13.3 and 13.4). In repeatedly treated subjects, PFS was 32.0 months for all (B), 34.5 months for GEP NET (C), and 11.9 months for other NET (D). Objective response rates (ORR) were 33.9%, 40.6%, 54.2%, and 0% for populations A, B, C, and D, respectively. A high number of complete responses (16.1%, 18.8%, and 25.0% for populations A, B, and C) were observed, 78% of which were ongoing at the end of observation. No serious adverse event and

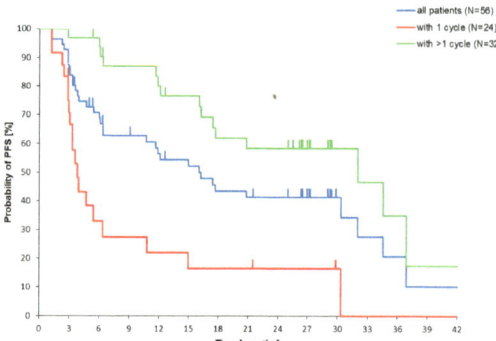

Fig. 13.3 Kaplan-Meier estimates of PFS in per protocol patients depending on number of ^{177}Lu-edotreotide PRRT cycles [7]

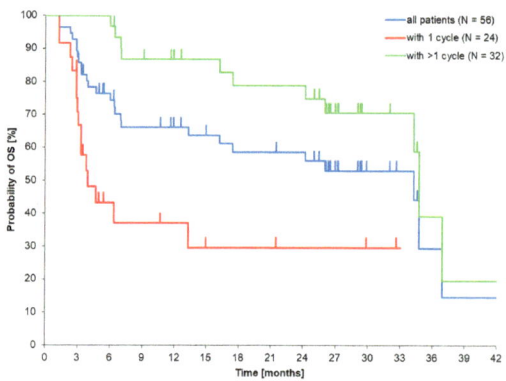

Fig. 13.4 Kaplan-Meier estimates of overall survival in PP patients depending on number of ^{177}Lu-edotreotide PRRT cycles [7]

only a single case of self-limited grade 3 haematotoxicity was observed (1.8%). No evidence for renal toxicity was found, although 34.4% of subjects had mild renal impairment at baseline. In addition, a long-term safety follow-up of patients included in the retrospective study showed no lasting relevant haematotoxic effects and no long-term renal toxicity for up to 6 years after first PRRT. These data show that ^{177}Lu-edotreotide is an agent for PRRT with the unusual potential to induce objective responses, and lasting disease control in progressive NETS, even when administered in moderate doses. A particularly high therapeutic index is suggested by the observed safety profile which includes subjects with preceding reduced bone marrow or renal function. At the present time, it is standard practice to provide renal protection with a 2.5% lysine/arginine infusion which is given concomitantly with the PRRT infusion.

Patients with G1 and G2 GEP NETS often present late with metastatic disease. Until recently, somatostatin analogues and the molecularly targeted drugs sunitinib and everolimus have provided the mainstays of treatment. These treatments usually result in disease stabilisation for a limited period of time. In the RADIANT-3 trial, everolimus achieved a PFS of 11 months in pancreatic NETS and a similar PFS was achieved in midgut and pulmonary NETS in the RADIANT-4 trial [8, 9]. Peptide receptor radionuclide therapy has recently emerged as a novel treatment option, with a PFS of 28.4 months in G1 and G2 mid-gut NETS being achieved in the NETTER-1 trial [10]. This Phase III study has resulted in the regulatory approval of ^{177}Lu c.a.-DOTATATE for G1 and G2 NETS.

Following on from the Bad Berka study [7], ITM has initiated a Phase III pivotal clinical trial. COMPETE is a prospective, randomised, open-label multi-centre Phase III study to evaluate the safety and efficacy of ^{177}Lu n.c.a.-edotreotide in comparison to everolimus in patients with G1 and G2 GEP NETs. The patients have progressive, somatostatin receptor (SSTR) positive disease on SSTR imaging. Uniquely, patients may be included as first-line therapy. There are 3 sub-studies which focus on ^{177}Lu-edotreotide dosimetry and pharmacokinetics. These sub-studies are of great importance in the development of a per-

sonalised, precision therapy approach to the management of patients with PRRT. In addition, ^{177}Lu is uniquely non-carrier-added, which means that it is a pure radionuclide of high specific activity.

The study is ongoing with a target recruitment of 300 patients. A total of 200 patients will receive 4 cycles of ^{177}Lu-edotreotide (7.5 GBq/cycle) every 3 months or until disease progression and 100 patients will receive everolimus 10 mg daily for 24 months or until disease progression. The study duration is 24 months with 5 years follow-up for OS. The primary end-point is PFS as assessed by RECIST 1.1. Key secondary end-points include safety and tolerability, dosimetry, ORR, OS and quality of life (Fig. 13.5). Patients with G3 neuroendocrine neoplasms (Ki-67 > 20%) have more aggressive disease than the G1 and G2 NETs. In 2017, the WHO subdivided G3 NENs into well-differentiated G3 neuroendocrine tumours (NETs) and poorly differentiated neuroendocrine carcinomas (NECs) [11]. A retrospective study of PRRT in G3 NENs has been reported by Professor Baum's group in Bad Berka [12]. Sixty-nine patients were treated with either ^{177}Lu- or ^{90}Y-labelled somatostatin analogues (DOTATATE or DOTATOC). This was a heterogeneous group of patients both in terms of disease and treatment. Overall, the median PFS was 9.6 months and the median OS was 19.9 months. When the patients were sub-into grouped into NETs with a Ki-67 index of ≤55%, the median PFS was 11 months and the OS 24 months. For NECs with a Ki-67

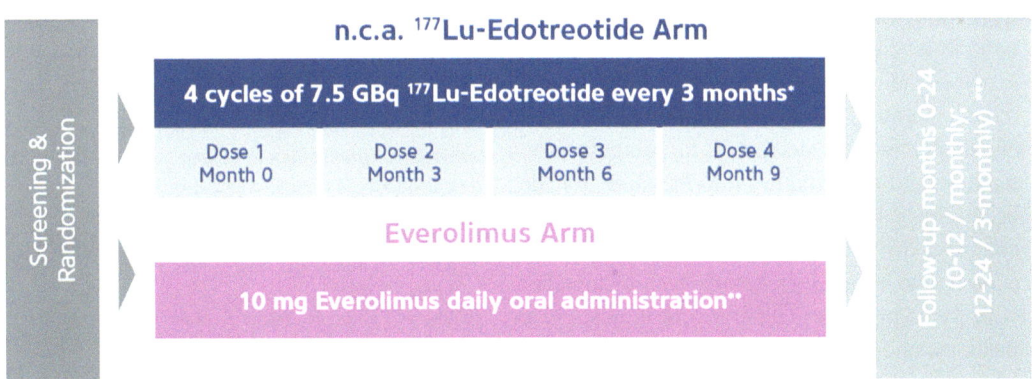

Fig. 13.5 COMPETE study. Study subjects are randomised 2:1 between 4 × 12 weekly cycles of 177Lu-edotreotide vs. 10 mg daily Everolimus, followed up for 24 months for PFS and 5 years for OS

index of ≥55%, the median PFS was 4 months and the median OS was 7 months. In the patients who had positive SSTR imaging but negative ^{18}F-FDG uptake, the prognosis was dramatically better. Other retrospective studies have also reported beneficial responses to PRRT in G3 NEN, particularly those with a Ki-67 index of ≤55% [13–15]. These low-grade G3 NETs are of particular interest for further clinical development. The high-grade G3 NECs (Ki-67 ≥ 55%) respond relatively poorly to PRRT. These tumours might benefit from combination therapies, particularly with DNA repair enzyme inhibitors.

13.4 Conclusion and Acknowledgements

Beyond the radionuclide targeted treatment of GEP NETs, a number of new targeted therapies have been introduced or are under development to treat serious oncological diseases such as castrate-resistant prostate cancer, pancreatic ductal adenocarcinoma and brain tumours. No-carrier-added Lutetium-177 is an excellent platform for development of these innovative treatment options. In addition to the in-house manufacture of radiopharmaceuticals by ITM, the radionuclide is in use in a number of investigational medicinal products, which are currently undergoing clinical trials worldwide.

The relationship that has been developed between ITM and Professor Baum goes back to the early days of ITM's foundation in 2004. During this time, the company has developed into a world-leading radiotheranostics company with a strong radioisotope manufacturing group and more recently a rapidly expanding clinical oncologics group, dedicated to bringing new radiotheranostics products into the clinic for the benefit of patients. Professor Baum's legacy will continue, driven by the many nuclear medicine experts who have been mentored by him, together with the many other collaborators in academia, medicine and industry. ITM is continuing to collaborate with Professor Baum's successors to drive the field of radiotheranostics onwards. Areas of development include the development

of ^{177}Lu-zolendonate for osteoblastic bone cancer, novel PSMA targeted therapies for prostate cancer and folate receptor alpha targeted therapies. Professor Baum is one of the early pioneers in radiotheranostics, being one of the key individuals who have developed radiotheranostics into the exciting, rapidly developing field in oncology that it is today. He has been a great collaborative colleague to ITM. That is a great legacy.

References

1. Fani, Melpomeni; Good, S.; Maecke, Helmut R in Handbook of Nuclear Chemistry: Radiochemistry and Radiopharmaceutical Chemistry in Life Sciences, 2011, Volume 4. Chapter 8. pp. 2143–2178.: Radiometals (non-Tc, non-Re) and Bifunctional Labeling Chemistry.
2. NuDat 2.8. https://www.nndc.bnl.gov/nudat2/.
3. Hofaman MS, Violet J, Hicks RJ, Ferdinandus J, et al. [177]Lu]-PSMA-617 radionuclide treatment in patients with metastatic castration-resistant prostate cancer (LuPSMA trial): a single-centre, single-arm, phase 2 study. Lancet Oncol. 2018;19(6):825–33.
4. Loktev A, Lindner T, Burger EA, Altmann A, et al. Development of fibroblast activation protein–targeted radiotracers with improved tumor retention. J Nucl Med. 2019;60:1421–9.
5. Forrer F, Uusijärvi H, Waldherr C, Cremonesi M, Bernhart P, Mueller-Brand J, Maecke HR. A comparison of 111In-DOTATOC and 111In-DOTATATE: biodistribution and dosimetry in the same patients with metastatic neuroendocrine tumours. Eur J Nucl Med Mol Imaging. 2004;31:1257–62.
6. Schuchardt C, Kulkarni HR, Prasad V, Zachert C, Müller D, Baum RP. The Bad Berka dose protocol: comparative results of dosimetry in peptide receptor radionuclide therapy using ^{177}Lu-DOTATATE, ^{177}Lu-DOTANOC, and ^{177}Lu-DOTATOC. Resent Res Cancer Res. 2013;194:519–36.
7. Baum RP, Kluge AW, Kulkarni H, et al. ^{177}Lu-DOTA][0]–D-Phe[1]-Tyr[3]-Octreotide (^{177}Lu-DOTATOC) for peptide receptor radiotherapy in patients with advanced neuroendocrine tumours: a phase-II study. Theranostics. 2016;6(4):501–10.
8. Yao JC, Shah MH, Ito T, et al. Everolimus for advanced pancreatic neuroendocrine tumors. N Engl J Med. 2011;364:514–23.
9. Yao JC, Fazio N, Singh S, et al. Everolimus for the treatment of advanced non-functional neuroendocrine tumours of the lung or gastrointestinal tract (RADIAT-4): a randomised, placebo controlled, phase 3 study. Lancet. 2016;387:968.

10. Strosberg J, El-Haddad G, Wolin E, et al. Phase 3 trial of ^{177}Lu-DOTATATE for midgut neuroendocrine tumors. N Engl J Med. 2017;376(2):125–35.

11. Rindi G, Klimstra DS, Abedi-Ardekani B, et al. A common classification framework for neuroendocrine neoplasms: an International Agency for Cancer Research (IACR) and World Health Organisation (WHO) expert consensus proposal. Mod Pathol. 2018;31:1770–86.

12. Zhang J, Kulkarni HR, Singh A, et al. Peptide receptor radionuclide therapy in grade 3 neuroendocrine neoplasms: safety and survival analysis in 69 patients. J Nucl Med. 2019;60:377–85.

13. Carlsen EA, Fazio N, Granberg D, et al. Peptide receptor radionuclide therapy in gastroenteropancreatic NEN G3: a multicenter cohort study. Endocr Relat Cancer. 2019;26(2):227–39.

14. Nicolini S, Severi S, Ianniello A, et al. Investigation of receptor radionuclide therapy with ^{177}Lu-DOTATATE in patients with GEP-NEN and a high Ki-67 proliferation index. Eur J Nucl Med Mol Imaging. 2018;45(6):923–30.

15. Thang SP, Lung MS, Kong G, et al. Peptide receptor radionuclide therapy (PRRT) in European neuroendocrine tumour society (ENETS) grade 3 (G3) neuroendocrine neoplasia (NEN)—a single institution retrospective analysis. Eur J Nucl Med Mol Imaging. 2018;45(2):262–77.

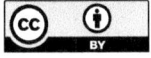

Fighting for PET in German
Oncological Guidelines and for Its
Reimbursement by Statutory
Health Insurances

14

Dirk Hellwig

Introducing new medical procedures into the broad care system is a particular challenge that Richard Baum has accepted. I have been pleased to accompany him for some time on this long journey, which will be described here.

The recognition of the clinical relevance of a diagnostic procedure is best documented when it is recommended in an interdisciplinary guideline. Until this was the case for the first time in Germany for FDG-PET/CT in lung cancer, both the evidence from studies and the reimbursability had to be established in parallel.

Therefore, both the commitment in scientific task forces for guideline development as well as the participation in committees of the Joint Federal Committee (G-BA, "Gemeinsamer Bundesausschuss") in an advisory function were necessary, which we have provided on behalf of the German Society of Nuclear Medicine.

The starting point in Germany is that a distinction is essentially made between the outpatient and inpatient care sectors. In the inpatient sector, new examination and treatment methods may be used and reimbursed as long as they are not explicitly prohibited (prohibition proviso). For non-invasive diagnostic procedures, however, there is generally no additional reimbursement in the inpatient sector. In the outpatient sector, new examination and treatment methods can only be used and reimbursed if they are explicitly permitted (subject to permission). This assessment is the responsibility of the G-BA, a body made up of representatives of the statutory health insurance funds (GKV, "Gesetzliche Krankenversicherung") on the one hand and service providers, i.e., hospitals as well as physicians and dentists in practices for outpatient care on the other.

The G-BA's consultations on PET and PET/CT have a long history and are still good for headlines today. On 26.05.1998, the GKVs requested consultations on PET. On 26.02.2002, the consultations led to the exclusion of all outpatient PET procedures for patients with statutory health insurance, fundamentally making individual decisions and selective contracts between GKVs and service providers impossible. Since 2003, there have been applications to the G-BA from the GKV and the Federal Association of Statutory Health Insurance Physicians (KBV, "Kassenärztliche Bundesvereinigung") to review PET for all indications as mentioned in the drug approval of FDG.

The consultations in the G-BA were carried out comparably efficiently with a positive vote for useful indications of PET in lung cancer by decision of 20.12.2005. Richard Baum was intensively engaged at that time [1]. With this decision, FDG-PET could be included in the S3

D. Hellwig (✉)
Department of Nuclear Medicine, University Hospital Regensburg, Regensburg, Germany
e-mail: dirk.hellwig@klinik.uni-regensburg.de;
Dirk.Hellwig@ukr.de

V. Prasad (ed.), *Beyond Becquerel and Biology to Precision Radiomolecular Oncology: Festschrift in Honor of Richard P. Baum*, https://doi.org/10.1007/978-3-031-33533-4_14

guideline for lung cancer, on which we both participated as delegates of the German Society for Nuclear Medicine [2–4].

Shortly after the positive G-BA decision, a legal amendment with stricter requirements for health technology assessment (HTA) came into effect. The G-BA's consultation practice now preferred randomized trials for the comparative evaluation of diagnostic procedures. On 24.01.2006, the GKVs applied for a new consultation of PET, also in the already reviewed indication of lung cancer.

PET imaging for lung cancer was again assessed by the G-BA and finally included in outpatient care by decision of 18.01.2007. However, the introduction of a billing code for outpatient PET/CT for those with statutory health insurance (and thus the possibility of reimbursement) lasted until 01.01.2016, i.e., more than 10 years after the first positive decision.

As can be seen, the process of HTA in the G-BA is difficult. In contrast to other healthcare systems, HTA in Germany requires prospective comparative proof of relevance regarding patient-related outcomes such as mortality, morbidity or quality of life, even for diagnostic procedures. The comparison of diagnostic test performance or the frequency of changes in patient management is not sufficient for the G-BA, and certainly not from retrospective studies. When strictly applied, the stringent formal rules of the G-BA are hard to bear for a clinically active physician, so I have a certain understanding for Richard Baum's temperamental contribution in a session at which he criticized the consultations in a way not described here, so that he was exempted from further participation.

Over the years, it was possible to demonstrate the usefulness of FDG-PET/CT in Hodgkin's lymphoma, namely for the diagnosis of the viability of residual lymphomas after chemotherapy in order to decide on the need for radiotherapy, so that the G-BA actually included FDG-PET/CT for this indication on 21.10.2010. However, according to the subsequently amended legal framework, at that time it was also imperatively prescribed to exclude a method that had been consulted by the G-BA if the usefulness of this method could not be proven by means of the strict methodological requirements. This mechanism led to the exclusion of FDG-PET/CT also on 21.10.2010 (even in the inpatient sector) for all other lymphoma indications, such as initial staging and restaging after chemotherapy for aggressive lymphomas, even if this is an internationally accepted standard of care.

Only some partial indications, such as the interim staging of aggressive lymphomas after 2 to 4 cycles of chemotherapy, were possible due to ongoing studies under the special guidelines of a so-called suspension order ("Aussetzungsbeschluss").

As the legislature later recognized and corrected, the law at that time contained the risk of a type II statistical error (error of omission), i.e., not to find any usefulness in the testing, although this is actually present. The respective law was amended as of 01.01.2011, but the decisions on lymphomas from that time are still effective to a large extent and make our daily work more difficult.

After lengthy consultations, which cannot be presented here in an exhaustive manner, only a few PET/CT indications have so far been transferred to patient care and reimbursement in Germany.

The applications for HTA of PET and PET/CT were withdrawn by the previous applicants on 11.07.2018 and 20.09.2018, respectively, for all indications applied for except for the indications of PET in lung cancer, head and neck tumors, and malignant lymphomas. Following this withdrawal of the application, the G-BA decided on 20.11.2020 to largely discontinue the HTA of PET/CT. This termination of consultations is accompanied by the lifting of the categorical exclusion in the outpatient sector, but without the additional inclusion of further PET/CT indications.

Whether the termination of the consultation on PET/CT, which has been largely inconclusive for more than 20 years, is a systemic failure must now (status 21.11.2020) be assessed by the Federal Ministry of Health as the legal supervisor of the G-BA.

Perhaps the current "reset" offers the chance to bring urgently needed PET/CT indications into patient care and reimbursement by new targeted applications to the G-BA. This requires the cooperation of colleagues from the field of nuclear medicine who are as committed as Richard Baum can be for important tasks.

References

1. Baum RP, Hellwig D, Mezzetti M. Position of nuclear medicine modalities in the diagnostic workup of cancer patients: lung cancer. Q J Nucl Med Mol Imaging. 2004;48:119–42.

2. Goeckenjan G, Sitter H, Thomas M, et al. Prevention, diagnosis, therapy, and follow-up of lung cancer. Pneumologie. 2010;64(Suppl 2):e1–164.

3. Goeckenjan G, Sitter H, Thomas M, et al. Prevention, diagnosis, therapy, and follow-up of lung cancer: interdisciplinary guideline of the German Respiratory Society and the German Cancer Society. Pneumologie. 2011;65:39–59.

4. Hellwig D, Baum RP, Kirsch C. FDG-PET, PET/CT and conventional nuclear medicine procedures in the evaluation of lung cancer: a systematic review. Nuklearmedizin. 2009;48:59–69, quiz N58–59.

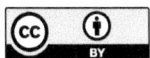

Precision Oncology with PSMA-Targeted α-Particle Therapy of mCRPC

15

Hossein Jadvar

15.1 Introduction

Metastatic castrate-resistant prostate cancer (mCRPC) is incurable. Patients with oligometastatic disease (typically defined as fewer than 3–5 metastases that are evident on imaging) may be candidates for metastasis-directed therapies (e.g., metastatectomy, stereotactic body radiotherapy). There have been major recent strides in approved therapeutic armamentarium in patients with multiple sites of mCRPC including the next-generation microtubule inhibitor, cabazitaxel, agents that target androgen axis, such as abiraterone acetate (androgen synthesis inhibitor) and enzalutamide (androgen receptor antagonist), sipuleucel-T immunotherapy (cancer vaccine), and α-particle therapy of bone lesions with $^{223}RaCl_2$.

(Chapter in: Beyond Becquerel and Biology to Precision Radiomolecular Oncology: Festschrift in Honor of Richard P. Baum).

H. Jadvar (✉)
Division of Nuclear Medicine and Molecular Imaging Center, Department of Radiology, Keck School of Medicine, University of Southern California, Los Angeles, CA, USA
e-mail: jadvar@med.usc.edu

15.2 Prostate-Specific Membrane Antigen as Biological Target

Prostate-specific membrane antigen (PSMA) is a promising target for diagnostics and therapy (theranostics) of prostate cancer. PSMA, also known as folate hydrolase I or glutamate carboxypeptidase II, is a type II, 750-amino-acid transmembrane protein (100–120 kDa), which is anchored in the secretory cells of prostate epithelium, small intestine, proximal renal tubule, salivary glands, and brain. In prostate cancer, PSMA is overexpressed in aggressive primary, recurrent and metastatic tumors and is correlated to androgen independence. PSMA is also overexpressed in neovasculature of many other tumors (e.g., kidney, bladder, pancreas, lung). There have been many designs for radiolabeled agents targeting the PSMA for PET imaging and targeted radionuclide therapy including ^{89}Zr- and ^{64}Cu-labeled anti-PSMA antibodies and antibody fragments, ^{64}Cu-labeled aptamers, and ^{11}C-, ^{18}F-, ^{68}Ga-, ^{64}Cu-, ^{44}Sc-, ^{86}Y-, ^{177}Lu-, ^{225}Ac-, ^{213}Bi-, ^{227}Th-, and $^{203}Pb/^{212}Pb$-labeled low molecular weight inhibitors of the external moiety of PSMA based on glutamate-urea-lysine dimers [1–8].

© The Author(s) 2024
V. Prasad (ed.), *Beyond Becquerel and Biology to Precision Radiomolecular Oncology: Festschrift in Honor of Richard P. Baum*, https://doi.org/10.1007/978-3-031-33533-4_15

15.3   PSMA PET

The most reported small molecule PSMA inhibitor is ^{68}Ga-PSMA-11 (also called HBED-CC) after its clinical introduction in 2012 by the group of investigators from Heidelberg, Germany [9]. Systematic review and meta-analysis studies have demonstrated the high diagnostic performance of ^{68}Ga-PSMA-11 in both initial staging and restaging of prostate cancer leading to major impact on clinical management in about half of the patients [10–14]. Moreover, in the clinical space of biochemical recurrence, several investigations have demonstrated the competitive advantage of ^{68}Ga-PSMA-11 over other relevant PET radiotracers (e.g., radiolabeled choline, ^{18}F-fluciclovine, ^{18}F-NaF) in detecting and localizing disease sites, particularly in the serum PSA levels below 1 ng/mL in which salvage therapy may be most clinically beneficial [15–17]. More recently, PSMA ligands radiolabeled with ^{18}F have been examined primarily due to the advantage of longer half-life (110 min for ^{18}F vs. 68 min for ^{68}Ga) which facilitates regional distribution of the radiotracer without the local need for a gallium generator or a cyclotron, leading to potentially widespread adoption after regulatory and reimbursement approvals [18–20].

15.4   PSMA β-Particle Radioligand Therapy

Apart from the apparent diagnostic advantage of small molecule PSMA inhibitor-based PET agents, these ligands may be radiolabeled to deliver targeted radionuclide therapy locally at the PSMA overexpressing disease sites, in accordance with the theranostic concept. There have been major recent strides in β-particle radioligand therapy with ^{177}Lu-PSMA-617 in patients with mCRPC that have yielded promising results. These mostly retrospective studies have generally demonstrated that ^{177}Lu-PSMA has low toxicity profile and is effective even in patients who have been pre-treated heavily and are refractory to standard therapies [21–31]. In a recent single-center prospective phase II clinical trial, 30 patients with high PSMA expression on ^{68}Ga-PSMA-11 PET/CT (defined as a site of metastatic disease with intensity significantly greater than normal liver – standardized uptake value [SUV]max of tumor involvement at least 1.5 times mean SUV of liver –, and no FDG-positive disease without high PSMA expression) received intravenously a mean radioactivity of 7.5 GBq per cycle of ^{177}Lu-PSMA-617 (up to 4 cycles at 6 weeks interval) [32]. The primary endpoint was PSA response according to the Prostate Cancer Clinical Trial Working Group criteria defined as a greater than 50% PSA decline from the pre-therapy baseline value. Seventeen of 30 patients (57%, 95% confidence interval [CI]; 37–75%) achieved a PSA decline of 50% or more. Objective response in nodal or visceral disease was noted in 82% of those patients with measurable disease. Grade 1 or 2 xerostomia, nausea, and fatigue were reported by 87%, 50%, and 50% of patients, respectively. Grade 3 or 4 thrombocytopenia was recorded in 13% of patients. These encouraging results received much publicity and led to development of procedure guidelines as an "unproven intervention in clinical practice in accordance with the best currently available knowledge" and paved the way for currently ongoing randomized clinical trials [33, 34].

TheraP trial (NCT03392428) is an open-label, 1:1 randomized, stratified, two-arm multicenter phase II trial (ANZUP 1603) designed to compare ^{177}Lu-PSMA-617 radioligand therapy (8.5 GBq decreasing by 0.5 GBq per cycle i.v. every 6 weeks, for up to a maximum of six cycles) to cabazitaxel (20 mg/m^2 i.v. every 3 weeks with prednisolone 10 mg daily orally, for a maximum of 10 cycles) in 200 patients [35]. The primary endpoint is PSA response with a number of other secondary endpoints including overall survival, progression-free survival (PFS), radiographic PFS, PSA PFS, etc. Eligibility criteria include prior docetaxel chemotherapy, rising PSA level, and no discordant FDG-avid PSMA-negative sites of disease. TheraP trial commenced in January 2018 and is currently ongoing with enrollment.

The *VISION trial* (NCT03511664) is an international, multicenter, 2:1 randomized, phase III trial comparing 177Lu-PSMA-617 radioligand therapy (7.4 GBq per cycle i.v. every 6 weeks for 4 to 6 cycles) plus best standard of care versus only best standard of care in patients with mCRPC who have PSMA-positive disease and have received at least one prior taxane and novel anti-androgen axis therapies [36]. The primary outcome measure is overall survival. The trial has concluded accrual of 814 patients. The favorable results of the trial have been published (Sartor O et al, N Eng J Med 2021; PMID: 34161051). Other notable trials include the *PRINCE trial* combining ^{177}Lu-PSMA-617 radioligand therapy with immunotherapy (pembroluzimab), *LuPARP trial* combining ^{177}Lu-PSMA-617 radioligand therapy with olaparib (DNA damage repair inhibitor), *UpFrontPSMA trial* that compares upfront ^{177}Lu-PSMA-617 and anti-androgen therapy followed by docetaxel versus only anti-androgen therapy and docetaxel, and *LuTectomy trial* in patients with high risk localized prostate cancer and high PSMA expression who will receive 1–2 cycles of ^{177}Lu-PSMA-617 followed in 6–8 weeks with radical prostatectomy and pelvic lymph node dissection.

15.5 PSMA α-Particle Radioligand Therapy

Alpha particle is a positively charged helium ion with typical kinetic energy of 5 MeV, a high linear energy transfer of about 80 keV/mm, and a short path travel (50–80 mm). α-particles can deposit large amount of energy locally that may lead to cellular apoptosis, independent of cellular oxygenation, through catastrophic double-strand DNA breaks in the nucleus [37–39].

15.5.1 Actinium-225

Actinium-225 (^{225}Ac) is a useful α-emailer in targeted radionuclide therapy. It has a half-life of 9.9 days and decays to [209]Bi (half-life of 1.9×10^{19} years) through net production of 4 α-particles with energies in the range of 5.8–8.4 MeV at tissue travel distance of 47–85 μm, 2

β-particles, and γ emissions at 218 KeV and 440 KeV. [225]Ac may be sourced from [229]Th with current worldwide production of approximately 68 GBq per year which is anticipated to grow [40–42].

There are several preclinical studies that have demonstrated the potential utility of [225]Ac for targeted therapy in various malignancies including prostate cancer [43]. Kelly et al. showed that a single dose of 148 kBq [225]Ac conjugated to albumin-binding prostate-specific membrane antigen (PSMA)-targeting RPS-074 ([225]Ac-RPS-074) in LNCaP xenograft mouse model of human prostate cancer induced a complete response in 6 of 7 tumors without major toxic effects [44]. More recently, researchers reported on a useful mouse model of human metastatic prostate cancer by injecting C4–2 cells into the left ventricle of immunodeficient male NSG mice which was then used to evaluate the effectiveness of [225]Ac-PSMA-617 at various disease stages [45]. This preclinical study suggested that early [225]Ac-PSMA-617 intervention may be efficacious in the setting of widespread metastatic prostate cancer. Delivery to tumor may also be accomplished by loading [225]Ac into PEGylated liposomes targeted to mouse antihuman PSMA J591 antibody or A10 PSMA aptamer [46]. Liposomes when loaded with [225]Ac or other α-emitters are attractive delivery systems since they can be decorated in different ways selectively to enhance therapeutic efficacy [47].

There has been much interest in the potential efficacy of [225]Ac-labeled PSMA-targeted in the treatment of patients with mCRPC [48]. The results of these small case series have been encouraging with remarkably favorable responses in individual patients albeit at a potential cost of xerostomia [49] (Fig. 15.1). Kratochwil and colleagues reported on dosimetry estimates and empiric dose finding for targeted therapy of mCRPC with [225]Ac-PSMA-617 [50]. They found that a treatment activity of 100 kBq/kg of [225]Ac-PSMA-617 per cycle every 8 weeks was an apparent optimal trade-off between toxicity and biochemical efficacy. Swimmer-plot analysis has indicated favorable duration of tumor control even in the prognostically unfavorable clinical

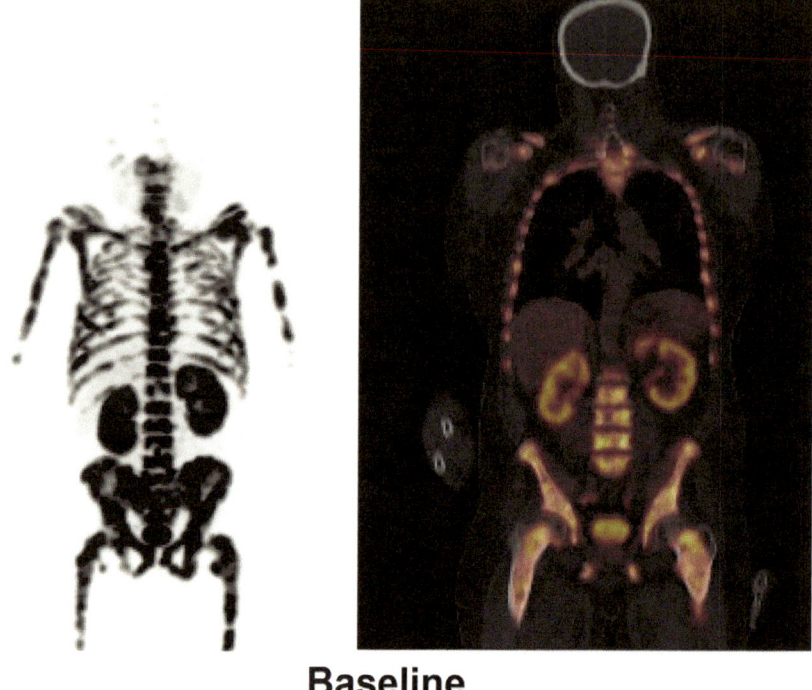

Baseline

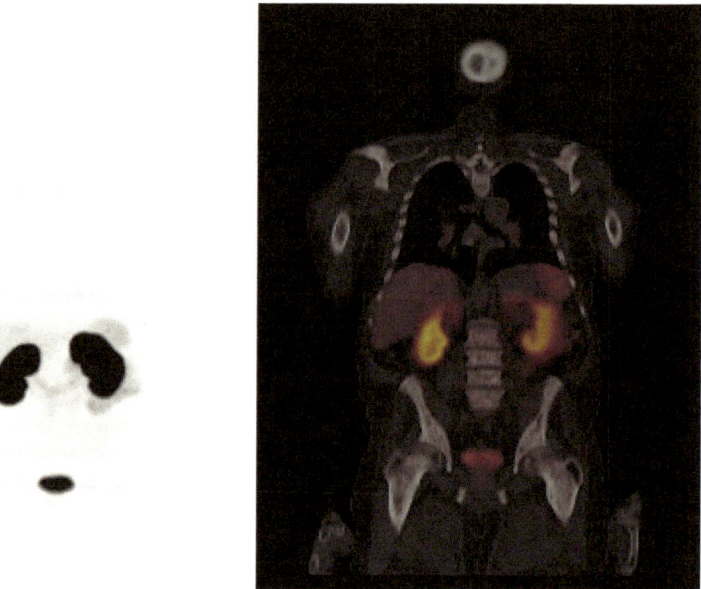

Post-Treatment

Fig. 15.1 67-year-old male with a history of prostate cancer (Gleason score 4 + 5) who was initially treated with prostatectomy and androgen deprivation therapy now presenting with extensive castration-resistant skeletal metastases. The upper panel shows baseline ^{68}Ga-PSMA-11 PET (left) and fused PET/CT (right) before treatment. The lower panel shows ^{68}Ga-PSMA-11 PET (left) and fused PET/CT (right) after 3 cycles of therapy with [225]Ac-PSMA-617. The post-therapy scans demonstrate remarkable response to radioligand therapy. The serum PSA declined from a baseline of 474.63 ng/mL to a post-treatment value of 0.14 ng/mL. There were no significant changes in hemoglobin and platelet counts and the glomerular filtration rate. (Courtesy of Dr. Mike Sathekge, University of Pretoria and Steve Biko Academic Hospital, South Africa)

setting of mCRPC with xerostomia as the main cause for discontinuation of therapy [51]. Kratochwil et al. also recently reported on their observation that patients who were resistant to ^{225}Ac-PSMA-617 often harbored mutations in DNA-damage repair and checkpoint genes suggesting that combination treatment with poly(ADP-ribose)-polymerase (PARP) inhibitors might be efficacious [52].

Recently, Khreish and colleagues reported on a retrospective study of tandem therapy of mCRPC with ^{225}Ac-PSMA-617/^{177}Lu-PSMA-617 [53]. This limited study showed that a single course of tandem therapy with low activity ^{225}Ac-PSMA-617 (range 1.5–7.9 MBq) following a full-activity ^{177}Lu-PSMA-617 (range 5.0–1.6 GBq) may be therapeutically efficacious with minimal additional adverse events such as xerostomia. Rathke et al. suggested that ^{225}Ac-PSMA-617 therapy may exert both an inflammatory and a direct radiation effect on the salivary glands that may lead to slavery gland dysfunction and xerostomia [54].

15.5.2 Bismuth-213

Bismuth-213 (^{213}Bi) is an α-emitter that has received attention for potential clinical use. ^{213}Bi emits both α (~92.7%) and β (~7.3%) particles with a relatively short half-life of 46 min. The 8.375 MeV α particle that is emitted by ^{213}Po along the decay path of ^{213}Bi comprises more than 98% of the α-particle energy from ^{213}Bi disintegration [55]. The decay cascade also includes 26.1% probability of 440 KeV γ-ray emission that enable imaging.

An in-vitro and LNCaP xenograft animal model study of two PSMA targeted α-radioligands (^{213}Bi-PSMA I&T and ^{213}Bi-JVZ-008) confirmed α-particle induced double-strand DNA damage [56]. An investigation using a prostate cancer animal model compared ^{213}Bi-DOTA-PESIN (DOTA-PEG(4)-bombesin) and ^{213}Bi-AMBA (DO3A-CH(2)CO-8-aminooctanoyl-Q-W-A-V-G-H-L-M-NH(2)) with ^{177}Lu-DOTA-PESIN reported that α-particle agent therapy was more efficacious than the counterpart β-particle agent

therapy [57]. McDevitt and colleagues used ^{213}Bi-J591 targeted to PSMA directed against androgen-sensitive LNCaP spheroids resulting in significantly improved median tumor-free survival [58].

Sathekge et al. from South Africa presented a case report of a patient with mCRPC who demonstrated exceptional response to ^{213}Bi-PSMA-617 therapy [59]. Kratochwil et al. estimated the dosimetry with ^{213}Bi-PSMA-617 based on extrapolation of ^{68}Ga-PSMA-617 PET imaging data to half-life of ^{213}Bi and compared the results to those for ^{225}Ac-PSMA-617 [60]. These authors concluded that the higher perfusion-dependent off-target radiation and the shorter physical half-life of ^{213}Bi in comparison to the longer biological half-life of PSMA-617 in dose-limiting organs renders ^{213}Bi as a second-choice radiolabel for PSMA-targeted α-particle therapy.

15.5.3 Thorium-227

Thorium-227 (^{227}Th) is another α-emitting radio-isotope that is gaining traction in targeted radionuclide therapy of cancer. It has a half-life of 19 days decaying first to ^{223}Ra and then follows the decay of ^{223}Ra. Hammer et al. described the preclinical efficacy of ^{227}Th-PSMA conjugates in PDX models of prostate cancer which prompted a currently ongoing phase I trial in patients with mCRPC (NCT03724747) [61]. This trial is being conducted by Bayer Inc. using the investigational drug ^{227}Th-PSMA targeted conjugate, BAY 2315497.

15.5.4 Lead-212

Lead-212 (^{212}Pb) is a β-emitter (half-life 10.64 h) and serves as an in-vivo nanogenerator of ^{212}Bi (half-life 1.01 h) which decays to stable ^{208}Pb via α-particle emission. Yong and Brechbiel have published comprehensive reviews of potential utility of ^{212}Pb in targeted α-particle therapy of cancer [62, 63]. In a recently reported preclinical study, the small molecular PSMA ligand, ^{212}Pb-

NG001, was compared to the commonly used DOTA-based PSMA agent in mice bearing C4–2 human prostate cancer xenografts [64]. While both agents had similar binding, cellular internalization, and tumor uptake, the ^{212}Pb-NG001 compound displayed 2.5-fold lower kidney uptake than the DOTA-conjugated compound. The researchers from the Johns Hopkins University reported recently on a proof-of-concept therapy study of dose-dependent inhibition of human prostate tumor growth in PSMA+ tumors implanted in animal hosts [65]. The tumor evolution could also be monitored with scintigraphy using the surrogate radionuclide, ^{203}Pb (half-life 51.9 h, $\gamma = 279$ KeV) using single-photon computed tomography, supporting the notion of ^{203}Pb/^{212}Pb as a suitable theranostic radionuclide pair [66].

15.5.5 Terbium-149

Terbium-149 (^{149}Tb) is an α-emitter (16.7%) and positron emitter (83.3%) with a half-life of 4.1 h, produced with commercial cyclotrons using a proton beam with energies up to 70 MeV, and can be useful clinically for targeted radionuclide therapy [67]. Umbricht et al. investigated ^{149}Tb-PSMA-617 for targeted α-therapy of mice bearing PSMA-positive PC-3 xenograft tumors [68]. When compared to control untreated mice, the median lifetime of treated mice was almost twice longer than that in untreated mice. The positron emission also allowed imaging localization of tumor sites with PET/CT. Of note, Muller and colleagues have also reported on first-in-human study of PET imaging of prostate cancer with ^{152}Tb-PSMA-617 and on targeted radionuclide therapy of mouse model of human prostate cancer with the β-particle emitting agent ^{161}Tb-PSMA-617 [69, 70].

15.6   Summary

The research and development with α-particle emitting PSMA targeted agents will provide new pathways for safe and effective therapy of meta-static prostate cancer. These novel agents when used in sequence or in combination with β-particle PSMA-based therapy or other standard drug regimens are anticipated to significantly improve the outcome of patients not only in terms of overall survival but also in terms of quality-of-life measures.

References

1. Rahbar K, Afshar-Oromieh A, Jadvar H, Ahamadzadehfar H. PSMA theranostics: current status and future directions. Mol Imaging. 2018;17:153601211877606.
2. Arsenault F, Beauregard JM, Pouliot F. Prostate-specific membrane antigen for prostate cancer theranostics: from imaging to targeted therapy. Curr Opin Support Palliat Care. 2018;12:359–65.
3. Kulkarni HR, Singh A, Langbein T, et al. Theranostics of prostate cancer: from molecular imaging to precision molecular radiotherapy targeting the prostate specific membrane antigen. Br J Radiol. 2018;91:20180308.
4. Wustermann T, Haberkorn U, Babich J, Mier W. Targeting prostate cancer: prostate-specific membrane antigen based diagnosis and therapy. Med Res Rev. 2019;39:40–69.
5. Awang ZH, Essler M, Ahmadzadehfar H. Radioligand therapy of metastatic castration-resistant prostate cancer: current approaches. Radiat Oncol. 2018;13:98.
6. Ahamadzadehfar H, Wegen S, Yordanova A, et al. Overall survival and response pattern of castration-resistant metastatic prostate cancer to multiple cycles of radioligand therapy using [^{177}Lu]Lu-PSMA-617. Eur J Nucl Med Mol Imaging. 2017;44:1448–54.
7. Farolfi A, Fendler W, Iravani A, et al. Theranostics for advanced prostate cancer: current indications and future developments. Eur Urol Oncol. 2019;2:152–62.
8. Lutje S, Heskamp S, Cornelissen AS, et al. PSMA ligands for radionuclide imaging and therapy of prostate cancer: clinical status. Theranostics. 2015;5:1388–401.
9. Eder M, Schafer M, Bauder-Wust U, et al. ^{68}Ga-complex lipophilicity and the targeting property of a urea-based PSMA inhibitor for PET imaging. Bioconjug Chem. 2012;23:688–97.
10. Hope TA, Goodman JZ, Allen IE, et al. Systematic review and metaanalysis of ^{68}Ga-PSMA-11 PET accuracy for detection of prostate cancer validated by histopathology. J Nucl Med. 2019;60:786–93.
11. Han S, Woo S, Kim YJ, Suh CH. Impact of ^{68}Ga-PSMA PET on the management of patients with prostate cancer: a systematic review and meta-analysis. Eur Urol. 2018;74:179–90.
12. Von Eyben FE, Picchio M, von Eyben R, et al. ^{68}Ga-labeled prostate-specific membrane antigen

ligand positron emission tomography/computed tomography for prostate cancer: a systematic review and meta-analysis. Eur Urol Focus. 2018;4:686–93.

13. Lenzo NP, Meyrick D, Turner JH. Review of Gallium-68 PET/CT imaging in the management of prostate cancer. Diagnostics (Basel). 2018;8(1):E16.

14. Eapen RS, Nzenza TC, Murphy DG, et al. PSMA PET applications in the prostate cancer journey: from diagnosis to theranostics. World J Urol. 37:1255–61.

15. Zhou J, Gou Z, Wu R, et al. Comparison of PSMA-PET/CT, choline PET/CT, NaF PET/CT, MRI, and bone scintigraphy in the diagnosis of bone metastases in patients with prostate cancer: systematic review and meta-analysis. Skeletal Radiol. 2019;48:1915–24.

16. Calais J, Ceci F, Eiber M, et al. [18F]-fluciclovine PET-CT and [68Ga]-PSMA-11 PET-CT in patients with early biochemical recurrence after prostatectomy: a prospective, single-center, single-arm, comparative imaging trial. Lancet Oncol. 2019;20:1286–94.

17. Treglia G, Pereira Mestre R, Ferrari M, et al. Radiolabeled choline versus PSMA PET/CT in prostate cancer restaging: a meta-analysis. Am J Nucl Med Mol Imaging. 2019;9:127–39.

18. Giesel FL, Knorr K, Spohn F, et al. Detection efficacy of [18F]-PSMA-1007 PET/CT in 251 patients with biochemical recurrence of prostate cancer after radical prostatectomy. J Nucl Med. 2019;60:362–8.

19. Eiber M, Kronke M, Wurzer A, et al. 18F-rhPSMA-7 positron emission tomography for the detection of biochemical recurrence of prostate cancer following radical prostatectomy. J Nucl Med. 2019;18:e684. [Epub ahead of print].

20. Chen Y, Pullamvhatla M, Foss CA, et al. 2-(3-{1-Carboxy-5-[(6-[18F]fluoro-pyridine-3-carbonyl)-amino]-pentyl}-ureido)-pentanedioic acid, [18F]DCFPyL, a PSMA-based PET imaging agent for prostate cancer. Clin Cancer Res. 2011;17:7645–53.

21. Yadav MP, Ballal S, Shaoo RK, et al. Radioligand therapy with ^{177}Lu-PSMA for metastatic castration-resistant prostate cancer: a systematic review and meta-analysis. AJR Am J Roentgenol. 2019;213:275–85.

22. Baum RP, Kulkarni HR, Schuchardt C, et al. ^{177}Lu-labeled prostate-specific membrane antigen Radioligand therapy of metastatic castration-resistant prostate cancer: safety and efficacy. J Nucl Med. 2016;57:1006–13.

23. Kim YJ, Kim YI. Therapeutic responses and survival effects of ^{177}Lu-PSMA-617 Radioligand therapy in metastatic castrate-resistant prostate cancer: a meta-analysis. Clin Nucl Med. 2018;43:728–73.

24. Ahmadzadehfar H, Rahbar K, Essler M, Biersack HJ. PSMA-based theranostics: a step-by-step practical approach to diagnosis and therapy for mCRPC patients. Semin Nucl Med. 2020;50:98–109.

25. Rahbar K, Ahmadzadehfar H, Kratochwil C, et al. German multicenter study investigating ^{177}Lu-PSMA-617 radioligand therapy in advanced prostate cancer patients. J Nucl Med. 2017;58:85–90.

26. Beheshti M, Heinzel A, von Mallek D, et al. Prostate-specific membrane antigen radioligand therapy of prostate cancer. Q J Nucl Med Mol Imaging. 2019;63:29–36.

27. Siva S, Udovicich C, Tran B, et al. Expanding the role of small-molecule PSMA ligands beyond PET staging of prostate cancer. Nat Rev Urol. 2020;17:107–18.

28. Virgolini I, Decristoforo C, Haug A, et al. Current status of theranostics in prostate cancer. Eur J Nucl Med Mol Imaging. 2018;45:471–95.

29. Ferdinandus J, Violet J, Sandhu S, Hofman MS. Prostate-specific membrane antigen theranostics: therapy with lutetium-177. Curr Opin Urol. 2018;28:197–204.

30. Emmett L, Willowson K, Violet J, et al. Lutetium-177 PSMA radionuclide therapy for men with prostate cancer: a review of the current literature and discussion of practical aspects of therapy. J Med Radiat Sci. 2017;64:52–60.

31. Kulkarni HR, Singh A, Schuchardt C, et al. PSMA-based radioligand therapy for metastatic castration-resistant prostate cancer: the Bad Berka experience since 2013. J Nucl Med. 2016;57(Suppl 3):97S–104S.

32. Hofman MS, Violet J, Hicks RJ, et al. [177Lu]-PSMA-617 radionuclide treatment in patients with metastatic castration-resistant prostate cancer (LuPSMA trial): a single-center, single-arm, phase 2 study. Lancet Oncol. 2018;19:825–33.

33. Kratochwil C, Fendler WP, Eiber M, et al. EANM procedure guidelines for radionuclide therapy with ^{177}Lu-labelled PSMA-ligands (^{177}Lu-PSMA-RLT). Eur J Nucl Med Mol Imaging. 2019;46:2536–44.

34. Iravani A, Violet J, Azad A, Hofman MS. Leutetium-177 prostate-specific membrane antigen (PSMA) theranostics: practical nuances and intricacies. Prostate Cancer Prostatic Dis. 2020;23:38–52.

35. Hofman MS, Emmett L, Violet J, et al. TheraP: a randomized phase 2 trial of ^{177}Lu-PSMA-617 theranostic treatment vs cabazitaxel in progressive metastatic castration-resistant prostate cancer (clinical trial protocol ANZUP 1603). BJU Int. 2019;124(Suppl 1):5–13.

36. Rahbar K, Bodei L, Morris MJ. Is the vision of radioligand therapy for prostate cancer becoming a reality? An overview of the phase III VISION trial and its importance for the future of theranostics. J Nucl Med. 2019;60:1504–6.

37. De Vincentis G, Gerritsen W, Gschwend JE, et al. Advances in targeted alpha therapy of prostate cancer. Ann Oncol. 2019;30:1728–39.

38. Chakravarty R, Siamof CM, Dash A, Cai W. Targeted a-therapy of prostate cancer using radiolabeled PSMA inhibitors: a game changer in nuclear medicine. Am J Nucl Med Mol Imaging. 2018;20:247–67.

39. Jadvar H. Targeted a-therapy in cancer management: synopsis of preclinical and clinical studies. Cancer Biother Radiopharm. 2020;35:475. [Epub ahead of print].

40. Morgenstern A, Apostolidis C, Kratochwil C, et al. An overview of targeted alpha therapy with [225]Actinium and [213]Bismuth. Curr Radiopharm. 2018;11:200–8.

41. Mulford DA, Scheinberg DA, Jurcic JG. The promise of targeted α-particle therapy. J Nucl Med. 2005;46:198S–204S.

42. Harvey JT. NorthStar perspectives for actinium-225 production at commercial scale. Curr Radiopharm. 2018;11:180–91.

43. Scheinberg DA, McDevitt MR. Actinium-225 in targeted alpha-particle therapeutic applications. Curr Radiopharm. 2011;4:306–20.

44. Kelly JM, Amor-Coarasa A, Ponnala S, et al. A single dose of [225]Ac-RPS-074 induces a complete tumor response in LNCaP xenograft model. J Nucl Med. 2018;60:649. [Epub ahead of print].

45. Stuparu AD, Meyer CAL, Evans-Axelsson SL, et al. Targeted alpha therapy in a systemic mouse model of prostate cancer—a feasibility study. Theranostics. 2020;10:2612. [Epub ahead of print].

46. Bandekar A, Zhu C, Jindal R, et al. Anti-prostate-specific membrane antigen liposomes loaded with [225]Ac for potential targeted antivascular a-particle therapy of cancer. J Nucl Med. 2014;55:107–14.

47. Chang MY, Seiderman J, Sofou S. Enhanced loading efficiency and retention of [225]Ac in rigid liposomes for potential targeted therapy of micrometastases. Bioconjug Chem. 2008;19:1274–982.

48. Kratochwil C, Haberkorn U, Giesel FL. [225]Ac-PSMA-617 for therapy of prostate cancer. Semin Nucl Med. 2020;50:133–40.

49. Kratochwil C, Bruchertseifer F, Giesel FL, et al. [225]Ac-PSMA-617 for PSMA-targeted α-radiation therapy of metastatic castration resistant prostate cancer. J Nucl Med. 2016;57:1941–4.

50. Kratochwil C, Bruchertseifer F, Rathke H, et al. Targeted a-therapy of metastatic castration-resistant prostate cancer with [225]Ac-PSMA-617: dosimetry estimates and empiric dose finding. J Nucl Med. 2017;58:1624–31.

51. Kratochwil C, Bruchertseifer F, Rathke H, et al. Targeted a-therapy of metastatic castration-resistant prostate cancer with [225]Ac-PSMA-617: swimmers-plot analysis suggests efficacy regarding duration of tumor control. J Nucl Med. 2018;59:795–802.

52. Kratochwil C, Giesel FL, Heussel CP, et al. Patients resistant against PSMA-targeting alpha-radiation therapy often harbor mutations in DNA-repair associated genes. J Nucl Med. 2020;61:683. [Epub ahead of print].

53. Khreish F, Ebert N, Ries M, et al. [225]Ac-PSMA-617/^{177}Lu-PSMA-617 tandem therapy of metastatic castration-resistant prostate cancer: pilot experience. Eur J Nucl Med Mol Imaging. 2020;47:721–8.

54. Rathke H, Kratochwil C, Hohenberger R, et al. Initial experience performing sialendoscopy for salivary gland protection in patients undergoing [225]Ac-PSMA-617 RLT. Eur J Nucl Med Mol Imaging. 2019;46:139–47.

55. Morgenstern A, Bruchertseifer F, Apostolidis C. Targeted alpha therapy with [213]Bi. Curr Radiopharm. 2011;4:295–305.

56. Nonnekens J, Chatalic KL, Molkenboer-Kuenen JD, et al. [213]Bi-labeled prostate-specific membrane antigen targeting agents induce DNA double-strand breaks in prostate cancer xenografts. Cancer Biother Radiopharm. 2017;32:67–73.

57. Wild D, Frischknerdt M, Zhang H, et al. Alpha- and beta-particle radiopeptide therapy in a human prostate cancer model ([213]Bi-DOTA-PESIN and [213]Bi-AMBA versus 177Lu-DOTA-PESIN). Cancer Res. 2011;71:1009–18.

58. McDevitt MR, Barendswaard E, Ma D, et al. An alpha-particle emitting antibody ([[213]Bi]J591) for radioimmunotherapy of prostate cancer. Cancer Res. 2000;60:6095–100.

59. Sathekge M, Knoesen O, Meckel M, et al. [213]Bi-PSMA-617 targeted alpha-radionuclide therapy in metastatic castration-resistant prostate cancer. Eur J Nucl Med Mol Imaging. 2017;44:1099–100.

60. Kratochwil C, Schmidt K, Afshar-Oromieh A, et al. Targeted alpha therapy of mCRPC: dosimetry estimates of [213]Bismuth-PSMA-617. Eur J Nucl Med Mol Imaging. 2018;45:31–7.

61. Hammer S, Hagemann UB, Zitzmann-Kolbe S, et al. Preclinical efficacy of a PSMA-targeted thorium-227 conjugate (PSMA-TTC), a targeted alpha therapy for prostate cancer. Clin Cancer Res. 2019;26:1985. [Epub ahead of print].

62. Yong K, Brechbiel MW. Application of [212]Pb for targeted a-particle therapy (TAT): pre-clinical and mechanistic understanding through to clinical translation. AIMS Med Sci. 2015;2:228–45.

63. Yong K, Brechbiel MW. Towards translation of [212]Pb as a clinical therapeutic; getting the lead in! Dalton Trans. 2011;40:6068–76.

64. Stenberg VY, Juzeniene A, Chen Q, et al. Preparation of the alpha-emitting prostate-specific membrane antigen targeted radioligand [212]Pb-NG001 for prostate cancer. J Labelled Comp Radiopharm. 2020;63:129–43.

65. Banerjee SR, Minn I, Kumar V, et al. Preclinical evaluation of [203/212]Pb-labeled low-molecular weight compounds for targeted radiopharmaceutical therapy of prostate cancer. J Nucl Med. 2020;61:80–8.

66. Dos Santos JC, Schafer M, Bauder-Wust U, et al. Development and dosimetry of [203]Pb/[212]Pb-labeled PSMA ligands: bringing the lead into PSMA-targeted alpha therapy. Eur J Nucl Med Mol Imaging. 2019;46:1081–91.

67. Muller C, Singh A, Umbricht CA, et al. Preclinical investigations and first-in-human application of [152]Tb-PSMA-617 for PET/CT imaging of prostate cancer. EJNMMI Res. 2019;9:68.

68. Umbricht CA, Koster U, Bernhardt P, et al. Alpha-PET for prostate cancer: preclinical investigation using [149]Tb-PSMA-617. Sci Rep. 2019;9:17800.

69. Muller C, Umbricht CA, Gracheva N, et al. Terbium-161 for PSMA-targeted radionuclide ther-

apy of prostate cancer. Eur J Nucl Med Mol Imaging. 2019;46:1919–30.

70. Muller C, Vermeulen C, Koster U, et al. Alpha-PET with terbium-149: evidence and perspectives for radio-theragnostics. EJNMMI Radiopharm Chem. 2017;1:5. https://doi.org/10.1186/s41181-016-0008-2.

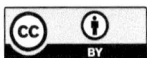

From Radioimmunodetection to Radiomolecular Precision Oncology Via Radionanotargeting by Intelligent Multidisciplinary Radiotheragnostic Nanoparticles

16

Kalevi Kairemo

I have been honoured to know Prof. Dr. Richard P. Baum (later Richard) for more than 30 years. Our first encounters happened at the end of 1980s when we both worked with Tc-99m- and In-111-labelled monoclonal antibodies [1–11]. Prof. Dr. Richard P. Baum was then in Frankfurt a Main. Our first meetings took place in European and American Nuclear Medicine conferences or Special monoclonal antibody meetings either in Princeton or San Diego. Typically, Richard Baum was suggesting radical improvements to my work and convincing that his work is much better; anyway, we both made substantial contributions to this field. We started fully new therapies, found new applications and indications, wrote reviews, etc. I considered Richard's criticism most often as a compliment, because I had caused a reaction. I really felt honoured when Prof. Dr. Richard P. Baum after one Society of Nuclear Medicine conference asked me to show my slides, because he could not attend my presentation. In spite of his criticism, I really did not consider Richard Baum as a competitor because my scientific environment and resources in Helsinki were modest as compared to those Richard was able to gain in

Germany. In some occasions, I remember Richard Baum state early 1990s the Americans being "years behind us". We were actively interacting with each other in many, many conferences, but never really made collaborative research.

We were both active in this field ever since, but moved to smaller molecules. We both introduced new concepts, especially Richard. I started to talk about *immuno-PET* in mid-1990s instead of complex radioimmunodetection methods [11]. I also screened a new field of *radionanotargeting,* gene therapy with radionuclides (Fig. 16.1). A long story [12–14] in brief was that this therapy would not be feasible based on my subcellular dosimetry results. But I did not fully get rid of new radioimmunodetection methods, because I introduced new methods, e.g. *radioimmunosynovectomy* in 1990s as well [15]. At this time Richard was very active with peptides, e.g. with his extensive IRIST (International Research Group in Immunoscintigraphy and Immunotherapy) activities. I worked late 1990s in Norway (Norwegian University of Science and Technology).

In the early 2000s I was active in Sweden (Uppsala University Hospital Akademiska), travelling weekly back home to Finland. While I was creating the Uppsala Nuclear Medicine Clinic, Richard was creating Zentralklinik Bad Berka (ZBB) which was early selected as the ENETS Center of Excellence. Simultaneously, I also started a Biotech company in Finland specializing in targeted drug delivery with tumour target-

Festschrift in Honor of Prof. Dr. Richard P. Baum.

K. Kairemo (✉)
Department of Nuclear Medicine & Theragnostics,
Docrates Cancer Center, Helsinki, Finland

V. Prasad (ed.), *Beyond Becquerel and Biology to Precision Radiomolecular Oncology: Festschrift in Honor of Richard P. Baum*, https://doi.org/10.1007/978-3-031-33533-4_16

Nanotargeting oligonucleotide radiotherapy

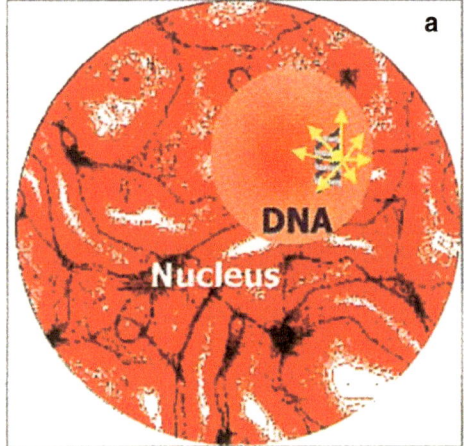

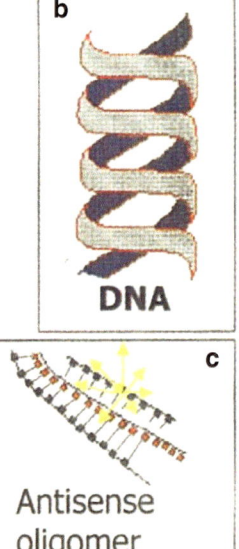

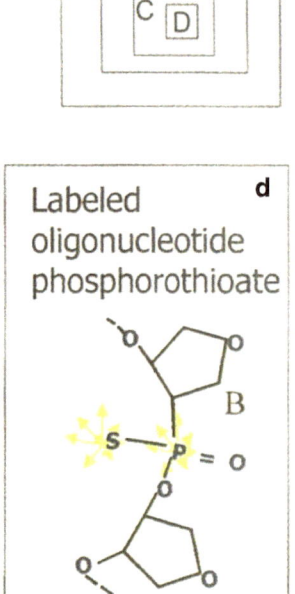

Fig. 16.1 Principle of radionanotargeting with antisense oligonucleotides. Nucleus in a cell schematically (a). 3-D presentation of a DNA double strand (b). Possible triplex formation of an antisense oligonucleotide in a close vicinity of DNA double strand (c). Sulphur (S) or phosphorus (P) atoms are substituted with radioactive 35S-, 32P- or 33P-atoms in oligonucleotide phosphorothioates (d). Oligonucleotide radiotherapy in mid 1990s from [14].

Nanotargeting describes nanometer scale events by antibodies or antisense oligonucleotides. Radioactive sulphur or phosphorus atoms substitute the same atoms in oligonucleotide phosphorothioates, and emitted radiation affects structures close to the binding site of the targeting molecule. Antisense oligonucleotides serve as vehicles for radionuclides, enhancing targeting efficacy

ing phage display peptides. We made progress in this field. Due to "financial toxicity" this new multidisciplinary targeting approach was never applied in clinical trials, even though I had funding for it. My hands were tied because of IPR development, hardly published anything for more than 5 years [16]. In Finland, I developed imaging applications for pharmaceutical industry [17]. Table 16.1 summarizes in nutshell the characteristics of multidisciplinary nanoparticles for theragnostic purposes. It is obvious from Table 16.1 that radionuclide methods will allow most clinical radiotheragnostic applications.

After serving as Clinical Director at Advanced Accelerator Applications (AAA) SA in France, I returned to Helsinki in 2009. Then it was the time for Docrates Cancer Center (DCC), the first full-service private oncology clinic in Nordic countries. Because Uppsala was the Neuroendocrinology Center in Nordic countries,

I was able to start this activity again in Finland and participate at AAA in designing the LutaThera trial. I also went to Bad Berka to attend the 10-year anniversary of Zentralklinik Bad Berka (ZBB) and for the second time, to present voxel-based dosimetry in the first World Congress on Gallium-68 and Peptide Receptor Radionuclide Therapy (PRRNT) (June 23–26, 2011). In Bad Berka I demonstrated voxel-based dosimetry data in clinical routine [18], the key characteristics are shown in Fig. 16.2.

At Docrates Cancer Center my focus has been development of molecular radiotherapy (later theragnostics) and nuclear medicine. For developing an international cancer centre where patients travel from other countries, special methods should be developed. The methods may be related to response evaluation, such as early response or response prediction. Early response is required to see the possible effect for expensive

Table 16.1 Summary of the differences between imaging modalities and their possibilities for nanoparticle applications

Imaging modality	Spatial resolution	Depth	Temporal resolution	Sensitivity (mol/L)	Molecular probe	Nanoparticle design	Clinical applicability
PET	1–2 mm	No limit	10 s–min	10^{-11}–10^{-12}	ng	Label outside, in the membrane, or inside (radionuclide)	E, S, A, P
SPECT	0.5–1 mm	No limit	Min	10^{-10}–10^{-11}	ng	Label outside, in the membrane, or inside(radionuclide)	E, S, A, P
Bio-luminescence	3–5 mm	1–2 mm	Sec–min	10^{-15}–10^{-17}	g–mg	Label inside (or outside), luminescent compound	S, A, P
Fluorescence	2–3 mm	<1 mm	Sec–min	10^{-9}–10^{-12}	g–mg	Label outside or inside, fluorescent compound	S, A, P
MRI	25–100 µm	No limit	Min–hours	10^{-3}–10^{-5}	g–mg	Label outside, in the membrane, or inside, paramagnetic atom, particles	E, P
CT	50–200 µm	No limit	Min	10^{-1}–10^{-4}	N/A	Label inside (or outside), contrast media	–
Ultrasound	50–500 µm	mm–cm	Sec–min	10^{-1}–10^{-4}	g–mg	Label inside, gas-filled particles	E, P

The method characteristics spatial resolution, depth resolution, temporal resolution, sensitivity, and the amount of needed molecular probe are modified from the data in the literature. A active targeting, E external imaging, P passive targeting, S surgery (modified/updated from Kairemo et al., Curr Radiopharm 2008)

DOSE

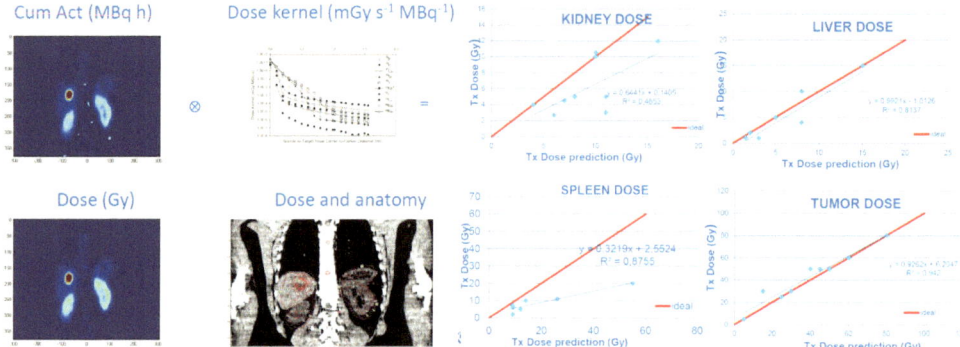

Fig. 16.2 Principle of voxel-based dosimetry for clinical routine. Serial 3D SPECT data allow voxel half-life calculations, which are multiplied by radionuclide characteristics (dose point kernels) in order to obtain absorbed radiation doses in Gy's. With hybrid imaging (SPECT/CT) Gy's can be located anatomically. This method suits also for dose prediction. On the right it is shown in seven patients that tumor and liver doses can be predicted from pre-therapeutic voxel-based dosimetric data using diagnostic doses. The prediction overestimated kidney and spleen doses. (Presented in 2011. Partly published in [18])

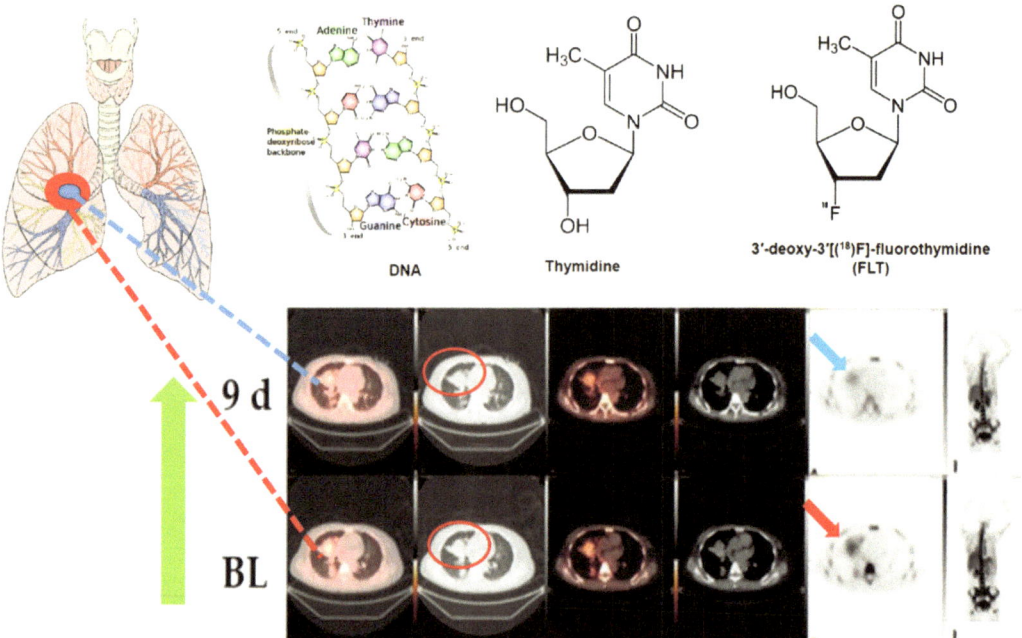

Fig. 16.3 Example of early response assessment in a new targeted therapy for lung cancer. Radiolabelled nucleotide analogue for DNA acts as surrogate marker for cellular proliferation rapidly. Here, a clear response is seen in 9 days. (Presented in the Graphical Abstract of [19])

or sophisticated therapies as early as possible (example Fig. 16.3). Prediction is more important, but more difficult. The world literature is full of prognostic factors, but no real prediction methods exist.

The atmosphere between me and Richard P. Baum has never been competitive, actually, the other way around, stimulating, supportive and synergistic. Our paths have crossed elsewhere as well and in many circumstances. I

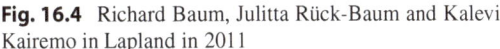

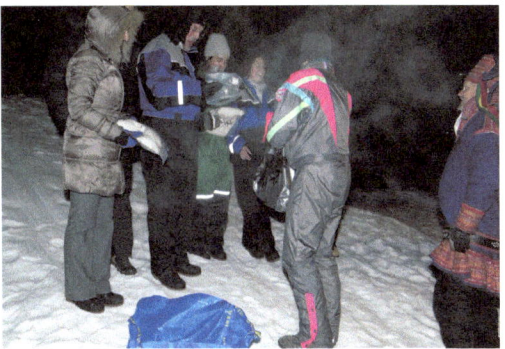

Fig. 16.4 Richard Baum, Julitta Rück-Baum and Kalevi Kairemo in Lapland in 2011

Fig. 16.5 Richard Baum (in blue) receiving the second Prize in the WC of Tandem Skiing. (From Kalevi Kairemo, in grey/ red) in Lapland in 2012

became very much involved with World Association of Radiopharmaceutical Therapy (WARMTH) since 2007 in Mongolia, by attending every WARMTH conference ever since like Richard. In the role of WARMTH President, Richard and his wife Julitta Rück-Baum visited Finnish Lapland 1 year before Levi Conference in Autumn 2011 (Fig. 16.4). I was in Richard's very first Theragnostics World Conference in summer 2011 as mentioned earlier [18].

Besides being active in the Scientific program, Richard is typically very active in the social program. In the seventh ICRT meeting in Levi 2012 Richard received the second prize in Tandem Ski Competition between the seven Continents (Fig. 16.5). And the Oenophilous Dinners, wine from participating countries, is a wonderful invention. Membership fee is three Italian Euros. Wife Julitta kept records of these events (Fig. 16.6).

The Richard's own landmark, the Bad Berka's ENETS Center of Excellence, Institute for Molecular Radiotherapy, later Theragnostics and Precision Oncology, is a unique hospital, based on Prof. Dr. Richard P. Baum's dreams to become a fantastic reality. Richard's own science has been outstanding, typically first injections of new theragnostics tracers, such as the Uppsala affibody molecules [20], new peptides and peptidomimetic compounds in neuroendocrine neoplasms and prostate cancer [21–23]. Richard is known all over the world, he has been a speaker in numerous conferences in every continent. A

picture taken in Teheran at Asia Oceania Congress of Nuclear Medicine and Biology where I am together with RPB and JRB and two Iranian organizers (Fig. 16.7). The theragnostics work requires very much from the clinician. Knowledge of numerous subspecialties is almost essential, I learned when developing my small clinic in Helsinki a lot about external beam radiation therapy, response assessment and development of response criteria for many cancers [24–27].

Thousands of patients from all over the world have got cured in ZBB, only because of Richard's hard work, perseverance and sustainability. The results are extraordinary and there is more to come [28, 29]. I have really been inspired by this and I once again feel really honoured by knowing this great man.

Finally, we have found each other in publications [30, 31]. I know that Richard knows Latin and that he is a friend of deeper understanding and philosophy. So am I, I am a great friend of genealogy. It was written in the stars, that I would become a nuclear medicine physician. *Per aspera ad astra.* One of my ancestors was Helena von Qvanten (since eight generations) verifying that my family was related with quanta (quantum) before they were even discovered in physics [32]. Another strange omen is my relation to the ancient Danish Kings (28 generations back) [32]. The last one, Knud IV was canonized and a church was erected in Odense in 1086 at the site of his violent death. Odense is a famous place, because of scientists such as the great Finn (E.

Fig. 16.6 Oenophilous
Dinner in Lapland 2012

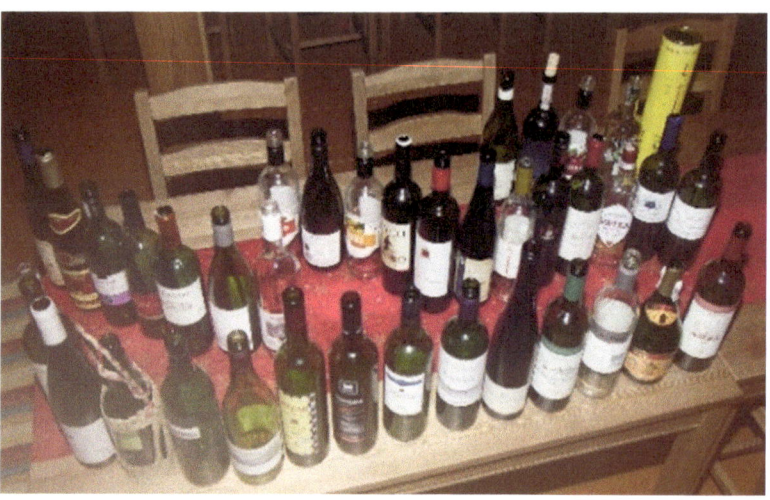

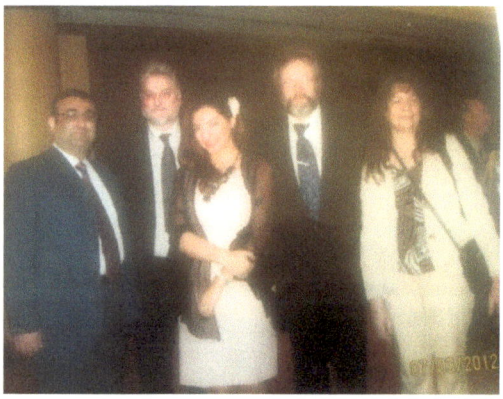

Fig. 16.7 The author and RPB and Julitta with Iranian hosts at AONMB Congress in Teheran

von Eyben [30]) and Fairytales by Hans Christian Andersen. Actually, the German Fairytale Route (Deutsche Märchestrasse) starts from Hanau, nahe bei Frankfurt (am Main) and ends in Bremen, also connecting my and Richard's *alma maters*. My first school abroad was in Bremen in 1973 (Gymnasium an der Parsevalstrasse).

I wish Prof. Dr. Richard P. Baum, the former Chairman and Clinical Director of the Center for Radiomolecular Precision Oncology in Zentralklinik Bad Berka, great success for his new academic initiative in International Centers for Precision Oncology (ICPO).

Sincerely yours
Kalevi Kairemo
Helsinki, January 2020

References

1. Baum RP, Hertel A, Lorenz M, Schwarz A, Encke A, Hör G. 99Tcm-labelled anti-CEA monoclonal antibody for tumour immunoscintigraphy: first clinical results. Nucl Med Commun. 1989;10(5):345–52. Erratum in: Nucl Med Commun 1989 Oct;10(10):772–3.
2. Baum RP. Immunoscintigraphy as a diagnostic tool in pancreatic cancer. Hepatogastroenterology. 1989;36(6):459–61.   Erratum   in: Hepatogastroenterology 1990 Feb;37(1):154.
3. Baum RP, Adams S, Kiefer J, Niesen A, Knecht R, Howaldt HP, Hertel A, Adamietz IA, Sykes T, Boniface GR, et al. A novel technetium-99m labeled monoclonal antibody (174H.64) for staging head and neck cancer by immuno-SPECT. Acta Oncol. 1993;32(7–8):747–51.
4. Baum RP, Niesen A, Hertel A, Adams S, Kojouharoff G, Goldenberg DM, Hör G. Initial clinical results with technetium-99m-labeled LL2 monoclonal antibody fragment in the radioimmunodetection of B-cell lymphomas. Cancer. 1994;73(3 Suppl):896–9.
5. Baum   RP,   Brümmendorf TH.   Radioimmunolocalization   of   primary and metastatic breast cancer. Q J Nucl Med. 1998;42(1):33–42. Review.
6. Kairemo KJA, Hopsu EV. Diagnosis of tumors of the parotid gland with anti-CEA immunoscintigraphy. AJR Am J Roentgenol. 1990;154(6):1259–62.
7. Kairemo KJA, Hopsu EV. Imaging of pharyngeal and laryngeal carcinomas with indium-111-labeled monoclonal anti-CEA antibodies. Laryngoscope. 1990;100(10 Pt 1):1077–82.
8. Kairemo KJA, Wiklund TA, Liewendahl K, Miettinen M, Heikkonen JJ, Virkkunen PJ, Aronen HJ, Blomqvist CP. Imaging of soft-tissue sarcomas with indium-111-labeled monoclonal antimyosin Fab fragments. J Nucl Med. 1990;31(1):23–31.

9. ^{99m}Tc-labeled monoclonal antibody (BW 431/26) reacting with carcinoembryonic antigen in breast cancer. Cancer Res. 1990;50:949s–54s.

10. Kairemo KJA, Aronen HJ, Liewendahl K, Paavonen T, Heikkonen JJ, Virkkunen P, Mäki-Hokkonen H, Karonen SL, Brownell AL, Mäntylä MJ. Radioimmunoimaging of non-small cell lung cancer with ^{111}In- and ^{99m}Tc-labeled monoclonal anti-CEA-antibodies. Acta Oncol. 1993;32(7–8):771–8.

11. Kairemo KJA. Positron emission tomography of monoclonal antibodies. Acta Oncol. 1993;32(7–8):825–30. Review.

12. Kairemo KJA, Tenhunen M, Jekunen AP. Oligoradionuclidetherapy using radiolabelled antisense oligodeoxynucleotide phosphorothioates. Anticancer Drug Des. 1996;11(6):439–49.

13. Kairemo KJA, Tenhunen M, Jekunen AP. Gene therapy using antisense oligodeoxynucleotides labeled with auger-emitting radionuclides. Cancer Gene Ther. 1998;5(6):408–12.

14. Kairemo KJA, Jekunen AP, Tenhunen M. Dosimetry and optimization of in vivo targeting with radiolabeled antisense oligodeoxynucleotides: oligonucleotide radiotherapy. Methods Enzymol. 2000;314:506–24.

15. Kairemo KJA, Strömberg S, Nikula TK, Karonen SL. Expression profile of vascular cell adhesion molecule-1 (CD106) in inflammatory foci using rhenium-188 labelled monoclonal antibody in mice. Cell Adhes Commun. 1998;5(4):325–33.

16. Penate Medina O, Haikola M, Tahtinen M, Simpura I, Kaukinen S, Valtanen H, Zhu Y, Kuosmanen S, Cao W, Reunanen J, Nurminen T, Saris PE, Smith-Jones P, Bradbury M, Larson SM, Kairemo K. Liposomal tumor targeting in drug delivery utilizing MMP-2- and MMP-9-binding ligands. J Drug Deliv. 2011;2011:160515. Epub 2010 Dec 29. https://doi.org/10.1155/2011/160515.

17. Kairemo KJA, Tähtinen M. Radiolabeled compounds in the development of cytotoxic agents. Curr Pharm Des. 2004;10(24):2923–34. Review.

18. Kairemo K, Kangasmäki A. 4D SPECT/CT acquisition for 3D dose calculation and dose planning in (177)Lu-peptide receptor radionuclide therapy: applications for clinical routine. Recent Results Cancer Res. 2013;194:537–50. https://doi.org/10.1007/978-3-642-27994-2_31.

19. Kairemo K, Santos EB, Macapinlac HA, Subbiah V. Early response assessment to targeted therapy using 3′-deoxy-3′[(^{18})F]-Fluorothymidine (^{18}F-FLT) PET/CT in lung cancer. Diagnostics. 2020;10(1):26.

20. Baum RP, Prasad V, Müller D, Schuchardt C, Orlova A, Wennborg A, Tolmachev V, Feldwisch J. Molecular imaging of HER2-expressing malignant tumors in breast cancer patients using synthetic ^{111}In- or ^{68}Ga-labeled affibody molecules. J Nucl Med. 2010;51(6):892–7. Epub 2010 May 19. https://doi.org/10.2967/jnumed.109.073239.

21. Baum RP, Kulkarni HR, Carreras C. Peptides and receptors in image-guided therapy: theranostics for neuroendocrine neoplasms. Semin Nucl Med.

2012;42(3):190–207. https://doi.org/10.1053/j.semnuclmed.2012.01.002.

22. Baum RP, Kulkarni HR, Müller D, Satz S, Danthi N, Kim YS, Brechbiel MW. First-in-human study demonstrating tumor-angiogenesis by PET/CT imaging with (68)Ga-NODAGA-THERANOST, a high-affinity Peptidomimetic for $\alpha v \beta 3$ integrin receptor targeting. Cancer Biother Radiopharm. 2015;30(4):152–9. https://doi.org/10.1089/cbr.2014.1747.

23. Baum RP, Kulkarni HR, Schuchardt C, Singh A, Wirtz M, Wiessalla S, Schottelius M, Mueller D, Klette I, Wester HJ. 177Lu-labeled prostate-specific membrane antigen radioligand therapy of metastatic castration-resistant prostate cancer: safety and efficacy. J Nucl Med. 2016;57(7):1006–13. Epub 2016 Jan 21. https://doi.org/10.2967/jnumed.115.168443.

24. Kairemo KJ. PET/computed tomography for radiation therapy planning of prostate cancer. PET Clin. 2017;12(2):257–67. Epub 2017 Jan 31. Review. https://doi.org/10.1016/j.cpet.2016.12.003.

25. Kairemo K, Joensuu T. Radium-223-dichloride in castration resistant metastatic prostate cancer-preliminary results of the response evaluation using F-18-fluoride PET/CT. Diagnostics (Basel). 2015;5(4):413–27. https://doi.org/10.3390/diagnostics5040413.

26. Kairemo K, Ravizzini GC, Macapinlac HA, Subbiah V. An assessment of early response to targeted therapy via molecular imaging: a pilot study of 3′-deoxy-3′[(18)F]-fluorothymidine positron emission tomography ^{18}F-FLT PET/CT in prostate adenocarcinoma. Diagnostics (Basel). 2017;7(2):E20. https://doi.org/10.3390/diagnostics7020020.

27. Kairemo K, Rohren EM, Anderson PM, Ravizzini G, Rao A, Macapinlac HA, Subbiah V. Development of sodium fluoride PET response criteria for solid tumours (NAFCIST) in a clinical trial of radium-223 in osteosarcoma: from RECIST to PERCIST to NAFCIST. ESMO Open. 2019;4(1):e000439. https://doi.org/10.1136/esmoopen-2018-000439. eCollection.2019.

28. Baum RP, Singh A, Schuchardt C, Kulkarni HR, Klette I, Wiessalla S, Osterkamp F, Reineke U, Smerling C. ^{177}Lu-3BP-227 for Neurotensin receptor 1-targeted therapy of metastatic pancreatic adenocarcinoma: first clinical results. J Nucl Med. 2018;59(5):809–14. Epub 2017 Oct 12. https://doi.org/10.2967/jnumed.117.193847.

29. Baum RP, Kulkarni HR, Singh A, Kaemmerer D, Mueller D, Prasad V, Hommann M, Robiller FC, Niepsch K, Franz H, Jochems A, Lambin P, Hörsch D. Results and adverse events of personalized peptide receptor radionuclide therapy with ^{90}Yttrium and ^{177}Lutetium in 1048 patients with neuroendocrine neoplasms. Oncotarget. 2018;9(24):16932–50.

30. von Eyben FE, Singh A, Zhang J, Nipsch K, Meyrick D, Lenzo N, Kairemo K, Joensuu T, Virgolini I, Soydal C, Kulkarni HR, Baum RP. ^{177}Lu-PSMA radioligand therapy of predominant lymph node metastatic prostate cancer. Oncotarget. 2019;10(25):2451–61.

31. Tulchinsky M, Baum RP, Bennet KG, Freeman LM, Jong I, Kairemo K, Marcus CS, Moadel RM, Suman P. Well-founded recommendations for radio-active iodine treatment of differentiated thyroid cancer require balanced study of benefits and harms. J Clin Oncol. 2018;36(18):1887–8. Epub 2018 May 3. https://doi.org/10.1200/JCO.2018.78.5972.

32. Rantala O-P. Henrik Trapp, esi-isät ja jälkeläiset (Henrik Trapp, ancestors and descendants). Helsinki; 2019. p. 163.

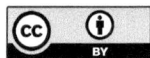

Nuclear Medicine and Surgery on the Way to Personalized Medicine. Ten Years of Clinical and Translational Oncology and Research

17

Daniel Kaemmerer

Surgery with a complete tumor removal is the only therapeutic option with a curative approach in a neuroendocrine tumor disease. Recurrent abdominal surgery is associated with inflammation, altered anatomy, and scar tissue and can be challenging [1]. Additionally, tumor lesions can be really small, invisible, or not palpable by the surgeon's fingers. For that reason, an intraoperative diagnostic tool is necessary because the prior imaging (scintigraphy, PET/CT) has a reduced sensitivity with lower tumor size. Sufficient, preoperative, and intraoperative imaging can provide the surgeon with valuable assistance and also significantly simplify the surgical procedure. Depending on the intraoperative findings, the surgical intervention can be expanded or even significantly reduced.

For several decades, nuclear medicine has offered surgery through the PET probes an intraoperative technology that offers these needs. Adams and Baum et al. 2000 report on one of the first PET probe applications in a patient with neuroendocrine neoplasia (NEN) [2]. In 2012, Kaemmerer et al. published data of a first pilot study using a hand-held pet-probe for the diagnostic of a NEN intraoperatively [3]. The data showed a significantly higher rate of tumor detection than the pre-operative Somatostatin-receptor PET/CT (SSTR-PET/CT) and even the surgical palpation (94% vs. 69% vs. 50%) respectively). Sadowski et al. 2015 confirmed the results of Kaemmerer et al. and they showed the suitability of the PET probe for SI-NEN, mesenteric lymph node metastases, and also for multilocular tumors. Not suitable are cases with a pancreatic primary tumor with liver metastases due to relatively high tumor to background counts [1]. In conclusion, the PET probe appears to be a useful tool for the surgeon in patients with small SI tumors, lymph node metastases, and multiple previous operations. New radiotracers will certainly continue to expand the range of applications to other tumor entities in the future. The Netter-1 study proved peptide-related radionuclid therapy (PRRT) in the therapies of neuroendocrine neoplasia. Depending on the initial somatostatin-receptor (SST) distribution and the SUVmax, excellent therapy results can be achieved.

Several studies independently presented the suitability of all 3 SST-peptides for the diagnosis of NEN and presented a significant immunohistochemical correlation between the PET parameters ex vivo and the histological SST receptors of the tumors in vivo [4–6].

Additionally, these studies showed that SST-PET/CT results allow conclusions for tumor biology (e.g., differentiation, tumor response), because high SST receptor expression is usually associated with good tumor differentiation and

D. Kaemmerer (✉)
Department of General and Visceral Surgery,
Zentralklinik Bad Berka, Bad Berka, Germany
e-mail: Daniel.Kaemmerer@zentralklinik.de

© The Author(s) 2024

V. Prasad (ed.), *Beyond Becquerel and Biology to Precision Radiomolecular Oncology: Festschrift in Honor of Richard P. Baum*, https://doi.org/10.1007/978-3-031-33533-4_17

excellent PRRT response. As often said by Prof. RP. Baum, if a tumor has been shown to have good receptor expression, then it is suitable for both receptor-based imaging and PRRT. This "Theranostic"concept is transferable to other tumor entities.

Our research group investigated also other receptors as new tools for further diagnostic and therapeutic approaches. Endothelin-receptor A expression as well as chemokine receptor CXCR4 were evaluated in a large set of NEN [7, 8]. Tumor cells and tumor stroma of NEN were characterized by a very low endothelin-A-expression whereas CXCR4-expression directly correlated with Ki-67 and was more expressed in undifferentiated neuroendocrine carcinoma. With a wide CXCR4-distribution of high-proliferative neuroendocrine tumors and carcinoma the CXCR4 was a very interesting target for diagnostic and therapy. With the cyclic peptide CPCR4–2 labeled with [68]Gallium an excellent tracer was developed by the Munich group of Prof. Wester [9]. As expected, the well-differentiated tumors showed no CXCR4 expression, so that imaging was also negative. In contrast, high-proliferative tumors were characterized by preclinically seen high CXCR4-receptor expression, so that the CXCR4-based imaging detected the high-proliferative tumor lesions. The authors recommended [68Ga] Pentixafor PET/CT as non-invasive read-out possibility of CXCR4 endoradiotherapy in advanced SST-negative tumors [10]. CXCR4-imaging presented a bone marrow toxicity as limitation. Later on, this side effect was used for molecular diagnosis of multiple myeloma patients [11]. Our group also presented preclinical data of strong CXCR4 expression in MALT lymphoma patients [12, 13]. New data published by Haug AR. demonstrated a more than 90% and an excellent imaging of the lymphomas by PET/MRT [14].

A high SST expression allows a PRRT, for this reason the SST expression of SCLC was examined as a treatment option. In our preclinical data SST expression was found to be expressed in almost 25% of the cases, so SST-based radionuclide therapy seemed suitable. This therapeutic approach was implemented by an external working group (Lapa C. Würzburg, Germany). Data published by Lapa C. et al. show that the SST-based PRRT is feasible as limited therapy option for very advanced SCLC patients [15].

Finally, theranostic proof of concept works in different tumor entities and seems to be a milestone on the way to personalized medicine. This way of treatment was strongly influenced by Prof. RP. Baum and made decisive progress.

With the Netter-1 study the PRRT in SI-NEN stage IV demonstrated superiority over SSA mono therapy [16, 17]. Different studies presented data of PRRT with other neuroendocrine tumor primaries. Alsadik et al. showed PRRT data of pancreatic neuroendocrine tumors and reported complete response rates of 2–6% and partial response up to 60% by an overall survival of 53 months and a progression-free survival of 34 months [18].

The removal of local advanced pancreatic neuroendocrine tumors is often limited by vessel involvement. In the last years, several studies presented excellent data which PRRT as a neoadjuvant approach to downsize and downstage tumors receiving resectability. The first case was published by our group and the neoadjuvant PRRT was performed by RP. Baum [19]. Later on, Esther I van Vliet published a series of neoadjuvant-treated pancreatic neuroendocrine tumor cases with an impressive median PFS of 69 months [20].

The resection of the primary tumors in stage IV neuroendocrine tumor patients is still discussed. But how about the primary resection in SST-positive expressed neuroendocrine tumor patients stage IV, treated with PRRT? Bertani et al. presented data with a median PFS of 70 vs. 30 months (HR 5.1; $p = 0.002$) and a median OS of 112 vs. 65 months (HR 1.13; $p = 0.011$) with a benefit for the primary resected patients [21]. Kaemmerer et al. published the largest European study with beneficial results for SI- and pancreatic neuroendocrine tumor patients with a resected primary tumor prior to PRRT with mOS of 142 vs. 80 months (HR 2.91; $p < 0.001$) and a mOS of 140 vs. 58 months (HR 1.86; $p = 0.002$) respectivly [22]. Finally, these data underline the synergistic effects of well-performed surgery and responsible nuclear medicine treatment.

Thank you Richard for more than 10 years of fruitful collaboration, outstanding collegiality, empathetic 24-h patients management, and many inspiring clinical and translational oncological research projects.

References

1. Sadowski SM, et al. Feasibility of radio-guided surgery with (6)(8)gallium-DOTATATE in patients with gastro-Entero-pancreatic neuroendocrine tumors. Ann Surg Oncol. 2015;22(Suppl 3):S676–82. https://doi.org/10.1245/s10434-015-4857-9.

2. Adams S, Baum RP. Intraoperative use of gamma-detecting probes to localize neuroendocrine tumors. Q J Nucl Med. 2000;44:59–67.

3. Kaemmerer D, et al. Radioguided surgery in neuroendocrine tumors using Ga-68-labeled somatostatin analogs: a pilot study. Clin Nucl Med. 2012;37:142–7. https://doi.org/10.1097/RLU.0b013e3182291de8.

4. Haug AR, et al. Quantification of immunohistochemical expression of somatostatin receptors in neuroendocrine tumors using 68Ga-DOTATATE PET/CT. Radiologe. 2010;50:349–54. https://doi.org/10.1007/s00117-009-1972-2.

5. Miederer M, et al. Correlation of immunohistopathological expression of somatostatin receptor 2 with standardised uptake values in 68Ga-DOTATOC PET/CT. Eur J Nucl Med Mol Imaging. 2009;36:48–52. https://doi.org/10.1007/s00259-008-0944-5.

6. Kaemmerer D, et al. Molecular imaging with (6)(8)Ga-SSTR PET/CT and correlation to immunohistochemistry of somatostatin receptors in neuroendocrine tumours. Eur J Nucl Med Mol Imaging. 2011;38:1659–68. https://doi.org/10.1007/s00259-011-1846-5.

7. Lupp A, et al. Reassessment of endothelin receptor a expression in normal and neoplastic human tissues using the novel rabbit monoclonal antibody UMB-8. Peptides. 2015;66:19–25. https://doi.org/10.1016/j.peptides.2015.02.005.

8. Kaemmerer D, et al. Differential expression and prognostic value of the chemokine receptor CXCR4 in bronchopulmonary neuroendocrine neoplasms. Oncotarget. 2015;6:3346–58. https://doi.org/10.18632/oncotarget.3242.

9. Gourni E, et al. PET of CXCR4 expression by a (68)Ga-labeled highly specific targeted contrast agent. J Nucl Med. 2011;52:1803–10. https://doi.org/10.2967/jnumed.111.098798.

10. Werner RA, et al. Imaging of chemokine receptor 4 expression in neuroendocrine tumors - a triple tracer comparative approach. Theranostics. 2017;7:1489–98. https://doi.org/10.7150/thno.18754.

11. Pan Q, et al. Chemokine receptor-4 targeted PET/CT with (68)Ga-Pentixafor in assessment of newly diagnosed multiple myeloma: comparison to (18)F-FDG PET/CT. Eur J Nucl Med Mol Imaging. 2020;47:537–46. https://doi.org/10.1007/s00259-019-04605-z.

12. Stollberg S, et al. Erratum to: differential somatostatin and CXCR4 chemokine receptor expression in MALT-type lymphoma of gastric and extragastric origin. J Cancer Res Clin Oncol. 2017;143:187. https://doi.org/10.1007/s00432-016-2312-3.

13. Stollberg S, et al. Differential somatostatin and CXCR4 chemokine receptor expression in MALT-type lymphoma of gastric and extragastric origin. J Cancer Res Clin Oncol. 2016;142:2239–47. https://doi.org/10.1007/s00432-016-2220-6.

14. Haug AR, et al. Prospective non-invasive evaluation of CXCR4 expression for the diagnosis of MALT lymphoma using [(68)Ga]Ga-Pentixafor-PET/MRI. Theranostics. 2019;9:3653–8. https://doi.org/10.7150/thno.31032.

15. Lapa C, et al. Somatostatin receptor expression in small cell lung cancer as a prognostic marker and a target for peptide receptor radionuclide therapy. Oncotarget. 2016;7:20033–40. https://doi.org/10.18632/oncotarget.7706.

16. Strosberg J, et al. Phase 3 trial of (177)Lu-Dotatate for midgut neuroendocrine tumors. N Engl J Med. 2017;376:125–35. https://doi.org/10.1056/NEJMoa1607427.

17. Strosberg J, Krenning E. 177Lu-Dotatate for midgut neuroendocrine tumors. N Engl J Med. 2017;376:1391–2. https://doi.org/10.1056/NEJMc1701616.

18. Alsadik S, Yusuf S, Al-Nahhas A. Peptide receptor radionuclide therapy for pancreatic neuroendocrine Tumours. Curr Radiopharm. 2019;12:126–34. https://doi.org/10.2174/1874471012666190201164132.

19. Kaemmerer D, et al. Neoadjuvant peptide receptor radionuclide therapy for an inoperable neuroendocrine pancreatic tumor. World J Gastroenterol. 2009;15:5867–70. https://doi.org/10.3748/wjg.15.5867.

20. van Vliet EI, et al. Neoadjuvant treatment of nonfunctioning pancreatic neuroendocrine tumors with [177Lu-DOTA0,Tyr3]Octreotate. J Nucl Med. 2015;56:1647–53. https://doi.org/10.2967/jnumed.115.158899.

21. Bertani E, et al. Resection of the primary tumor followed by peptide receptor radionuclide therapy as upfront strategy for the treatment of G1-G2 pancreatic neuroendocrine tumors with Unresectable liver metastases. Ann Surg Oncol. 2016;23:981–9. https://doi.org/10.1245/s10434-016-5550-3.

22. Kaemmerer D, et al. Prior resection of the primary tumor prolongs survival after peptide receptor radionuclide therapy of advanced neuroendocrine neoplasms. Ann Surg. 2019;274:e45. https://doi.org/10.1097/SLA.0000000000003237.

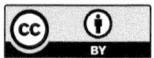

PSMA Radioligand Therapy: A Revolution in the Precision Radiomolecular Oncology of Prostate Cancer

Harshad R. Kulkarni

The incidence of prostate cancer is ever increasing. After various time intervals, the disease almost always becomes resistant to the standard hormone treatment (castration-resistant prostate cancer, CRPC). Most patients with CRPC either already have metastases at diagnosis or develop them during the early months of follow-up, which is associated with a relatively poor prognosis. The taxane-based chemotherapy for metastatic CRPC (mCRPC), first line with docetaxel and second line using cabazitaxel, are associated with a high incidence of adverse effects. The novel androgen-axis drugs (NAAD) used after chemotherapy are androgen biosynthesis inhibitor abiraterone acetate (combined with prednisolone), the androgen receptor blockers enzalutamide as well as the newer generation apalutamide and darolutamide. However, these treatment regimens only provide a meager survival benefit in mCRPC. Radium-223 targets only the osteoblastic metastases and does not treat nodal or visceral metastases. Therefore, there has been an unmet need for targeted therapy.

Indeed, rightly called by Prof. Baum as molecule of the decade, prostate-specific membrane antigen (PSMA) is a glutamate carboxypeptidase II overexpressed in prostate cancer. Although it has been identified many decades ago, PSMA

was targeted by Prof. Pomper's group for the first time in vivo using a urea-based compound targeting PSMA for diagnosis [1]. A milestone in precision oncology was theranostics of mCRPC based on molecular imaging using PET/CT with ^{68}Ga-labeled PSMA ligands and molecular radiotherapy using PSMA-targeted radioligand therapy (PRLT) with beta-emitter (like Lutetium-177, ^{177}Lu) and alpha-emitter (like Actinium-225, ^{225}Ac)-based PSMA ligands [2–5]. PRLT involves selective targeting of PSMA using the radioligand, which then after specific binding, internalizes and retains within the tumor cell, causing the cell-killing.

^{177}Lu-PRLT was first performed at Zentralklinik Bad Berka in February 2013 using ^{177}Lu-labeled DOTAGA-FFK(Sub-KuE) – developed by Prof. Wester's research group at the Technical University Munich (Fig. 18.1). Following this, PRLT was performed using the ^{177}Lu-labeled therapeutic PSMA ligand (DOTAGA-(I-y)fk(Sub-KuE), also called PSMA I&T, for "imaging and therapy") in a large cohort of patients. The comprehensive experience over the past 8 years using different radioligands since then indicates that PRLT is highly effective for the treatment of mCRPC, even in advanced cases, and potentially lends a significant benefit to overall and progression-free survival. Additionally, significant improvement in clinical symptoms and excellent palliation of pain can be achieved. It is safe and very well tolerated with minimal

H. R. Kulkarni (✉)
Department of Nuclear Medicine, Zentralklinik Bad Berka, Bad Berka, Germany
e-mail: harshad.kulkarni@zentralklinik.de

© The Author(s) 2024
V. Prasad (ed.), *Beyond Becquerel and Biology to Precision Radiomolecular Oncology: Festschrift in Honor of Richard P. Baum*, https://doi.org/10.1007/978-3-031-33533-4_18

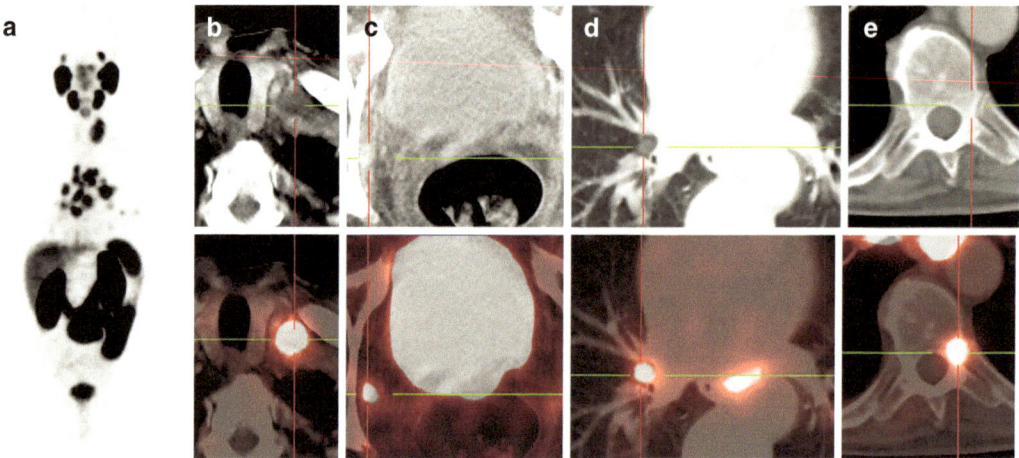

Fig. 18.1 This 68-year-old patient with acinar prostate adenocarcinoma of the left lateral lobe with infiltration of the periprostatic tissue, initial tumor classification pT3a pN0 (0/5) L1 V1 PR1, Gleason score 6 (3 + 3), first diagnosed in 10/2004, status post surgery, radiotherapy, hormone-, and chemotherapy presented with increase in PSA (63.41 ng/mL from previously 10.35 ng/mL) for follow-up. The ^{68}Ga-PSMA PET/CT demonstrated progression of disease with high PSMA expression in numerous new mediastinal and abdominal lymph node involvement, multiple pulmonary and trifocal osseous metastases, thereby confirming the indication for PSMA radioligand therapy (PRLT). He was the first patient treated at our center in February 2013 using ^{177}Lu- DOTAGA-FFK(Sub-KuE). (**a**, maximum intensity projection (MIP) image of ^{68}Ga-PSMA PET/CT; **b**, **c**, **d**, **e**, corresponding axial CT (upper panel) and fused PET/CT (lower panel); **b**, left retroclavicular lymph node; **c**, right obturator lymph node; **d**, pulmonary metastasis; **e**, bone metastasis)

and acceptable adverse effects, including in patients with single kidney/renal insufficiency as well as previously compromised bone marrow function, for example, due to diffuse metastases [3–6]. ^{68}Ga-PSMA PET/CT can be used for appropriate selection and follow-up of patients undergoing PRLT through the application of the concept of theranostics – we treat what we see, and we see what we treat.

The patients currently receive PRLT under individual compassionate basis after exhaustion of the standard treatment options, i.e., following chemotherapy and NAAD. However, at this stage, the disease is already at a very advanced stage and possibly with aggressive mutants. Therefore, these patients are already at a disadvantage, receiving PRLT as a last-ditch effort. We demonstrated for the first time the benefit of providing earlier ^{177}Lu PRLT to patients with metastatic prostate cancer [7]. The median overall survival in all patients was 27 months. Patients previously treated with chemotherapy had a significantly shorter survival (median of 19 months) than those not having received chemotherapy (38 months). Survival was also shorter in patients with previous radium-223 (^{223}Ra) treatment (17 months). On the other hand, prior surgical or radiation treatment of the primary tumor had no significant effect on overall survival. Patients demonstrating a PSA decline of more than 50% after at least two PRLT cycles, lived significantly longer (38 months). In fact, additional treatment with newer antiandrogen agents Abiraterone or Enzalutamide in combination with ^{177}Lu PRLT also prolonged survival. PRLT is a promising therapy with encouraging outcomes and minimal associated toxicity, also chemotherapy-naïve patient cohorts [8]. First retrospective data from an earlier application of Lu-177 PSMA in the hormone-sensitive stage of the disease showed even better response rates [9]. In 11 patients with metastatic prostate cancer without previous antihormonal therapy or orchiectomy (so-called "de novo RLT") could be a PSA drop >50% in 9/11 patients (82%) and tumor control (DCR) can be achieved in 100% of patients (CR 1/11, PR 4/11,

SD 6/11). First-line therapy was associated with the longest survival (all patients alive at 55 months).

We had addressed the issue of potential salivary gland toxicity in two of the initial patients treated with PRLT. The salivary glands were cooled using a special radiotherapy shield. However, no significant difference was observed in the salivary gland uptake in these patients, as compared to those treated without salivary gland protection. This can be explained by a rather non-specific tracer accumulation and a possible reflex hyperperfusion, which negates the whole purpose of trying to reduce the uptake due to vasoconstriction [10]. Indeed, a systemic analysis failed to prove the benefit of external salivary gland cooling using icepacks, as a means of salivary gland protection [11]. In 2018, our group could demonstrate the first proof-of-concept of a non-specific tracer accumulation, where injection of botulinum toxin into a parotid gland achieved a 64% decrease in ^{68}Ga-PSMA uptake ipsilaterally (Fig. 18.2, [12]).

In our experience of about 500 patients treated with around 2000 cycles of ^{177}Lu-PRLT over almost 8 years, there has been no significant xerostomia when using ^{177}Lu alone. Although ^{177}Lu is relatively safe, there are treatment failures, especially in more advanced tumors. Alpha emitters like ^{225}Ac are more potent as they cause more frequent DNA double-strand breaks due to their high linear energy transfer as compared to beta emitters like ^{177}Lu. However, xerostomia is a limiting adverse effect of ^{225}Ac-PRLT, due to which patients discontinue the treatment [13]. In January 2018, we successfully administered the first tandem PSMA radioligand therapy, applying a combination of ^{225}Ac-PSMA-617 and ^{177}Lu-PSMA-617, in a patient who had progressed under ^{177}Lu-PSMA-617 monotherapy (Fig. 18.2). The proposal was that administering a relatively lower radioactivity of the alpha emitter ^{225}Ac-PSMA-617 to that already reported by the Heidelberg group [13], in addition to the beta emitter, might minimize the potential xerostomia because of the salivary gland irradiation by the alpha particles, while at the same time probably prove therapeutically effective (synergistic emission characteristics). In a very promising first analysis, 13/16 patients (82%) showed a bio-

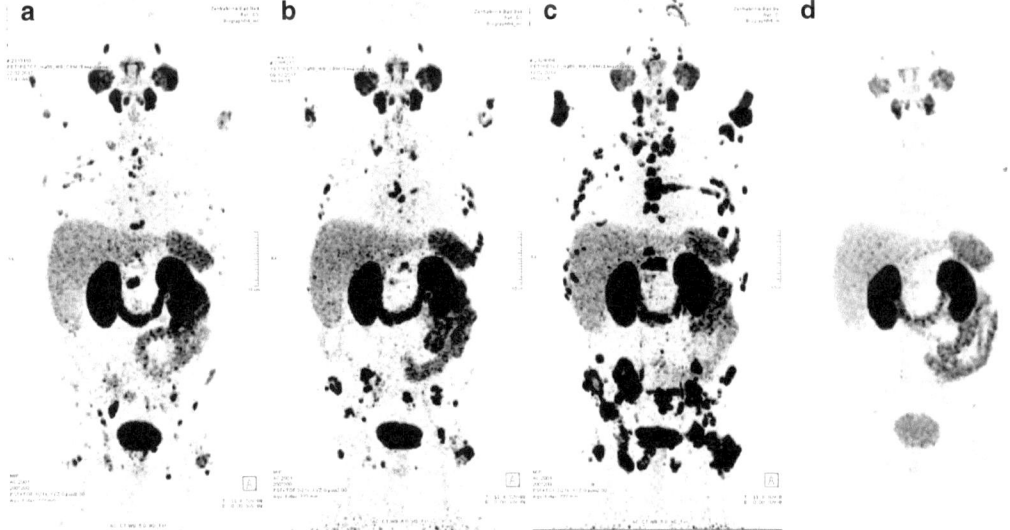

Fig. 18.2 A 56-year-old patient with Gleason 9 metastatic castration-resistant prostate cancer s.p. cabazitaxel and enzalutamide progressed under ^{177}Lu-PRLT. (**a, b, c, d**, MIP images of ^{68}Ga-PSMA PET/CT; **a, b, c** demonstrate progression before first PRLT (**a**, PSA 0.93 ng/mL), after 2nd (**b**, PSA 11.2 ng/mL) and after third PRLR (**c**, PSA 137 ng/mL). After administration of the first tandem PRLT in January 2018 using a combination of 4.5 GBq ^{177}Lu- and 5 MBq of ^{225}Ac-PSMA-617. A good response to TANDEM PRLT was observed with partial remission of the multiple metastases. It is important to note that the PSA does not correlate with the tumor burden

chemical response. In 3 cases, there was a PSA drop>99% [14]. The pain symptoms improved significantly in 8/16 patients with one very impressive improvement of the Karnofsky index (this, at the time of first presentation, wheelchair-bound patient, drove 1200 km himself for the second treatment). No serious xerostomia (but moderate and tolerable) was observed, which could have otherwise caused the treatment to be discontinued. Thus, tandem PRLT could be demonstrated as a fair compromise between effectiveness and side effects of alpha PRLT alone.

Like any other strategy in oncology, the stress should be on combination therapies, best selected depending upon tumor- and patient-specific factors. Quite early on in combination with PRLT, we treated 1 patient with an aggressive treatment-resistant prostate cancer with immune checkpoint inhibitor Nivolumab, and another was treated with the PARP inhibitor Olaparib. However, both these patients experienced severe side effects – esophagitis and bone-marrow suppression, respectively, causing treatment discontinuation. Indeed, a recent report suggests promise of this strategy in selected patients [15].

In a pilot study, we reported for the first time, a high frequency (35.8%) of germline mutations in a larger patient cohort referred for PRLT. The CHEK2 germline mutations seemed to be associated with the best PSA response. The treatment outcome appeared to not correlate with the presence of radiosensitizer (FANCA, BRCA1, ATR) or historically prognosis-determining (HOXB13 or BRCA2) germline gene variants [16]. The future of PRLT and precision radiomolecular oncology of prostate cancer lies in pharmacogenomics, metabolomics, and radiomics with the aim of selecting the right therapy at the right time for the patient.

Thank you, Prof. Baum, for the support, encouragement, and privilege of working with you. A great visionary, brilliant clinician, and an immaculate teacher and orator, your lectures have had long-lasting impression on thousands of minds like mine. Always up to date with preclinical research to promote clinical translation, there is always this strive to take the field of theranostics forward and to go out of the way to find the best possible treatment for the individual patient – *'Aut viam inveniam aut faciam'* probably sums up the motto of your life!

References

1. Pomper MG, Musachio JL, Zhang J, et al. 11C-MCG: synthesis, uptake selectivity, and primate PET of a probe for glutamate carboxypeptidase II (NAALADase). Mol Imaging. 2002;1:96–101.
2. Weineisen M, Schottelius M, Simecek J, Baum RP, Yildiz A, Beykan S, Kulkarni HR, Lassmann M, Klette I, Eiber M, Schwaiger M, Wester HJ. 68Ga- and 177Lu- labeled PSMA I&T: optimization of a PSMA-targeted Theranostic concept and first proof-of-concept human studies. J Nucl Med. 2015;56(8):1169–76.
3. Baum RP, Kulkarni HR, Schuchardt C, Singh A, Wirtz M, Wiessalla S, Schottelius M, Mueller D, Klette I, Wester HJ. 177Lu-labeled prostate-specific membrane antigen radioligand therapy of metastatic castration-resistant prostate cancer: safety and efficacy. J Nucl Med. 2016 Jul;57(7):1006–13.
4. Kulkarni HR, Singh A, Schuchardt C, Niepsch K, Sayeg M, Leshch Y, Wester HJ, Baum RP. PSMA-based Radioligand therapy for metastatic castration-resistant prostate cancer: the Bad Berka experience since 2013. J Nucl Med. 2016 Oct;57(Suppl 3):97S–104S.
5. Kulkarni HR, Singh A, Langbein T, Schuchardt C, Mueller D, Zhang J, Lehmann C, Baum RP. Theranostics of prostate cancer: from molecular imaging to precision molecular radiotherapy targeting the prostate specific membrane antigen. Br J Radiol. 2018;91(1091):20180308.
6. Zhang J, Kulkarni HR, Singh A, Schuchardt C, Niepsch K, Langbein T, Baum RP. Lu-177 PSMA-617 Radioligand therapy in metastatic castration-resistant prostate cancer patients with a single functioning kidney. J Nucl Med. 2019;60(11):1579–86.
7. Kulkarni HR, Schuchardt C, Singh A, Langbein T, Baum RP. Early initiation of Lu-177 PSMA radioligand therapy prolongs overall survival in metastatic prostate cancer. J Nucl Med. 2018;59(Suppl 1):529.
8. Barber TW, Singh A, Kulkarni HR, Niepsch K, Billah B, Baum RP. Clinical outcomes of 177Lu-PSMA radioligand therapy in earlier and later phases of metastatic castration-resistant prostate cancer grouped by previous Taxane chemotherapy. J Nucl Med. 2019;60(7):955–62.
9. Kulkarni HR, Zhang J, Singh A, et al. De novo radioligand therapy using Lu-177 labelled PSMA small molecules in patients with metastatic prostate cancer. Eur J Nucl Med Mol Imaging. 2018;45(Suppl 01):126.
10. Langbein T, Chaussé G, Baum RP. Salivary gland toxicity of PSMA Radioligand therapy: relevance and preventive strategies. J Nucl Med. 2018;59(8):1172–3.

11. van Kalmthout L, Lam M, de Keizer B, Braat A. Impact of external cooling on PSMA uptake in salivary glands [abstract]. Eur J Nucl Med Mol Imaging. 2017;44(suppl 2):328.
12. Baum RP, Langbein T, Singh A, et al. Injection of botulinum toxin for preventing salivary gland toxicity after PSMA radioligand therapy: an empirical proof of a promising concept. Nucl Med Mol Imaging. 2018;52:80–1.
13. Kratochwil C, Bruchertseifer F, Giesel FL, et al. ^{225}Ac-PSMA-617 for PSMA-targeted α-radiation therapy of metastatic castration-resistant prostate cancer. J Nucl Med. 2016;57:1941–4.
14. Kulkarni H, Schuchardt C, Langbein T, et al. First clinical and dosimetry results of tandem alpha-Beta PSMA Radioligand therapy (TABPRLT) using a combination of ac-225 and Lu-177 labelled PSMA-617 for progressive end-stage metastatic prostate cancer. Eur J Nucl Med Mol Imaging. 2018;45(Suppl. 01):110.
15. Prasad V, Zengerling F, Steinacker JP, Bolenz C, Beer M, Wiegel T, Eiber M, Fleshner N, Beer AJ. First experiences with Lu-177 PSMA therapy in combination with Pembrolizumab or after pretreatment with Olaparib in single patients. J Nucl Med. 2020;62:975. Epub ahead of print.
16. Baum RP, Prasad VP, Singh A, Zhang J, Sartor O, Kulkarni HR. Germline gene variants and therapy response in patients referred for radioligand therapy with 177Lu-PSMA: a huge step towards pharmacogenomics in Theranostics of prostate cancer. J Nucl Med. 2020;61(Suppl 1):1272.

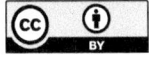

The Role of Individuals for Innovation: The Nuclear Medicine Biotope

Andreas Kluge

Biomedical research, not unlike any other research, should be driven ideally by the intention to solve a problem. In basic science, the aim of good biomedical research is to understand the principles underlying physiology in health and disease, as a pre-requisite to identify targets, tools, and mechanisms suitable for a possible intervention. When it comes to clinical medicine, research—apart from purely epidemiological investigations—typically aims to satisfy so-called "unmet needs" for better diagnosis, prevention, or therapy of diseases.

Nuclear medicine, the opera of the sciences, nowadays combines the possibility to quantitatively investigate—once a suitable radiopharmaceutical tracer is available—virtually any physiological process, and to translate such diagnostic method into a therapeutic intervention by simple isotope exchange. The basis of the signal, pharmacological interactions of a tracer with its molecular target, irrespective of whether receptor, transport system, or enzyme, combined with radioactive decay, the most sensitive, reproducible, and quantifiable detection system in nature, allows in connection with current SPECT and PET camera systems to detect, measure, and analyze physiology of the host in health and disease on one hand, as well as pharmacokinetics and pharmacology of the radiopharmaceutical on the other.

Nuclear medicine, though, has been in its beginnings a purely therapeutic discipline, when Saul Hertz in 1941 first used artificially manufactured ^{130}Iodine to treat hyperthyroidism [1, 2], followed in 1946 by Samuel Seidlin treating metastasized thyroid cancer with ^{131}Iodine [3].

Only in 1951 it became possible to actually localize radioactivity inside the body using the "rectilinear scanner" invented by Benedict Cassen, a simple scintillation counter moving linearly over the body allowing to correlate count rates to two-dimensional anatomical coordinates at the body surface [4]. To the present day, therefore, camera systems in nuclear medicine continue to be referred to as "scanners".

The unique feature of nuclear medicine, providing its right to exist as an independent diagnostic discipline besides radiology, is the possibility to investigate physiological processes, rather than only anatomical structures. What is now generally known as molecular imaging, exemplified by standard techniques such as functional uptake, perfusion, or excretion studies, required the introduction of time, as the fourth dimension into signal acquisition. In order to achieve this, the detection of signal changes over time, as well as a sufficiently large detector area, allowing to detect regional variances in radioactivity in a given field of view was necessary. In

A. Kluge (✉)
ABX—CRO Advanced Pharmaceutical Services, Forschungsgesellschaft m.b.H, Dresden, Germany
e-mail: kluge@abx-cro.com

V. Prasad (ed.), *Beyond Becquerel and Biology to Precision Radiomolecular Oncology: Festschrift in Honor of Richard P. Baum*, https://doi.org/10.1007/978-3-031-33533-4_19

1958, Hal Anger solved the problem, to first "focus" photons using a parallel collimator, and then detect their presence using scintillation crystals. An intelligent array of photomultipliers enabled an unprecedented localization of photons with sufficient timely and spatial resolution, creating an image of the underlying object in the detector plane [5]. This device, today known in honor of its inventor as Anger camera, enabled for the first time dynamic imaging studies of functional phenomena *in vivo*. Nuclear medicine found its feet. To the present day, Anger's basic concept of photon detection by scintillation crystals coupled to photomultipliers remains the standard layout of current SPECT and PET systems.

When represented in a two-dimensional detector plane, though, photons originating in different planes of the body cannot be differentiated. For a more appropriate anatomical allocation of the photon signal, the resolution of the third dimension was required. The physician David Kuhl and the engineer Roy Edwards pioneered tomographic medical imaging, introducing the concept of "rotational scanning" in 1958 [6]. Their work involved the development of basic methodologies for acquisition, reconstruction, and display of data, acquired with multiple rotating detectors, allowing to generate a three-dimensional image. It took until 1964, when sufficient computational power became available, until the first human SPECT scans of brain and body could be performed [7]. Computer-filtered back projection replaced the initial optical back projection.

Only in 1971 X-ray computed tomography was introduced by Godfrey Hounsfield also for morphological imaging, for which he received a Nobel prize in 1979 [8]. It is unclear, whether or not Hounsfield knew Kuhl's and Edward's prior work.

On their way through the tissue, photons undergo attenuation and scatter, which both degrade image quality, and hence the precision of anatomical allocation of a photon source in the body, even when using three-dimensional SPECT imaging. Photons originating from annihilation of a positron with an electron, though, have the peculiarity to occur as pairs, leaving the spot of annihilation in an angle of 180° with a high energy of 511 MeV. These features allow localization of an annihilation event in the body based on simultaneous – "coincident" – activation of opposite scintillation detectors, which avoids the need for "focusing" by collimation, as in SPECT, a procedure, which excludes 99.99% of available photons in the body from contributing to image generation. Accordingly, positron emission tomography (PET) has a much higher sensitivity, better spatial resolution, and quantitative accuracy, compared to SPECT. The basic scanner layout for tomographic positron imaging by coincidence detection was—again – initially conceived by David Kuhl in the 1960s.

In 1973, the first clinically used PET scanner was built at the UCLA by Edward Hoffman, Michael Ter-Pogossian, and Michael Phelps, initially for brain imaging only, followed by a first whole-body scanner in 1977 [9]. With this achievement, PET was established as a general methodology to non-invasively image and quantitatively measure physiological phenomena in vivo. To fully exploit the potential of the new methodology, dedicated positron-emitting radiopharmaceuticals were needed, as well as methodologies, to analyze and interpret the now truly four-dimensional complex data sets, which then consumed the performance of the most powerful computer systems available at the time, a likable feature nuclear medicine has retained to the present day. Two handful of PET institutions in Japan, Europe, and the USA developed into the drivers of method development which attracted the most talented, creatively thinking scientists from any discipline and all over the world. Not surprisingly most of these institutions were run by scientists, mostly physicists and chemists, rather than physicians, who tend—often hindered by a widespread professional conceit—to be less able to create truly interdisciplinary teams at eye level. Where until the 1990s nuclear medicine was often condescendingly referred to as "Unclear Medicine", holistically thinking scientific visionaries like Terry Jones, Michael Welsh, Bengt Langström, Jun Hatazawa, Adriaan Lammertsma,

André Luxen, or Richard Baum have established today's perception of nuclear medicine as the embodiment of precision medicine per se.

For imaging of physiology, radiolabeled tracer molecules—rather than just elemental radionuclides such as [131]iodine, [133]xenon, [67]gallium, or [201]thallium—were required. The basic methodologies to introduce radionuclides into organic molecules, though, had yet to be developed. Alfred P. Wolf at Brookhaven, together with his co-workers Tatsuo Ido, Joanna Fowler, Michael Welsh, and Gerhard Stöcklin developed the first methods to introduce [14]carbon [10], [11]carbon [11] and later [18]fluorine into chemical syntheses [12], which all of a sudden enabled covalent radiolabeling of any organic molecule—at least theoretically.

These methods were soon widely used, in order to explore derivatives of simple biomolecules as potential tracers, to address the carbohydrate, the nucleic acid, and protein metabolism. Ido, Fowler, and Wolf in 1976 first synthesized ^{18}F-fluorodesoxy-glucose (FDG) [13], Hiroshi Fukuda and Ren Iwata explored ^{18}F-fluorodesoxy-mannose [14], Anthony Shields and John Grierson explored ^{18}F-fluoro-thymidine [15], while Stöcklin [16] Kiichi Ishiwata, and others explored amino acids, from which ^{18}F-fluoroethyl-tyrosine (FET) [17] and ^{18}F-fluoro-DOPA [18] made their way into clinical medicine.

On the other side, the possibility to label pharmacologically active substances, in order to study drug biodistribution, metabolism, and more importantly, receptor occupancy *in vivo* was soon perceived. Marieannik and Bernard Mazière in Orsay, Henry N. Wagner, J. James Frost, and Robert Dannels in Baltimore, Philipp Elsinga and Aren van Waarde in Groningen, Joanna Fowler, Nora Volkow, and Stephen Dewie in Brookhaven, Lars Farde, Christer Halldin, and Bengt Langström in Sweden, Kazuhiko Yanai and Tatsuhaki Watanabe in Sendai or Olof Solin in Turku all deserve credit for having developed and introduced the basic methodologies for PET *in vivo* pharmacology.

The analysis of four-dimensional functional imaging data required new methods. The neuroscientist Albert Gjedde and the mathematician

Clifford Patlak developed independently (1981 and 1983) graphical methods to analyze the pharmacokinetics of tracers involving irreversible uptake, such as FDG, now known as Gjedde-Patlak [19, 20] plot. For tracers binding reversibly to receptors and enzymes – as most pharmacologically active substances do – Jean Logan from Joanna Fowler's group found in 1990 a graphical method to estimate the distribution volume from plasma activity curves, which allows to determine receptor occupancy. This method is now referred to as the Logan plot [21].

In order to comprehensively characterize the biological behavior of a physiological substrate or a drug, not only the binding characteristics to their receptors *in vivo*, i.e., binding constants, are of interest, but also pharmacokinetic properties, such as biodistribution, penetration of the blood-brain barrier, plasma protein binding, the relationship of plasma concentration and receptor occupancy, as well as kinetics and pattern of metabolization and excretion. Once a positron-emitter-labeled analog is available, all these questions can be addressed in a single experiment. Since in particular metabolic pathways may differ considerably between animal models and humans, it is of high interest to get early information from the human target species.

Mats Bergström and Bengt Langström from Uppsala were the first to suggest in 2003 the concept of PET microdosing for the development of new drugs [22]. Microdosing means the administration of less than 100 µg or 30 nMol of a substance, which is generally assumed to be pharmacologically inactive. As the mass dose of PET tracers is nearly always below this margin, new compounds can mostly be administered to humans in the context of PET microdosing studies, also referred to as phase 0 studies, with a significantly reduced toxicological characterization. Such a method allows to verify expected substance properties, and on the other hand to recognize possible development roadblocks, such as unexpectedly high protein binding, fast metabolization, or lacking brain uptake, early on during the development process. Nowadays, many new drug candidates intended for CNS indications and beyond contain fluorine atoms, in order to allow a quantitative characterization of pharmacology in vivo using chemically identical ^{18}F-analogs in PET microdosing studies.

In contrast, for routine diagnostics in clinical medicine, a universal PET tracer is desirable, which allows to detect physiological abnormalities in the body, without the need for advanced data processing. In other words, producing a foolproof signal. Such a tracer is ^{18}F-FDG. In 1976, the physician Abass Alavi was the first to administer ^{18}F-FDG, synthesized by Joanna Fowler, to two healthy human volunteers, which were scanned on the UCLA scanner [23].

Today, ^{18}F-FDG is the by far most frequently used PET radiopharmaceutical, accounting for more than 90% of an estimated more than four million PET scans conducted around the world annually. This broad clinical adoption of PET imaging would not have been possible without a remarkable industrialization of all aspects of production and distribution for the very short-lived PET radiopharmaceuticals.

Introducing a robust stereospecific, high-yield radiosynthesis for carrier-free FDG, Kurt Hamacher in 1986 laid the ground for this development. The method—using an aminopolyether, the legendary Kryptofix 222, as phase transfer catalyst for [18]F—has revolutionized the preparation of ^{18}F-labeled tracers in general, and laid the ground for commercial high-volume routine preparation of PET radiopharmaceuticals [24]. The high radiation exposure associated with the handling of positron-emitters had early on stimulated the automated production of PET radiopharmaceuticals. In 1986, JW Brodack, Michael Kilbourn, and Michael Welsh were the first to use an adapted commercial lab automation system for the preparation of a PET radiopharmaceutical [25]. In the 1990s, Bruno Nebeling, Jean-Luc Morelle, and later Vincent Tadino designed the first dedicated automated synthesizer modules for [18]F- and ^{11}C-labeling reactions, and commercialized these successfully. In parallel, new commercial players were created to make available materials for isotope production, pharmaceutical grade chemicals for GMP radiosynthesis, as well as radiopharmacy networks, able to provide reliable manufacturing and distribution of PET

radiopharmaceuticals, opening the possibility to operate clinical PET imaging sites without an own radiopharmacy. Today manufacturing PET radiopharmaceuticals is a several hundred-million-euro business, with strong competition, which has led to a remarkably complete geographical coverage of tracer supply in the developed countries.

The production of the required positron-emitting radionuclides does—in contrast to most single photon emitters—not require a nuclear reactor as neutron or proton beam source, which involves always a massive investment, typically only amenable to governments or large monopolistic utility companies, but is possible using smaller scale particle accelerators, the cyclotrons.

The basic design of the cyclotron was conceived by Leo Szilard already in 1929 [26], and reduced to practice independently by Ernest Lawrence in 1931 in Berkeley [27], who in 1939 received a Nobel prize for it, 1935 by Nishina and Nishikawa in Japan, 1937 by George Gamov and Igor Kurtchatov in Russia, and 1943 by Walther Bothe and Wolfgang Gentner in Germany. The times and the names indicate that the primary motivation for their research was not at all medical in nature. Nevertheless, having experienced the non-medical applications of their work, most of these brilliant physicists, many of which Nobel laureates, became driving forces to establish peaceful applications of radioactivity.

In this spirit, the Brookhaven National Laboratory (BNL) was founded in 1947, which stimulated the establishment of similar nuclear research institutions in many countries around the world, and initially educated many of their leading scientists. At the international level, the IAEA with its mission "atoms for peace" was created in 1957.

With the increasing installation of PET scanners in academia, the need for positron-emitting radionuclides ideally produced in the vicinity of the scanner, grew. Rather than large-scale research installations, small self-shielded cyclotrons, amenable to medical institutions, were needed. Newly created companies, started by academic physicists active in the field served this need. In 1983 Michael Phelps, together with Ronald Nutt, and Terry Douglass founded CTI, which—besides cyclotrons – later also manufactured PET scanners, and considerably contributed to the clinical establishment of the methodology. CTI was acquired by SIEMENS in 2005. In 1986, Yves Jongen of Louvain founded IBA, which remains a leading independent manufacturer of medical cyclotrons.

To the present day, however, the mainstay of diagnostic procedures in nuclear medicine is being conducted using ^{99m}Technetium as a radiolabel. From an estimated 40 million annual diagnostic procedures globally, approximately 85% involve ^{99m}Tc-labeled radiopharmaceuticals. Ironically, the development of this radionuclide was only by chance.

When Walt Tucker and Margaret Greene, chemists at BNL, tried in the late 1950s to chromatographically isolate ^{132}Iodine – which they believed might be favorable for diagnostic procedures in view of a 2-h short half-life – from ^{132}Tellurium out of reactor fission products, they found it to be contaminated with ^{99}Molybdenum, which decayed to ^{99m}Technetium. Due to the chemical similarity of the ^{132}Te/^{132}I and ^{99}Mo/^{99m}Tc nuclide pairs, they could recycle their methodology to create the first ^{99}Mo/^{99m}Tc generator, which they nicknamed a "moly cow", since the mother nuclide ^{99}Mo stays immobilized on the alumina generator column, from which pure ^{99m}Tc can be eluted by physiological saline for further use [28]. When trying to apply for a patent, the patent office replied visionarily, "We are not aware of a potential market for ^{99m}Tc great enough to encourage one to undertake the risk of patenting".

Powell "Jim" Richards, though, the head of isotope production at BNL recognized, that ^{99m}Tc had—compared to all other accessible nuclides at the time—by far the best physical properties for medical imaging with the just invented Anger camera. The photon emission of 140 keV had a sufficient tissue penetration, and was at the same time low enough, to allow efficient collimation for "focusing". The comparatively short half-life minimized radiation exposure for the patient, and in addition, the difference in half-lives between parent and daughter nuclide (66 vs. 6 h) allowed to ship the generator to hospitals, allowing to generate the radionuclide for diagnostic practice on the spot, which could create accessibility.

Richards and Suresh Srivastava, who later substantially refined the generator technology and technetium labeling [29], started lobbying the medical and scientific community for the nuclide. Richards first presented on ^{99m}Tc in 1960 at the *seventh Electronic and Nuclear Symposium* in Rome. On his way, he met Paul V. Harper, from the newly founded Argonne Cancer Research Hospital in Chicago, who ordered in 1961 the first ^{99}Mo/^{99m}Tc generator from BNL. He introduced ^{99m}Tc for blood flow measurements of liver and kidney. In the same year Harper could also demonstrate the use of ^{99m}Tc for imaging thyroid and brain tumors, a more than welcome alternative to pneumoencephalography in the pre-CT era [30]. His methods—obviously satisfying an unmet need—were soon widely adopted. By 1967 BNL had to transfer the production of the ^{99}Mo/^{99m}Tc generator to commercial providers, able to industrially scale manufacturing, in order to keep up with the rising clinical demand. Today, the key role of the trio ^{99m}Tc, Richards, and Harper for establishing nuclear medicine as a medical specialty in its own right is widely recognized.

In order to extend the use of the physically favorable ^{99m}Technetium to biological targets, not addressable by virtue of perfusion or their avidity for the iodine-like properties of the element, Richards started in the mid-1960s his search for ways to use technetium ^{99m}Tc as a radiolabel for more complex tracers. As metals do not form covalent bonds, complexation agents were required, allowing to bind the radiometal to pharmacophores, intended to bind to a biological target. However, the chemistry proved to be tricky. Only in 1970 William Eckelman and Richards succeeded to identify DTPA as a universal complexing agent for ^{99m}Technetium, which was subsequently used to radiolabel not only multiple pharmacophores with ^{99m}Technetium, but also with other radiometals such as ^{111}Indium [31].

The general possibility to label pharmacophores with radiometals stimulated the research to enable internal radiotherapy with beta-emitting radiometals, extending the principles of ^{131}I-radioiodine therapy, to targets not addressable with elemental [131]I.

Donald Hnatowich, as well as Sally and Gerald DeNardo in the 1980s, were among the first to consider [90]Yttrium as an alternative to ^{131}I for labeling pharmacophores for therapeutic purposes [32]. After initial dissatisfactory attempts with DTPA, which produced unstable complexes, Shrikant Deshpande and Sally Denardo in 1989 finally identified DOTA as a suitable chelator for [90]Y [33].

DOTA offered for the first time the possibility to form stable complexes not only with ^{90}Y, but also with other tri-valent radiometals such as [177]Lutetium, a beta-emitter with shorter particle path length in tissue, featuring an imageable gamma emission, alpha-emitters such as [225]Actinium, and at the same time diagnostic nuclides for SPECT and PET, like [111]Indium, [68]Gallium, or [64]Copper.

Only with the introduction of DOTA, as a multivalent chelator suitable to complex diagnostic and therapeutic nuclides alike, nuclear medicine finally became technically able to unfold its full theranostic potential. Pharmacophores as diverse as monoclonal antibodies, peptides, small molecules, or nanobodies have since been labeled for PET and SPECT imaging, as well as for therapeutic administration with either beta- or alpha-emitters. Theoretically, any given pharmacophore can—by exchange of the radiolabel—be multiply used as a targeting agent to diagnostically identify target expression, to measure target engagement, and then to plan and administer a therapeutic intervention, using a therapeutic payload.

The general access to today's most popular theranostic nuclide pair ^{68}Ga and ^{177}Lu, both efficiently complexed by DOTA, was paved by Frank Rösch and Konstantin Zhernosekov from Mainz, who translated what Tucker and Green had done for ^{99m}Tc into the PET world, making available the [68]Ge/^{68}Ga generator [34], allowing on-site production of positron-labeled tracers without a cyclotron, and devising – together with Nicolai A. Lebedev from Dubna—an efficient and reli-able way to produce carrier-free ^{177}Lu, today's standard therapy radionuclide [35].

David Goldenberg is credited to have first used antibodies as targeting agents in 1977 [36]. It took until the late 1990s that peptide ligands were explored for diagnosis and treatment by many groups. The somatostatin receptor system, well known from established peptide therapeutics for neuroendocrine tumors, served as a model to pave the way for many other receptor systems, today addressed by most diverse peptide therapeutics under development. Claude Reubi, Helmut Maecke, and Marion de Jong paved the way for pharmacology and chemistry. Jan Müller-Brand in Basel, Dik Kwekkeboom and Eric Krenning in Rotterdam, as well as Richard Baum in Bad Berka were among the earliest clinical adopters of the method [37–39], and later continued the development of this new therapy modality in academia for the benefit of their patients on their own, in the absence of any industrial interest for many years.

Thanks to important progress in instrumentation, it is now possible to also quantitatively reconstruct SPECT, yielding information in terms of Bq/mL tissue, which is a prerequisite for accurate detection and dosimetry of therapeutic nuclides *in vivo*, most of which are single photon emitters. Bruce Hasegawa is credited for having first suggested to combine SPECT and CT imaging to acquire simultaneous SPECT/CT, allowing for voxel-based scatter and attenuation correction [40]. Hidehiro Iida from Osaka [41], as well as Dale Bailey from Sydney [42] practically implemented the absolute quantification of SPECT images ("QSPECT") in the years 2000, with which it is now possible not only to image and localize, but also to quantitatively measure the radiation absorbed dose, conveyed by a therapeutic radiopharmaceutical to a tumor in Gray (Gy), as established in external field radiation therapy. It took until the years 2010, though, that the major camera manufacturers started implementing this methodology into their SPECT scanners, as they feared, their PET camera business—much higher priced in reason of the possibility to quantify the image data—might suffer.

With these achievements the basic technical toolbox of nuclear medicine as a universal diagnostic and therapeutic discipline was complete.

Nevertheless, PET instrumentation has since seen quantum leaps in sensitivity and resolution. The introduction of simultaneous PET/CT by Thomas Beyer and David Townsend in 2000 has increased the sensitivity of PET by a factor of 40 compared to the initial UCLA instrument [43]. Time-of-flight detection further improved the signal-to-noise ratio of the PET images [44]. The development of a total body PET scanner, driven by Simon Cherry and colleagues, now allows to further increase the sensitivity of PET by a factor of 100, allowing to reduce activity doses of diagnostic radiopharmaceuticals accordingly, without any loss in image quality [45]. Provided, however, that the budgets involved in health care—not only for instrumentation—will not prohibit a wider adoption.

Last but not least: PET/MRI. Its development has been much more of a technical challenge than the PET/CT, considering the need to harmonize mutually incompatible magnetic and scintillation detector systems in a very small space, and to come up with attenuation correction methods based on an MRI, rather than a CT image, to which Bernd Pichler from Tübingen provided key contributions. Now, after years of enthusiastic search by the scientific community for the "killer application", with series of own symposia conducted in the pre-pandemic era, the unique clinical value of PET/MRI becomes increasingly clear in situations, where a detailed morphological or perfusion information are needed in addition to molecular information [46].

With the complete methodology of nuclear medicine available today, we have become able to read the book of life, at least its physiological basis. We may need artificial intelligence to master the flood of information and to decipher its meaning in the future, but we will always need academic teachers, and great humans, able to welcome new members to the community, and spread the flame of curiosity.

Thank you, Richard.

References

1. Hertz S, Roberts A. Radioactive iodine in the study of thyroid physiology: VII. The Use of radioactive iodine therapy in hyperthyroidism. JAMA. 1946;131(2):81–6.
2. Fahey FH, Grant FD, Thrall JH. Saul Hertz, MD, and the birth of radionuclide therapy. EJNMMI Phys. 2017;4:15.
3. Seidlin SM, Marinelly LD, Oshry E. Radioactive iodine therapy; effect on functioning metastases of adenocarcinoma of the thyroid. JAMA. 1946;132(14):838–47.
4. Cassen B, Curtis L, Reed C, Libby R. Instrumentation for 131I use in medical studies. Nucleonics. 1951;9:46–50.
5. Anger HO. Scintillation camera. Rev Sci Instrm. 1958;29:27–33.
6. Kuhl DE. Rotational scanning of the liver. Radiology. 1958;71:875–6.
7. Kuhl DE, Edwards RQ. Image separation radioisotope scanning. Radiology. 1963;80:653–61.
8. Hounsfield GH. Computerizes transverse axial scanning tomography. I. Description of the system. Br J Radiol. 1973;68:166–73.
9. Ter-Pogossian MM, Phelps ME, Hoffman EJ, Mullani NA. A positron-emission transaxial tomography for nuclear imaging PETT. Radiology. 1975;114:89–98.
10. Wolf A, Redvanly C, Anderson R. Benzene-12C from the neutron irradiation of the clathrate with ammonia-cal nickel cyanide. Nature. 1955;176:831.
11. Stöcklin G, Wolf A. Phase dependence of carbon-11 recoil products in ethane and propane: evidence for methylene insertion. J Am Chem Soc. 1963;85:229.
12. Hoyte RM, Lin SS, Christman DR, Wolf AP. Organic radiopharmaceuticals labeled with short-lived nuclides. 2. 18F-labeled phanylalanines. J Nucl Med. 1971;12(6):280–6.
13. Ido T, Wan CN, Fowler JS, Wolf AP. Fluorination with molecular fluorine. A convenient synthesis of 2-deoxy-2-fluoro-D-glucose. J Org Chem. 1977;42:2341–2.
14. Fukuda H, Matsuzawa T, Abe Y, Ido T. Experimental study for cancer diagnosis with positron-labeled fluorinated glucose analgos: 18F-2-fluoro-2-deoxy--D-mannose: a new tracer for cancer detection. Eur J Nucl Med. 1982;7:294–7.
15. Shields AF, Grierson JR, Kozawa SM, Zheng M. Development of labled thymidine analogs for imaging tumor proliferation. Nucl Med Biol. 1996;23:17–22.
16. Coenen HH, Stöcklin G. Evaluation of radiohalogenated amino acid analogues aspotential tracers for PET and SPECT studies of protein synthesis. Radioisot Klinik Forschung. 1988;18:402–40.
17. Wester HJ, Dittmar C, Herz M, Stöcklin G. Synthesisand biological evaluation of O-2-[F-18] fluoroethyl-L-tyrosine ([18F]FET). Nuklearmedizin. 1997;36:A75.

18. Namavari M, Bishop A, Satyamurthy, Barrio JR. Regioselective radiofluorodestannylation with [18F]F2 and [18F]CH3COOF: a high yield synthesis of 6-[18F]fluoro-l-dopa. Appl Radiat Isot. 1992;43:989–96.
19. Gjedde A. High- and low-affinity transport of D-glucose from blood to brain. J Neurochem. 1981;36:1463–71.
20. Patlak CS, Blasberg RG, Fenstermacher JD. Graphical evaluation of blood-to brain transfer constants from multiple-time uptake data. J Cereb Blood Flow Metab. 1983;3:1–7.
21. Logan J, Fowler JS, Volkow, Gatley SJ. Graphical analysis of reversible radioligand binding from time-activity measurements applied to [N-11C-methyl]-(−)-cocaine PET studies in human subjects. J Cereb Blood Flow Metab. 1990;10:740–7.
22. Bergström M, Grahnén A, Långström B. Positron emission tomography micro dosing: a new concept with application in tracer and early clinical drug development. Eur J Clin Pharmacol. 2003;59:357–66.
23. Reivich M, Kuhl D, Wolf A, Sokoloff L. Measurement of local cerebral glucose metabolism in man with 18F-2-fluoro-2-deoxy-d-glucose. Acta Neurol Scand. 1977;64:190–1.
24. Hamacher K, Coenen HH, Stöcklin G. Efficient stereospecific synthesis of no-carrier-added 2-[18F]-fluoro-2-deoxy-D-glucose using aminopolyether supported nucleophilic substitution. J Nucl Med. 1986;27(2):235–8.
25. Brodack JW, Kilbourn MR, Welch MJ, Katzenellenbogen JA. Application of robotics to radiopharmaceutical preparation: controlled synthesis of fluorine-18 16 alpha-fluoroestra-diol −17 beta. J Nucl Med. 1986;27(5):714–21.
26. Telegdi VL. Szilard as inventor: accelerators and more. Phys Today. 2000;53:25.
27. Lawrence EO, Edlefsen NE. On the production of high speed protons. Science. 1930;72:376.
28. Tucker WD, Greene MW, Weiss AJ, Murenhoff A. Methods of preparation of some carrierfree radio-isotopes involving sorption on alumina. BNL 3746. Trans Am Nocl Soc. 1958;1:160.
29. Srivastava SC, Meinken G, Smith TD, Richards P. Problems associated with stannous 99mTc-radiopharmaceuticals. Int J Appl Radiat Isot. 1977;28:83–95.
30. Harper PV, Lathrop KA, Jiminez F, Gottschalk A. Technetium 99m as a scanning agent. Radiology. 1965;85:101–9.
31. Eckelman W, Richards P. Instant 99mTc-DTPA. J Nucl Med. 1970;11:761.
32. Hnatowich DJ, Virzi F, Doherty PW. DTPA-Coupled Antibodies Labeled with Yttrium-90. J Nucl Med. 1985;26:503–9.
33. Deshpande SV, DeNardo SJ, Kukis DL, Meares CF. Yttrium-90-Labeled monoclonal antibody for therapy: labeling by a new Macrocycic bifunctional chelating agent. J Nucl Med. 1990;31:473–47.
34. Zhernosekov KP, Filosofov DV, Baum RP, Rösch F. Processing of generator-produced 68Ga for medical application. J Nucl Med. 2007;48(10):1741–8.
35. Lebedev NA, Novgorodov AF, Misiak R, Brockmann J, Rösch F. Radiochemical separation of no-carrier-added 177Lu as produced via the 176Yb(n,gamma)177Yb-->177Lu process. Appl Radiat Isot. 2000;53(3):421–5.
36. Primus FJ, Macdonald R, Goldenberg DM, Hansen HJ. Localization of GW-39 human tumors in hamsters by affinity-purified antibody to carcinoembryonic antigen. Cancer Res. 1977;37(5):1544–7.
37. Krenning EP, Kwekkeboom DJ, Oei HY, Lamberts SW. Somatostatin receptor imaging of endocrine gastrointestinal tumors. Schweiz Med Wochenschr. 1992;122:634–7.
38. Otte A, Jermann E, Behe M, Maecke HR. DOTATOC: a powerful new tool for receptor-mediated radionu-clide therapy. Eur J Nucl Med. 1997;24(7):792–5.
39. de Jong M, Krenning E. New advances in peptide receptor radionuclide therapy. J Nucl Med. 2002;5:617–20.
40. Hasegawa BH, Lang TF, Brown JK, Ramanathan C. Object-specific attenuation correction of SPECT with correlated dual-energy x-ray CT. IEEE Trans Nucl Sci. 1993;40(4):1242–52.
41. Kim KW, Varrone A, Watabe H, Lida H. Contribution of scatter and attenuation compensation to SPECT images of nonuniformly distributed brain activities. J Nucl Med. 2003;44(4):512–9.
42. Willowson K, Bailey DL, Baldock C. Quantitative SPECT reconstruction using CT-derived corrections. Phys Med Biol. 2008;53(12):3099–122.
43. Beyer T, Townsend DW, Brun T, Nutt R. A combined PET/CT scanner for clinical oncology. J Nucl Med. 2000;41:1369–79.
44. Karb JS, Surti S, Daube-Witherspoon ME, Muehllehner G. Benefit of time-of-flight in PET: experimental and clinical results. J Nucl Med. 2008;49(3):462–70.
45. Cherry SR, Badawi RD, Karp JS, Jones T. Total-body imaging: Transforming the role of positron emission tomography. Sci Transl Med. 2017;9:eaaf6169.
46. Bailey DL, Pichler BJ, Gückel B, Beyer T. Combined PET/MRI: from status quo to status go. Summary report of the fifth international workshop on PET/MR imaging. Mol Imaging Biol. 2016;18:637–50.

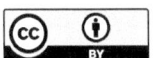

Working at Isotopentherapiestation D3: A Daily Challenge or Adventure Never Stops

Coline Lehmann

My first day of work as a resident in the Dept. of Nuclear Medicine—Center for PET/CT in Bad Berka was on 01.08.2008. I applied for this job in springtime that year and shortly thereafter I had the job interview with Prof. Dr. med. Richard Baum. I remember we were sitting together in a very unspectacularly room, beside this I had a very nice talk with him and expressed my wish to become a nuclear medicine and that I'd love to have the opportunity to work in his department. Of course I previously got some information about working there and I was more than willing to overcome the daily travel of 150 km. After gaining experience in internal medicine by working as a student for years on several internal wards as well as doing the doctoral thesis in endocrinology together with my great motivation I got the job in the end. Before my job interview, in the beginning of May 2008 the "10 Years Anniversary PET and Nuclear Medicine Bad Berka (1998-2008) International Symposium - Molecular Diagnosis and Therapy of Cancer in Nuclear Medicine" took place in Bad Berka. So I got the chance already to get a first real impression in this exciting discipline of medicine and also get to know some of my future colleagues.

The Radio-Isotopentherapiestation became my workplace from the first day on.

The Klinik für Molekulare Radiotherapie in Bad Berka offers 22 beds after reconstruction and expansion for patients who will be treated with all possible nuclear medicine therapies with nuclides. This patient-friendly ward has modern 2-bedroom and 2 1-bedroom facilities. You also find friendly and highly specialized nursing staff caring for their patients.

The focus of treatments is on the therapy of thyroid diseases as well as neuroendocrine tumors (NET) or metastasized castration-resistant prostate cancer since February 2013. Radioimmunotherapy (e.g., in lymphomas and colorectal cancers) is also part of the treatment spectrum. With in total 6248 realized peptide receptor radionuclide therapies (PRRT) with (90) Y- and/or (177)Lu-labeled peptides since 16.2.1997 and 1312 therapies since 18.06.2013 in prostate cancer under the direction of Prof. Dr. med. R.P. Baum, The Klinik für Molekulare Radiotherapie in Bad Berka is a worldwide leading center and offers an excellent expertise in this field. In our opinion for example PRRT should only be performed at specialized centers, as NET patients need highly individualized interdisciplinary treatment and long-term care.

As a new resident I had to work in the thyroid ambulance as well as at the ward. In the morning I had to learn all about the pitfalls of thyroid diagnostics and therapy and in the afternoon the focus was on neuroendocrine tumors and their treatment.

C. Lehmann (✉)
Institute for Diagnostic and Interventional Radiology, SRH Wald-Klinikum Gera GmbH, Gera, Germany

© The Author(s) 2024
V. Prasad (ed.), *Beyond Becquerel and Biology to Precision Radiomolecular Oncology: Festschrift in Honor of Richard P. Baum*, https://doi.org/10.1007/978-3-031-33533-4_20

A small, well-organized, and experienced team of doctors is taking care of the well-regulated processes and the realization of the treatments.

During their internship all new doctors have the daily clinical routine with the patients' administration and detailed case histories with a focus on the classification of the sometimes rare case histories and the multimorbidity of the patients.

One key aspect which I want to emphasize is the treatment of international patients. The percentage of foreign patients (more than 50 different nationalities) was increasing month after month during the last years. Due to this fact many logistical and organizational problems have occurred. In 2012 the Kommission für Krankenhaushygiene und Infektionsprävention (KRINKO) updated the hygiene measurements concerning infection and colonization with multiresistant gram-negative rods. They recommended a pre-emptive isolation of patients coming out of countries with higher prevalence to avoid a 4-MRGN-infection. After careful consideration only a few exceptions were tolerated in very limited cases. This was leading several times into acute occupancy problems at the ward. As being the physician responsible for hygiene matters, a very close collaboration with the department for labor and hygiene was often really helpful and led to efficient solutions in all hygienic relevant questions. Furthermore, this collaboration was also very important concerning another big issue in dealing with our patients.

In the context of realization of Lutetium-177 (Lu)-labeled prostate-specific membrane antigen radioligand therapy (Lu-PRLT) for patients with metastatic castration-resistant prostate cancer (mCRPC), the patients more frequently exhibit a worsening in clinical status as well as a labor constellation which lead into a direct need to apply red blood cell concentrate. The clinical indication for giving a red blood cell infusion is depending on several facts like age, gender, case history and clinical state of the patient as well as sort and cause of the anemia. It is also addicted to previous treatments and so the need for transfusion was increasing. Prescribed by law, all medi-

cal facilities which use blood products have to name a lead consultant for transfusion who is responsible for all tasks concerning transfusion. In the bigger centers you have to name also a transfusion practitioner, who is taking care of all procedures which are announced from the lead consultant for transfusion or the transfusion panel.

When you look at the increasing numbers of transfusion and also want to secure a constant high quality in these procedures it was just a logical step to become the transfusion practitioner of the department.

In the context of the function as a radiation safety officer, you're not only the direct contact person for all instructions and briefings, you are also responsible for the different questions from patients and their family. Most of the patients never had any contact to nuclear medicine or only limited experience to diagnostics in nuclear medicine and are completely inexperienced to how to behave at an isotopentherapiestation.

This generates an extensive need of clarification.

Even when you're really careful and cautious, you can have unwanted contaminations in extreme rare cases. Also here, the radiation safety officer is an advisor as well as a coordinator. Some years ago we had a case of a bigger contamination which required the attention of the complete staff and all our physicians to clear up the situation in forensic detail. Presumably several small contaminations occurred during work in the ward with Lu-177, some were found at the floor, one at the top of the nurse and supposably there was also a contamination on the printed label of the nuclide which is in the patient files. With the result that the hands of the doctors and the nurses had been contaminated as well. In the end the contamination was recognized but you could detect small amounts of radioactivity all over the ward, in the hot labor, on hands, shoes, even in the patient files. Due to not identified new contaminated sources you got repeatedly new starting points of measurable activity. The complete staff and all radiation safety officers had to take measures with decontamination procedures for 2 days.

As a result of the radioligand therapy with Lu-177 labeled PSMA antagonists for patients with prostate cancer in 2013 another therapy option was established, the so-called alpha therapy with Bismut-213 in December 2016 which switched to Actinium-225 in February 2018.

The establishment of new treatments is always a big challenge for all people involved. You have to plan, analyze, and calculate all logistical problems into detail to avoid problems later. With a high amount of calculation and preparation work done by our physicians, you try to anticipate future outcomes and once established you get trained on the theory. Starting at the point of delivery of the radioisotope and ending in the radioactive waste management, you have to discuss all topics related. You also need to train your staff, generate new SOPs, clarify administrative problems like text modules, for example, for letters, etc. and of course every detail has to be clear before the new nuklid is ready to be used in a suitable patient. Due to the increasing use of Actinium-225 as a single treatment as well as the so-called Tandem therapy (when you administer two different radiopeptides in one session) in combination with Lu-177, we saw also more severe clinical cases with multimorbidity.

The number of patients coming to us for therapy was again rising.

My personal treatment record for 1 day was 18 treatments in 9 patients, which were performed as Tandem therapy in patients suffering from metastasized prostate cancer.

This achievement is only possible when you are part of such a highly skilled and motivated team. It is also very important to have regular multidisciplinary meetings (with the radiopharmacy, the technical assistants, the secretaries, study nurses, etc.).

Another focus is especially regarding the dosimetry scans, performed after the therapies which are of the utmost significance for the patients, you always have to ensure a very close teamwork of all people involved to make the whole procedure possible. To achieve these results, you're on the phone for a big part of the day, coordinating the workflow. It needs all hands on deck to reach such high numbers of treatments.

When I think back to my work since 2008 till 2019, many situations have impressed me. As a new resident I was full of respect of the diversity of tumor diseases of these patients, their often long life of suffering and their thankfulness that we could help them. This was especially thanks to the Bad Berka system. Over so many years a complex procedure evolved. It needed month after month of job training to understand this system. So many different staff members took care of such a big amount of things, everything had to run like clockwork, so in the end another happy patient could leave the ward. Thanks to the extremely high motivation on a daily base of the staff members we were able to achieve these results.

Until my very last day there my personal highlights which fascinated me the most were the ward rounds with Prof. Dr. med. Baum. It is really amazing how somebody could have such a memory, he caught every detail, was able to build interactions which not everybody is able to do, seeing facts which most people would miss out.

Every ward round with him was a big lesson for me. Even when you were overloaded with work you dropped everything and joined him for rounds as this was such a big opportunity to learn from him!

There was never enough time to do everything. There was always a very high standard of care and although our goal was to do everything perfect, it was almost impossible. We worked very long days and often left the clinic late in the evening.

And after becoming a specialist you had to do on-call duties on top of the daily work and as a senior physician you had to be on call half of the month. For a while we had to admit patients on Saturdays because of the workload during the week. The Mondays were too full to admit patients because of the scheduled therapies and administration.

Nevertheless, my personal motivation has always been very high. I was proud to be a member of this team and to have the ability to make a contribution to this work and to learn in reverse so many things. When you compare it with a university institution, we as a relatively small hospital reached so many milestones.

With this approach the Klinik für Molekulare Radiotherapie is able to look back to 7560 therapies in 2059 patients in total over the last 22 years.

The whole team can be proud of their individual contribution so we were able to reach these milestones!

An expertise, which is really unique.

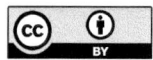

Theranostics in Australia: The Importance of Vision and Training, and the Power of Collaboration

Nat Lenzo

Nuclear medicine began as a therapeutic onco-logical specialty over 75 years ago principally on the back of the discovery, and then widespread adoption, of Iodine-131 as an effective and safe treatment for differentiated thyroid cancer [1]. With a half-life of just over 8 days, this physical attribute meant that Iodine-131 could be centrally produced by neutron bombardment of tellerium in a reactor and then distributed widely to patients. Thus, dissemination of this therapy occurred over the ensuing years throughout the world, including into Australia.

In Australia, the first nuclear reactor was con-structed, in the late 1950s, at Lucas Heights in the outskirts of Sydney [2], and following its com-missioning, began producing not only Iodine-131 for therapeutic nuclear medicine, but also other neutron-rich radioisotopes such as technetium-99m for diagnostic nuclear medicine. In the 1960s through to the 1980s, nuclear medicine in Australia transitioned into a predominantly diag-nostic specialty heavily focused on technetium-99m, and to a lesser degree, the imported cyclotron produced radioisotopes gallium-67 and

thallium-201. Almost 50 years after the initial reactor, a replacement nuclear (OPAL—Open Pool Australian Lightwater) reactor was commis-sioned at Lucas Heights in 2007.

The first national medical cyclotron was estab-lished in Camperdown, Sydney, in the early 1990s [2]. This cyclotron was situated across the road from one of the first PET scanners in Australia at the Royal Prince Alfred Hospital in Sydney. Smaller cyclotrons were subsequently set up in the 1990s at the Austin Hospital and then at the Peter MacCallum Cancer Institute in Melbourne. With the introduction of this technology came the early foray into positron emission tomography utilising cyclotron-produced radioisotopes, predominantly Fluorine-18. These developments expanded the diagnostic capability of nuclear medicine. By the end of the 1990s, there were over 160 nuclear medicine sites with over 300 gamma cameras in public institutions, private hospitals and suburban practices in Australia. Only three PET cameras were in operation at the end of the 1990s. By 2020, however, PET had grown to over 80 centres across Australia with cyclotrons now present in every state and territory apart from Tasmania and the Australian Capital Territory.

With the development of nuclear medicine practice, the Australian and New Zealand Association of Nuclear Medicine (ANZSNM) was founded in 1969, and around the same time, the Australian and New Zealand Association of Physicians in Nuclear Medicine (ANZAPNM),

N. Lenzo (✉)
GenesisCare (Theranostics and Molecular Imaging), Perth, WA, Australia

Fiona Stanley Hospital, Murdoch, WA, Australia

Notre Dame University Australia, Fremantle, WA, Australia
e-mail: Nat.Lenzo@genesiscare.com

V. Prasad (ed.), *Beyond Becquerel and Biology to Precision Radiomolecular Oncology: Festschrift in Honor of Richard P. Baum*, https://doi.org/10.1007/978-3-031-33533-4_21

more recently known as the Australasian Association of Nuclear Medicine Specialists, also came into existence. Over the 1970s and 1980s, training in nuclear medicine for medical graduates developed into structured programmes under the direction and supervision of the Royal Colleges of both radiology and medicine (Royal Australian and New Zealand College of Radiologists—RANZCR; Royal Australasian College of Physicians—RACP). The structure evolved such that training could be obtained either as part of a 4 + 2 year programme within the postgraduate radiology training programme or part of the 6 year postgraduate physician (internal medicine) training programme. As part of the 6-year radiology training programme, nuclear medicine comprised the last 2 years of training after completing 4 core years in radiology training. This allowed such trained practitioners to be dual qualified in both general radiology and in nuclear medicine. Positron Emission Tomography (PET) accreditation was incorporated into core nuclear medicine training in Australia in the early 2000s. Advanced training in nuclear medicine is supervised by a joint committee made up from representatives from the RANZCR and the RACP. There are now over 40 accredited training sites for nuclear medicine and PET sites around Australia in both public and private practice settings.

Within the physician stream, advanced training in nuclear medicine comprised of a minimum of 2 core years of nuclear medicine +1 elective year. Advanced training in nuclear medicine commenced after completing a minimum of 3 years of basic physician training post-intern year and passing the rigorous basic physician written and clinical exams. It is possible also in the physician training stream to specialise in two subspecialities of internal medicine by completing a minimum of 2 core years of nuclear medicine training and then an additional 2 core training years in a separate medical specialty (e.g. medical oncology, respiratory medicine, cardiology, endocrinology). This pathway allows physicians to become dual qualified in two subspecialties, a pathway very relevant to current and future theranostic practice.

Since the 1990s, there has been a resurgence in interest in therapeutic nuclear oncology and the development of significant expertise in this area in Australia. This has occurred for several reasons. Australia still has a relatively large number of nuclear physicians trained via the physician route under the clinical internal medicine model. These nuclear physicians have traditionally gravitated more to academic institutions and academic endeavours rather than the dual-trained radiologist/nuclear physicians who, due to their breadth of diagnostic capabilities and expertise, are highly sought after for private radiology practice. The length and rigour of training, the emphasis on research and evidence-based medicine in an academic teaching hospital environment and the hands-on clinical nature of internal medicine physician training subsequently led to a number of Australian nuclear physicians developing further subspecialty interest in therapeutic nuclear oncology. Dual-trained radiologists/nuclear physicians by and large were more comfortable and interested in the imaging aspects of nuclear medicine practice, rather the clinical, hands-on-patient, therapeutic practice.

The well-equipped and well-funded public Australian teaching hospitals working closely with excellent partnering tertiary universities allowed new techniques and radioisotope-based therapies to be developed such as Yttrium-90 SIR (Selective Internal Radiation) spheres at Royal Perth Hospital (Prof Bruce Gray, University of Western Australia) [3–6] and Iodine-131 rituximab at Fremantle Hospital (Prof Harvey Turner, University of Western Australia) [7–10]. The Australian Therapeutic Goods Administration Special Access Scheme allowed (and continues to allow) for compassionate use of in-hospital radiopharmacy-produced agents thus facilitating early use and adoption of both diagnostic and therapeutic agents long before formal regulatory approval occurred (e.g. Gallium-68 DOTATATE and Lutetium-177 DOTATATE for imaging and treating neuroendocrine tumours) [11–16]. Through this mechanism, a number of investigator-initiated single and multiple site studies could be and were performed. This coupled with the vision, drive and passion of a number of key individuals such as Prof Rod Hicks, Prof Andrew Scott and Prof Paul Donnelly meant that over the last 25 years institutions, such as the

Peter MacCallum Cancer Institute and the University of Melbourne, have driven discovery of new agents and have evolved to become world-class centres of translational research and clinical excellence in the fields of diagnostic and therapeutic nuclear oncology.

In the early 2000s, the introduction of PET in Australia necessitated, for the first time, the development of a collaborative multi-site, inter-state approach towards data capture and data management in Australian nuclear medicine practice. This programme, called the Australian prospective multicentre PET data collection project, was mandated by the Australian federal government as they pursued objective data for justification for the introduction and reimbursement of PET into the national medical system. This programme utilised a change of management measure (developed by Prof Rod Hicks at the Peter MacCallum) [16] to determine the clinical impact of the new diagnostic modality of PET. The Australian PET data collection project [17] collected a large amount of high-quality data on multiple cancer types which confirmed the clinical utility of PET. The project led to multiple publications [18–22] and eventually the widespread reimbursement of PET by the Australian Federal government from 2004. This programme, I believe, was the nidus for what we are now seeing with the collaborative networks that have started in the last few years in both the public and private sectors. The Australian PET data collection project brought different institutions together for a common aim, and despite some initial difficulties and some latter controversy [23], overall, the programme proved the power of the collective, collaborative network.

Apart from physician resources, university-trained nuclear medicine technologist, physicist, radiochemist and radiopharmacy services have been available at all teaching hospital nuclear medicine departments since the 1980s. This has been critical to foster high-quality clinical and research work. Interest in peptide, chelation and metal chemistry at a number of universities, but in particular the University of Melbourne, has been critical for the development of novel theranostic agents such as sartate [24, 25] now licenced to Clarity Pharmaceuticals (Sydney,

Australia). The government-funded Australian Nuclear Science and Technology Organisation (ANSTO) has also supported therapeutic nuclear oncology, most notably in recent years with the licencing of technology from Germany allowing for local production of Lutetium-177 in the replacement OPAL reactor. The premier government-backed scientific research organisation within Australia (CSIRO) has also committed, in the last 5 years, to research endeavours in this area developing a theranostics division within the organisation. The Australian Government itself has recognized the importance in supporting and developing the field of theranostics and through Australian Research Council and the Modern Manufacturing Initiative has committed tens of millions of dollars in the last 2–3 years to develop collaborative inititatives between public and private institutions in Australia in the areas of alpha particle therapy and novel radiometal PET pharmaceuticals.

Within the public and academic sector, ARTNET (Australasian Radiopharmaceutical Trials Network) was developed in 2014 as a joint initiative of the AANMS and the ANZSNM to address the need for a formal research network in Australia for collaborative multicentre clinical trials using radiopharmaceuticals for imaging and therapy. ARTNET provides advice on appropriate facilities for clinical trials, helps with protocol design if required, provides equipment and site validation and facilitates large-scale data collection. ARTNET has an executive committee which is responsible for overall governance, strategic planning and financial management of ARTNET and a scientific committee with wide representation from around Australia that oversees the scientific research activities of the network and reports to the committee. A similar network has recently been developed by the initially Australian, but now multinational, company GenesisCare. GenesisCare is one of the largest private oncology service provider in the world with over 150 cancer clinics throughout Australia, the UK and Spain. The GenesisCare network has a number of sites that provide imaging and therapy infrastructure for clinical trials as well as routine care of patients. This network differs from ARTNET in that GenesisCare also incorporates trial sites outside of Australia, has its own site research management within each jurisdiction (state or country) and has an overarching global contract research organisation liaising with pharma to facilitate efficient execution of mainly pharma-sponsored trials both within and outside of the GenesisCare trial network, thus linking both private and public institutions to achieve the aim of providing responsive high-quality research output. The network also works with external contract research organisations bringing pharma sponsored trials to the network. Due to the cost effectiveness of performing trial work in Australia, the high quality of research performed and the research and development tax incentives for overseas sponsors provided by the Australian government, there has been much interest from pharmaceutical companies to use this network as well as other Australian institutions, to perform, in particular, first-in-human, phase I and phase II theranostic trials in Australia.

Ultimately the aims of these networks, both in the public and private domains, are to obtain high-quality clinical trial evidence as quickly as possible to make the case for, or against, new theranostic agents. An additional benefit of a clinical network of sites utilising standardised protocols across the network is the ability to obtain high-quality real-world registry data as well as become an effective means to pursue post-marketing (phase IV) drug surveillance when the new theranostic agents are eventually approved and come into more widespread clinical use. This network registry approach has already yielded clinically significant findings for compassionate Lutetium-177 PSMA use in the Australian setting [26–29].

The success of this network approach is demonstrated in the speed of recruitment to trials, the high-quality, robust data collected, and the impact of the publications stemming from the data. The Pro-PSMA Study [30] and Thera-P study [31] looking at Gallium-68 PSMA and Lutetium-177 PSMA-617, respectively, are testament to this approach. This has had the consequence of further trial funding being successfully obtained for the newly initiated, Novartis-sponsored, ENZA-P

and Upfront trials. An added benefit of the network is by providing exposure in a controlled setting; this allows for the development of familiarity, experience and expertise across the whole nuclear medicine department, not only in running clinical trials but more importantly, in learning how to safely manage oncology patients. Thus, expertise in clinical decision-making and symptom management is developed on the back of the clinical trial. This will place the physicians and the departments involved in a position of knowledge and heightened clinical expertise for when these agents eventually become reimbursed and more freely available. Ultimately, this bodes well for the profession as it ensures patient safety and solidifies trust in the nuclear oncologist and the nuclear medicine department treating the patient.

In this chapter, I have hoped to guide you through the multiple reasons why Australia, like Germany, is currently one of the leaders in provision of cutting-edge techniques and new research in the areas of diagnostic and therapeutic nuclear medicine. A well-trained, academically focused work force, well-equipped facilities, attractive regulatory framework, supportive government nuclear and research science organisations and a strong commitment by practitioners in the field to develop well-organised collaborative networks with the aim of obtaining high-quality and robust data in a timely fashion are the combination of factors that have led to Australian nuclear medicine's current position in the world of theranostics and therapeutic nuclear oncology.

Potential Conflicts of Interest Dr. Lenzo is an employee and minority shareholder of GenesisCare. Dr Lenzo is also the founder and major shareholder in Cyclowest.

References

1. Beierwaltes WH. The history of the use of radioactive iodine. Semin Nucl Med. 1979;9(3):151–5.
2. Barnes RK. The National Medical Cyclotron–An Australian Experience in Technology; 1997. p. 76–9. www.osti.gov/etdeweb/servlets/purl/611850.
3. Gray BN, Burton MA, Kelleher DK, Anderson J, Klemp P. Selective internal radiation (SIR) therapy for treatment of liver metastases: measurement of

response rate. J Surg Oncol. 1989;42(3):192–6. https://doi.org/10.1002/jso.2930420313.

4. Gray BN, Anderson JE, Burton MA, van Hazel G, Codde J, Morgan C, Klemp P. Regression of liver metastases following treatment with yttrium-90 microspheres. Aust N Z J Surg. 1992;62(2):105–10. https://doi.org/10.1111/j.1445-2197.1992.tb00006.x.

5. Burton MA, Gray BN. Adjuvant internal radiation therapy in a model of colorectal cancer-derived hepatic metastases. Br J Cancer. 1995;71(2):322–5. https://doi.org/10.1038/bjc.1995.64.

6. Gray B, Van Hazel G, Hope M, Burton M, Moroz P, Anderson J, Gebski V. Randomised trial of SIR-spheres plus chemotherapy vs. chemotherapy alone for treating patients with liver metastases from primary large bowel cancer. Ann Oncol. 2001;12(12):1711–20. https://doi.org/10.1023/a:1013569329846.

7. Turner JH, Martindale AA, Boucek J, Claringbold PG, Leahy MF. 131I-anti CD20 radioimmunotherapy of relapsed or refractory non-Hodgkins lymphoma: a phase II clinical trial of a nonmyeloablative dose regimen of chimeric rituximab radiolabeled in a hospital. Cancer Biother Radiopharm. 2003;18(4):513–24. https://doi.org/10.1089/108497803322287583.

8. Leahy MF, Seymour JF, Hicks RJ, Turner JH. Multicenter phase II clinical study of iodine-131-rituximab radioimmunotherapy in relapsed or refractory indolent non-Hodgkin's lymphoma. J Clin Oncol. 2006;24(27):4418–25. Epub 2006 Aug 28. https://doi.org/10.1200/JCO.2005.05.3470.

9. Leahy MF, Turner JH. Radioimmunotherapy of relapsed indolent non-Hodgkin lymphoma with 131I-rituximab in routine clinical practice: 10-year single-institution experience of 142 consecutive patients. Blood. 2011;117(1):45–52. Epub 2010 Sep 23. https://doi.org/10.1182/blood-2010-02-269753.

10. McQuillan AD, Macdonald WB, Turner JH. Phase II study of first-line (131)I-rituximab radioimmunotherapy in follicular non-Hodgkin lymphoma and prognostic (18)F-fluorodeoxyglucose positron emission tomography. Leuk Lymphoma. 2015;56(5):1271–7. Epub 2014 Aug 19. https://doi.org/10.3109/10428194.2014.949260.

11. Hicks RJ. Use of molecular targeted agents for the diagnosis, staging and therapy of neuroendocrine malignancy. Cancer Imaging. 2010;10(1A):S83–91. https://doi.org/10.1102/1470-7330.2010.9007.

12. Claringbold PG, Brayshaw PA, Price RA, Turner JH. Phase II study of radiopeptide 177Lu-octreotate and capecitabine therapy of progressive disseminated neuroendocrine tumours. Eur J Nucl Med Mol Imaging. 2011;38(2):302–11. Epub 2010 Oct 30. https://doi.org/10.1007/s00259-010-1631-x.

13. Claringbold PG, Price RA, Turner JH. Phase I-II study of radiopeptide 177Lu-octreotate in combination with capecitabine and temozolomide in advanced low-grade neuroendocrine tumors. Cancer Biother Radiopharm. 2012;27(9):561–9. Epub 2012 Oct 18. https://doi.org/10.1089/cbr.2012.1276.

14. Claringbold PG, Turner JH. Pancreatic neuroendocrine tumor control: durable objective response to combination 177Lu-Octreotate-Capecitabine-Temozolomide Radiopeptide chemotherapy. Neuroendocrinology. 2016;103(5):432–9. Epub 2015 Jun 10. https://doi.org/10.1159/000434723.

15. Kong G, Hicks RJ. Peptide receptor radiotherapy: current approaches and future directions. Curr Treat Options in Oncol. 2019;20(10):77. https://doi.org/10.1007/s11864-019-0677-7.

16. Kalff V, Hicks RJ, MacManus MP, Binns DS, McKenzie AF, Ware RE, Hogg A, Ball DL. Clinical impact of (18)F fluorodeoxyglucose positron emission tomography in patients with non-small-cell lung cancer: a prospective study. J Clin Oncol. 2001;19(1):111–8. https://doi.org/10.1200/JCO.2001.19.1.111.

17. Scott A, Rowe C, Allman K, Lenzo N, Hicks R, Stuckey J, Lin P, Kelly B, Kirkwood I, Ramshaw J, Macfarlane D, Fulham M. Australian prospective multicentre PET data collection project—impact of FDG PET in oncology, epilepsy and cardiac patients. J Nucl Med. 2007;48(supplement 2):185.

18. Scott AM, Gunawardana DH, Kelley B, Stuckey JG, Byrne AJ, Ramshaw JE, Fulham MJ. PET changes management and improves prognostic stratification in patients with recurrent colorectal cancer: results of a multicenter prospective study. J Nucl Med. 2008;49(9):1451–7. Epub 2008 Aug 14. https://doi.org/10.2967/jnumed.108.051615.

19. Scott AM, Gunawardana DH, Bartholomeusz D, Ramshaw JE, Lin P. PET changes management and improves prognostic stratification in patients with head and neck cancer: results of a multicenter prospective study. J Nucl Med. 2008;49(10):1593–600. Epub 2008 Sep 15. https://doi.org/10.2967/jnumed.108.053660.

20. Chatterton BE, Ho Shon I, Baldey A, Lenzo N, Patrikeos A, Kelley B, Wong D, Ramshaw JE, Scott AM. Positron emission tomography changes management and prognostic stratification in patients with oesophageal cancer: results of a multicentre prospective study. Eur J Nucl Med Mol Imaging. 2009;36(3):354–61. Epub 2008 Oct 18. https://doi.org/10.1007/s00259-008-0959-y.

21. Scott AM, Gunawardana DH, Wong J, Kirkwood I, Hicks RJ, Ho Shon I, Ramshaw JE, Robins P. Positron emission tomography changes management, improves prognostic stratification and is superior to gallium scintigraphy in patients with low-grade lymphoma: results of a multicentre prospective study. Eur J Nucl Med Mol Imaging. 2009;36(3):347–53. Epub 2008 Oct 18. https://doi.org/10.1007/s00259-008-0958-z.

22. Fulham MJ, Carter J, Baldey A, Hicks RJ, Ramshaw JE, Gibson M. The impact of PET-CT in suspected recurrent ovarian cancer: a prospective multi-Centre study as part of the Australian PET data collection project. Gynecol Oncol. 2009;112(3):462–8. Epub 2009 Jan 15. https://doi.org/10.1016/j.ygyno.2008.08.027.

23. Ware RE, Francis HW, Read KE. The Australian government's review of positron emission tomography: evidence-based policy-making in action. Med J Aust. 2004;180(12):627–32. https://doi.org/10.5694/j.1326-5377.2004.tb06125.x.

24. Paterson BM, Roselt P, Denoyer D, Cullinane C, Binns D, Noonan W, Jeffery CM, Price RI, White JM, Hicks RJ, Donnelly PS. PET imaging of tumours with a 64Cu labeled macrobicyclic cage amine ligand tethered to Tyr3-octreotate. Dalton Trans. 2014;43(3):1386–96. Epub 2013 Nov 7. https://doi.org/10.1039/c3dt52647j.

25. Cullinane C, Jeffery CM, Roselt PD, van Dam EM, Jackson S, Kuan K, Jackson P, Binns D, van Zuylekom J, Harris MJ, Hicks RJ, Donnelly PS. Peptide receptor radionuclide therapy with (67)Cu-CuSarTATE is highly efficacious against a somatostatin-positive neuroendocrine tumor model. J Nucl Med. 2020;61(12):1800–5. Epub 2020 May 15. https://doi.org/10.2967/jnumed.120.243543.

26. von Eyben FE, Singh A, Zhang J, Nipsch K, Meyrick D, Lenzo N, Kairemo K, Joensuu T, Virgolini I, Soydal C, Kulkarni HR, Baum RP. (177)Lu-PSMA radioligand therapy of predominant lymph node metastatic prostate cancer. Oncotarget. 2019;10(25):2451–61. https://doi.org/10.18632/oncotarget.26789.

27. Gallyamov M, Meyrick D, Barley J, Lenzo N. Renal outcomes of radioligand therapy: experience of (177) lutetium-prostate-specific membrane antigen ligand therapy in metastatic castrate-resistant prostate cancer. Clin Kidney J. 2019;13(6):1049–55. https://doi.org/10.1093/ckj/sfz101.

28. Meyrick D, Gallyamov M, Sabarimurugan S, Falzone N, Lenzo N. Real-world data analysis of efficacy and survival after Lutetium-177 labelled PSMA ligand therapy in metastatic castration-resistant prostate cancer. Target Oncol. 2021;16:369. Online ahead of print. https://doi.org/10.1007/s11523-021-00801-w.

29. Kesavan M, Meyrick D, Gallyamov M, Turner JH, Yeo S, Cardaci G, Lenzo NP. Efficacy and haematological toxicity of palliative radioligand therapy of metastatic castrate-resistant prostate cancer with Lutetium-177 labeled prostate specific membrane antigen in heavily pre-treated patients. Diagnostics. 2021;11:515.

30. Hofman MS, Lawrentschuk N, Francis RJ, Tang C, Vela I, Thomas P, Rutherford N, Martin JM, Frydenberg M, Shakher R, Wong LM, Taubman K, Ting Lee S, Hsiao E, Roach P, Nottage M, Kirkwood I, Hayne D, Link E, Marusic P, Matera A, Herschtal A, Iravani A, Hicks RJ, Williams S, Murphy DG, proPSMA Study Group Collaborators. Prostate-specific membrane antigen PET-CT in patients with high-risk prostate cancer before curative-intent surgery or radiotherapy (proPSMA): a prospective, randomised, multicentre study. Lancet. 2020;395(10231):1208–16. Epub 2020 Mar 22. https://doi.org/10.1016/S0140-6736(20)30314-7.

31. Hofman MS, Emmett L, Sandhu S, Iravani A, Joshua AM, Goh JC, Pattison DA, Tan TH, Kirkwood ID, Ng S, Francis RJ, Gedye C, Rutherford NK, Weickhardt A, Scott AM, Lee ST, Kwan EM, Azad AA, Ramdave S, Redfern AD, Macdonald W, Guminski A, Hsiao E, Chua W, Lin P, Zhang AY, MM MJ, Stockler MR, Violet JA, Williams SG, Martin AJ, Davis ID, TheraP Trial Investigators and the Australian and New Zealand Urogenital and Prostate Cancer Trials Group. [(177) Lu]Lu-PSMA-617 versus cabazitaxel in patients with metastatic castration-resistant prostate cancer (TheraP): a randomised, open-label, phase 2 trial. Lancet. 2021;397(10276):797–804. Epub 2021 Feb 11. https://doi.org/10.1016/S0140-6736(21)00237-3.

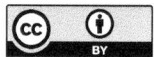

Berthold A. Nock and Theodosia Maina

22.1 Introduction

Advances in molecular biology and basic cancer research have documented the expression of "footprint" biomolecules on the surface of tumor cells, as for example antigens, peptide receptors, or enzymes [1–3]. This finding offers the opportunity to direct the respective radionuclide carriers to these biomolecular targets on cancer sites after injection to patients. Accordingly, radiolabeled antibodies, peptides or enzyme inhibitors will deliver gamma (e.g., ^{99m}Tc, ^{111}In) or positron emitters (e.g., ^{68}Ga, ^{64}Cu) to tumor sites with a high specificity for SPECT and PET imaging, respectively. Molecular imaging consequently represents a powerful tool for initial diagnosis, assessment of disease spread and patient stratification for the step which may follow next, namely, radionuclide therapy. The latter is accomplished by applying the same molecular probe which this time will deliver cytotoxic payloads to tumor sites by means of particle-emitting radionuclides, such as Auger electron (^{111}In), beta (^{177}Lu, $^{64/67}$Cu), or alpha (^{213}Bi, ^{225}Ac) emitters. Again, molecular imaging with the respective diagnostic counterpart will be instrumental not only for the preceding dosimetry and therapy planning but most importantly for monitoring therapeutic responses and disease progression. Hence, diagnosis and therapy—theranostics—may be elegantly combined in the management of cancer patients allowing for a personalized approach with maximized benefits. Furthermore, molecular imaging is essential for sparing patients from ineffective and toxic therapies which will only deteriorate quality of life without offering any tangible benefits [4–10].

All abovementioned classes of compounds have shown successful application paradigms in clinical nuclear medicine, but in the current chapter we shall focus on radiolabeled peptide analogs [3]. Peptides are native substances regulating a plethora of functions in the human body via specific interaction with protein receptors located on the cell membrane of target cells. Peptide receptors belong to the superfamily of G-protein coupled receptors (GPCRs) characterized by seven transmembrane domains and are essential for the transduction of extracellular messages within the cell [11, 12]. Most drugs of classical pharmacology are directed against GPCRs. Thus, native peptides as well as synthetic anti-GPCR drugs (peptidic or not) represent an abundant source of chemical entities that may serve as motifs for the development of radionuclide peptide-like carriers directed to GPCRs on tumors [13–15].

Amongst the attractive features of peptides for clinical application, one can cite their low immunogenicity, fast reaching the target after injection, rapid clearance from the body, most often prefer-

B. A. Nock · T. Maina (✉)
Molecular Radiopharmacy, INRASTES, NCSR
"Demokritos", Athens, Greece

V. Prasad (ed.), *Beyond Becquerel and Biology to Precision Radiomolecular Oncology: Festschrift in Honor of Richard P. Baum*, https://doi.org/10.1007/978-3-031-33533-4_22

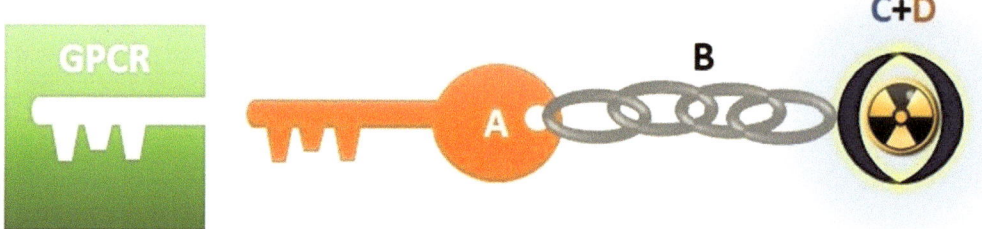

Fig. 22.1 Radiolabeled bioconjugate comprising the peptide part (**A**), the linker (**B**), and the chelator (**C**) stably binding the radiometal (**D**); the radiopeptide localizes on tumor sites through specific interaction with the GPCR target residing on tumor cells

ably via the kidneys and the urinary system. Moreover, peptides have turned out to be resilient during chemical and radiochemical manipulations, and can be synthesized and modified with relative ease, as compared with other vectors, as for example antibodies. A major problem in their use is associated with their notorious propensity to proteolytic degradation mainly by a class of enzymes hydrolyzing peptide bonds, that is, peptidases (vide infra). Further concerns during the development of peptide analogs for use in nuclear medicine are the high-density expression of the GPCR target in physiological tissues and organs of the body as well as the adverse effects elicited in patients after injection of peptide agonists and activation of their cognate receptor [3, 15, 16].

Peptide-based radionuclide carriers used in nuclear medicine usually comprise the following major segments (Fig. 22.1): the peptide fragment (A), recognizing and interacting with the cognate GPCR target on cancer cells, the metal chelator (C) binding the radiometal of choice (D) while coupled to the peptide chain either directly or via the linker or spacer (B), keeping the metal-chelate and the peptide segments apart from each other and often serving as a pharmacokinetic modifier [8, 15, 17, 18].

22.2 Peptides and GPCR Targets on Tumors

The rationale behind the clinical success of theranostic radiopeptides in the management of human tumors relies one hand on the high density and high incidence expression of the cognate GPCR target on tumor cells and on the other on the lack or minimal expression of the target in healthy surrounding tissue [3]. The list of Table 22.1 includes major peptide families used as motifs in the development of theranostic radiopeptides and the tumor classes where they are overexpressed.

Thus far, the research activities of Molecular Radiopharmacy at NCSR "Demokritos" (MR-NCSRD) have been directed toward the development and preclinical screening of radiopeptides from the somatostatin, bombesin (BBN)/gastrin-releasing peptide (GRP), cholecystokinin (CCK)/gastrin and neurotensin (NT) peptide families (Table 22.1), for eventual clinical assessment in patients. The problems and difficulties during this effort will be briefly discussed in individual sections in this chapter.

Although the GPCR targets of the above-mentioned peptide families are abundantly present in the tumors indicated in the table, they are also physiologically expressed in certain tissues and organs of the body complicating the application of diagnosis and therapy. Thus, the somatostatin subtype 2 receptor (SST_2R) [19–23] and the gastrin-releasing peptide receptor (GRPR) [24–31] are expressed in high numbers in the human pancreas, the cholecystokinin subtype 2 receptors (CCK_2Rs) [32–38] are abundantly found in the gastric mucosa and neurotensin subtype 1 receptors (NTS_1Rs) [39–44] in the intestines. Moreover, radiopeptide excretion via the kidneys may be delayed in some cases due to tubular reabsorption mechanisms, imposing dosimetric restrictions for radionuclide therapy [45].

Table 22.1 Peptides and target receptors on tumors; the clinically relevant subtypes are marked in bold

Peptide	Receptor	Tumor expression
Somatostatin	SST_1R, **SST_2R**, SST_3R, SST_4R, SST_5R	NET, NHL, melanoma, BC, MTC, SCLC
Bombesin/ GRP	$BB_1R/$ NMBR, **$BB_2R/$ GRPR**, BB_3R	PC, BC, SCLC, colorectal cancer, glioblastoma, gastrinoma, GIST
CCK/gastrin	CCK_1R, **CCK_2R**	MTC, SCLC, astrocytoma, stromal ovarian cancer, GIST
Neurotensin	**NTS_1R**, NTS_2R, NTS_3R	SCLC, PDAC, Ewing sarcoma, meningioma, astrocytoma
Substance P	**NK_1R**, NK_2R, NK_3R	Glioblastoma, astrocytoma, SCLC, MTC, BC
NPY	**NPY_1R**, **NPY_2R**, **NPY_4R**, NPY_5R	PC, renal cell carcinoma, ovarian adenocarcinoma, neuroblastoma, paraganglioma, GIST
VIP	**$VPAC_1R$**, $VPAC_2R$	SCLC, colorectal cancer, BC, gastrinoma, PC
α-MSH	**$MC_{1-5}R$**	Melanoma

NET neuroendocrine tumor, *NHL* non-Hodgkin's lymphoma, *BC* breast cancer, *MTC* medullary thyroid carcinoma, *SCLC* small cell lung cancer, *GRP* gastrin-releasing peptide, *PC* prostate cancer, *GIST* gastrointestinal stromal tumors, *PDAC* pancreatic ductal adenocarcinoma, *LHRH* luteinizing hormone-releasing hormone, *NPY* neuropeptide Y, *VIP* vasoactive intestinal peptide, *α-MSH* α-melanocyte-stimulating hormone

These handicaps may be addressed by structural modifications of the peptide chain and/or the linker. Other approaches have been adopted as well. For example, faster washout of BBN-like radiopeptide agonists from physiological GRPR-rich organs, such as the pancreas, can be achieved by the application of GRPR-antagonists instead [46, 47]. Such a switch from agonist- to antagonist-based radiopeptides offers the additional advantage of circumventing the problem of adverse effects elicited after GRPR activation. Finally, reduction of renal accumulation can be effectively tackled by applying kidney protection regimens. For example, infusion of the plasma expander gelofusine alone or in combination with basic amino acid cocktails has been shown to significantly reduce the renal uptake of anti-SST_2R theranostic radiopeptides [45, 48, 49].

22.3   Radiometals and Their Chelators in Cancer Theranostics

A list of the most clinically relevant radiometals employed in cancer theranostics with the aid of radiopeptides is provided in Table 22.2, including subgroups of radiometals for SPECT, PET and for radionuclide therapy, along with their nuclear characteristics and modes of production [17, 18, 50]. Radiometals used in MR-NCSRD facilities are: ^{99m}Tc, ^{111}In and ^{177}Lu; for the development of ^{68}Ga-radiopeptides for PET, we have used the ^{67}Ga surrogates ($t_{1/2}$: 78.3 h, decay: EC/100%— 887.7, 393.5, 184.6, 93.3/keV, cyclotron produced).

The pre-eminent diagnostic radionuclide in nuclear medicine has been and still is ^{99m}Tc, owing to its excellent nuclear properties, wide and cost-effective availability in high specific activity and high purity via commercial ^{99}Mo/^{99m}Tc generators [51–53]. The versatile coordination chemistry of ^{99m}Tc, seen often both as a blessing and a curse, offers exciting options for the development of new chelating systems and for "revisiting" existing ones for molecular imaging applications. The ^{99m}Tc-based peptide radioligands developed at MR-NCSRD for diagnosis of human tumors with SPECT and SPECT/CT have involved acyclic tetraamines for binding of the radiometal. Such tetraamine donor arrangements have been shown to form monocationic octahedral *trans*-dioxo-Tc-chelates, which are hydrophilic and in vivo robust (Fig. 22.2) [54, 55]. Several somatostatin, BBN, gastrin and NT analogs have been coupled to 6-R-1,4,8,11-tetraazaundecane (R: a bifunctional anchor, such as a carboxylic group) and labeled with ^{99m}Tc. During biological evaluation in preclinical models a few analogs displayed excellent profiles qualifying for further clinical testing as well. It should be noted that due to the "lanthanide con-

Table 22.2 Radiometals for PET and SPECT imaging and for radionuclide therapy

Modality	Radionuclide	Half-life	Decay mode (%)	$E_\gamma/E_\beta/E_\alpha$ (keV)	Production
SPECT	^{99m}Tc	6.02 h	γ, IC (100%)	141	^{99}Mo/^{99m}Tc generator
	^{111}In	67.2 h	Auger e$^-$, EC (100%)	172, 247	Cyclotron
PET	^{68}Ga	67.8 min	β^+ (90%), EC (10%)	820, 1895	^{68}Ge/^{68}Ga generator
	^{64}Cu	12.7 h	β^+ (18%), β^- (39%), EC (43%)	653	Reactor
	^{89}Zr	78.4 h	β^+ (23%), EC (77%)	396	Cyclotron
Therapy	^{177}Lu	6.7 d	β^- (79%), γ (21%)	174, 249, 385, 497	Reactor
	^{90}Y	64.1 h	β^- (100%)	2270	^{90}Sr/^{90}Y generator
	^{213}Bi	45.6 min	β^- (97.8%), α (2.2%)	5500, 5900 8320	^{225}Ac/^{213}Bi generator
	^{225}Ac	9.920 d	α (100%)	5935	^{229}Th/^{225}Ac generator, reactor, cyclotron
	^{67}Cu	61.8 h	β^- (100%)	570	Accelerator

EC electron capture, *IC* internal conversion, E_γ photon energy, E_β β energy, E_α α energy

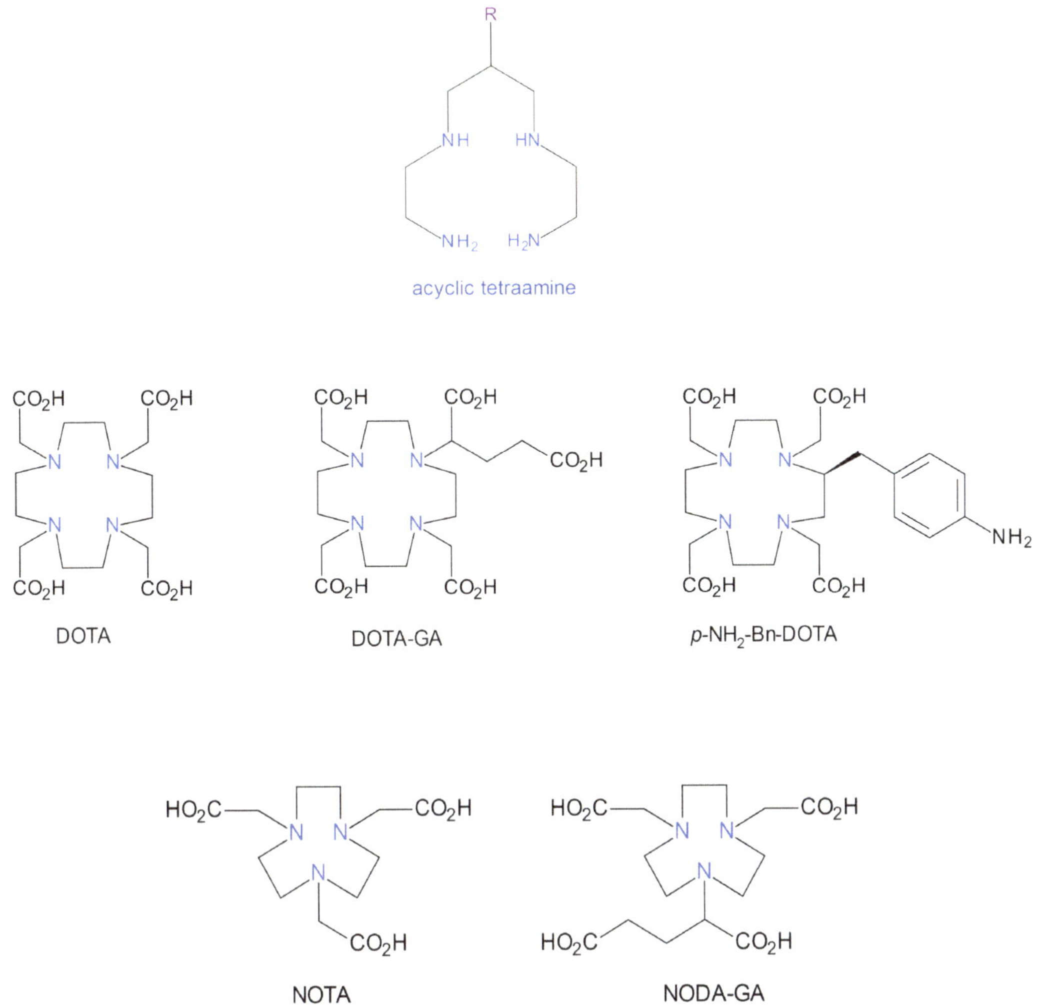

Fig. 22.2 Bifunctional chelators used for labeling peptides with ^{99m}Tc (acyclic tetraamines) and the trivalent metals ^{111}In, ^{177}Lu and $^{67/68}$Ga at MR-NCSRD (the polyamino-polycarboxylic-macrocycles DOTA, NOTA and their bifunctional versions)

traction" the atomic radii of technetium and its third row congener rhenium are almost identical and their compounds exhibit similar physico-chemical and structural characteristics [56]. Rhenium, besides serving as a surrogate for technetium during chemical investigations, is of special relevance to nuclear medicine by means of two important therapeutic radionuclides, ^{186}Re ($t_{1/2}$: 90.6 h, decay: β^- 2120 keV/γ 155 keV, reactor produced) and ^{188}Re ($t_{1/2}$: 17 h, decay: EC/100% - 887.7, 393.5, 184.6, 93.3 /keV, ^{188}W/^{188}Re generator) [57]. This fact provides the exciting prospect of routine preparations of matched ^{99m}Tc/diagnostic–$^{186/188}$Re/therapeutic radiopharmaceutical pairs in hospital radiopharmacy departments.

The trivalent radionuclides listed in Table 22.2 form stable complexes with the polyamino-polycarboxylic-macrocycles DOTA (1,4,7,10-tetraazacyclododecane-1,4,7,10-tetraacetic acid), NOTA (1,4,7-triazacyclononane-N,N',N''-triacetic acid) and their bifunctional versions (Fig. 22.2) [17, 18, 50]. The majority of the peptide analogs developed at MR-NCSRD have been derivatized with the so called universal chelator DOTA, because it provides the unique option of labeling peptides with $^{67/68}$Ga (for PET), ^{111}In (for SPECT) and ^{177}Lu (for radionuclide therapy) without the need for developing analogs carrying a different chelator for each application. It should be noted however that, owing to the differences in the coordination chemistries across these radiometals, the forming radiopeptides may differ in their charge, lipophilicity and other physicochemical features. As a result, significant differences may be observed in several biological responses, including receptor affinity, metabolic stability and pharmacokinetics [58–60]. The use of theranostic radionuclides (e.g., ^{64}Cu) [61, 62], or theranostic radioisotopes of the same element (e.g., $^{149/152/155/161}$Tb, or $^{44/47}$Sc) [63–65] represents an attractive alternative in this respect. Selection of the appropriate radionuclide for each application depends on several important factors, such as advantageous nuclear characteristics, availability and cost [50].

22.4 Metabolic Stability of Radiopeptides: The Pep-Protect Concept

A major hurdle in the development of peptide drugs, including peptide radiopharmaceuticals, is their susceptibility to enzymes hydrolyzing the peptide bond, known as peptidases [13, 14]. Peptidases are abundantly present in the biological milieu and are found in the blood solute, the extracellular matrix, within cells, as well as anchored on epithelial cell membranes in many organs and tissues of the body. Omnipresent peptidases are actually orchestrating the action of native peptides, cooperating with other enzymes to release the active peptide from precursor molecules and degrading it thereafter to biologically inert fragments [66]. In nuclear medicine applications, the peptide radiopharmaceutical is intravenously injected to patients and rapidly—within minutes—reaches the GPCR-targets on tumor sites owing to its small size. The integrity of the radiopeptide within this time window is very essential for its "safe" arrival to tumor sites and subsequent uptake by cancer cells. Such integrity may be seriously challenged by peptidases

encountered by the radiopeptide on the way to the target, which may act quite fast and devastatingly (Fig. 22.3) [67].

In fact, several studies using in vitro incubation of radiopeptides in plasma or serum have shown the swift action of peptidases found in the blood solute, such as angiotensin-converting enzyme (ACE) [66, 68, 69]. Recently, the leading role of neprilysin (NEP) in the rapid in vivo degradation of radioligands originating from numerous peptide families has been revealed by chromatographic analysis of blood samples collected after injection in the living organism [67]. Interestingly, the above-mentioned central role of NEP had been largely disregarded, because its presence in plasma or serum is minimal. Instead, NEP is anchored on vasculature walls and epithelial cell membranes of several tissues and organs of the body, such as lungs, intestines and kidneys, in high local concentrations [70, 71]. The fast degrading action of NEP, ACE and/or other proteases, encountered by the radiopeptide after entering the circulation allows only a small portion of the intact analog to reach and eventually interact with the GPCR target on tumor sites. Hence, tumor uptake is compromised, directly impairing image quality and/or therapeutic index.

One way to address the problem of metabolic instability is via structural modifications of the peptide sequence, such as replacements of key amino acids by their D- or beta-congeners or by other synthetic residues, cyclization, reduction or methylation of known cleavage sites, or even substitution of peptide bonds by their 1,2,3-triazole isosteres [13, 14, 72]. All these methods are time- and resources-intensive. At the same time, improvements of metabolic stability by structural interventions very often occur at the cost of other biological characteristics, important for the optimal performance of radiopeptide analogs, such as receptor affinity, internalization rate and pharmacokinetics.

We have recently proposed the co-administration of a single or twin protease inhibitor with the radiopeptide to "protect" it from the attacking proteases (NEP and/or ACE) and "serve" for safer delivery at tumor sites, the so-called pep-protect concept (Fig. 22.3) [67]. We

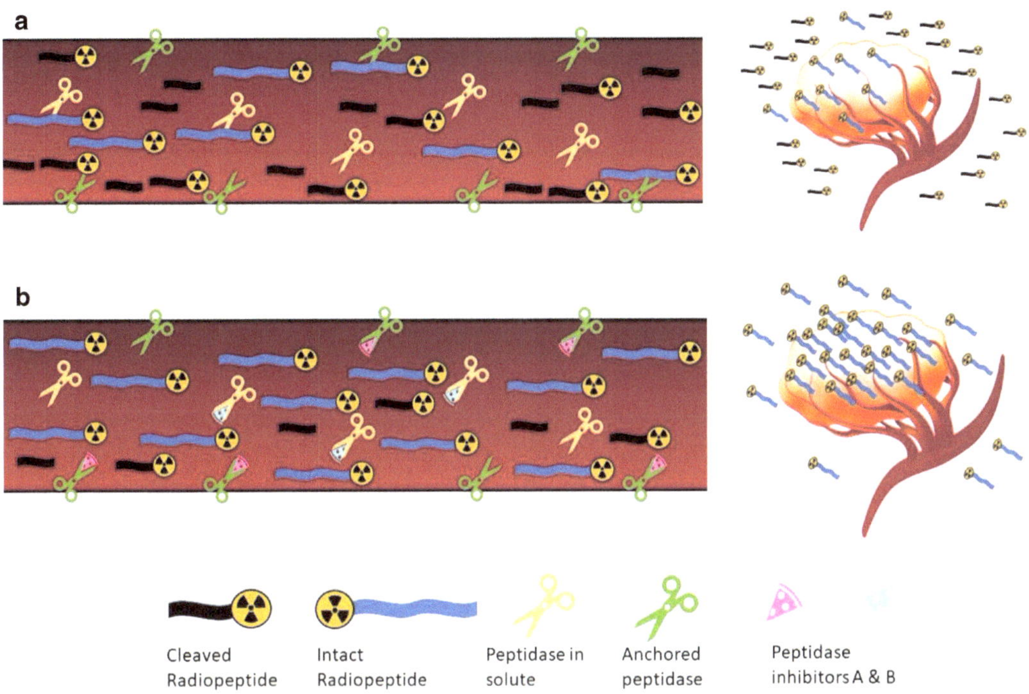

Cleaved Radiopeptide	Intact Radiopeptide	Peptidase in solute	Anchored peptidase	Peptidase inhibitors A & B

Fig. 22.3 (**a**) Upon entry into the blood stream, a biodegradable radiopeptide is attacked by peptidases, such as wall-anchored neprilysin (green) and/or angiotensin-converting enzyme in the solute (yellow). Thus, only a few intact radiopeptide molecules are delivered to tumor sites, compromising tumor uptake. (**b**) Coinjection of suitable peptidase(s)-inhibitor(s), such as phosphoramidon, or thiorphan (pink) and/or lisinopril (turquoise), leads to an increase of the number of intact radiopeptide molecules that will be delivered to tumor sites, enhancing the localization of the radiolabel to malignant lesions. This will eventually translate into improved imaging quality and/or therapeutic index

have shown that administration of a NEP-inhibitor (or a precursor thereof), such as phosphoramidon [73], thiorphan [70], or sacubitrilat [74], can stabilize biodegradable radiopeptides from the somatostatin [67], BBN [60, 72, 75–80], gastrin [66, 81–84] and NT [69] families, translating into notable increases of tumor targeting in experimental animal models. In a few cases, combination of a NEP and an ACE-inhibitor, such as lisinopril, is required for maximum effect [69, 82, 83]. This simple and elegant concept warrants further validation in the clinic. The availability of registered and over-the-counter NEP [70, 74] and ACE [85] inhibitors that have been used for years for a series of medical conditions is a valuable asset in this respect. It should be noted that the first promising results on the efficacy and safety of the pep-protect approach have been very recently reported for radiolabeled gastrin in a small number of medullary thyroid carcinoma patients (MTC) [86]. These results will pave the way for broader application of the pep-protect concept in nuclear oncology.

22.5   Radiopeptide Agonists and Antagonists

The first peptide motifs used for the development of peptide radiopharmaceuticals were native peptides, acting as agonists at their cognate receptors on target cells and thereby regulating several functions of the body. Accordingly, the synthetic cyclic octapeptide somatostatin analog octreotide and its derivatives targeting the SST_2R on neuroendocrine tumor (NET) cells preserve the ability of the parent hormone to induce the SST_2R internalization after binding and to transduce pharmacological responses further within the cell [87]. The ability of radioagonists to internalize has long been considered as an essential prerequisite for high uptake and prolonged retention of radiopeptides on tumor sites, enhancing diagnostic signal and therapeutic responses [88]. Surprisingly though, radiolabeled SST_2R-antagonists showed significantly higher in vitro uptake in target cells and in experimental tumors in animal models [89, 90]. It was shown that these analogs were able to bind to a significant larger SST_2R population (both in active and inactive state) on target cells remaining bound on the cell surface for long periods of time. Another unexpected feature of SST_2R radioantagonists was their notably faster clearance from physiological tissues compared to agonists. All above-mentioned clinically attractive qualities were subsequently demonstrated in patients as well [47].

Unlike somatostatin which exerts inhibitory effects on target cells, other native peptides after binding and activation of their cognate receptor elicit potent pharmacological responses mainly in the gut and the nervous system [91–93]. Accordingly, intravenous administration of even small amounts of such peptides and their analogs may turn out to be very unpleasant and even dangerous to patients. For example, during clinical testing of BBN-like radioligands in prostate cancer patients, severe effects from the gastrointestinal system were recorded raising serious biosafety concerns in the nuclear medicine community [94]. It should be added that several GPCR agonists in addition exert proliferative action on cancer cells. Consequently, large libraries of synthetic GPCR antagonists have been developed in previous decades as anticancer drugs [95]. This plethora of well-established motifs represents an invaluable asset to radiopharmacists engaged in the design of antagonist-based radiopeptides. Usually, truncation of C-terminal residues and other chemical manipulations, like alkylamidation or esterification of the C-terminal carboxylic group, has proven to be an efficient means to generate receptor-antagonists from agonist precursors.

In recent years, a wide range of radiolabeled GRPR antagonists have been introduced as potential theranostic agents in the management of prostate and breast cancers with relative success [46]. In most cases, prolonged tumor retention and rapid background clearance could be established both in animal models and in humans. None of the adverse effects elicited by the administration of BBN-like radioligands was observed, further favoring the application of antagonists in the clinic. It should be noted that antagonists display better metabolic stability and are more subtype selective compared to agonists too. A list of the major GPCR-radioagonists and antagonists developed at MR-NCSRD is shown in Table 22.3, divided by receptor target [46, 77, 82, 84, 96–136].

It is interesting to mention as well recent experience at MR-NCSRD from the gastrin and NT radioligands. Gastrin analogs elicit adverse effects after intravenous injection to patients, which have been well-known to clinicians from the broadly applied provocative pentagastrin test [91]. Nevertheless, a wide range of radiolabeled CCK_2R-radiotracers have been developed over the years, a few of which have been clinically tested [115–117]. A non-peptidic CCK_2R-radioantagonist, ^{99m}Tc-DGA1 has been recently introduced by us in a head-to-head comparison with the clinically tested agonist ^{99m}Tc-Demogastrin 2, showing promising qualities for targeting CCK_2R-positive lesions in MTC patients [123]. Further studies with peptide−/peptidomimetic-based CCK_2R-radioantagonists will reveal potential benefits of their use compared to agonists. Several efforts have also been directed toward the development of NT-based radiopeptides to target NTS_1R-positive tumors, such as pancreatic ductal adenocarcinoma (PDAC), or small-cell lung cancer (SCLC), with very moderate success thus far. A major handicap of NTS_1R-directed radiopeptides is related to the very poor metabolic stability of NT and its analogs in vivo, the loss of internalization capability of structurally modified analogs thereof with enhanced stability and the often high kidney retention. We have shown first promising results

Table 22.3 List of major GPCR radioligands developed at MR-NCSRD, divided by receptor family groups and in subgroups of agonists and antagonists, including references

GPCR-family/subtype	Name	Structure	Radiometal	References
$SST_{1-5}R$	PanSS-28	[DOTA]LTT-SS28	^{111}In	[108]
	PanSS-14	[DOTA]SS14-based	^{111}In	[109, 110]
SST_2R	Demotates	[N$_4$-X]Tate	^{99m}Tc	[111–114]
	DATA-Tide	[DATA]Tide	$^{67/68}$Ga	[107]
GRPR	*Agonists*			
	Demobesins	[N'$_4$/N$_4$-X]BBN/BBN(6-14)	^{99m}Tc	[99, 105]
	Demomedins	[N'$_4$/N$_4$-X]GRP(17-27)	^{99m}Tc	[77, 101, 103]
	GRP-based	[DOTA]GRP(17-27)/GRP(13-27)	^{111}In	[100]
	Antagonists			
	Demobesins	[N'$_4$/N$_4$-X,DPhe^6,Leu-NHEt^{13}]BBN(6-13)	^{99m}Tc	[97, 104, 106]
	SB3	[DOTA,DPhe^6,Leu-NHEt^{13}]BBN(6-13)	$^{67/68}$Ga, ^{111}In, ^{177}Lu	[46, 60, 78, 79, 134]
	NeoBOMB1	[DOTA,DPhe^6,His^{12}-NH-CH[CH$_2$-NH-CH[CH$_2$-CH(CH$_3$)$_2$]$_2$]BBN(6-12)	$^{67/68}$Ga, ^{111}In, ^{177}Lu	[98, 133, 135, 136]
CCK_2R	*Agonists*			
	Demogastrins	[N'$_4$/N$_4$-X-DGlu^1]MG	^{99m}Tc	[82, 115–117]
	SGs	[DOTA-X-DGlu^1]MG/MG(10-17)	^{111}In	[81, 83, 84, 86]
	Antagonists			
	DGA1	[N$_4$-X]Z360	^{99m}Tc	[123]
NTS_1R	Demotensins	[N$_4$-X]NT(8-13)-based	^{99m}Tc	[69, 118–120]

DOTA 1,4,7,10-tetraazacyclododecane-1,4,7,10-tetraacetic acid, *LTT-SS28* [Ser^1,Leu^8,DTrp^{22},Tyr^{25}]SS28, *SS28* H-Ser-Ala-Asn-Ser-Asn-Pro-Ala-Leu-Ala-Pro-Arg-Glu-Arg-Lys-Ala-Gly-c[Cys-Lys-Asn-Phe-Phe-Trp-Lys-Thr-Phe-Thr-Ser-Cys]-OH, *SS14* Ala-Gly-c[Cys-Lys-Asn-Phe-Phe-Trp-Lys-Thr-Phe-Thr-Ser-Cys-OH], *X* linker or spacer, *N$_4$* 6-(carboxy)-1,4,8,11-tetraazaundecane, *Tate* H-DPhe-c[Cys-Tyr-DTrp-Lys-Thr-Cys]-Thr-ol), *DATA* 6-amino-1,4-diazepine-triacetic acid, *Tide* H-DPhe-c[Cys-Tyr-DTrp-Lys-Thr-Cys]-Thr-ol), *N'$_4$* 6-{*p*-[(carboxymethoxy)acetyl]aminobenzyl}-1,4,8,11-tetraazaundecane), *BBN* Pyr-Gln-Arg-Leu-Gly-Asn-Gln-Trp-Ala-Val-Gly-His-Leu-Met-NH$_2$, *GRP* H-Val-Pro-Leu-Pro-Ala-Gly-Gly-Gly-Thr-Val-Leu-Thr-Lys-Met-Tyr-Pro-Arg-Gly-Asn-His-Trp-Ala-Val-Gly-His-Leu-Met-NH$_2$, *MG0* [DOTA-DGlu^1]minigastrin, mini-gastrin: H-Leu-(Glu)$_5$-Ala-Tyr-Gly-Trp-Met-Asp-Phe-NH$_2$, *[DGlu]MG(10–17)* H-DGlu-Ala-Tyr-Gly-Trp-Met-Asp-Phe-NH$_2$, *Z360* Nastorazepide, 3-[[[[(3R)-5-Cyclohexyl-1-(3,3-dimethyl-2-oxobutyl)-2,3,4,5-tetrahydro-2-oxo-1H-1,5-benzodiazepin-3-yl]amino]carbonyl]amino]benzoic acid, *NT* H-Pyr-Leu-Tyr-Glu-Asn-Lys-Pro-Arg-Arg-Pro-Tyr-Ile-Leu-OH

for clinical translation by the application of a ^{99m}Tc-labeled NT(8–13) analog in combination with the pep-protect concept [118–122]. By minimal structural interventions and protease-inhibition regimens, we could observe preservation of full internalization capacity of the radiotracer in NTS₁R-positive cells and stabilization in peripheral mice blood, translating into high uptake in experimental NTS₁R-positive tumors and rapid background clearance in mice [69]. Recently, a non-peptidic NTS₁R-antagonist has been used as a motif for the generation of a library of radiolabeled analogs for cancer theranostics. Surprisingly, these agents displayed high internalization rates in target cells despite their antagonistic profile during functional assays, such as Ca^{2+}-mobilization. The clinical value of this class of compounds remains to be confirmed [124–126].

22.6   Radiopeptide Candidates for Clinical Translation

The preclinical evaluation of new radiopeptides in cell and animal models is an essential step to identify best candidates for translation in patients [127]. Proof-of-principle studies are indeed very crucial to verify that the promising profile of a peptide radioligand acquired in mice can accurately depict its actual performance in cancer patients. Discrepancies may occur from interspecies differences at both the molecular and the macroscopic levels [128, 129]. For example, newly developed radioligands may be able to distinguish between the mouse and the human receptor target and thus, uptake and clearance from tissues physiologically expressing the receptor may differ. On the other hand, tumor induction, localization and propagation in mice models are distinctly different than spontaneous carcinogenesis events occurring in patients. Furthermore, the rate of several physiological functions vary between mice and men, partly due to differences of body weight, eventually affect-

ing bioavailability, tumor uptake and background clearance. Accordingly, results from proof-of-principle studies in a small number of patients are necessary for first assessments of a new agent's clinical value, qualifying or disqualifying it for broader clinical validation and potentially for subsequent radiopharmaceutical development [130]. The last step is expected to last for years, is highly costly and requires considerable managerial and regulatory expertise which is usually provided by pharmaceutical industry. Hence, pilot studies are invaluable in cutting down costs, time and efforts to the minimum, by addressing translational concerns and further narrowing down choices to justifiable candidates.

Until recently, license for performing pilot translational studies with diagnostic peptide-radioligands required approval by the clinical center's ethical committee after submission of a summary of the compound specifications. The latter included information on the synthesis and radiolabeling of the new agent, along with data on its efficacy during preclinical testing in cells and mice models expressing the GPCR target. Information on biosafety practically comprised acute single dose toxicity study in one animal species, usually mice. At a later stage, approval of the clinical protocol was additionally requested from national authorities. Under the latter status, we were able to get official clearance and perform first translational studies of the somatostatin-based ^{99m}Tc-Demotate 1 in NET patients and the neurotensin-based ^{99m}Tc-Demotensin 6 in pancreatic, lung and other type cancer patients in cooperation with the University Clinics, Innsbruck, Austria [112, 113, 118]. Likewise, pilot studies have been conducted for the gastrin-based ^{99m}Tc-Demogastrin 2 applying SPECT/CT initially at the University Clinics Marburg in Germany [117] and subsequently at Erasmus MC, Rotterdam, The Netherlands (Table 22.3) [115, 116]. Soon thereafter in an increasing number of EU countries, starting with the UK, approvals required much more detailed and thorough information on new compounds of GMP grade, as for example more extended toxicology studies. We had the opportunity to follow the newly imposed regulations during a pilot study on the BBN-like radiotracer ^{99m}Tc-Demobesin 4 in a small number of prostate cancer patients in St. Bartholomew's Hospital, London, UK [99]. The compilation of all necessary efficacy and safety data as well as the availability of sufficient amounts of GMP-grade tracer required strong support from a sponsor, in this case "Cancer Research UK."

Clearly, in most EU countries, regulations for clinical studies have been becoming stricter over recent years, requiring license not only from ethical committees of clinical centers, but also from national or even from European authorities, such as European Medicines Agency (EMEA), especially in case of multicenter clinical trials. Consequently, both high-quality GMP-grade radiotracers and extensive efficacy and safety documentation have become mandatory [130–132]. At the same time, in a few EU countries, it is still possible to carry out pilot studies with new compounds locally in a small number of patients, under certain provisions. For example, in Germany, the decision to conduct a diagnostic peptide-radio-ligand proof-of-principle study can be based on the opinion of the referring oncologist as the best choice for the patients' respective clinical conditions. The new agent should be administered in compliance with the German Medicinal Products Act (section 13, subsection 2b), the 1964 Declaration of Helsinki, and the responsible regulatory body and under the compassionate-use clause of the German Medicinal Products Act (Federal Institute for Drugs and Medical Devices, "Compassionate use" programs, http://www.bfarm.de/EN/Drugs/licensing/clinicalTrials/compUse/_node). Following this pathway, we have recently performed such clinical studies in Bad Berka with two promising diagnostic ^{68}Ga-labeled GRPR-antagonists, ^{68}Ga-SB3 [46] and ^{68}Ga-NeoBOMB1 [133], and PET/CT in a small number of prostate and breast cancer patients with very positive outcomes. Accordingly, ^{68}Ga-SB3 is further evaluated in Erasmus MC, Rotterdam, The Netherlands, in early stage therapy naïve prostate cancer patients [134]. It should be noted that positive results on ^{68}Ga-NeoBOMB1 in prostate cancer patients are being further acquired in Erasmus MC, Rotterdam, The Netherlands, as well as in gastrointestinal stromal tumor (GIST) patients at Innsbruck University Hospital, Austria [135]. These results have attracted the interest of the private sector, currently supporting the performance of multi-center clinical studies aiming at radiopharmaceutical development and registration [136].

Acknowledgments We wish to thank so many colleagues and friends who have been supporting us in a multitude of ways since our early days at MR-NCSRD. Special thanks to Prof. H. Maecke (University Hospital Basel, Switzerland), who first initiated us in the field of radiopeptides, Prof. J.C. Reubi (Institute of Pathology, University of Berne, Switzerland) for excellent cooperation and inspiring discussions on exciting aspects of GPCR pharmacology, Prof. C. Decristoforo (University Hospital Innsbruck, Austria) and Prof. S. Mather (St. Bartholomew's Hospital, London, UK) for their cooperation in translational studies of our first products. Special thanks to Prof. M. de Jong and her team at Erasmus MC, Rotterdam, for a most fruitful cooperation for more than 20 years now and of course, Prof. E. P. Krenning (currently at Cyclotron Rotterdam BV, Erasmus MC), who has generously, firmly and unfailingly supported us in so many ways all this time. Special thanks as well to PiChem (Gratz, Austria) for a long and enduring cooperation and reliable provision of excellent quality peptide and peptidomimetic analogs.

Last but not least, we wish to thank Prof. Baum, Richard, for his enthusiastic inspiration of the clinical translation of two very important GRPR-antagonist-based ^{68}Ga-radiotracers for prostate and breast cancer diagnosis with PET/CT (Fig. 22.4). Richard, we know you since 2000 when you were visiting Greece within a COST Meeting. We then showed you our preclinical results of the first ^{99m}Tc-based GRPR-antagonist, ^{99m}Tc-Demobesin 1, in PC-3 tumor-bearing animals. Since that moment, you have been reminding us on every opportunity to provide you with the ^{68}Ga-version of ^{99m}Tc-Demobesin 1 the soonest possible and you would not let go – fortunately. Your strongly expressed willingness to test such agent in prostate and breast cancer patients applying PET/CT in Bad Berka, has been the impetus for

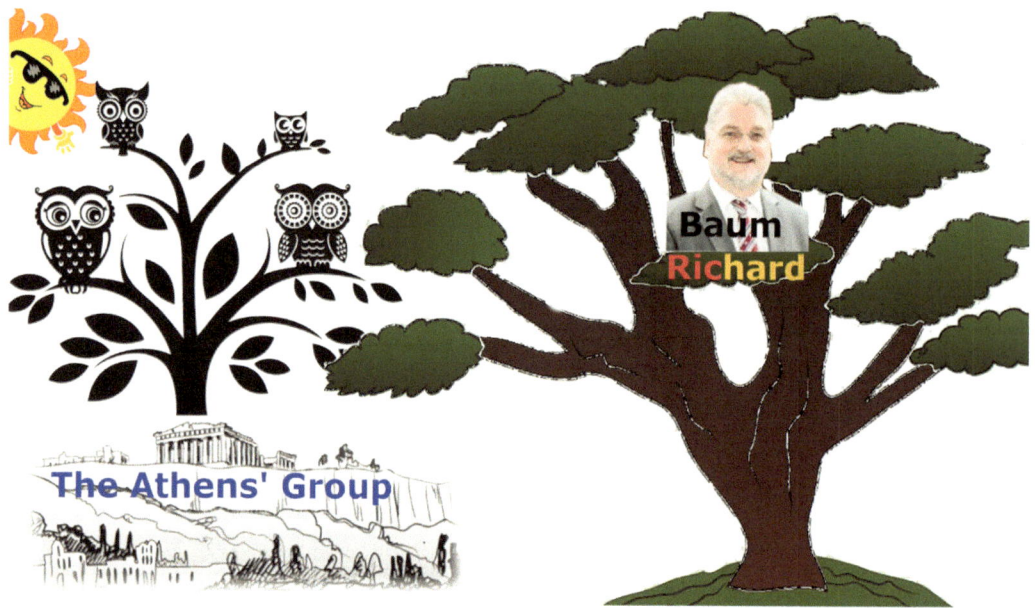

Fig. 22.4 The fruitful Athens (design, preclinical) ⇔ Bad Berka (clinical) interaction: Baum's (tree's) branches reaching out as far as Athens to interact with the local owl group

the successful development of ^{68}Ga-SB3 and ^{68}Ga-NeoBOMB1. Eventually, the first clinical testing of both ^{68}Ga-SB3 and ^{68}Ga-NeoBOMB1 was indeed performed by you and your team in Bad Berka. Thank you!.

References

1. Chen R, Snyder M. Systems biology: personalized medicine for the future? Curr Opin Pharmacol. 2012;12(5):623–8.
2. Herrmann K, Schwaiger M, Lewis JS, Solomon SB, McNeil BJ, Baumann M, Gambhir SS, Hricak H, Weissleder R. Radiotheranostics: a roadmap for future development. Lancet Oncol. 2020;21(3):e146–e56.
3. Reubi JC. Peptide receptors as molecular targets for cancer diagnosis and therapy. Endocr Rev. 2003;24(4):389–427.
4. Oberg K. Molecular imaging radiotherapy: Theranostics for personalized patient management of neuroendocrine tumors (NETs). Theranostics. 2012;2(5):448–58.
5. Zhang J, Singh A, Kulkarni HR, Schuchardt C, Müller D, Wester HJ, Maina T, Rösch F, van der Meulen NP, Müller C, Mäcke H, Baum RP. From bench to bedside-the Bad Berka experience with first-in-human studies. Semin Nucl Med. 2019;49(5):422–37.
6. Baum RP, Kulkarni HR. THERANOSTICS: from molecular imaging using Ga-68 labeled tracers and PET/CT to personalized radionuclide therapy—the Bad Berka experience. Theranostics. 2012;2(5):437–47.
7. Baum RP, Kulkarni HR, Carreras C. Peptides and receptors in image-guided therapy: theranostics for neuroendocrine neoplasms. Semin Nucl Med. 2012;42(3):190–207.
8. Fani M, Maecke HR, Okarvi SM. Radiolabeled peptides: valuable tools for the detection and treatment of cancer. Theranostics. 2012;2(5):481–501.
9. Fani M, Maecke HR. Radiopharmaceutical development of radiolabelled peptides. Eur J Nucl Med Mol Imaging. 2012;39(Suppl. 1):S11–30.
10. Farolfi A, Lima GM, Oyen W, Fanti S. Molecular imaging and theranostics—a multidisciplinary approach. Semin Nucl Med. 2019;49(4):247–54.
11. Alexander SPH, Christopoulos A, Davenport AP, Kelly E, Mathie A, Peters JA, Veale EL, Armstrong JF, Faccenda E, Harding SD, Pawson AJ, Sharman JL, Southan C, Davies JA, Collaborators C. THE CONCISE GUIDE TO PHARMACOLOGY 2019/20: G protein-coupled receptors. Br J Pharmacol. 2019;176(Suppl. 1):S21–S141.
12. Chan HCS, Li Y, Dahoun T, Vogel H, Yuan S. New binding sites, new opportunities for GPCR drug discovery. Trends Biochem Sci. 2019;44(4):312–30.
13. Vlieghe P, Lisowski V, Martinez J, Khrestchatisky M. Synthetic therapeutic peptides: science and market. Drug Discov Today. 2010;15(1–2):40–56.
14. Erak M, Bellmann-Sickert K, Els-Heindl S, Beck-Sickinger AG. Peptide chemistry toolbox—trans-

forming natural peptides into peptide therapeutics. Bioorg Med Chem. 2018;26(10):2759–65.

15. Chatalic KL, Kwekkeboom DJ, de Jong M. Radiopeptides for imaging and therapy: a radiant future. J Nucl Med. 2015;56(12):1809–12.

16. Maina T, Nock BA, Kulkarni H, Singh A, Baum RP. Theranostic prospects of gastrin-releasing peptide receptor-radioantagonists in oncology. PET Clin. 2017;12(3):297–309.

17. Kostelnik TI, Orvig C. Radioactive main group and rare earth metals for imaging and therapy. Chem Rev. 2019;119(2):902–56.

18. Cutler CS, Hennkens HM, Sisay N, Huclier-Markai S, Jurisson SS. Radiometals for combined imaging and therapy. Chem Rev. 2013;113(2):858–83.

19. Reubi JC, Schaer JC, Markwalder R, Waser B, Horisberger U, Laissue J. Distribution of somatostatin receptors in normal and neoplastic human tissues: recent advances and potential relevance. Yale J Biol Med. 1997;70(5–6):471–9.

20. Reubi JC, Kappeler A, Waser B, Schonbrunn A, Laissue J. Immunohistochemical localization of somatostatin receptor sst$_{2A}$ in human pancreatic islets. J Clin Endocrinol Metab. 1998;83(10):3746–9.

21. Reubi JC, Kappeler A, Waser B, Laissue J, Hipkin RW, Schonbrunn A. Immunohistochemical localization of somatostatin receptors sst$_{2A}$ in human tumors. Am J Pathol. 1998;153(1):233–45.

22. Reubi JC. Somatostatin and other peptide receptors as tools for tumor diagnosis and treatment. Neuroendocrinology. 2004;80(Suppl 1):51–6.

23. Reubi JC. Relevance of somatostatin receptors and other peptide receptors in pathology. Endocr Pathol. 1997;8(1):11–20.

24. Reubi JC, Wenger S, Schmuckli-Maurer J, Schaer JC, Gugger M. Bombesin receptor subtypes in human cancers: detection with the universal radioligand ^{125}I-[D-Tyr^6, beta-Ala^{11}, Phe^{13}, Nle^{14}] bombesin(6-14). Clin Cancer Res. 2002;8(4):1139–46.

25. Körner M, Waser B, Rehmann R, Reubi JC. Early over-expression of GRP receptors in prostatic carcinogenesis. Prostate. 2014;74(2):217–24.

26. Markwalder R, Reubi JC. Gastrin-releasing peptide receptors in the human prostate: relation to neoplastic transformation. Cancer Res. 1999;59(5):1152–9.

27. Beer M, Montani M, Gerhardt J, Wild PJ, Hany TF, Hermanns T, Muntener M, Kristiansen G. Profiling gastrin-releasing peptide receptor in prostate tissues: clinical implications and molecular correlates. Prostate. 2012;72(3):318–25.

28. Gugger M, Reubi JC. Gastrin-releasing peptide receptors in non-neoplastic and neoplastic human breast. Am J Pathol. 1999;155(6):2067–76.

29. Mattei J, Achcar RD, Cano CH, Macedo BR, Meurer L, Batlle BS, Groshong SD, Kulczynski JM, Roesler R, Dal Lago L, Brunetto AT, Schwartsmann G. Gastrin-releasing peptide receptor expression in lung cancer. Arch Pathol Lab Med. 2014;138(1):98–104.

30. Reubi JC, Körner M, Waser B, Mazzucchelli L, Guillou L. High expression of peptide receptors as a novel target in gastrointestinal stromal tumours. Eur J Nucl Med Mol Imaging. 2004;31(6):803–10.

31. Fleischmann A, Laderach U, Friess H, Buechler MW, Reubi JC. Bombesin receptors in distinct tissue compartments of human pancreatic diseases. Lab Invest. 2000;80(12):1807–17.

32. Reubi JC, Waser B. Unexpected high incidence of cholecystokinin-B/gastrin receptors in human medullary thyroid carcinomas. Int J Cancer. 1996;67(5):644–7.

33. Sethi T, Herget T, Wu SV, Walsh JH, Rozengurt E. CCKA and CCKB receptors are expressed in small cell lung cancer lines and mediate Ca^{2+} mobilization and clonal growth. Cancer Res. 1993;53(21):5208–13.

34. Reubi JC, Waser B, Gugger M, Friess H, Kleeff J, Kayed H, Buchler MW, Laissue JA. Distribution of CCK1 and CCK2 receptors in normal and diseased human pancreatic tissue. Gastroenterology. 2003;125(1):98–106.

35. Reubi JC, Schaer JC, Waser B. Cholecystokinin (CCK)-A and CCK-B/gastrin receptors in human tumors. Cancer Res. 1997;57(7):1377–86.

36. Hur K, Kwak MK, Lee HJ, Park DJ, Lee HK, Lee HS, Kim WH, Michaeli D, Yang HK. Expression of gastrin and its receptor in human gastric cancer tissues. J Cancer Res Clin Oncol. 2006;132(2):85–91.

37. Körner M, Waser B, Reubi JC, Miller LJ. CCK$_2$ receptor splice variant with intron 4 retention in human gastrointestinal and lung tumours. J Cell Mol Med. 2010;14(4):933–43.

38. Hayakawa Y, Jin G, Wang H, Chen X, Westphalen CB, Asfaha S, Renz BW, Ariyama H, Dubeykovskaya ZA, Takemoto Y, Lee Y, Muley A, Tailor Y, Chen D, Muthupalani S, Fox JG, Shulkes A, Worthley DL, Takaishi S, Wang TC. CCK$_2$R identifies and regulates gastric antral stem cell states and carcinogenesis. Gut. 2015;64(4):544–53.

39. Kitabgi P. Targeting neurotensin receptors with agonists and antagonists for therapeutic purposes. Curr Opin Drug Discov Devel. 2002;5(5):764–76.

40. Evers BM. Neurotensin and growth of normal and neoplastic tissues. Peptides. 2006;27(10):2424–33.

41. Evers BM, Ishizuka J, Chung DH, Townsend CM Jr, Thompson JC. Neurotensin expression and release in human colon cancers. Ann Surg. 1992;216(4):423–30. Discussion 30-1

42. Reubi JC, Waser B, Friess H, Büchler M, Laissue J. Neurotensin receptors: a new marker for human ductal pancreatic adenocarcinoma. Gut. 1998;42(4):546–50.

43. Reubi JC, Waser B, Schaer JC, Laissue JA. Neurotensin receptors in human neoplasms: high incidence in Ewing's sarcomas. Int J Cancer. 1999;82(2):213–8.

44. Nikolaou S, Qiu S, Fiorentino F, Simillis C, Rasheed S, Tekkis P, Kontovounisios C. The role of neuroten-

sin and its receptors in non-gastrointestinal cancers: a review. Cell Commun Signal. 2020;18(1):68.

45. Gotthardt M, van Eerd-Vismale J, Oyen WJ, de Jong M, Zhang H, Rolleman E, Maecke HR, Béhé M, Boerman O. Indication for different mechanisms of kidney uptake of radiolabeled peptides. J Nucl Med. 2007;48(4):596–601.

46. Maina T, Bergsma H, Kulkarni HR, Mueller D, Charalambidis D, Krenning EP, Nock BA, de Jong M, Baum RP. Preclinical and first clinical experience with the gastrin-releasing peptide receptor-antagonist [68Ga]SB3 and PET/CT. Eur J Nucl Med Mol Imaging. 2016;43(5):964–73.

47. Fani M, Nicolas GP, Wild D. Somatostatin receptor antagonists for imaging and therapy. J Nucl Med. 2017;58(Suppl. 2):61S.

48. Melis M, Bijster M, de Visser M, Konijnenberg MW, de Swart J, Rolleman EJ, Boerman OC, Krenning EP, de Jong M. Dose-response effect of gelofusine on renal uptake and retention of radiolabelled octreotate in rats with CA20948 tumours. Eur J Nucl Med Mol Imaging. 2009;36(12):1968–76.

49. Melis M, Krenning EP, Bernard BF, de Visser M, Rolleman E, de Jong M. Renal uptake and retention of radiolabeled somatostatin, bombesin, neurotensin, minigastrin and CCK analogues: species and gender differences. Nucl Med Biol. 2007;34(6):633–41.

50. Mikolajczak R, van der Meulen NP, Lapi SE. Radiometals for imaging and theranostics, current production, and future perspectives. J Labelled Comp Radiopharm. 2019;62(10):615–34.

51. Nock B, Maina T. Tetraamine-coupled peptides and resulting 99mTc-radioligands: an effective route for receptor-targeted diagnostic imaging of human tumors. Curr Top Med Chem. 2012;12(23):2655–67.

52. Dilworth JR, Parrott SJ. The biomedical chemistry of technetium and rhenium. Chem Soc Rev. 1998;27:43–5.

53. Schwochau K. Technetium radiopharmaceuticals - fundamentals, synthesis, structure, and development. Angew Chem Int Ed. 1994;33:2258–67.

54. Mantegazzi DIE, Lerch P, Nicoló F, Chapuis G. Preparation and crystal-structure of polymeric lithium[dioxoTc(V)tetraazaundecane]-bis(trifluoromethanesulfonate) complex. Inorg Chim Acta. 1990;176:99–105.

55. Blauenstein P, Pfeiffer G, Schubiger PA, Anderegg G, Zollinger K, May K, Proso Z, Ianovici E, Lerch P. Chemical and biological properties of a cationic Tc-tetraamine complex. Int J Appl Radiat Isot. 1985;36(4):315–7.

56. Parker DRP. Synthesis and characterization of stable rhenium(V) dioxo complexes with acyclic tetraamine ligands, [LReO2]+. Inorg Chem. 1988;27:4127–30.

57. Deutsch E, Libson K, Vanderheyden JL, Ketring AR, Maxon HR. The chemistry of rhenium and technetium as related to the use of isotopes of these elements in therapeutic and diagnostic nuclear medicine. Int J Rad Appl Instrum B. 1986;13(4):465–77.

58. Fani M, Braun F, Waser B, Beetschen K, Cescato R, Erchegyi J, Rivier JE, Weber WA, Maecke HR, Reubi JC. Unexpected sensitivity of sst2 antagonists to N-terminal radiometal modifications. J Nucl Med. 2012;53(9):1481–9.

59. Fani M, Del Pozzo L, Abiraj K, Mansi R, Tamma ML, Cescato R, Waser B, Weber WA, Reubi JC, Maecke HR. PET of somatostatin receptor-positive tumors using 64Cu- and 68Ga-somatostatin antagonists: the chelate makes the difference. J Nucl Med. 2011;52(7):1110–8.

60. Lymperis E, Kaloudi A, Sallegger W, Bakker IL, Krenning EP, de Jong M, Maina T, Nock BA. Radiometal-dependent biological profile of the radiolabeled gastrin-releasing peptide receptor antagonist SB3 in cancer theranostics: metabolic and biodistribution patterns defined by neprilysin. Bioconjug Chem. 2018;29(5):1774–84.

61. Wadas TJ, Wong EH, Weisman GR, Anderson CJ. Copper chelation chemistry and its role in copper radiopharmaceuticals. Curr Pharm Des. 2007;13(1):3–16.

62. Cai Z, Anderson CJ. Chelators for copper radionuclides in positron emission tomography radiopharmaceuticals. J Labelled Comp Radiopharm. 2014;57(4):224–30.

63. Müller C, Domnanich KA, Umbricht CA, van der Meulen NP. Scandium and terbium radionuclides for radiotheranostics: current state of development towards clinical application. Br J Radiol. 2018;91(1091):20180074.

64. Notni J, Wester HJ. Re-thinking the role of radiometal isotopes: towards a future concept for theranostic radiopharmaceuticals. J Labelled Comp Radiopharm. 2018;61(3):141–53.

65. Talip Z, Favaretto C, Geistlich S, Meulen NPV. A step-by-step guide for the novel radiometal production for medical applications: case studies with 68Ga, 44Sc, 177Lu and 161Tb. Molecules. 2020;25(4):966.

66. Kaloudi A, Nock BA, Krenning EP, Maina T, de Jong M. Radiolabeled gastrin/CCK analogs in tumor diagnosis: towards higher stability and improved tumor targeting. Q J Nucl Med Mol Imaging. 2015;59(3):287–302.

67. Nock BA, Maina T, Krenning EP, de Jong M. "To serve and protect": enzyme inhibitors as radiopeptide escorts promote tumor targeting. J Nucl Med. 2014;55(1):121–7.

68. Ocak M, Helbok A, Rangger C, Peitl PK, Nock BA, Morelli G, Eek A, Sosabowski JK, Breeman WA, Reubi JC, Decristoforo C. Comparison of biological stability and metabolism of CCK2 receptor targeting peptides, a collaborative project under COST BM0607. Eur J Nucl Med Mol Imaging. 2011;38(8):1426–35.

69. Kanellopoulos P, Kaloudi A, Jong M, Krenning EP, Nock BA, Maina T. Key-protease inhibition regimens promote tumor targeting of neurotensin radioligands. Pharmaceutics. 2020;12(6):528.

70. Roques BP. Zinc metallopeptidases: active site structure and design of selective and mixed inhibitors: new approaches in the search for analgesics and anti-hypertensives. Biochem Soc Trans. 1993;21(Pt 3):678–85.

71. Roques BP, Noble F, Dauge V, Fournie-Zaluski MC, Beaumont A. Neutral endopeptidase 24.11: structure, inhibition, and experimental and clinical pharmacology. Pharmacol Rev. 1993;45(1):87–146.

72. Maina T, Kaloudi A, Valverde IE, Mindt TL, Nock BA. Amide-to-triazole switch vs. in vivo NEP-inhibition approaches to promote radiopeptide targeting of GRPR-positive tumors. Nucl Med Biol. 2017;52:57–62.

73. Suda H, Aoyagi T, Takeuchi T, Umezawa H. Letter: a thermolysin inhibitor produced by actinomycetes: Phosphoramidon. J Antibiot (Tokyo). 1973;26(10):621–3.

74. McMurray JJ, Packer M, Desai AS, Gong J, Lefkowitz MP, Rizkala AR, Rouleau JL, Shi VC, Solomon SD, Swedberg K, Zile MR, Investigators P-H, Committees. Angiotensin-neprilysin inhibition versus enalapril in heart failure. N Engl J Med. 2014;371(11):993–1004.

75. Mitran B, Rinne SS, Konijnenberg MW, Maina T, Nock BA, Altai M, Vorobyeva A, Larhed M, Tolmachev V, de Jong M, Rosenstrom U, Orlova A. Trastuzumab cotreatment improves survival of mice with PC-3 prostate cancer xenografts treated with the GRPR antagonist ^{177}Lu-DOTAGA-PEG$_2$-RM26. Int J Cancer. 2019;145:3347.

76. Lymperis E, Kaloudi A, Kanellopoulos P, Krenning EP, de Jong M, Maina T, Nock BA. Comparative evaluation of the new GRPR-antagonist ^{111}In-SB9 and ^{111}In-AMBA in prostate cancer models: implications of in vivo stability. J Labelled Comp Radiopharm. 2019;62(10):646–55.

77. Kaloudi A, Lymperis E, Kanellopoulos P, Waser B, de Jong M, Krenning EP, Reubi JC, Nock BA, Maina T. Localization of ^{99m}Tc-GRP analogs in GRPR-expressing tumors: effects of peptide length and neprilysin inhibition on biological responses. Pharmaceuticals (Basel). 2019;12(1):42.

78. Lymperis E, Kaloudi A, Kanellopoulos P, de Jong M, Krenning EP, Nock BA, Maina T. Comparing Gly^{11}/dAla^{11}-replacement vs. the in-situ neprilysin-inhibition approach on the tumor-targeting efficacy of the ^{111}In-SB3/^{111}In-SB4 radiotracer pair. Molecules. 2019;24(6):1015.

79. Bakker IL, van Tiel ST, Haeck J, Doeswijk GN, de Blois E, Segbers M, Maina T, Nock BA, de Jong M, Dalm SU. In vivo stabilized SB3, an attractive GRPR antagonist, for pre- and intra-operative imaging for prostate cancer. Mol Imaging Biol. 2018;20(6):973–83.

80. Chatalic KL, Konijnenberg M, Nonnekens J, de Blois E, Hoeben S, de Ridder C, Brunel L, Fehrentz JA, Martinez J, van Gent DC, Nock BA, Maina T, van Weerden WM, de Jong M. In vivo stabilization of a gastrin-releasing peptide receptor antagonist

enhances PET imaging and radionuclide therapy of prostate cancer in preclinical studies. Theranostics. 2016;6(1):104–17.

81. Kaloudi A, Nock BA, Lymperis E, Krenning EP, de Jong M, Maina T. Improving the in vivo profile of minigastrin radiotracers: a comparative study involving the neutral endopeptidase inhibitor phosphoramidon. Cancer Biother Radiopharm. 2016;31(1):20–8.

82. Kaloudi A, Nock BA, Lymperis E, Krenning EP, de Jong M, Maina T. ^{99m}Tc-labeled gastrins of varying peptide chain length: distinct impact of NEP/ACE-inhibition on stability and tumor uptake in mice. Nucl Med Biol. 2016;43(6):347–54.

83. Kaloudi A, Nock BA, Lymperis E, Valkema R, Krenning EP, de Jong M, Maina T. Impact of clinically tested NEP/ACE inhibitors on tumor uptake of [^{111}In-DOTA]MG11-first estimates for clinical translation. EJNMMI Res. 2016;6(1):15.

84. Kaloudi A, Nock BA, Lymperis E, Sallegger W, Krenning EP, de Jong M, Maina T. In vivo inhibition of neutral endopeptidase enhances the diagnostic potential of truncated gastrin ^{111}In-radioligands. Nucl Med Biol. 2015;42(11):824–32.

85. Millar JA, Derkx FH, McLean K, Reid JL. Pharmacodynamics of converting enzyme inhibition: the cardiovascular, endocrine and autonomic effects of MK421 (enalapril) and MK521. Br J Clin Pharmacol. 1982;14(3):347–55.

86. Valkema RFA, Maina T, Nock BA, de Blois E, Melis ML, Konijnenberg MW, Koolen SLW, Peeters RP, de Herder WW, de Jong M. Clinical translation of the PepProtect: a novel method to improve the detection of cancer and metastases by peptide scanning under the protection of enzyme inhibitors. Eur J Nucl Med Mol Imaging. 2019;46(Suppl. 1):S701–2.

87. Cescato R, Schulz S, Waser B, Eltschinger V, Rivier JE, Wester HJ, Culler M, Ginj M, Liu Q, Schonbrunn A, Reubi JC. Internalization of sst$_2$, sst$_3$, and sst$_5$ receptors: effects of somatostatin agonists and antagonists. J Nucl Med. 2006;47(3):502–11.

88. de Jong M, Breeman WA, Kwekkeboom DJ, Valkema R, Krenning EP. Tumor imaging and therapy using radiolabeled somatostatin analogues. Acc Chem Res. 2009;42(7):873–80.

89. Cescato R, Erchegyi J, Waser B, Piccand V, Maecke HR, Rivier JE, Reubi JC. Design and in vitro characterization of highly sst$_2$-selective somatostatin antagonists suitable for radiotargeting. J Med Chem. 2008;51(13):4030–7.

90. Ginj M, Zhang H, Waser B, Cescato R, Wild D, Wang X, Erchegyi J, Rivier J, Macke HR, Reubi JC. Radiolabeled somatostatin receptor antagonists are preferable to agonists for in vivo peptide receptor targeting of tumors. Proc Natl Acad Sci U S A. 2006;103(44):16436–41.

91. Ubl P, Gincu T, Keilani M, Ponhold L, Crevenna R, Niederle B, Hacker M, Li S. Comparison of side effects of pentagastrin test and calcium stimulation test in patients with increased basal calcito-

nin concentration: the gender-specific differences. Endocrine. 2014;46(3):549–53.

92. Bruzzone R, Tamburrano G, Lala A, Mauceri M, Annibale B, Severi C, de Magistris L, Leonetti F, Delle FG. Effect of bombesin on plasma insulin, pancreatic glucagon, and gut glucagon in man. J Clin Endocrinol Metab. 1983;56(4):643–7.

93. Bitar KN, Zhu XX. Expression of bombesin-receptor subtypes and their differential regulation of colonic smooth muscle contraction. Gastroenterology. 1993;105(6):1672–80.

94. Bodei L, Ferrari M, Nunn A, Llull J, Cremonesi M, Martano L, Laurora G, Scardino E, Tiberini S, Bufi G, Eaton S, de Cobelli O, Paganelli G. ^{177}Lu-AMBA bombesin analogue in hormone refractory prostate cancer patients: a phase I escalation study with single-cycle administrations. Eur J Nucl Med Mol Imaging. 2007;34(Suppl. 2):S221.

95. de Castiglione R, Gozzini L. Bombesin receptor antagonists. Crit Rev Oncol Hematol. 1996;24(2):117–51.

96. Maina T, Nock BA. From bench to bed: new gastrin-releasing peptide receptor-directed radioligands and their use in prostate cancer. PET Clin. 2017;12(2):205–17.

97. Nock BA, Charalambidis D, Sallegger W, Waser B, Mansi R, Nicolas GP, Ketani E, Nikolopoulou A, Fani M, Reubi JC, Maina T. New gastrin releasing peptide receptor-directed [^{99m}Tc]Demobesin 1 mimics: synthesis and comparative evaluation. J Med Chem. 2018;61(7):3138–50.

98. Kaloudi A, Lymperis E, Giarika A, Dalm S, Orlandi F, Barbato D, Tedesco M, Maina T, de Jong M, Nock BA. NeoBOMB1, a GRPR-antagonist for breast cancer theragnostics: first results of a preclinical study with [^{67}Ga]NeoBOMB1 in T-47D cells and tumor-bearing mice. Molecules. 2017;22(11):1950.

99. Mather SJ, Nock BA, Maina T, Gibson V, Ellison D, Murray I, Sobnack R, Colebrook S, Wan S, Halberrt G, Szysko T, Powles T, Avril N. GRP receptor imaging of prostate cancer using [^{99m}Tc]Demobesin 4: a first-in-man study. Mol Imaging Biol. 2014;16(6):888–95.

100. Marsouvanidis PJ, Maina T, Sallegger W, Krenning EP, de Jong M, Nock BA. Tumor diagnosis with new ^{111}In-radioligands based on truncated human gastrin releasing peptide sequences: synthesis and preclinical comparison. J Med Chem. 2013;56(21):8579–87.

101. Marsouvanidis PJ, Maina T, Sallegger W, Krenning EP, de Jong M, Nock BA. ^{99m}Tc radiotracers based on human GRP(18-27): synthesis and comparative evaluation. J Nucl Med. 2013;54(10):1797–803.

102. Marsouvanidis PJ, Nock BA, Hajjaj B, Fehrentz JA, Brunel L, M'Kadmi C, van der Graaf L, Krenning EP, Maina T, Martinez J, de Jong M. Gastrin releasing peptide receptor-directed radioligands based on a bombesin antagonist: synthesis, ^{111}In-labeling, and preclinical profile. J Med Chem. 2013;56(6):2374–84.

103. Nock BA, Cescato R, Ketani E, Waser B, Reubi JC, Maina T. [^{99m}Tc]Demomedin C, a radioligand based on human gastrin releasing peptide(18-27): synthesis and preclinical evaluation in gastrin releasing peptide receptor-expressing models. J Med Chem. 2012;55(19):8364–74.

104. Cescato R, Maina T, Nock B, Nikolopoulou A, Charalambidis D, Piccand V, Reubi JC. Bombesin receptor antagonists may be preferable to agonists for tumor targeting. J Nucl Med. 2008;49(2):318–26.

105. Nock BA, Nikolopoulou A, Galanis A, Cordopatis P, Waser B, Reubi JC, Maina T. Potent bombesin-like peptides for GRP-receptor targeting of tumors with ^{99m}Tc: a preclinical study. J Med Chem. 2005;48(1):100–10.

106. Nock B, Nikolopoulou A, Chiotellis E, Loudos G, Maintas D, Reubi JC, Maina T. [^{99m}Tc]Demobesin 1, a novel potent bombesin analogue for GRP receptor-targeted tumour imaging. Eur J Nucl Med Mol Imaging. 2003;30(2):247–58.

107. Nock BA, Kaloudi A, Nagel J, Sinnes JP, Roesch F, Maina T. Novel bifunctional DATA chelator for quick access to site-directed PET Ga-68-radiotracers: preclinical proof-of-principle with [Tyr^3]octreotide. Dalton Trans. 2017;46(42):14584–90.

108. Maina T, Cescato R, Waser B, Tatsi A, Kaloudi A, Krenning EP, de Jong M, Nock BA, Reubi JC. [^{111}In-DOTA]LTT-SS28, a first pansomatostatin radioligand for in vivo targeting of somatostatin receptor-positive tumors. J Med Chem. 2014;57(15):6564–71.

109. Tatsi A, Maina T, Cescato R, Waser B, Krenning EP, de Jong M, Cordopatis P, Reubi JC, Nock BA. [DOTA]Somatostatin-14 analogs and their ^{111}In-radioligands: effects of decreasing ring-size on sst$_{1-5}$ profile, stability and tumor targeting. Eur J Med Chem. 2014;73:30–7.

110. Tatsi A, Maina T, Cescato R, Waser B, Krenning EP, de Jong M, Cordopatis P, Reubi JC, Nock BA. [^{111}In-DOTA]Somatostatin-14 analogs as potential pansomatostatin-like radiotracers - first results of a preclinical study. EJNMMI Res. 2012;2(1):25.

111. Maina T, Nock BA, Cordopatis P, Bernard BF, Breeman WA, van Gameren A, van den Berg R, Reubi JC, Krenning EP, de Jong M. [^{99m}Tc]Demotate 2 in the detection of sst$_2$-positive tumours: a preclinical comparison with [^{111}In]DOTA-Tate. Eur J Nucl Med Mol Imaging. 2006;33(7):831–40.

112. Gabriel M, Decristoforo C, Maina T, Nock B, von-Guggenberg E, Cordopatis P, Moncayo R. ^{99m}Tc-N$_4$-[Tyr^3]octreotate versus ^{99m}Tc-EDDA/HYNIC-[Tyr^3] octreotide: an intrapatient comparison of two novel technetium-99m labeled tracers for somatostatin receptor scintigraphy. Cancer Biother Radiopharm. 2004;19(1):73–9.

113. Decristoforo C, Maina T, Nock B, Gabriel M, Cordopatis P, Moncayo R. ^{99m}Tc-Demotate 1: first data in tumour patients-results of a pilot/phase I study. Eur J Nucl Med Mol Imaging. 2003;30(9):1211–9.

114. Maina T, Nock B, Nikolopoulou A, Sotiriou P, Loudos G, Maintas D, Cordopatis P, Chiotellis E. [^{99m}Tc]Demotate, a new ^{99m}Tc-based [Tyr^3] octreotate analogue for the detection of somatostatin receptor-positive tumours: synthesis and preclinical results. Eur J Nucl Med Mol Imaging. 2002;29(6):742–53.

115. Fröberg AC, de Jong M, Nock BA, Breeman WA, Erion JL, Maina T, Verdijsseldonck M, de Herder WW, van der Lugt A, Kooij PP, Krenning EP. Comparison of three radiolabelled peptide analogues for CCK-2 receptor scintigraphy in medullary thyroid carcinoma. Eur J Nucl Med Mol Imaging. 2009;36(8):1265–72.

116. Breeman WA, Fröberg AC, de Blois E, van Gameren A, Melis M, de Jong M, Maina T, Nock BA, Erion JL, Macke HR, Krenning EP. Optimised labeling, preclinical and initial clinical aspects of CCK-2 receptor-targeting with 3 radiolabeled peptides. Nucl Med Biol. 2008;35(8):839–49.

117. Nock BA, Maina T, Béhé M, Nikolopoulou A, Gotthardt M, Schmitt JS, Behr TM, Macke HR. CCK-2/gastrin receptor-targeted tumor imaging with ^{99m}Tc-labeled minigastrin analogs. J Nucl Med. 2005;46(10):1727–36.

118. Gabriel M, Decristoforo C, Woll E, Eisterer W, Nock B, Maina T, Moncayo R, Virgolini I. [^{99m}Tc] Demotensin VI: biodistribution and initial clinical results in tumor patients of a pilot/phase I study. Cancer Biother Radiopharm. 2011;26(5):557–63.

119. Maina T, Nikolopoulou A, Stathopoulou E, Galanis AS, Cordopatis P, Nock BA. [^{99m}Tc]Demotensin 5 and 6 in the NTS1-R-targeted imaging of tumours: synthesis and preclinical results. Eur J Nucl Med Mol Imaging. 2007;34(11):1804–14.

120. Nock BA, Nikolopoulou A, Reubi JC, Maes V, Conrath P, Tourwé D, Maina T. Toward stable N$_4$-modified neurotensins for NTS1-receptor-targeted tumor imaging with ^{99m}Tc. J Med Chem. 2006;49(15):4767–76.

121. Buchegger F, Bonvin F, Kosinski M, Schaffland AO, Prior J, Reubi JC, Blauenstein P, Tourwé D, Garcia Garayoa E, Bischof DA. Radiolabeled neurotensin analog, ^{99m}Tc-NT-XI, evaluated in ductal pancreatic adenocarcinoma patients. J Nucl Med. 2003;44(10):1649–54.

122. Fröberg AC, Verdijsseldonck MC, Melis M, Bakker H, Krenning EP. Use of neurotensin analogue IN-111-DTPA-neurotensin (IN-111-MP2530) in diagnosis of pancreatic adenocarcinoma. Eur J Nucl Med Mol Imaging. 2004;31(Suppl. 2):S392.

123. Kaloudi A, Kanellopoulos P, Radolf T, Chepurny OG, Rouchota M, Loudos G, Andreae F, Holz GG, Nock BA, Maina T. [^{99m}Tc]Tc-DGA1, a promising CCK$_2$R-antagonist-based tracer for tumor diagnosis with single-photon emission computed tomography. Mol Pharm. 2020;17:3116–28.

124. Schulz J, Rohracker M, Stiebler M, Goldschmidt J, Grosser OS, Osterkamp F, Pethe A, Reineke U, Smerling C, Amthauer H. Comparative evaluation of the biodistribution profiles of a series of nonpeptidic neurotensin receptor-1 antagonists reveals a promising candidate for theranostic applications. J Nucl Med. 2016;57(7):1120–3.

125. Schulz J, Rohracker M, Stiebler M, Goldschmidt J, Stober F, Noriega M, Pethe A, Lukas M, Osterkamp F, Reineke U, Hohne A, Smerling C, Amthauer H. Proof of therapeutic efficacy of a ^{177}Lu-labeled neurotensin receptor 1 antagonist in a colon carcinoma xenograft model. J Nucl Med. 2017;58(6):936–41.

126. Baum RP, Singh A, Schuchardt C, Kulkarni HR, Klette I, Wiessalla S, Osterkamp F, Reineke U, Smerling C. ^{177}Lu-3BP-227 for neurotensin receptor 1-targeted therapy of metastatic pancreatic adenocarcinoma: first clinical results. J Nucl Med. 2018;59(5):809–14.

127. de Jong M, Mather S, Maina T. Preclinical in vivo cancer tudies, straightway to patients? Q J Nucl Med Mol Imaging. 2017;61(2):145–52.

128. Maina T, Nock BA, Zhang H, Nikolopoulou A, Waser B, Reubi JC, Maecke HR. Species differences of bombesin analog interactions with GRP-R define the choice of animal models in the development of GRP-R-targeting drugs. J Nucl Med. 2005;46(5):823–30.

129. de Jong M, Maina T. Of mice and humans: are they the same?—Implications in cancer translational research. J Nucl Med. 2010;51(4):501–4.

130. Kolenc-Peitl P, Rangger C, Garnuszek P, Mikolajczak R, Hubalewska-Dydejczyk A, Maina T, Erba P, Decristoforo C. Clinical translation of theranostic radiopharmaceuticals: current regulatory status and recent examples. J Labelled Comp Radiopharm. 2019;62(10):673–83.

131. Maina T, Konijnenberg MW, Kolenc-Peitl P, Garnuszek P, Nock BA, Kaloudi A, Kroselj M, Zaletel K, Maecke H, Mansi R, Erba P, von Guggenberg E, Hubalewska-Dydejczyk A, Mikolajczak R, Decristoforo C. Preclinical pharmacokinetics, biodistribution, radiation dosimetry and toxicity studies required for regulatory approval of a phase I clinical trial with ^{111}In-CP04 in medullary thyroid carcinoma patients. Eur J Pharm Sci. 2016;91:236–42.

132. Pawlak D, Rangger C, Kolenc-Peitl P, Garnuszek P, Maurin M, Ihli L, Kroselj M, Maina T, Maecke H, Erba P, Kremser L, Hubalewska-Dydejczyk A, Mikolajczak R, Decristoforo C. From preclinical development to clinical application: kit formulation for radiolabelling the minigastrin analogue CP04 with In-111 for a first-in-human clinical trial. Eur J Pharm Sci. 2016;85:1–9.

133. Nock BA, Kaloudi A, Lymperis E, Giarika A, Kulkarni HR, Klette I, Singh A, Krenning EP, de Jong M, Maina T, Baum RP. Theranostic perspectives in prostate cancer with the gastrin-releasing peptide receptor antagonist NeoBOMB1: preclinical and first clinical results. J Nucl Med. 2017;58(1):75–80.

134. Bakker IL, van Leenders GJLH, Segbers M, Fröberg AC, Dalm YK, Veenland J, Konijnenberg M,

Busstra MB, Verzijlbergen JF, Schoots J, de Blois E, van Weerden WM, Maina T, Nock B, de Jong M. Correlation of clinical GRP receptor PET imaging of prostate cancer to receptor expression status. Eur J Nucl Med Mol Imaging. 2017;44(Suppl. 2):S147.

135. Gruber L, Jimenez-Franco LD, Decristoforo C, Uprimny C, Glatting G, Hohenberger P, Schoenberg SO, Reindl W, Orlandi F, Mariani M, Jaschke W, Virgolini IJ. MITIGATE-NeoBOMB1, a phase I/IIa study to evaluate safety, pharmacokinetics and preliminary imaging of ^{68}Ga-NeoBOMB1, a gastrin-releasing peptide receptor antagonist, in GIST patients. J Nucl Med. 2020;61:1749.

136. Djaileb LMC, van der Veldt A, Virgolini I, Cortes F, Demange A, Orlandi F, Wegener A. Preliminary diagnostic performance of [^{68}Ga]-NeoBOMB1 in patients with gastrin-releasing peptide receptor-positive breast, prostate, colorectal or lung tumors (NeoFIND). J Nucl Med. 2020;61(Suppl. 1):346.

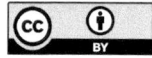

Cristina Müller and Nicholas P. van der Meulen

23.1 Introduction

Currently, the concept of radiotheragnotics—referring to *ther*apy and dia*gnosis*—is well implemented at many nuclear medicine entities worldwide [1]. In this context, various tumor-targeting agents, labeled with diagnostic and therapeutic radionuclides, are currently being used for nuclear imaging and radionuclide therapy, respectively. Since PET has become the imaging methodology of choice, ^{68}Ga has become the most important radiometal for imaging purposes, whereas radionuclide therapy is mostly performed with ^{177}Lu, a medium-energy β$^-$-particle emitter [2]. The co-emission of a low percentage of γ-radiation also enables its use for pre-therapeutic dosimetry purposes.

While the concept of ^{68}Ga/^{177}Lu-radiotheragnostics using somatostatin receptor-targeted peptides has shown promise for the treatment of neuroendocrine tumors [3], more recently, PSMA-targeted small molecules have

been extensively investigated with this pair of radionuclides for patients suffering from metastatic castration-resistant prostate cancer (mCRPC) [4, 5].

At Paul Scherrer Institute (PSI), we have focused on the concept of using radionuclides of the same element (i.e., radioisotopes) with the aim to prepare chemically identical radiopharmaceuticals for both imaging and therapy. In this regard, we have performed extensive work with the scandium family and set up the production of scandium-44 using the research cyclotron at PSI [6]. Prof. Richard Baum's group was the first worldwide to use the cyclotron-produced scandium-44 for a patient scan with [^{44}Sc]Sc-DOTATOC [7]. This was the start of our fruitful collaboration with Prof. Baum and colleagues at Zentralklinik Bad Berka, Germany.

A major focus of our work at PSI over the last decade has been the production and investigation of the terbium "sisters." Terbium comprises four radioisotopes of interest for nuclear imaging, using single photon emission computed tomography (SPECT; terbium-155) and positron emission tomography (PET; terbium-152), respectively, as well as for α-particle (terbium-149) and β$^-$-particle-based (terbium-161) radionuclide therapy [8]. The production and a preliminary preclinical application of all four terbium sisters was demonstrated in a collaborative study between the Paul Scherrer Institute (PSI) and ISOLDE/CERN, Geneva, Switzerland, and

C. Müller (✉)
Center for Radiopharmaceutical Sciences ETH-PSI,
Paul Scherrer Institute, Villigen-PSI, Switzerland
e-mail: cristina.mueller@psi.ch

N. P. van der Meulen
Center for Radiopharmaceutical Sciences ETH-PSI,
Paul Scherrer Institute, Villigen-PSI, Switzerland

Laboratory of Radiochemistry, Paul Scherrer
Institute, Villigen-PSI, Switzerland

© The Author(s) 2024
V. Prasad (ed.), *Beyond Becquerel and Biology to Precision Radiomolecular Oncology: Festschrift
in Honor of Richard P. Baum*, https://doi.org/10.1007/978-3-031-33533-4_23

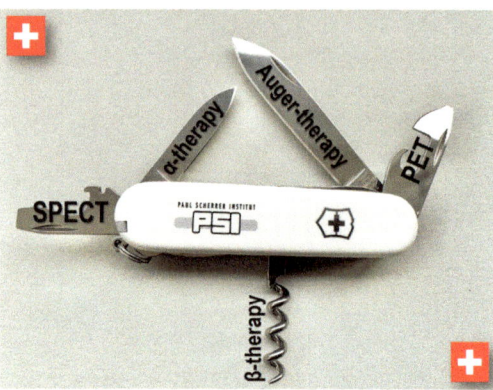

Fig. 23.1 Terbium represented by "PSI's Swiss Army Knife"—one tool for multiple functions of the terbium sisters in nuclear medicine

published in 2012 [9]. Terbium-161 was produced at PSI according to the method previously published by Lehenberger et al. [10], while the three other terbium sisters were obtained by spallation reaction and subsequent online mass separation at CERN, followed by chemical separation at PSI [9]. The activity obtained was low; however, it was possible to perform proof-of-concept SPECT and PET imaging experiments and α- and β⁻-radionuclide therapy in a small number of mice [9]. The unique feature of terbium raised the idea of calling it a "Swiss Army Knife" (originated from Prof. R. Schibli, head of Center of Radiopharmaceutical Sciences at PSI), as it combines all functions of nuclear medicine in just one element like a Swiss army knife—a multifunctional device. In order to specify the origin of the quadruplet of terbium radioisotopes for nuclear medicine applications more precisely, the term has been modified to "PSI's Swiss Army Knife" (Fig. 23.1).

Each of the four terbium sisters was investigated more in depth by our research groups at PSI and in collaboration with internal and external partners. In this chapter, we briefly summarize the achievements in the field of research with the four terbium sisters.

23.2   The PET Sister: Terbium-152

PET is the preferred imaging modality over SPECT due to the higher resolution and increased sensitivity as demonstrated by the high-quality PET scans obtained with ^{68}Ga-labeled somatostatin analogues, which has basically replaced the use of ^{111}In-octreotide for SPECT [11, 12]. Terbium-152 is the only radiolanthanide that emits β⁺-particles useful for PET imaging without co-emission of α- or β⁻-particles. Although the β⁺-energy is quite high (E$β^+_{av}$ = 1140 keV, I = 20.3%) and the decay accompanied by several γ-ray emissions, it was our goal to demonstrate the concept of "bench-to-bedside" with this particular terbium sister (Scheme 23.1).

Terbium-152 was used to label to DOTANOC and the radiopeptide was employed in a proof-of-concept PET imaging study in AR42J tumor-bearing mice [13]. In collaboration with the university hospital of Lausanne (CHUV), Switzerland, a microPET-based dosimetry study was performed in tumor-bearing mice using a ^{152}Tb-labeled antibody fragment ([^{152}Tb]Tb-CHX-DTPA-scFv78-Fc) [14]. Finally, [^{152}Tb]Tb-PSMA-617 was also employed for PET imaging of a prostate cancer mouse model for comparison of the distribution with its ^{177}Lu-labeled counterpart (Fig. 23.2) [15].

Terbium-152 was the first of all four terbium sisters to be used for a clinical application in a patient [15, 16]. [^{152}Tb]Tb-DOTATOC, prepared at Zentralklinik Bad Berka, Germany, was administered to a 67-year-old patient with metastatic well-differentiated functional neuroendocrine neoplasm of the ileum, presented for restaging 8 years after the sixth cycle of peptide receptor radionuclide therapy (PRRT) [16]. PET images visualized even the smaller metastases, with increased tumor-to-background contrast over time. The relatively long half-life of terbium-152 ($T_{1/2}$ = 17.5 h) made it feasible to scan the patient over an extended period, a feature which would be useful for dosimetry purposes

Scheme 23.1 The terbium-152 sister's personality. (Figurine ©Ekaterina Zimodro/123RF)

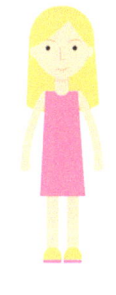

Tb 152

17.5 h

ε
β⁺ 2.8…
γ 344;
586;
271…

PET

Characteristics

- She is shy, but very pretty.
- She hasn't traveled a lot, but she has already met with Prof. R. Baum.
- She is proud, as she was the first of the terbium sisters to have worked in a hospital.
- She is not very popular, but the work with Prof. R. Baum has made her famous.

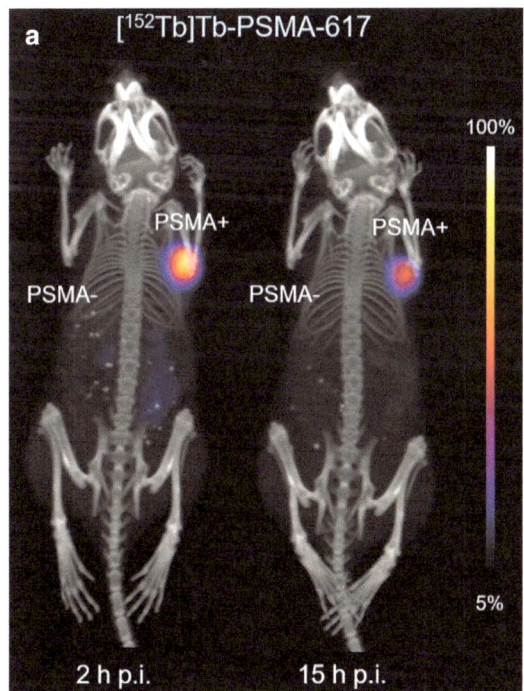

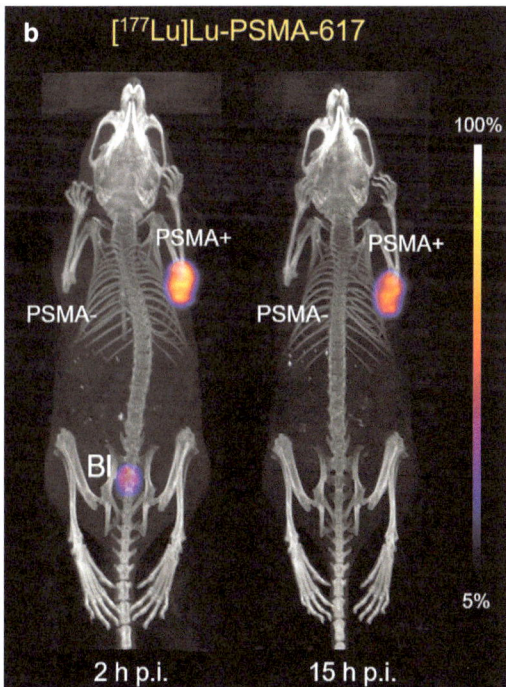

Fig. 23.2 Nuclear images shown as maximum intensity projections of PC-3 PIP/flu tumor-bearing mice at 2 h and 15 h *post injection* of the radioligand. (**a**) PET/CT scans of a mouse injected with [^{152}Tb]Tb-PSMA-617 and (**b**) SPECT/CT scan of a mouse injected with [^{177}Lu]Lu-PSMA-617. *PSMA+* PSMA-positive PC-3 PIP tumor, *PSMA−* PSMA-negative PC-3 flu tumor, *Bl* urinary bladder. (This figure was reproduced from Müller et al. 2019 EJNMMI Res [15])

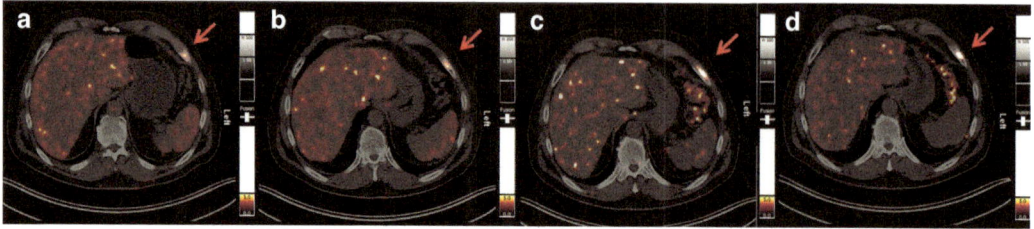

Fig. 23.3 PET/CT scans, shown as transversal slices through the upper abdomen at the level of the liver and spleen, obtained over time. (**a**) PET/CT scan acquired at 50 min, (**b**) 2.0 h, (**c**) 18.5 h, and (**d**) 25 h, respectively, after injection of 140 MBq [^{152}Tb]Tb-PSMA-617. The images clearly demonstrated a PSMA-avid bone metastasis in the ventrolateral part of the left seventh rib (red arrow), where maximum uptake was determined at 18.5 h and 25 h *post injection*. (This figure was reproduced from Müller et al. 2019 EJNMMI Res [15])

prior to radiolanthanide-based radionuclide therapy [16]. In a subsequent attempt to demonstrate the potential of performing clinical PET, terbium-152 was shipped to Zentralklinik Bad Berka, Germany, where it was used for the labeling of PSMA-617 [15]. [^{152}Tb]Tb-PSMA-617 was administered to a patient suffering from mCRPC, and the resultant PET scans were of diagnostic quality (Fig. 23.3). In particular, the images obtained at late time points enabled the visualization of the same metastatic lesions and of the local recurrent tumor as previously detected by [^{68}Ga]Ga-PSMA-11 [15].

The production of this radionuclide is challenging and, hence, the chances to make it available in large quantities in the near future rather small. Nevertheless, the clinical application of terbium-152 conducted by Prof. Richard Baum and his team paved the way towards translating terbium sisters to clinical application [15, 16].

23.3 The SPECT Sister: Terbium-155

SPECT imaging is still the most commonly used nuclear imaging technology, because of the established technetium-^{99m} kits and imaging protocols for multiple applications [17]. ^{111}In has served as a diagnostic match to yttrium-90 and lutetium-177 for many years [18]. Although PET imaging using gallium-68 has become the preferred technology for diagnostic imaging using tumor-targeted peptides and small molecules, there are still many nuclear medicine sites worldwide without PET scanners. Importantly, the technology of SPECT has improved over the years, enabling the generation of SPECT images of decent quality [19]. In this context, terbium-155 ($E\gamma = 86$ keV $I = 32\%$; 105 keV, $I = 25\%$) may have a role to play in future, as another diagnostic lanthanide match to therapeutic radiolanthanides (Scheme 23.2). Due to its long half-life ($T_{1/2} = 5.32$ days), it may be useful for pre-therapeutic dosimetry and/or have a role to play for labeling of long-circulating tumor-targeting agents including albumin-binding small molecules and antibodies.

The excellent imaging capability of this novel SPECT nuclide has been demonstrated preclinically with a series of biomolecules of interest at PSI [20]. It included an albumin-binding DOTA-folate ligand, a minigastrin analogue and a L1-CAM-targeting antibody, as well as the clinically employed DOTATOC. Current investigations at PSI are focused on the production of terbium-155 via various nuclear reactions using a cyclotron as a potential option to make it more freely available and in sufficient quantities for future clinical application.

Scheme 23.2 The terbium-155 sister's personality. (Figurine ©Ekaterina Zimodro/123RF)

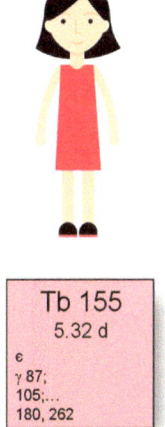

SPECT

Characteristics

- She has lots of potential, but is not yet well experienced in research.
- She has not traveled a lot, even though she would be strong enough to do so.
- She likes her terbium-161 sister, but is jealous of her terbium-152 sister.

Tb 155
5.32 d

ε
γ 87;
105;...
180, 262

23.4 The Alpha Therapy Sister: Terbium-149

Targeted α-radionuclide therapy (TAT) has garnered interest due to the promising results recently obtained with ^{225}Ac-based radioligand therapy (RLT) of mCRPC patients [21–24]. An open question refers to potential long-term undesired side effects to the kidneys and other radiosensitive organs and tissue, in which the (α- and β⁻-particle-emitting) daughter nuclides of actinium-225 may accumulate. On the other hand, it was found to be superior over the use of bismuth-213 with regard to the therapeutic index for the treatment of mCRPC patients [25]. Terbium-149 may be an alternative α-particle emitter to the currently employed actinium-225 and bismuth-213, respectively (Scheme 23.3). Terbium-149's half-life of 4.1 h lies between those of bismuth-213 ($T_{1/2}$ = 45 min) and actinium-225 ($T_{1/2}$ = 9.9 days). Importantly, the daughter nuclides do not emit α-particles, which may be advantageous with regard to the safety profile of this radionuclide. Even though several production routes were proposed [26], the preparation of substantial quantities of this radionuclide remains a major challenge and would require the construction of dedicated facilities, including mass separation, required to avoid the production of a mixture of terbium radioisotopes.

From an application perspective, there are a limited number of preclinical studies with terbium-149 reported in the literature [27, 28]. Beyer et al. performed preclinical experiments, in which ^{149}Tb-labeled rituximab was applied to sterilize single circulating cancer cells in a leukemia mouse model [27]. The treatment led to almost complete remission of mice over a period of 4 months, while untreated control mice developed tumor disease and had to be euthanized as a consequence [27]. At PSI, we have investigated terbium-149 in a proof-of-concept study using a DOTA-folate conjugate in a small number of KB tumor-bearing mice [28]. A dose-dependent inhibition of the tumor growth was observed and, as a consequence, an increased survival time of treated mice as compared to untreated controls [28]. More recently, we were able to conduct a study to investigate [^{149}Tb]Tb-PSMA-617 with several groups of PC-3 PIP tumor-bearing mice [29]. The resulting tumor growth curves revealed a favorable effect of two injections (2 × 3 MBq) as compared to only one injection (1 × 6 MBq). The study indicated the need for more frequent injections, which would most likely also be the case in a clinical setting. Terbium-149 is particularly attractive due to the emission of β⁺-particles (E$\beta^+_{average}$ = 730 keV, I = 7.1%), which enables PET imaging and would allow the monitoring of applied α-therapy [29]. This has been exemplified using [^{149}Tb]Tb-DOTANOC and a mouse model of somatostatin-expressing tumors (Fig. 23.4) [30].

Scheme 23.3 The terbium-149 sister's personality. (Figurine ©Ekaterina Zimodro/123RF)

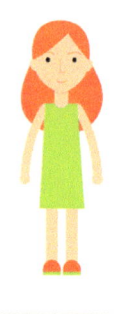

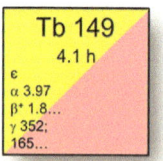

Tb 149
4.1 h
ε
α 3.97
β⁺ 1.8…
γ 352;
165…

Alpha Therapy

Characteristics

- She is red-haired and the strongest of all the terbium sisters.
- She is curious, yet shy and retiring and prefers staying close to where she was born, since traveling weakens her.
- She is increasing in popularity, because of her outstanding capabilities which make her particularly attractive.

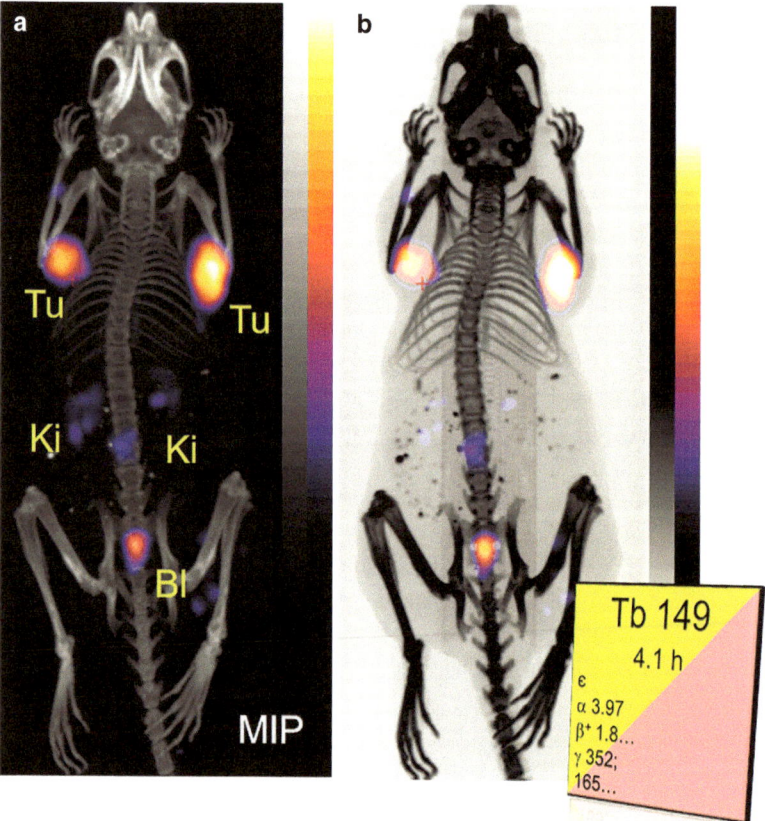

Fig. 23.4 PET/CT images of an AR42J tumor-bearing mouse 2 h after injection of [^{149}Tb]Tb-DOTANOC (7 MBq). (**a, b**) Maximal intensity projections (MIP) showing distinct accumulation of radioactivity in tumor xenografts (Tu) and residual radioactivity in kidneys (Ki) and urinary bladder (Bl). (This figure was reproduced from Müller et al. 2016 EJNMMI Radiopharm Chem [30])

23.5 The Beta Therapy^{PLUS} Sister (β⁻/Conversion/Auger-e⁻): Terbium-161

Lutetium-177 is an almost ideal β⁻-particle-emitting radionuclide for targeted radionuclide therapy [2]. While it was initially employed with receptor-targeted peptides such as somatostatin analogues [31], it has recently found widespread application in combination with small-molecular-weight PSMA targeting agents [32–34]. The medium energy β⁻-particles (Eβ⁻$_{average}$ = 134 keV; $T_{1/2}$ = 6.65 days) was determined to be favorable for the treatment of smaller metastases, while preventing radionephrotoxicity previously observed when using yttrium-90, which emits high-energy β⁻-particles [35]. Moreover, the co-emission of γ-radiation (Eγ = 113 keV, I = 6.2% and 208 keV, I = 10.4%) enables visualization of the radioligand's tissue distribution using SPECT.

The concept of using terbium-161 may be seen as a beta therapy^{PLUS} approach: this implies that terbium-161 shares largely all the characteristics of lutetium-177; however, it provides additional features which may make it more effective in cancer therapy (Scheme 23.4).

More specifically, the decay properties of terbium-161 are almost identical to those of lutetium-177 in terms of the β⁻-energy (Eβ⁻$_{average}$ = 154 keV) and half-life ($T_{1/2}$ = 6.953 days, recently determined by Duran et al. [36]). Like lutetium-177, ter-

bium-161 also emits γ-radiation useful for SPECT imaging. Terbium-161 may, however, have significant advantages with regard to the emission of low-energy electrons. It emits a substantial number of conversion and Auger electrons, which may be of particular value regarding the absorbed dose to single tumor cells. According to published calculations, the mean absorbed dose to small spheres (diameter: 10–20 μm) would increase approximately three to fourfold when using terbium-161 instead of lutetium-177 [37–40].

The comparison between the effects of terbium-161 and lutetium-177 was performed for the first time in a study using a DOTA-folate ligand [41]. More recently, another comparison was also performed with PSMA-617. It was experimentally demonstrated that [^{161}Tb]Tb-PSMA-617 was more effective in the killing of tumor cells in vitro compared to [^{177}Lu]Lu-PSMA-617 (Fig. 23.5) [42].

Extensive investigations were performed with human phantoms by Prof. Peter Bernhardt, University of Gothenburg, Sweden, in order to develop a reconstruction code which enables the preparation of high-quality images based on the γ-radiation emitted by terbium-161 (unpublished data). The first SPECT scan using [^{161}Tb]Tb-DOTATOC in a patient with neuroendocrine cancer was performed recently by Prof. Baum at Zentralklinik Bad Berka (unpublished data).

Scheme 23.4 The terbium-161 sister's personality. (Figurine ©Ekaterina Zimodro/123RF)

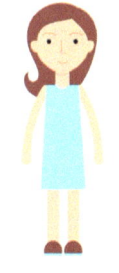

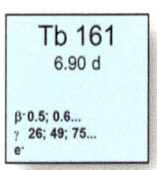

Tb 161
6.90 d

β⁻ 0.5; 0.6...
γ 26; 49; 75...
e⁻

Beta Therapy^{PLUS}

Characteristics

- She is the most mature and experienced in research among all terbium sisters.
- She has traveled to several sites and met with physicists, chemists and biologists, and also met with Prof. R. Baum.
- She is very strong, curious and hard-working.
- She has become popular in recent years and many people are interested in working with her.

Fig. 23.5 Results of an in vitro study demonstrating the favorable effect of terbium-161 over lutetium-177. The bars represent the percentage of PC-3 PIP tumor cell viability after exposure to [^{161}Tb]Tb-PSMA-617 and [^{177}Lu]Lu-PSMA-617, respectively, compared to untreated control cells (set to 100% viability; average ± SD). (This figure was reproduced from Müller et al. 2019 Eur J Nucl Med Mol Imaging [42])

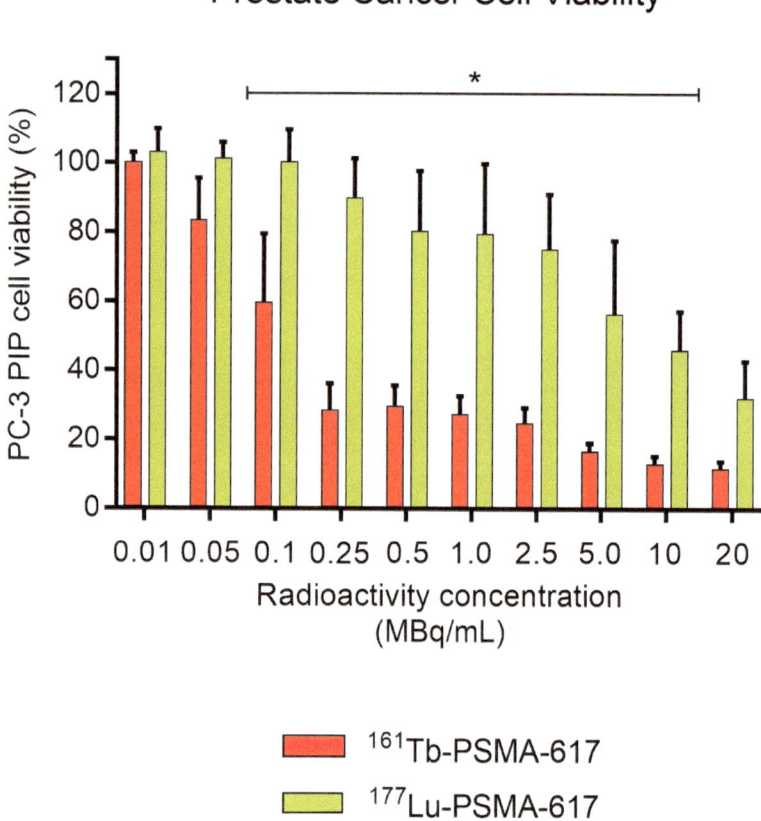

In contrast to the other three terbium sisters, terbium-161 can be produced in large quantities using the ^{160}Gd(n,γ)^{161}Gd → ^{161}Tb nuclear reaction in analogy to the no-carrier-added lutetium-177, as reported by Lehenberger et al. [10]. At PSI, we have developed the production method further over the years to make the radionuclide available at excellent quality that enables labeling of DOTA-functionalized biomolecules at molar activities >100 MBq/nmol [43]. The quantity that can be produced is limited to 20 GBq by the current restriction of the international air transport agency (IATA); however, this restriction is expected to be lifted soon. The current situation regarding the production opportunities is most promising in view of the feasibility to make the radionuclide available for clinical studies in the near future.

23.6 Conclusion and Outlook

Having focused on the investigation of "PSI's Swiss Army Knife" over the last decade, we have been approached with increased interest from researchers and physicians worldwide over the years. We have performed a number of preclinical studies with the terbium sisters at PSI in collaboration with external partners in Switzerland and abroad. These endeavors enabled the improvement of procedures and results on each level: (1) The production, including targetry and chemical separation, was optimized; (2) radiolabeling of biomolecules was achieved at high molar activities; (3) more detailed preclinical in vitro and in vivo investigations were performed with relevant quantities of activity; (4) human phantom studies were performed with terbium-

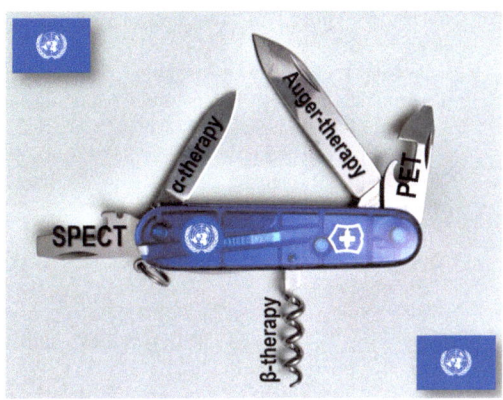

Fig. 23.6 "PSI's Swiss Army Knife" has become a "European Terbium Knife"—one tool for multiple functions of the terbium sisters in nuclear medicine

161 and (5) finally also proof-of-concept clinical applications were achieved with terbium-152 and terbium-161. Thanks to our collaborators in several countries throughout Europe, most prominently, Prof. Richard Baum, the "PSI's Swiss Army Knife" is becoming a tool of international interest beyond Switzerland and Europe, hence a "United Nations' Army Knife" (Fig. 23.6). Researchers and clinicians from all other continents including North and South America, Africa, Asia and Australia are interested in using the terbium sisters for nuclear medicine applications.

Based on the results we have achieved over the last decade investigating terbium sisters and according to numerous discussions with researchers and physicians from different fields, it is likely that terbium-161 will be translated to clinical application in the near future. This radionuclide may be also the first to be produced in large quantities for a worldwide application, as is currently the case for lutetium-177. While physicists were the first to propose terbium-161 as a valid alternative to lutetium-177, radiochemists developed the production routes and (radio)pharmacists and biologists experimentally demonstrated the superiority of this radionuclide in preclinical settings. Now, it is time for the nuclear medicine physicians and oncologists to demonstrate the benefit of low-energy electrons in the treatment of disseminated disease by means of clinical

studies. Since the production methods for the other three terbium sisters are more challenging and not yet established for large-scale production, success with regard to clinical translation will critically depend on the investment in production facilities.

Finally, it remains to be said that the terbium sisters owe their current popularity in the medical community to Prof. Richard Baum's efforts to support the translation from bench to bedside.

Our terbium sisters have just started their career in the community. They are still young and, consequently, full of dreams and desires for their future lives in the interdisciplinary environment of research and medical activities. We will continue educating and supporting them to make their future bright and successful and wish them all the best on their future career journey.

Acknowledgments The authors thank researchers and technical staff members at the Center for Radiopharmaceutical Sciences and the Laboratory of Radiochemistry at PSI for all the work and effort they have placed into the research with the terbium sisters. They would also like to thank all external collaborators, particularly Dr. Karl Johnston and his team at ISOLDE/CERN, Dr. Claude Bailat and his team at the Institute of Radiation Physics (IRA) Lausanne, Switzerland; Prof. Peter Bernhardt and his team at the University of Gothenburg, Sweden; Dr. Ulli Köster and his team at the reactor facility Institute Lau-Langevin, Grenoble, France and Dr. Jan Rijn Zeevaart and his team at the SAFARI-1 reactor facility at Necsa, Pelindaba, South Africa. The authors would like to thank Prof. Richard Baum and his team of physicians and medical physicists for their interest in the terbium sisters and are grateful for all the efforts of the nursing staff, as well as nuclear medicine technologists of the Theranostics Center for Molecular Radiotherapy and Precision Oncology for patient management at Zentralklinik Bad Berka, Germany.

Funding The research conducted with terbium sisters was supported by several funding institutions which are gratefully acknowledged: the Swiss National Science Foundation (SNSF: IZLIZ3_156800, 310030–156803); the Neuroendocrine Tumor Research Foundation (NETRF; Petersen Investigator Award 2018); the Personalized Health and Related Technology (PHRT-301), the Swiss Cancer Research Foundation (KFS-4678-02-2019-R) and the ENSAR2 (EU H2020 project N° 654002).

References

1. Jadvar H, Chen X, Cai W, Mahmood U. Radiotheranostics in cancer diagnosis and management. Radiology. 2018;286:388–400. https://doi.org/10.1148/radiol.2017170346.

2. Banerjee S, Pillai MR, Knapp FF. Lutetium-177 therapeutic radiopharmaceuticals: linking chemistry, radiochemistry, and practical applications. Chem Rev. 2015;115:2934–74. https://doi.org/10.1021/cr500171e.

3. Gabriel M, Decristoforo C, Kendler D, Dobrozemsky G, Heute D, Uprimny C, et al. ^{68}Ga-DOTA-Tyr^3-octreotide PET in neuroendocrine tumors: comparison with somatostatin receptor scintigraphy and CT. J Nucl Med. 2007;48:508–18.

4. Scarpa L, Buxbaum S, Kendler D, Fink K, Bektic J, Gruber L, et al. The ^{68}Ga/^{177}Lu theragnostic concept in PSMA targeting of castration-resistant prostate cancer: correlation of SUVmax values and absorbed dose estimates. Eur J Nucl Med Mol Imaging. 2017;44:788–800. https://doi.org/10.1007/s00259-016-3609-9.

5. Heinzel A, Boghos D, Mottaghy FM, Gärtner F, Essler M, von Mallek D, et al. ^{68}Ga-PSMA PET/CT for monitoring response to ^{177}Lu-PSMA-617 radioligand therapy in patients with metastatic castration-resistant prostate cancer. Eur J Nucl Med Mol Imaging. 2019;46:1054–62. https://doi.org/10.1007/s00259-019-4258-6.

6. van der Meulen NP, Bunka M, Domnanich KA, Müller C, Haller S, Vermeulen C, et al. Cyclotron production of ^{44}Sc: from bench to bedside. Nucl Med Biol. 2015;42:745–51. https://doi.org/10.1016/j.nucmedbio.2015.05.005.

7. Singh A, van der Meulen NP, Müller C, Klette I, Kulkarni HR, Türler A, et al. First-in-human PET/CT imaging of metastatic neuroendocrine neoplasms with cyclotron-produced ^{44}Sc-DOTATOC: a proof-of-concept study. Cancer Biother Radiopharm. 2017;32:124–32. https://doi.org/10.1089/cbr.2016.2173.

8. Müller C, Domnanich KA, Umbricht CA, van der Meulen NP. Scandium and terbium radionuclides for radiotheranostics: current state of development towards clinical application. Br J Radiol. 2018;91:20180074. https://doi.org/10.1259/bjr.20180074.

9. Müller C, Zhernosekov K, Köster U, Johnston K, Dorrer H, Hohn A, et al. A unique matched quadruplet of terbium radioisotopes for PET and SPECT and for a- and b$^-$-radionuclide therapy: an in vivo proof-of-concept study with a new receptor-targeted folate derivative. J Nucl Med. 2012;53:1951–9. https://doi.org/10.2967/jnumed.112.107540.

10. Lehenberger S, Barkhausen C, Cohrs S, Fischer E, Grünberg J, Hohn A, et al. The low-energy beta$^-$ and electron emitter ^{161}Tb as an alternative to ^{177}Lu for targeted radionuclide therapy. Nucl Med Biol. 2011;38:917–24. https://doi.org/10.1016/j.nucmedbio.2011.02.007.

11. Buchmann I, Henze M, Engelbrecht S, Eisenhut M, Runz A, Schäfer M, et al. Comparison of ^{68}Ga-DOTATOC PET and ^{111}In-DTPAOC (Octreoscan) SPECT in patients with neuroendocrine tumours. Eur J Nucl Med Mol Imaging. 2007;34:1617–26. https://doi.org/10.1007/s00259-007-0450-1.

12. Srirajaskanthan R, Kayani I, Quigley AM, Soh J, Caplin ME, Bomanji J. The role of ^{68}Ga-DOTATATE PET in patients with neuroendocrine tumors and negative or equivocal findings on ^{111}In-DTPA-octreotide scintigraphy. J Nucl Med. 2010;51:875–82. https://doi.org/10.2967/jnumed.109.066134.

13. Müller C, Vermeulen C, Johnston K, Köster U, Schmid R, Türler A, et al. Preclinical in vivo application of ^{152}Tb-DOTANOC: a radiolanthanide for PET imaging. EJNMMI Res. 2016;6:35. https://doi.org/10.1186/s13550-016-0189-4.

14. Cicone F, Gnesin S, Denoel T, Stora T, van der Meulen NP, Müller C, et al. Internal radiation dosimetry of a ^{152}Tb-labeled antibody in tumor-bearing mice. EJNMMI Res. 2019;9:53. https://doi.org/10.1186/s13550-019-0524-7.

15. Müller C, Singh A, Umbricht CA, Kulkarni HR, Johnston K, Benešová M, et al. Preclinical investigations and first-in-human application of ^{152}Tb-PSMA-617 for PET/CT imaging of prostate cancer. EJNMMI Res. 2019;9:68. https://doi.org/10.1186/s13550-019-0538-1.

16. Baum RP, Singh A, Benešová M, Vermeulen C, Gnesin S, Köster U, et al. Clinical evaluation of the radiolanthanide terbium-152: first-in-human PET/CT with ^{152}Tb-DOTATOC. Dalton Trans. 2017;46:14638–46. https://doi.org/10.1039/c7dt01936j.

17. Israel O, Pellet O, Biassoni L, De Palma D, Estrada-Lobato E, Gnanasegaran G, et al. Two decades of SPECT/CT - the coming of age of a technology: an updated review of literature evidence. Eur J Nucl Med Mol Imaging. 2019;46:1990–2012. https://doi.org/10.1007/s00259-019-04404-6.

18. Kwekkeboom DJ, Bakker WH, Kooij PP, Konijnenberg MW, Srinivasan A, Erion JL, et al. [^{177}Lu-DOTA^{0}Tyr^3]octreotate: comparison with [^{111}In-DTPA^0]octreotide in patients. Eur J Nucl Med. 2001;28:1319–25.

19. Ljungberg M, Pretorius PH. SPECT/CT: an update on technological developments and clinical applications. Br J Radiol. 2018;91:20160402. https://doi.org/10.1259/bjr.20160402.

20. Müller C, Fischer E, Behe M, Köster U, Dorrer H, Reber J, et al. Future prospects for SPECT imaging using the radiolanthanide terbium-155—production and preclinical evaluation in tumor-bearing mice. Nucl Med Biol. 2014;41(Suppl):e58–65. https://doi.org/10.1016/j.nucmedbio.2013.11.002.

21. Kratochwil C, Bruchertseifer F, Giesel FL, Apostolidis C, Haberkorn U, Morgenstern A. ^{225}Ac-PSMA-617 for PSMA targeting alpha-radiation therapy of 28

patients with mCRPC. Eur J Nucl Med Mol Imaging. 2016;43:S137.

22. Kratochwil C, Bruchertseifer F, Giesel FL, Weis M, Verburg FA, Mottaghy F, et al. ^{225}Ac-PSMA-617 for PSMA-targeted a-radiation therapy of metastatic castration-resistant prostate cancer. J Nucl Med. 2016;57:1941–4. https://doi.org/10.2967/jnumed.116.178673.

23. Kratochwil C, Bruchertseifer F, Rathke H, Hohenfellner M, Giesel FL, Haberkorn U, et al. Targeted alpha therapy of mCRPC with ^{225}Actinium-PSMA-617: swimmer-plot analysis suggests efficacy regarding duration of tumor-control. J Nucl Med. 2018;59:795. https://doi.org/10.2967/jnumed.117.203539.

24. Sathekge M, Bruchertseifer F, Knoesen O, Reyneke F, Lawal I, Lengana T, et al. ^{225}Ac-PSMA-617 in chemotherapy-naive patients with advanced prostate cancer: a pilot study. Eur J Nucl Med Mol Imaging. 2019;46:129–38. https://doi.org/10.1007/s00259-018-4167-0.

25. Kratochwil C, Schmidt K, Afshar-Oromieh A, Bruchertseifer F, Rathke H, Morgenstern A, et al. Targeted alpha therapy of mCRPC: dosimetry estimate of ^{213}Bismuth-PSMA-617. Eur J Nucl Med Mol Imaging. 2018;45:31–7. https://doi.org/10.1007/s00259-017-3817-y.

26. Beyer GJ, Comor JJ, Dakovic M, Soloviev D, Tamburella C, Hagebo E, et al. Production routes of the alpha emitting ^{149}Tb for medical application. Radiochim Acta. 2002;90:247–52. https://doi.org/10.1524/ract.2002.90.5_2002.247.

27. Beyer GJ, Miederer M, Vranjes-Duric S, Comor JJ, Kunzi G, Hartley O, et al. Targeted alpha therapy in vivo: direct evidence for single cancer cell kill using ^{149}Tb-rituximab. Eur J Nucl Med Mol Imaging. 2004;31:547–54. https://doi.org/10.1007/s00259-003-1413-9.

28. Müller C, Reber J, Haller S, Dorrer H, Köster U, Johnston K, et al. Folate receptor targeted alpha-therapy using terbium-149. Pharmaceuticals (Basel). 2014;7:353–65. https://doi.org/10.3390/ph7030353.

29. Umbricht CA, Köster U, Bernhardt P, Gracheva N, Johnston K, Schibli R, et al. Alpha-PET for prostate cancer: preclinical investigation using ^{149}Tb-PSMA-617. Sci Rep. 2019;9:17800. https://doi.org/10.1038/s41598-019-54150-w.

30. Müller C, Vermeulen C, Köster U, Johnston K, Türler A, Schibli R, et al. Alpha-PET with terbium-149: evidence and perspectives for radiotheragnostics. Eur J Nucl Med Mol Imaging Radiopharm Chem. 2017;1:5.

31. Strosberg J, El-Haddad G, Wolin E, Hendifar A, Yao J, Chasen B, et al. Phase 3 trial of ^{177}Lu-DOTATATE for midgut neuroendocrine tumors. N Engl J Med. 2017;376:125–35. https://doi.org/10.1056/NEJMoa1607427.

32. Baum RP, Kulkarni HR, Schuchardt C, Singh A, Wirtz M, Wiessalla S, et al. ^{177}Lu-labeled prostate-specific membrane antigen radioligand therapy of metastatic castration-resistant prostate cancer: safety and efficacy. J Nucl Med. 2016;57:1006–13. https://doi.org/10.2967/jnumed.115.168443.

33. Rahbar K, Ahmadzadehfar H, Kratochwil C, Haberkorn U, Schäfers M, Essler M, et al. German multicenter study investigating ^{177}Lu-PSMA-617 radioligand therapy in advanced prostate cancer patients. J Nucl Med. 2017;58:85–90. https://doi.org/10.2967/jnumed.116.183194.

34. Bräuer A, Grubert LS, Roll W, Schrader AJ, Schäfers M, Bögemann M, et al. ^{177}Lu-PSMA-617 radioligand therapy and outcome in patients with metastasized castration-resistant prostate cancer. Eur J Nucl Med Mol Imaging. 2017;44:1663–70. https://doi.org/10.1007/s00259-017-3751-z.

35. Valkema R, Pauwels SA, Kvols LK, Kwekkeboom DJ, Jamar F, de Jong M, et al. Long-term follow-up of renal function after peptide receptor radiation therapy with ^{90}Y-DOTA^0,Tyr^3-octreotide and ^{177}Lu-DOTA^0,Tyr^3-octreotate. J Nucl Med. 2005;46(Suppl 1):83S–91S.

36. Duran MT, Juget F, Nedjadi Y, Bochud F, Grundler PV, Gracheva N, et al. Determination of ^{161}Tb half-life by three measurement methods. Appl Radiat Isot. 2020;159:109085. https://doi.org/10.1016/j.apradiso.2020.109085.

37. Bernhardt P, Benjegard SA, Kolby L, Johanson V, Nilsson O, Ahlman H, et al. Dosimetric comparison of radionuclides for therapy of somatostatin receptor-expressing tumors. Int J Radiat Oncol Biol Phys. 2001;51:514–24.

38. Hindie E, Zanotti-Fregonara P, Quinto MA, Morgat C, Champion C. Dose deposits from ^{90}Y, ^{177}Lu, ^{111}In, and ^{161}Tb in micrometastases of various sizes: implications for radiopharmaceutical therapy. J Nucl Med. 2016;57:759–64. https://doi.org/10.2967/jnumed.115.170423.

39. Champion C, Quinto MA, Morgat C, Zanotti-Fregonara P, Hindie E. Comparison between three promising b⁻-emitting radionuclides, ^{67}Cu, ^{47}Sc and ^{161}Tb, with emphasis on doses delivered to minimal residual disease. Theranostics. 2016;6:1611–8. https://doi.org/10.7150/thno.15132.

40. Alcocer-Avila ME, Ferreira A, Quinto MA, Morgat C, Hindie E, Champion C. Radiation doses from ^{161}Tb and ^{177}Lu in single tumour cells and micrometastases. EJNMMI Phys. 2020;7:33. https://doi.org/10.1186/s40658-020-00301-2.

41. Müller C, Reber J, Haller S, Dorrer H, Bernhardt P, Zhernosekov K, et al. Direct in vitro and in vivo comparison of ^{161}Tb and ^{177}Lu using a tumour-targeting folate conjugate. Eur J Nucl Med Mol Imaging. 2014;41:476–85. https://doi.org/10.1007/s00259-013-2563-z.

42. Müller C, Umbricht CA, Gracheva N, Tschan VJ, Pellegrini G, Bernhardt P, et al. Terbium-161 for PSMA-targted radionuclide therapy of prostate cancer. Eur J Nucl Med Mol Imaging. 2019;46:1919. https://doi.org/10.1007/s00259-019-04345-0.

43. Gracheva N, Müller C, Talip Z, Heinitz S, Köster U, Zeevaart JR, et al. Production and characterization of no-carrier-added [161]Tb as an alternative to the clinically-applied ^{177}Lu for radionuclide therapy. EJNMMI Radiopharm Chem. 2019;4:12. https://doi.org/10.1186/s41181-019-0063-6.

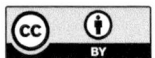

High-Performance Radiopharmacy: The Base for Precision Oncology

Dirk Müller, Alexander Fuchs, Yevgeniy Leshch, Peter Schulze, and Michael Pröhl

The Zentralklinik Bad Berka is a privately financed hospital, and it is not a university hospital. Since it is not located in the immediate vicinity of a large city, one could assume that it is rather an unspectacular clinic on the edge of a forest. Nevertheless, for many years, this hospital has been generating high-quality scientific publications [1–7].

Since the establishment of nuclear medicine in this hospital, thousands of patients have been treated with innovative radiopharmaceuticals. One has to ask oneself how such a hospital can examine so many patients with innovative radiopharmaceuticals that so many different scientific results are generated and published?

To answer these questions, one should look at the starting point of every nuclear medical exam-

D. Müller (✉)
ABX Advanced Biochemical Compounds, Radeberg, Germany

Zentralklinik Bad Berka, Bad Berka, Germany
e-mail: dirk.mueller@abx.de

A. Fuchs
Städtisches Klinikum Karlsruhe, Karlsruhe, Germany

Y. Leshch
Department of Nuclear Medicine, University Hospital Essen, Essen, Germany

P. Schulze
Bayer Weimar GmbH & Co., Weimar, Germany

M. Pröhl
Eckert and Ziegler Radiopharma, Braunschweig, Germany

ination or therapy: the production of drugs in a radiopharmacy.

If you look at the job descriptions for the position of radiochemists/pharmacists, often one finds a fully packed field of activity. Additionally, a wide range of radiotracers and its production is desired (Fig. 24.1).

It can partly be seen that neither the hot cells for the radiopharmaceutical production, nor the synthesis modules and analytical equipment, and also no budget is available. Only a few lead shields and shielded syringes. One asks again oneself how these tasks are to be fulfilled?

Very often both the personnel requirements, the financial and technical necessities are completely underestimated.

For example, the cost of synthesis of a new radiopharmaceutical is often incorrectly calculated, since the descriptions of the radiolabeling in the scientific papers are usually reduced to the essentials. A short sentence in the experimental part of the publication can therefore conceal an equipment requirement of more than 100,000 euros. A misinterpretation of these data leads very quickly to the failure of the project.

As an example, Fig. 24.2 lists the personnel requirements for routine production of innovative drugs. The more technology is required, the more personnel is required to maintain the technology.

Since the last decades, the role of nuclear medicine in precision oncology has been growing. More and more radiolabeled target-seeking

V. Prasad (ed.), *Beyond Becquerel and Biology to Precision Radiomolecular Oncology: Festschrift in Honor of Richard P. Baum*, https://doi.org/10.1007/978-3-031-33533-4_24

A Natural Scientist in a Department of
Nuclear Medicine
? ? ?

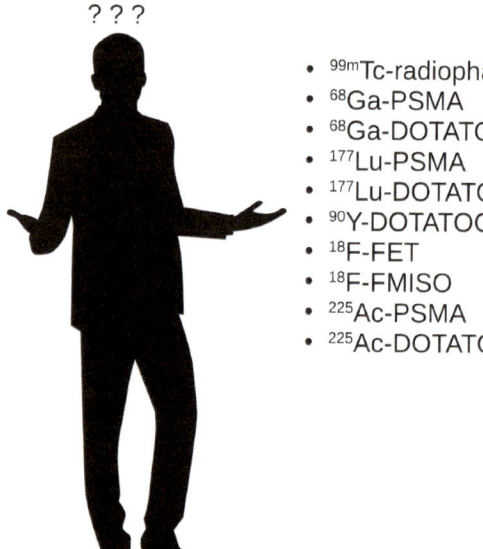

- Head of Production
- Head of Quality Control
- Qualified Person
- GMP- documentation
- Quality Assurance
- Radiation Safety Officer
- Medical Physicist
- Technical assistant for PET, SPECT, γ-cameras, animal-PET
- Order of radiopharmaceuticals
- Contact person for all technical questions
- Microbiological monitoring
- Environmental monitoring

- ^{99m}Tc-radiopharmaceuticals
- ^{68}Ga-PSMA
- ^{68}Ga-DOTATOC
- ^{177}Lu-PSMA
- ^{177}Lu-DOTATOC
- ^{90}Y-DOTATOC
- ^{18}F-FET
- ^{18}F-FMISO
- ^{225}Ac-PSMA
- ^{225}Ac-DOTATOC...

Fig. 24.1 Job descriptions for scientists in nuclear medicine flooded with tasks

Fig. 24.2 Personal requirements for the radiopharmaceutical production of innovative radiotracers

Production of innovative radiopharmaceuticals

• Personnel and financial costs are often underestimated	
• Head of Production	1
• Head of Quality Control	1
• Qualified Person	(1)
• GMP-documentation	
• Quality Assurance	1
• Radiation Safety Officer	
• Medical Physicist	(1 - 3)
• Technical assistant for PET, SPECT, γ-cameras, animal-PET	
• Order of radiopharmaceuticals	
• Contact person for all technical questions	1
• Microbiological monitoring	(1)
• Environmental monitoring	

drugs are basically available for use in clinical practice. The requirements for this is that a corresponding radiopharmacy can provide these innovative radiotracers. Thus, the radiopharmacy plays an important role in the application of modern radiopharmaceuticals to patients.

Let us get back to the question why so many innovative tracers can be routinely used in our hospital?

It is thanks to the farsightedness, the vision and understanding of the clinic management and above all to the Director of Nuclear Medicine, Professor Richard Baum, that the basic requirements for the production of radiopharmaceuticals were consistently created both technically and in terms of personnel.

This can be illustrated with a historical review. The radiopharmacy was completed in 1998.

The laboratory was equipped with 11 MeV Cyclotron, six hot cells, analytical equipment (analytical HPLCs, GC), and synthesis modules (Fig. 24.3).

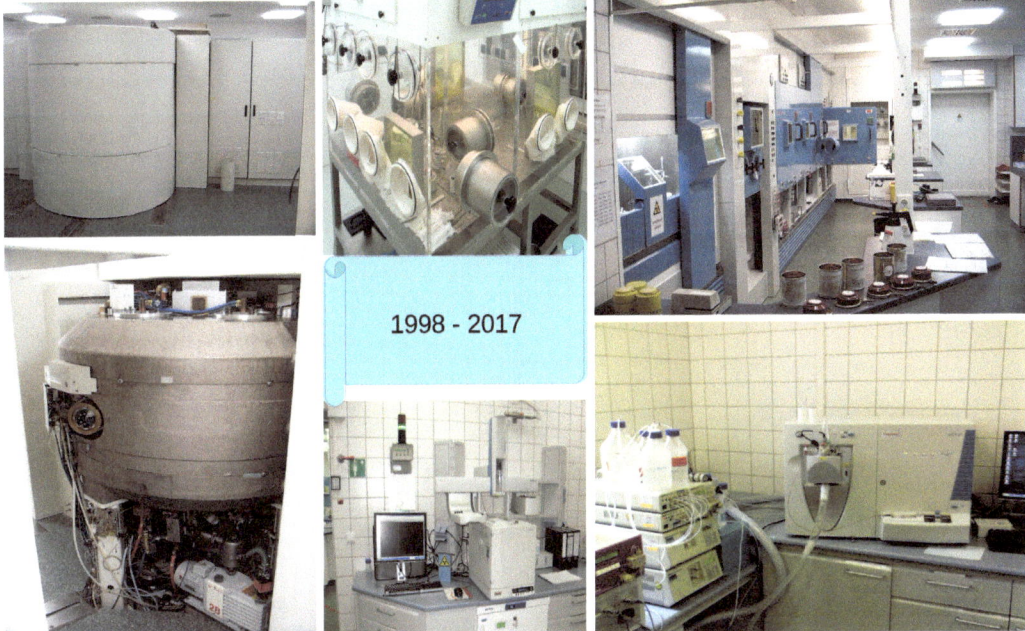

Fig. 24.3 Technical equipment in the Bad Berka Radiopharmacy (1998–2017)

In 1999, ^{18}F-FDG production and distribution started. Starting from 2000 ^{18}F-FDG was produced with a manufacturing authorization, and since 2003, ^{18}F-FDG was produced regularly during the night shift. At this time, two engineers, two chemists, and three medical technical assistants were working in our radiopharmacy. In 2004, the production of ^{68}Ga-DOTA-peptides and ^{177}Lu-DOTA-peptides started.

Figure 24.4 shows the production bench for the manual routine synthesis of ^{68}Ga-DOTA-peptides. The manual module has been slightly modified to reduce the radiation exposure of the hands of our staff.

The ^{68}Ga-labeling was carried out using the acetone-based labeling procedure which was created by Professor Frank Rösch, Dr. Tschernosekov et al. This method was the workhorse at this time [8].

In 2010, two synthesis runs were performed daily to care for our patients.

During this time, some synthesis processes have been developed and optimized.

Examples are:

- The combined cationic/anionic purification and labeling procedure for the labeling of fragile compounds with ^{68}Ga [9].
- The one-pot synthesis of ^{18}F-FEC [10].
- The cartridge-based purification of ^{18}F-FET [11].

In 2011, the NaCl-based ^{68}Ga-labeling method was discovered in our radiopharmacy and was subsequently used for the routine production of ^{68}Ga-labeled tracers as well as for the labeling of experimental peptides and other compounds. These results have been also published [12]. The ^{68}Ga-labeling procedure is shown schematically in Fig. 24.5. This scheme shows also the anionic labeling and the acetone-based ^{68}Ga-labeling procedure.

Furthermore, this method was immediately transferred to various automatic synthesis modules and was used for thousands of synthesis runs in our hospital for the radiopharmaceutical

2004
^{68}Ga-DOTATOC – First Routine Production

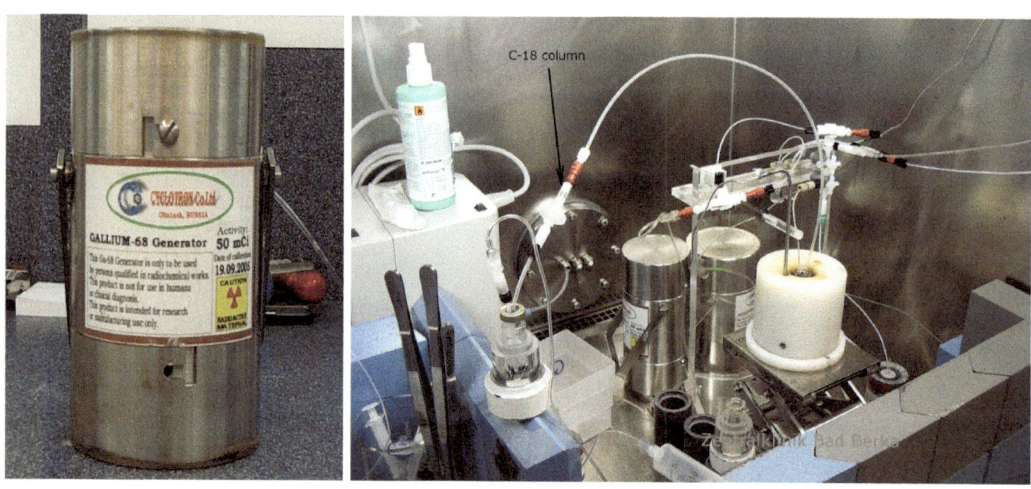

Fig. 24.4 Manual synthesis module for the production of ^{68}Ga-labeled DOTA-peptides

Fig. 24.5 Scheme of different ^{68}Ga-labeling procedures

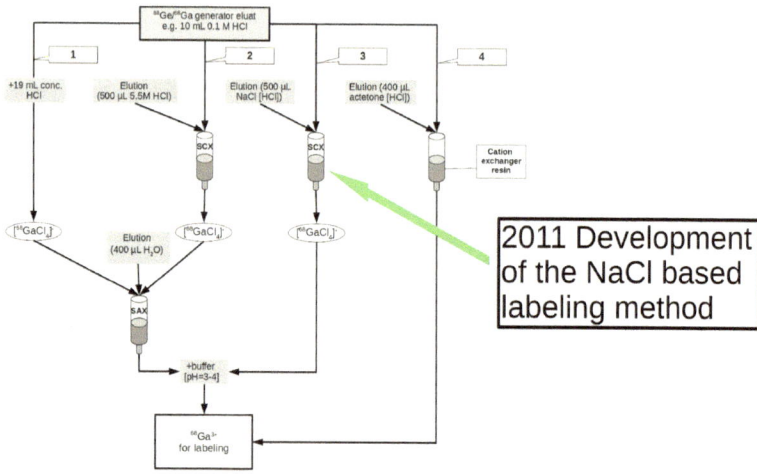

production of ^{68}Ga-DOTA-TOC and ^{68}Ga-PSMA [13] (Fig. 24.6).

Table 24.1 exemplarily shows an overview of some innovative radiotracers produced in the radiopharmacy for application to patients.

With this list of experimental tracers, the authors would like to highlight the outstanding pioneering work that Professor Richard Baum has done for the Nuclear Medicine Society.

The new radiopharmacy was built between 2014 and 2017. A new cyclotron with a solid tar-

get, an alpha laboratory, and new analytical equipment has been installed (Fig. 24.7).

At the same time, the routine production of alpha-emitting therapeutics in our radiopharmacy, the ^{225}Ac-labeled peptides, began. Additionally, first results from experimental data on the cyclotron-based production of ^{68}Ga could be collected and has been presented in 2019.

One of the most important topics is the fibroblast activation protein FAP which is expressed on cancer-associated fibroblasts. The concentra-

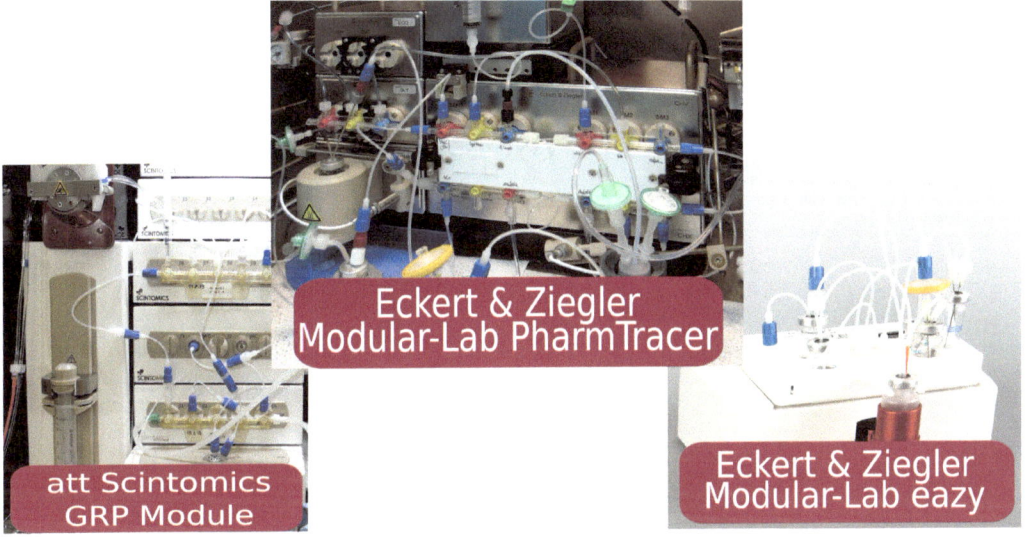

NaCl based labeling procedure used for the production of ⁶⁸Ga labeled petides - Adapted to different synthesis modules

Eckert & Ziegler Modular-Lab PharmTracer

att Scintomics GRP Module

Eckert & Ziegler Modular-Lab eazy

Fig. 24.6 Different automated synthesis modules for the production of ⁶⁸Ga compounds using the NaCl-based labeling procedure. This procedure was developed at the hospital Bad Berka by the author Dirk Müller

Table 24.1 A selection of experimentally applied radiotracers, which were used in the context of compassionate trials in the Zentralklinik Bad Berka

⁶⁸Ga-Affibody	⁶⁸Ga-MG-11
⁶⁸Ga-Sarabesin	¹¹¹In-affibody
⁶⁸Ga-Demobesin	¹¹¹In-PSMA-Minibody
⁶⁸Ga-neurotensin	⁴⁴Sc-DOTATOC
⁶⁸Ga-JR-10	¹⁵²Tb-DOTATOC
⁶⁸Ga-JR-11	¹⁵²Tb-PSMA
⁶⁸Ga-RGD	¹⁷⁷Lu-PSMA-Minibody
⁶⁸Ga-TRAP-RGD	¹⁷⁷Lu-Sabesin
⁶⁸Ga-MSH	¹⁷⁷Lu-JR-11
⁶⁸Ga-MAA	¹⁷⁷Lu-neurotensin
⁶⁸Ga-Exendin-4	¹⁷⁷Lu-LM-3
⁶⁸Ga-LM-3	¹⁷⁷Lu-BPAMD
⁶⁸Ga-PSMA-ALB6	¹⁷⁷Lu-DOTA-M-ZOL
⁶⁸Ga-BPAMD	¹⁷⁷Lu-PSMA-ALB6
⁶⁸Ga-FAP	¹⁷⁷Lu-FAP

tion in normal tissue is usually low. FAP is therefore a highly interesting target for radio-molecular imaging and therapy, and this could be a milestone in the history of nuclear medicine. A few quinoline-based PET tracers have been developed which act as FAP inhibitors (FAPIs). The study of the biodistribution of ⁶⁸Ga-labeled FAPIs showed an uptake which is comparable with ¹⁸F-FDG but also a significant washout effect between 1–3 h after injection [14].

Another approach, namely, the use of FAP-affine peptides such as the peptide FAP-2286, opens the opportunity for radio-molecular therapy due to significantly longer residence times. Furthermore, the PET tracers based on FAP-2286 seem to show a higher tumor uptake compared to ¹⁸F-FDG. FAP-2286 is a new and innovative compound of the company 3B-Pharma.

The following Figs. 24.8 and 24.9 show some HPLC results of the radiolabeling and synthesis of the radiopharmaceutical production of FAP tracers for the diagnosis and therapy for patients with different tumor diseases. Fig. 24.8 shows the HPLCs of the compound FAP-2286 labeled with ⁶⁸Ga, immediately after the labeling and 2 h later. Figure 24.9 shows the HPLCs of the ¹⁷⁷Lu-labeled peptide FAP-2286, again immediately after the labeling and after 2 and 24 h.

Finally the authors would like to thank Professor Baum for many, many years of close cooperation.

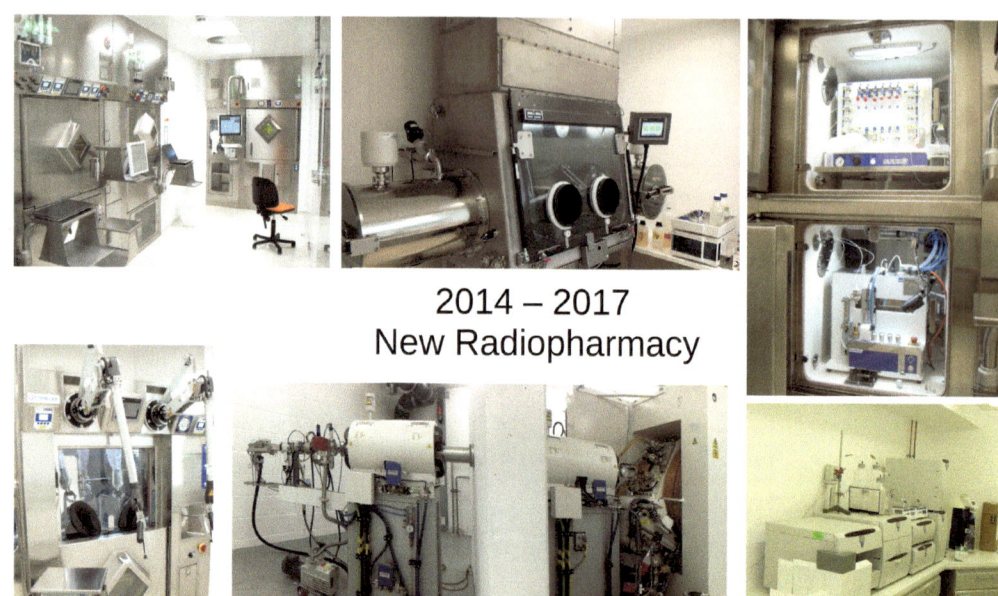

Fig. 24.7 The new radiopharmacy was built between 2014 and 2017

Fig. 24.8 Stability of ^{68}Ga-FAP-2286: HPLC of the final product, immediately after the labeling and after 2 h

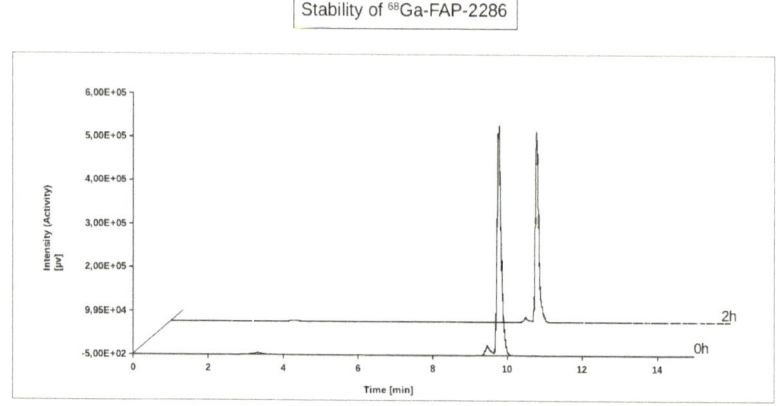

Fig. 24.9 Stability of ^{177}Lu-FAP-2286: HPLC of the final product, immediately after the labeling, after 2 and 24 h

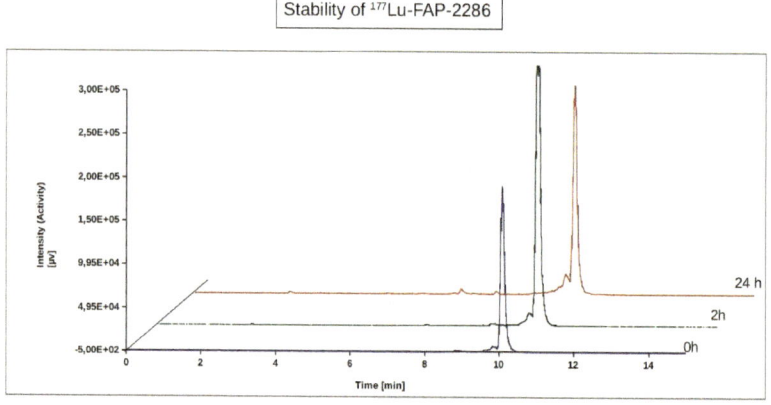

References

1. Hamm KD, Surber G, Schmücking M, Wurm RE, Aschenbach R, Kleinert G, Niesen A, Baum RP. Sterotactic radiation treatment planning and follow-up studies involving fused multimodality imaging. J Neurosurg. 2004;101(Suppl 3):326–33.
2. Prasad V, Baum RP. Biodistribution of the Ga-68 labeled somatostatin analogue DOTA-NOC in patients with neuroendocrine tumors: characterization of uptake in normal organs and tumor lesions. Q J Nucl Med Mol Imaging. 2010;54(1):61–7.
3. Fellner M, Baum RP, Kubicek V, Hermann P, Lukes I, Prasad V, et al. PET/CT imaging of osteoblastic bone metastases with ^{68}Ga-bisphosphonates: first human study. Eur J Nucl Med Mol Imaging. 2010;37(4):834.
4. Baum RP, Prasad V, Müller D, Schuchardt C, Orlova A, Wennborg A, et al. Molecular imaging of HER2-expressing malignant tumors in breast cancer patients using synthetic ^{111}In- or ^{68}Ga-labeled affibody molecules. J Nucl Med. 2010;51(6):892–7.
5. Mueller D, Kulkarni H, Baum RP, Odparlik A. Rapid synthesis of ^{68}Ga-labeled macroaggregated human serum albumin (MAA) for routine application in perfusion imaging using PET/CT. Appl Radiat Isot. 2017;122:72–7. https://doi.org/10.1016/j.apradiso.2017.01.003.
6. Baum RP, Kulkarni HR, Schuchardt C, Singh A, Wirtz M, Wiessalla S, Wester H-J. 177Lu-labeled prostate-specific membrane antigen radioligand therapy of metastatic castration-resistant prostate cancer: safety and efficacy. J Nucl Med. 2016;57(7):1006. https://doi.org/10.2967/jnumed.115.168443.
7. Wehrmann C, Senftleben S, Zachert C, Müller D, Baum RP. Results of individual patient dosimetry in peptide receptor radionuclide therapy with 177Lu DOTA-TATE and 177Lu DOTA-NOC. Cancer Biother Radiopharm. 2007;22(3):406–16. https://doi.org/10.1089/cbr.2006.325.
8. Zhernosekov KP, Filosofov DV, Baum RP, Aschoff P, Bihl H, Razbash AA, Jahn M, Jennewein M, Rösch F. Processing of generator produced ^{68}Ga for medical application. J Nucl Med. 2007;48:1741–8.
9. Müller D, Klette I, Baum RP. The combined cationic-anionic purification of the ^{68}Ge/^{68}Ga generator eluate for the labelling of fragile peptides, world. J Nucl Med. 2011;1(10):73–89.
10. Mueller D, Klette I, Kalb F, Baum R. One pot synthesis of [18F]-Fluoroethylcholine. J Nucl Med. 2010;51:1543.
11. Mueller D, Klette I, Kalb F, Baum RP. Synthesis of O-(2-[18F]fluoroethyl)-L-tyrosine based on a cartridge purification method. Nucl Med Biol. 2011;38(5):653–8.
12. Mueller D, Klette I, Baum RP, Gottschaldt M, Schultz MK, Breeman W, a P. Simplified NaCl based (68)ga concentration and labeling procedure for rapid synthesis of (68)ga radiopharmaceuticals in high radiochemical purity. Bioconjug Chem. 2012;23(8):1712–7. https://doi.org/10.1021/bc300103t.
13. Schultz MK, Mueller D, Baum RP, Watkins LG, Breeman WAP. A new automated NaCl based robust method for routine production of gallium-68 labeled peptides. Appl Radiat Isot. 2013;76:46–54.
14. Giesel FL, Kratochwil C, Lindner T, Marschalek MM, Loktev A, Lehnert W, Debus J, Jäger D, Flechsig P, Altmann A, Mier W, Haberkorn U. ^{68}Ga-FAPI PET/CT: biodistribution and preliminary dosimetry estimate of 2 DOTA-containing FAP-targeting agents in patients with various cancers. J Nucl Med. 2019;60(3):386–92. https://doi.org/10.2967/jnumed.118.215913.

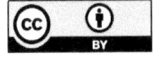

John O. Prior ⓘ, Marie Nicod Lalonde ⓘ, Niklaus Schaefer ⓘ, and Margret Schottelius ⓘ

Abbreviations

h-index	Hirsch index, a bibliometric index measuring both productivity and citation impact suggested in 2005 by the physicist Jorge E. Hirsch at University of California San Diego, USA, to measure the theoretical physicist's relative quality (https://en.wikipedia.org/wiki/H-index).
iCite	Tool to access bibliometrics associated to a portfolio accessible at https://icite.od.nih.gov
NETTER-1	Neuroendocrine Tumors Therapy study (NCT01578239)
NIH	National Institute of Health
PET	positron emission tomography
PRRT	peptide receptor radionuclide therapy
PSMA	prostate specific membrane antigen
PubMed®	Free search engine accessible at https://pubmed.ncbi.nlm.nih.gov/
RCR	relative citation ratio

J. O. Prior (✉) · M. Nicod Lalonde · N. Schaefer
Nuclear Medicine and Molecular Imaging
Department, Lausanne University Hospital and
University of Lausanne, Lausanne, Switzerland
e-mail: john.prior@chuv.ch;
marie.nicod-lalonde@chuv.ch;
niklaus.schaefer@chuv.ch

M. Schottelius
Nuclear Medicine and Molecular Imaging
Department, Lausanne University Hospital and
University of Lausanne, Lausanne, Switzerland

Translational Radiopharmaceutical Science
Laboratory, Lausanne University Hospital and
University of Lausanne, Lausanne, Switzerland
e-mail: margret.schottelius@chuv.ch

25.1 Introduction

In this work, we try to capture the footprint of Richard P. Baum in the scientific literature throughout his whole career, ranging from his first publication up to the time of this analysis (March 28, 2021). Since his scientific output encompasses many cited works, we limited our search to the Web of Science Database "Core Collection."

25.2 Material and Methods

We searched the Web of Science Database "Core Collection" to export the abstract and full reference list of all articles using the search term "Richard P. Baum" as author. Results were exported in CSV format and imported in the VOSviewer version 1.6.16 [1] (Leiden University, Leiden, Netherlands). VOSviewer has been

245

V. Prasad (ed.), *Beyond Becquerel and Biology to Precision Radiomolecular Oncology: Festschrift in Honor of Richard P. Baum*, https://doi.org/10.1007/978-3-031-33533-4_25

developed to visualize bibliometric networks and has already been used in over 500 articles cited in the literature [2, 3]. For the Relative citation Ratio (RCR) we used the iCite Database, which contains 26,482,789 articles in PubMed as of March 8, 2021 and which is freely available at https://icite.od.nih.gov, applying the methodology described by Hutchins et al. [4].

25.3   Results

The Web of Science search returned 715 publication records for Richard P. Baum as an author as of March 28, 2021 (https://www.webofscience.com/wos/woscc/general-summary?q=W3siZiI6IkRYT kciLCJ0IjoiMjMyOCJ9XQ). This results in a *h-index* of 51 for a *sum of times cited* totaling 11,247 (10,641 without self-citations) and 8020 *citing articles* (7837 without self-citations). The evaluation of the *sum of times cited per year* metrics is presented in Fig. 25.1, and the overall average citation per item is 15.73. In terms of number of publications per year, there has always been a sustained scientific production, with a steady increase during the last 20 years and an almost doubled publication output during the last decade (Fig. 25.1). In all these records, Richard P. Baum

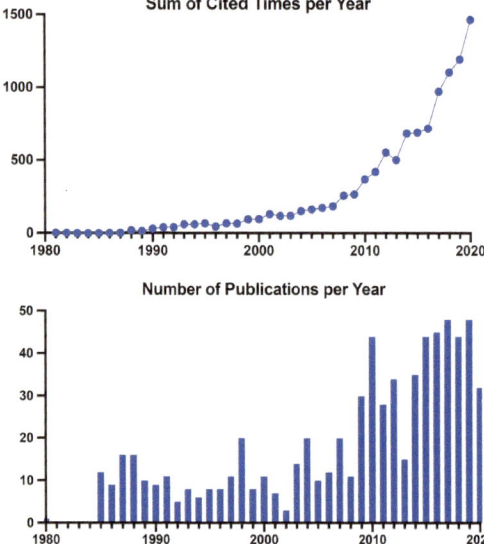

Fig. 25.1 Bar chart of the sum of times cited per year and the number of publications per year of Richard P. Baum over the 1981–2020 interval

was cited most often as last author (41%) and as first author (13%). Furthermore, he was corresponding author in 8% of the records. When examining the publication types, meeting abstracts, articles, and editorials constitute the majority of the records with 59%, 30%, and 4%, respectively, followed by reviews, proceeding papers, and review articles (each 4%, respectively).

Overall, eight articles were found to be highly cited in the field, as listed in Table 25.1. Alone, these eight articles are responsible for 3155 citation (28% of the total times cited) for an impressing average of 394.28 citation par article.

When all these 715 publications are grouped in five most frequent subject categories, most of the records were in Radiology and Nuclear Medicine Medical Imaging (n = 471 or 65%) and Oncology (*n* = 131 or 18%) as shown in Fig. 25.2. The country of origin of the publication records is shown in Fig. 25.3 for the seven most frequent countries.

The VOSviewer was used to display a co-occurrence network of terms extracted from the titles and abstracts of the selected publications as previously described [3]. The result is displayed in Fig. 25.4. The size of the circles displays the number of times the term was found in the title or the abstract. Furthermore, the terms that co-occur are located close to each other in the visualization. All terms were also grouped in three clusters of significant size. The details are given in the legend of Fig. 25.4. Using the same data, cluster density visualization was performed and allowed to better examine the co-occurrence terms with the weight of the color depending on the number of items belonging to that cluster (Fig. 25.5).

When examining the scientific themes development of Richard P. Baum over time, one can see that it started with monoclonal antibodies around year 2000, then moved to PET diagnosis around 2005 before evolving to peptide receptor radionuclide therapy of neuroendocrine tumors and its efficacy (2010) before moving on to PSMA therapy starting in 2015, as shown in the overlay visualization of Fig. 25.6. Finally, the last overlay visualization of Fig. 25.7 shows the number of average citations per co-occurrence term, demonstrating variation of up to fourfold among co-occurrence terms.

Table 25.1 Highly cited articles from Richard P. Baum totaling 3155 citation (3151 without self-citations) for an average of 394.28 citation par article

Year	Title	Reference	Total Citations	Average per Year	RCR
2017	Phase 3 trial of Lu-177-Dotatate for midgut neuroendocrine tumors	[5]	913	182.6	76.41
2010	FDG PET and PET/CT: EANM procedure guidelines for tumour PET imaging: Version 1.0	[6]	866	72.17	29.56
2013	The joint IAEA, EANM, and SNMMI practical guidance on peptide receptor radionuclide therapy (PRRNT) in neuroendocrine tumours	[7]	344	38.22	–
2017	German multicenter study investigating Lu-177-PSMA-617 Radioligand therapy in advanced prostate cancer patients	[8]	318	63.6	25.03
2016	Lu-177-labeled prostate-specific membrane antigen Radioligand therapy of metastatic castration-resistant prostate cancer: Safety and efficacy	[9]	232	38.67	6.79
2015	Ga-68- and Lu-177-labeled PSMA I&T: Optimization of a PSMA-targeted Theranostic concept and first proof-of-concept human studies	[10]	227	32.43	12.67
2015	Long-term tolerability of PRRT in 807 patients with neuroendocrine tumours: The value and limitations of clinical factors	[11]	174	24.86	10.31
2018	Health-related quality of life in patients with progressive midgut neuroendocrine tumors treated with Lu-177-Dotatate in the phase III NETTER-1 trial	[12]	81	20.25	9.89

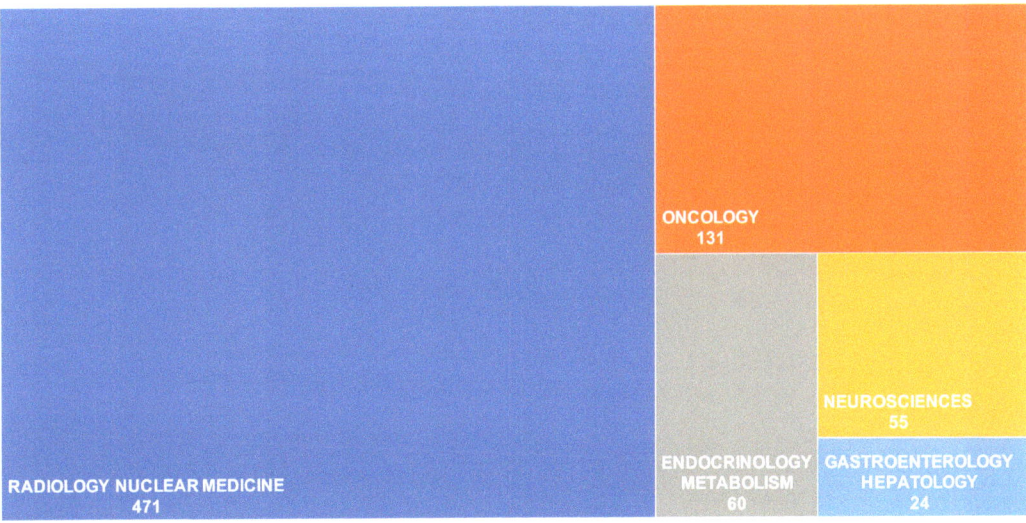

Fig. 25.2 Treemap visualization of Richard P. Baum 715 publication records grouped in five Web of Science categories

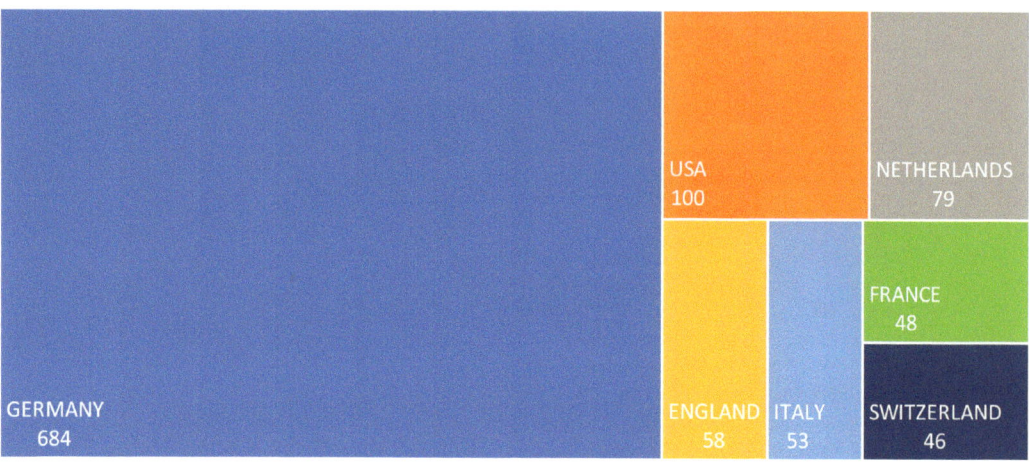

Fig. 25.3 Treemap visualization of Richard P. Baum articles grouped in seven countries of 715 records

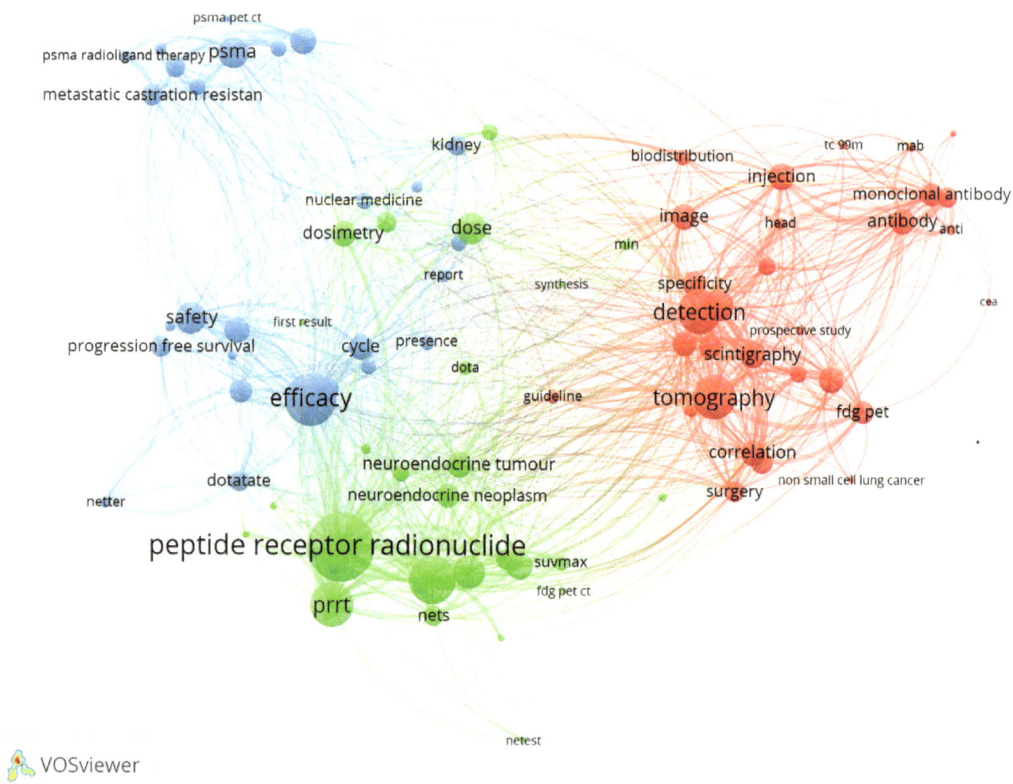

Fig. 25.4 Co-occurrence network of terms using the VOSviewer visualization software of terms extracted from the titles and abstracts of the selected 715 publications of Richard P. Baum. The size of the circles displays the number of times the term was found in the title or the abstract. The 85 terms that co-occur are located close to each other and grouped in three clusters of significant size (in green peptide receptor radionuclide therapy of neuroendocrine tumors, in blue efficacy and PSMA therapy and in red PET and detection). The 1000 strongest links are represented

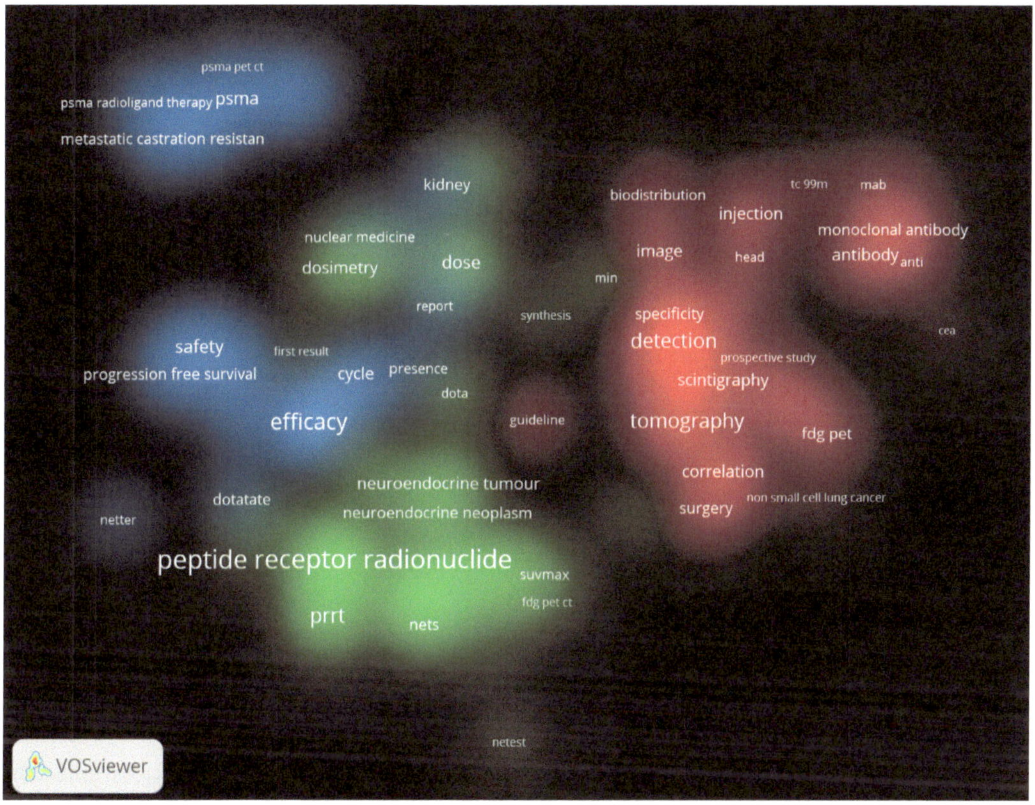

Fig. 25.5 Using the same data as in Fig. 25.4, this cluster density visualization displays the co-occurrence terms with weight of the color depending on the number of items belonging to that cluster (in green peptide receptor radionuclide therapy of neuroendocrine tumors, in blue efficacy and PSMA therapy and in red PET and detection)

To round off this analysis of Richard P. Baum's footprint in science, we were interested in one of the latest academic metrics available, the so-called Relative Citation Ratio (RCR), which is a different bibliometric assessment of scientific productivity as compared to the usual ones (journal's impact factor, h-index) to assess publications. With the RCR, the number of citations is compared to an expected citation rate of all articles derived from the same field [4]. Lately, this new metrics has been advocated as a more valid practice to identify influential papers across all disciplines. When applying this easy analysis in iCite (Fig. 25.8), one discovers that the median RCR of Richard P. Baum was 1.46 with a range from 0–76.41 (Fig. 25.8). This is above the 80th percentile of all articles in iCite with a RCR above 0 (19,859,778 publications as of March 8, 2021). Furthermore, most of his articles contained in PubMed and listed in iCites are above the 50th percentile of all the publications with a RCR above 0, which would correspond to a 50th percentile RCR of 0.37. Finally, Richard P. Baum has ten publications with a RCR above the 99th percentile of all PubMed articles (RCR > 7.98) and three above the 99.9th percentile (RCR > 23.62) with a maximum at 76.41. The RCR for the eight highly cited articles is also presented in Table 25.1.

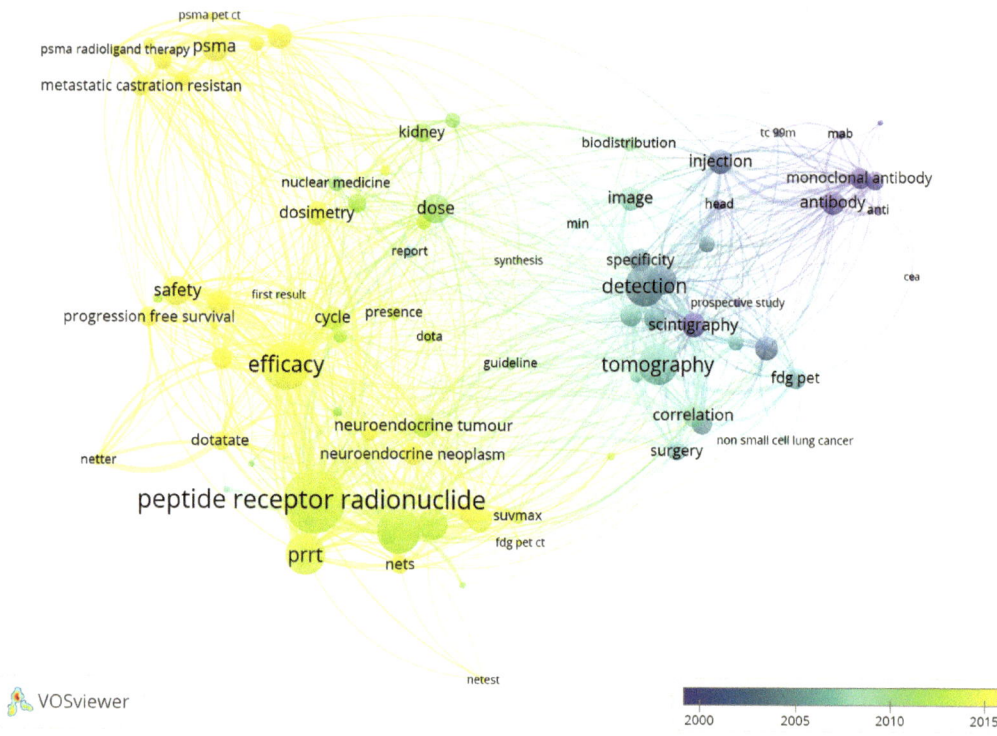

Fig. 25.6 Overlay visualization of the same co-occurrence cluster data showing the development over average citation year of Richard P. Baum publications, starting with monoclonal antibodies (around year 2000), then PET diagnosis (2005), peptide receptor radionuclide therapy of neuroendocrine tumors and its efficacy (2010) PSMA (starting 2015). The 1000 strongest links are represented

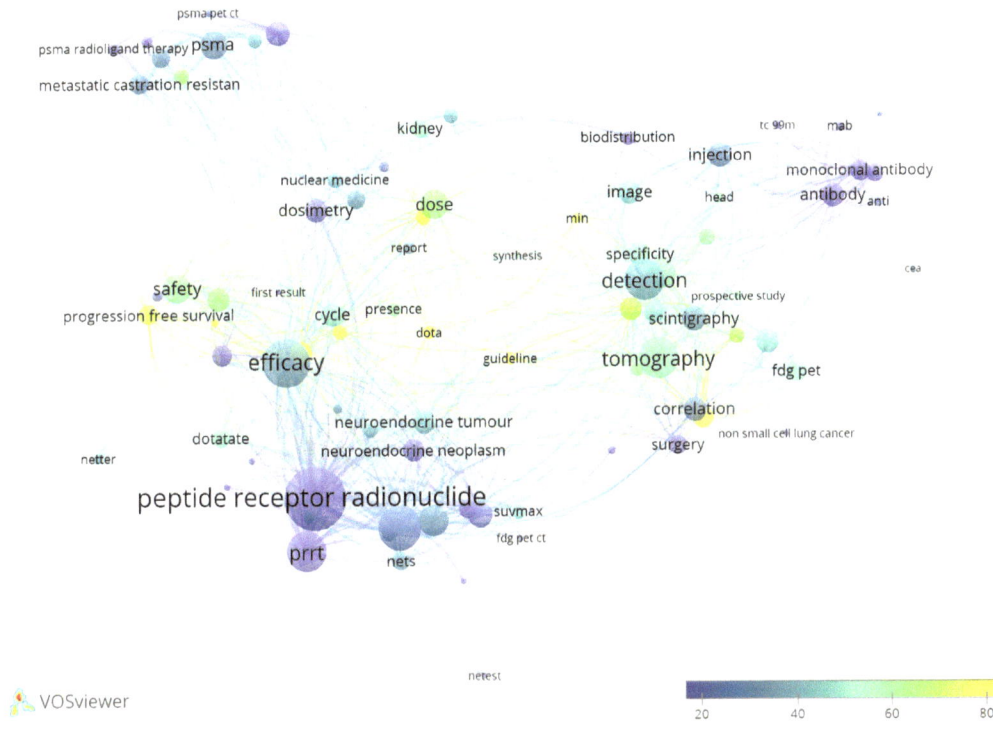

Fig. 25.7 Overlay visualization of the average citations per co-occurrence terms showing the number of times each term was cited in average in Richard P. Baum publications. The color scale shows between 20 and 80 citations per co-occurrence term

Fig. 25.8 Distribution of the Relative Citation Ratio (RCR) of Richard P. Baum articles contained in the iCite Database of the NIH accessible at https:// icite.od.nih.gov over the 1980–2020 period [4]. His median RCR is 1.46, which is above the 80th percentile of all publication contained in the iCite database. Most of his iCite Database publications (85%) are above the 50th percentile of all publications in the iCite Database which corresponds to a RCR of 0.37

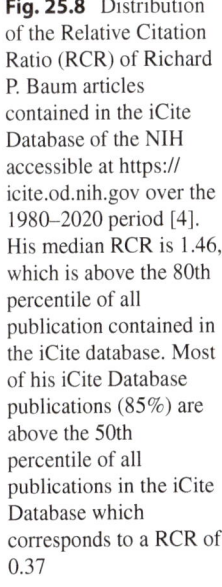

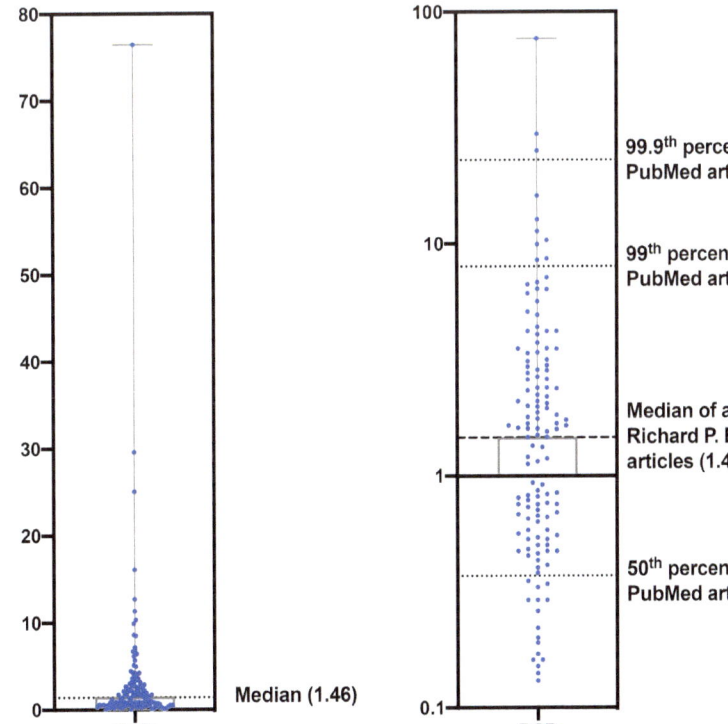

25.4 Discussion

The publication record of Richard P. Baum is truly impressive as outlined in the results section, leading to over 11,000 citations and 725 records in the Web of Science Database. Not only are his standard bibliometric metrics such as his h-index or the journal's impact factors excellent, but the latest more valid metrics of scientific productivity as the relative Citation ratio (RCR) is equally impressive with most of his articles being cited more often than half of the articles with a RCR in PubMed, with ten of his articles being even cited more often than 99% of all PubMed articles.

The results presented here constitute only a bibliometric analysis of the work of Richard P. Baum and is forcedly reducing his work to mere citations. On a personal note, one should say that knowing Richard is clearly superior to reading his work, as anyone who has interacted with him will agree that he has impressive interpersonal skills, making encounters with Richard highly memorable. With his presence, energy, positivism and eagerness to pragmatically solve the next scientific problems, he has always been one of the outstanding characters in our field – and it maybe not even be saying too much when characterizing him as a "Rockstar in Nuclear Medicine," also characterized by coming too late to a session and leaving early when getting bored. This honesty and clarity made him an excellent dinner conversation partner. His openness for exploiting novel routes and methods, which have led him to be oftentimes the first one (sometimes only one) to bring novel radiopharmaceuticals and radionuclides to his patients, cannot be captured appropriately with bibliometric metrics, showing us its limitations. Life is about stories, not about numbers.

As a limitation to our analysis, one should mention that the profile of Richard P. Baum in the Web of Science and PubMed databases was algorithmically generated, which means Richard P. Baum himself did not verify all founds records. Furthermore, as these databases are continuously updated, the number of citations in this chapter was found as of March 28, 2021 and will keep on increasing daily and forever, as long as new articles will cite the work of Richard P. Baum.

25.5 Conclusion

The present analysis outlined the scientific publication footprint of Richard P. Baum over the last four decades in the domain of nuclear medicine and therapy. He helped to shape the field of neuroendocrine tumors diagnosis and therapy, as well as prostate cancer radionuclide therapy. His scientific productivity was constant since 1980 and even doubled during the last decade. His works have been cited over 11,000 times in the literature and even when using the latest metrics of scientific productivity such as the relative citation rate, his bibliometric achievements remain outstanding and are only matched by very few authors among the many with a similarly long scientific career.

Acknowledgments/Conflict of Interest The authors declare that no conflict of interest exist.

References

1. VOSviewer Visualizing scientific landscapes: Leiden University. 2021. www.vosviewer.com/. Accessed 21 Mar 2021.
2. van Eck NJ, Waltman L. Software survey: VOSviewer, a computer program for bibliometric mapping. Scientometrics. 2010;84(2):523–38.
3. van Eck NJ, Waltman L. Visualizing bibliometric networks. In: Ding Y, Rousseau R, Wolfram D, editors. Measuring scholarly impact: methods and practice. Cham: Springer; 2014. p. 285–320.
4. Hutchins BI, Yuan X, Anderson JM, Santangelo GM. Relative citation ratio (RCR): a new metric that uses citation rates to measure influence at the article level. PLoS Biol. 2016;14(9):e1002541.
5. Strosberg J, El-Haddad G, Wolin E, Hendifar A, Yao J, Chasen B, et al. Phase 3 trial of Lu-177-Dotatate for midgut neuroendocrine tumors. N Engl J Med. 2017;376(2):125–35.
6. Boellaard R, O'Doherty MJ, Weber WA, Mottaghy FM, Lonsdale MN, Stroobants SG, et al. FDG PET and PET/CT: EANM procedure guidelines for tumour PET imaging: version 1.0. Eur J Nucl Med Mol Imaging. 2010;37(1):181–200.
7. Zaknun JJ, Bodei L, Mueller-Brand J, Pavel ME, Baum RP, Horsch D, et al. The joint IAEA, EANM, and SNMMI practical guidance on peptide receptor radionuclide therapy (PRRNT) in neuroendocrine tumours. Eur J Nucl Med Mol Imaging. 2013;40(5):800–16.
8. Rahbar K, Ahmadzadehfar H, Kratochwil C, Haberkorn U, Schafers M, Essler M, et al. German

multicenter study investigating Lu-177-PSMA-617 Radioligand therapy in advanced prostate cancer patients. J Nucl Med. 2017;58(1):85–90.

9. Baum RP, Kulkarni HR, Schuchardt C, Singh A, Wirtz M, Wiessalla S, et al. Lu-177-labeled prostate-specific membrane antigen Radioligand therapy of metastatic castration-resistant prostate cancer: safety and efficacy. J Nucl Med. 2016;57(7):1006–13.

10. Weineisen M, Schottelius M, Simecek J, Baum RP, Yildiz A, Beykan S, et al. Ga-68- and Lu-177-labeled PSMA I&T: optimization of a PSMA-targeted theranostic concept and first proof-of-concept human studies. J Nucl Med. 2015;56(8):1169–76.

11. Bodei L, Kidd M, Paganelli G, Grana CM, Drozdov I, Cremonesi M, et al. Long-term tolerability of PRRT in 807 patients with neuroendocrine tumours: the value and limitations of clinical factors. Eur J Nucl Med Mol Imaging. 2015;42(1):5–19.

12. Strosberg J, Wolin E, Chasen B, Kulke M, Bushnell D, Caplin M, et al. Health-related quality of life in patients with progressive midgut neuroendocrine tumors treated with Lu-177-Dotatate in the phase III NETTER-1 trial. J Clin Oncol. 2018;36(25):2578.

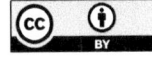

Therapy of Castration-Resistant
Prostate Cancer: Where Is the Place
of ^{225}Ac-PSMA?

26

Ismaheel O. Lawal, Alfred Morgenstern,
Otto Knoesen, Mariza Vorster,
Frank Bruchertseifer, and Mike M. Sathekge

26.1 Introduction

Over the past decade and a half, many life-prolonging therapy agents have been approved for the treatment of metastatic castration-resistant prostate cancer (mCRPC), the lethal form of prostate cancer. These therapy agents fall into four categories, including chemotherapy (docetaxel and cabazitaxel), androgen-signaling-targeted inhibitors (abiraterone and enzalutamide), immunotherapy (Sipuleucel-T), and bone-targeting agent for skeletal metastases (radium-223 dichloride- ^{223}RaCl$_2$) [1–6].

Extensive application of these life-prolonging agents has not translated into commensurate reduction in mortality of patients with mCRPC. Prostate cancer mortality has remained stable or even increased in some countries of the world [7]. The multitude of the available life-prolonging agents for mCRPC has introduced a new challenge of the sequence to apply them in patients' treatment. Longer survival advantage is conferred when an agent is applied earlier in the treatment cycle compared with its application later in the sequence of treatment. It is, therefore, not only necessary to select an agent that has survival benefit but also has tolerable side effects without associated negative impact on the quality of life earlier in the treatment sequence of mCRPC.

Radionuclide therapy targeting prostate-specific membrane antigen (PSMA), a transmembrane glycoprotein overexpressed on prostate cancer cells, has emerged as an attractive therapy option for men with mCRPC. PSMA radioligand therapy (PRLT) is more commonly applied using Lutetium-177-labeled PSMA (^{177}Lu-PSMA) [8]. ^{225}Ac-PSMA targeted therapy is an alternative PRLT agent for targeted alpha therapy (TAT), which is effective in the treatment of mCRPC, including patients who failed treatment with ^{177}Lu-PSMA. In this chapter, we aim to present an update on the evidence in support of the use of ^{225}Ac-PSMA as a TAT agent for mCRPC. We will review its effectiveness, safety

I. O. Lawal · M. Vorster · M. M. Sathekge (✉)
Department of Nuclear Medicine, University of Pretoria, Pretoria, South Africa

Nuclear Medicine Research Infrastructure (NuMeRI), Steve Biko Academic Hospital, Pretoria, South Africa
e-mail: mike.sathekge@up.ac.za

A. Morgenstern
Department of Nuclear Medicine, University of Pretoria, Pretoria, South Africa

European Commission, Joint Research Centre, Directorate of Nuclear Safety and Security, Karlsruhe, Germany

O. Knoesen
Nuclear Technology Products (NTP), Pelindaba, South Africa

F. Bruchertseifer
European Commission, Joint Research Centre, Directorate of Nuclear Safety and Security, Karlsruhe, Germany

V. Prasad (ed.), *Beyond Becquerel and Biology to Precision Radiomolecular Oncology: Festschrift in Honor of Richard P. Baum*, https://doi.org/10.1007/978-3-031-33533-4_26

profile, and its upfront application in the chemotherapy-naïve setting for the treatment of mCRPC.

26.2 ^{177}Lu-PSMA Versus ^{225}Ac-PSMA PRT in mCRPC

Many centers across the world now administer ^{177}Lu-PSMA therapy for PRLT of mCRPC. Consequently, several nuclear medicine societies have published guidance documents for safe application of ^{177}Lu-PSMA therapy as a last-line therapy option in men who have exhausted, refused, or do not qualify for therapy with the life-prolonging therapy agents [9–12]. Following the encouraging results from an early German multicenter study which showed good efficacy with minimal side effects [13], ^{177}Lu-PSMA has gained increasing acceptance as a viable treatment option in mCRPC [14]. Many studies have subsequently been published showing its efficacy and safety in different populations of patients with mCRPC including in men who are chemotherapy-naïve [15], have single functional kidney [16], have lymph node-predominant metastatic disease [17], and for rechallenge in patients who progressed after an initial response to ^{177}Lu-PSMA therapy [18]. In a prospective phase II trial, 57% of heavily pretreated men with mCRPC achieved a prostate-specific antigen (PSA) decline of 50% or more with a median progression-free survival (PFS) and overall survival (OS) of 7.6 months (95%CI: 6.3–9) and 13.5 months (95%CI: 10.4–22.7), respectively [19]. The most common side effects seen in the patients were hematologic toxicity and xerostomia [19]. In a recent meta-analysis of 17 studies of ^{177}Lu-PSMA treatment in men with mCRPC, 45% of patients had a PSA decline greater than 50% while an average of 74% of patients had any PSA decline [20].

It is evident from the preceding discussion that a significant proportion of patients with mCRPC may not respond to ^{177}Lu-PSMA therapy. Up to 37% of patients (95CI: 33.9–40.3) who initially respond to treatment will experi-

ence PSA progression in the short term [20]. These nonresponders, as well as the relapsing patients who may have exhausted or are unfit for the available life-prolonging agents, need alternative treatment options. ^{177}Lu decays by beta particle emission. Its beta particle can traverse between 20 to 60 cells [8]. This long path length of beta particles of ^{177}Lu precludes its use in certain patterns of disease, particularly diffuse prostate cancer metastasis to the bone marrow in a superscan pattern, as this may result in severe bone marrow toxicity in patients who may already have a compromised bone marrow reserve [21]. Also, the ability of beta emission ^{177}Lu to cause cellular damage is dependent on its penetration and the diameter of the tumor [22]. Dose deposited by ^{177}Lu beta emission decline significantly as the diameter of lesion reduces, making effective eradication of micrometastases with ^{177}Lu-PSMA an unrealizable goal [22, 23].

Actinium-225 (^{225}Ac) decays with a physical half-life of 9.9 days via a cascade of six short-lived radionuclide daughters to stable Bismuth-209 generating four alpha particles of energies ranging from 5.8 to 8.4 MeV and associated soft tissue range of 47 to 85 μm [24]. Alpha particles cause irreparable double-stranded DNA damage making them particularly effective in tumor kill. As they traverse the tumor, alpha particles deposit ionizing energy that is up to a thousandth times higher than the energy deposited by beta particles [25]. The short range in the tissue of alpha particles ensures the deposition of high energy within a small radius, about 110 KeV per micron distance traveled compared with about 0.2–0.5 KeV per micron deposited by beta particles [25]. Alpha particles cause direct DNA damage independent of free radical-induced indirect DNA damage that heavily relies on adequate tissue oxygen tension. ^{225}Ac-PSMA delivers a 14-fold higher radiation absorbed dose to the tumor compared with ^{223}RaCl$_2$ [26], another alpha-emitting radionuclide which prolongs the survival of patients with bone-predominant mCRPC [6]. The ability of ^{225}Ac-PSMA to be internalized by tumor cells [27], compared with ^{223}RaCl$_2$, which is adsorbed to areas of increased turnover surrounding the tumor deposit in the bone makes ^{223}Ac-PSMA theoretically better in causing an effective tumor killing than ^{223}RaCl$_2$.

26.3 Efficacy of ^{225}Ac-PSMA as a Last-Line Therapy of mCRPC

The prospect of ^{225}Ac-PSMA for TAT of mCRPC was first reported by Kratochwil et al. in two patients who had exhausted available therapy options [28]. One of these two patients had diffuse skeletal metastases in the typical superscan pattern that precluded therapy with ^{177}Lu-PSMA while the other patients with visceral metastases of prostate cancer showed no response to ^{177}Lu-PSMA. After treatment with ^{225}Ac-PSMA, PSA in both patients declined to below detectable limits while imaging findings returned to normal. No bone marrow toxicity was seen in either patient, including the patient with diffuse skeletal metastases. Xerostomia was the only treatment-related side effect reported by both patients [28]. These first cases not only show the first evidence supporting the efficacy of ^{225}Ac-PSMA in mCRPC but also lay the foundation of the type of patient who may benefit from this type of therapy as well as the efficacy of ^{225}Ac-PSMA in the post^{-177}Lu-PSMA setting.

In a study to define the optimum activity of ^{225}Ac-PSMA-617 and the dose delivered to critical organs which included 14 patients with mCRPC, Kratochwil and colleagues further reported mean doses of 2.3 Sv, 0.7 Sv and 0.05 Sv to salivary glands, kidneys, and red marrow, respectively, per MBq of administered ^{225}Ac-PSMA-617 assuming radiobiological effectiveness of five for the emitted alpha particles [29]. The corresponding mean doses to these same organs from their previous study in Gy/GBq of ^{177}Lu-PSMA-617 were 1.38, 0.75, and 0.03, respectively [30]. In this dosimetry study, patients received different activities of ^{225}Ac-PSMA-617, ranging from 50 to 200 kBq/kg body weight. Only one patient who received 200 KBq/kg had treatment-induced grade 2

hematotoxicity. Xerostomia was seen in the majority of patients treated with an activity of $\geq$100 KBq/kg. Administered activity of 150 to 200 KBq/kg was associated with good antitumor activity at the risk of increased treatment-induced toxicities leading to treatment discontinuation or de-escalation of administered activity. 100 KBq/kg of ^{225}Ac-PSMA-617 provided a compromise between effective antitumor activity and tolerable treatment-induced toxicity, mainly xerostomia. In patients who received more than one cycle of treatment, there was a progressive PSA decline when treatment was repeated after every 2 months. In contrast, when there was a delay in the administration of subsequent treatment cycles after an initial response, resistance develops without significant response to the subsequent treatment cycles [29]. Taken together, this study established xerostomia as the dose-limiting toxicity in TAT with ^{225}Ac-PSMA-617 showed the impact of the administered activity on the dynamics of antitumor activity and the appearance of toxicities, and the impact of timing of treatment cycles on PSA response [29].

In current routine medical practice, PRLT with either ^{177}Lu or ^{225}Ac-labeled PSMA is reserved for patients who have exhausted, declined, or are unfit for the life-prolonging approved therapy agents pending the availability of results of ongoing clinical trials evaluating the effectiveness and safety of PRLT in mCRPC and its comparative effectiveness versus the current standards of treatment. Treatment applied late in the sequence of therapy of mCRPC performs less well compared with the treatment given earlier in the therapy sequence. In the absence of a head-to-head comparison between ^{225}Ac-PSMA and the life-prolonging therapy agents for mCRPC, the Heidelberg group, in their most recent study on this subject, used a Swimmer-Plot analysis to compare the duration of tumor control by ^{225}Ac-PSMA-617 versus the currently used approved agents for mCRPC [31]. The median duration for any first-, second, third-, or fourth-line therapy, regardless of the drug, was 8.0, 7.0, 6.0, and 4.0 months, respectively. The median duration of abiraterone, docetaxel, enzalutamide, cabazitaxel, and $^{223}RaCl_2$, regardless of the time in the treatment sequence at which they were applied, were 10.0, 6.5, 6.5, 6.0, and 4.0 months, respectively. For ^{225}Ac-PSMA-617 applied as a last-line agent after patients have failed the approved agents, the median duration of tumor control was 9.0 months [31]. These results show the relative performance of TAT with ^{225}Ac-PSMA in a group of heavily pretreated patients, and in the absence of results from formal trials evaluating the comparative performance of ^{225}Ac-PSMA relative to the known life-prolonging agents, represent robust evidence in support of its use for mCRPC treatment.

In the largest series to date of men with mCRPC treated with ^{225}Ac-PSMA-617, Sathekge et al. reported a PSA decline of 50% or higher in 70% of patients treated after a median of three treatment cycles [32]. Imaging findings returned to normal in about 29% of patients. After a median follow-up period of 9 months (range = 2–22), 18% patients had died while disease had progressed in 32% of patients given an estimated PFS and OS of 15.2 months (95% CI: 13.1–17.4) and 18 months (95% CI: 16.2–19.9), respectively. This study provides the first published insight into the efficacy of ^{225}Ac-PSMA therapy in patients who are status post^{-177}Lu-PSMA therapy for mCRPC. Prior ^{177}Lu-PSMA therapy was associated with a shorter time to PSA progression. Median PFS in patients with prior ^{177}Lu-PSMA therapy was 5.1 months (95% CI: 3.8–6.5) compared with 16.5 months (95% CI: 14.3–18.7) in patients without therapy [32]. The negative association of prior ^{177}Lu-PSMA therapy with survival is especially significant, and it calls for proper selection of patients to either ^{177}Lu-PSMA or ^{225}Ac-PSMA therapy. ^{225}Ac-PSMA therapy will be better suited for patients with diffuse bone marrow metastasis or patients with limited baseline bone marrow reserve as the short range of the emitted alpha particles will result in a lesser absorbed dose to the limited red marrow compared with the longer-ranged beta particles of ^{177}Lu. Since beta particles of ^{177}Lu are incapable of an effective eradication of micrometastases due to the inverse relationship between the size of micrometastases and the

energy deposited in it [23], ^{225}Ac-PSMA may be more suitable for the treatment of smaller lesions especially if they are widespread compared with ^{177}Lu-PSMA.

Some factors have been found to significantly impact on survival of patients with mCRPC treated with ^{225}Ac-PSMA. In the study by Sathekge and colleagues, patients who had any PSA decline, PSA decline of 50% or more, and without prior history of chemotherapy had a significantly longer OS [32]. Factors found to be significantly associated with a longer PFS were any PSA decline, PSA decline of 50% or more, achieving an undetectable serum level following treatment, normalization of ^{68}Ga-PSMA PET/CT following treatment and absence of prior ^{177}Lu-PSMA therapy. Also, patients who do not respond to ^{225}Ac-PSMA therapy despite adequate expression of PSMA glycoprotein shown as intense tracer uptake in prostate cancer metastases on ^{68}Ga-PSMA PET/CT imaging have been reported to harbor mutations in genes responsible for the repair of DNA damage [33]. While mutations in DNA damage repair genes are generally believed to be advantageous in cancer therapy owing to the cell cycle arrest and apoptosis that is triggered by the failure to repair DNA damage [34], damage in some specific DNA repair pathways may, however, translate into radioresistant which may account for the prevalence of these mutations in patients who do not respond to ^{225}Ac-PSMA [35]. This finding is exciting and may justify combination therapy of ^{225}Ac-PSMA with radiosensitizers such as the inhibitors of poly ADP ribose polymerase (PARP inhibitors) in qualifying patients with mCRPC.

Sufficient expression of PSMA glycoprotein on prostate cancer lesions is an essential prerequisite to PRLT [10–12]. mCRPC lesions express higher levels of PSMA compared with hormone-sensitive prostate cancer lesions. In patients with mCRPC, there is significant heterogeneity in the expression of PSMA within and between lesions [36]. In lesions with heterogeneous PSMA expression, foci without PSMA expression may be outside of a 2 mm radius from foci with high expression of PSMA. The implication of this is that even with the longer path length of beta particles of ^{177}Lu that can travel an average distance of 2 mm in soft tissue, ^{177}Lu-PSMA treatment of such lesions will result in lack of radiation dose delivery to regions of no PSMA expression lying outside of the zone within which the "cross-fire effect" may be effective. This heterogeneity in target expression, even in lesions with intense PSMA expression, is more problematic in TAT where the path length of the alpha particle is below 0.01 mm. Unfortunately, the limited resolution of the PET system makes delineation of the within-lesion heterogeneity of PSMA expression impossible. Combined ^{18}F-FDG PET and ^{68}Ga-PSMA PET may be advantageous to fully characterize tumor behavior and target expression before submitting patients to PRLT [37]. Low PSMA expression or discordance between ^{68}Ga-PSMA PET and ^{18}F-FDG PET imaging portends poor treatment outcome [38, 39].

26.4 Toxicities of [225]Ac-PSMA for PRLT of mCRPC

The short path length of alpha particles ensures that energy deposition is limited to within cancer lesions with a relative sparing of surrounding normal tissues. PSMA expression is not exclusive to prostate cancer tissues. Normal tissues such as the salivary gland, renal tubular cells, lachrymal glands, and epithelial cells of the small bowel express PSMA as well [29, 40]. Off-target binding on radiolabeled PSMA ligand such as [225]Ac-PSMA is an important cause of treatment-related side effects in PRLT.

Xerostomia is the most common toxicity resulting from [225]Ac-PSMA therapy. Among all normal tissues that express PSMA, the salivary glands received the highest absorbed dose during [225]Ac-PSMA therapy [29]. There is an intense accumulation of radiolabeled PSMA ligand in the salivary gland due to specific and nonspecific bindings [41]. The first symptoms of xerostomia are seen within a few days after [225]Ac-PSMA infusion [29]. Partial recovery may occur in patients who receive limited cycles of treatment. More cycles of [225]Ac-PSMA therapy produce additive salivary gland damage resulting in severe

xerostomia. In one series, 10% of patients discontinued further [225]Ac-PSMA therapy due to intolerable xerostomia [31]. Severe xerostomia may sometimes be associated with dysgeusia causing anorexia and consequently, weight loss, fatigue, dyspepsia, and constipation [32]. Several interventions for either preventing or reducing the impact of xerostomia on patients' quality of life have been proposed [42]. These interventions include external cooling of the salivary gland to reduce dose delivery to them during therapy administration [43, 44]; injection of botulinum toxin into the salivary gland to induce vasospasm and hence dose reduction to the glands [45]; and sialendoscopy with dilatation, saline irrigation, and steroid injection to reduce radiation-induced inflammation in an attempt to prevent xerostomia [46]. To date, none of these interventions has been found sufficiently effective for noninvasive application in routine clinical practice.

Other approaches have been explored in mitigating the impact of [225]Ac-PSMA therapy on salivary gland function, mostly by reducing the activity the radioligand administered for therapy [22]. In the approach popularized by our group – the dynamic de-escalation approach, 8 MBq of [225]Ac-PSMA is administered for the first cycle of treatment. Response is evaluated by clinical evaluation, repeat ^{68}Ga-PSMA imaging findings, and level of PSA decline. Administered activity is reduced to 6 MBq in cycle 2 for responders. A similar re-evaluation is done before cycle 3, and administered activity is reduced to 4 MBq in responders. In essence, the activity of the therapeutic agent between 4 and 8 MBq is titrated against the volume of residual malignant disease to reduce the tumor sink effect that causes intense off-target radioligand uptake in normal tissues as the volume of malignant disease reduces. Using this approach, 85% of our most recent cohorts reported grade I/II xerostomia [32]. No treated patients had severe xerostomia (grade III), and no patient declined further treatment due to xerostomia. Other approaches to reducing the incidence and severity of xerostomia complicating PRLT include administering a cocktail of 4 GBq of ^{177}Lu-PSMA and 4 MBq [225]Ac-PSMA and administration of lower activity of [225]Ac-PSMA especially since the severity of xerostomia is proportional to the activity of the radioligand administered for therapy.

Hematologic toxicity may be seen in patients treated with [225]Ac-PSMA. No treatment-induced grave IV hematologic toxicity has been reported. In our series of 73 patients treated with a median of three cycles of [225]Ac-PSMA, we found grade I or II anemia, leucopenia and thrombocytopenia in 22, 7, and 6 patients, respectively [32]. We found grade III anemia, leucopenia, and thrombocytopenia in 5, 2, and 1 patient, respectively. We found no grade IV hematologic toxicity. The characteristics of the study population can explain this level of hematological toxicity. Out of 73 patients included, 28 (38%) of them had diffuse bone metastases with a superscan pattern, and 30 patients (41%) had a hemoglobin level of 10 g/dL or lower [32]. All patients who had any form of grade III hematologic toxicity had an abnormal hematologic profile at baseline assessment, indicating that these patients already had an impaired bone marrow function even before they were submitted to [225]Ac-PSMA therapy.

The kidneys are exposed to radiation dose from [225]Ac-PSMA due to the physiological expression of PSMA in the renal tubular cells and the renal route of excretion of the radioligand. Intravenous isotonic fluids such as normal saline (about 2 L of 0.9% NaCl) is coadministered with the radioligand to enhance its urinary excretion. A baseline ^{99m}Tc-MAG3 dynamic renal scintigraphy is necessary in patients with suspected obstructive uropathy who may benefit from ureteral stenting to relief obstruction prior to PRLT [11]. Intravenous frusemide may be necessary in addition to intravenous hydration in patients with dilated renal collecting system not associated with anatomic obstruction to enhance urinary flow rate and hence absorbed dose to the kidneys [11]. In our most recent series, any renal toxicity was seen in 23 patients – 32% of all patients (grade I or II =18, grade III = 3, and grade IV = 2) [32]. Again, all five patients who had either grade III or IV renal toxicity had a grade II renal toxicity at baseline assessment before therapy with [225]Ac-PSMA [32].

The lachrymal gland is another organ with high PSMA expression and at risk of radiation damage during PRLT. In our series, we reported grade I or II xerophthalmia in 5% of patients [32].

26.5 Upfront Application of [225]Ac-PSMA for Therapy of mCRPC in Chemotherapy-Naïve Patients

Docetaxel was the first agent to demonstrate a survival benefit in the treatment of mCRPC [1]. Cabazitaxel was shown in 2010 to have a survival benefit in men who progressed after docetaxel and has since been one of the second-line agents for the treatment of men with mCRPC [2]. Abiraterone and enzalutamide, two agents that act on the androgen signaling pathway, are other drugs with life-prolonging capabilities that are commonly applied in patients with mCRPC [3, 4]. In real-world practice, docetaxel was the most commonly used agent for first-line therapy of mCRPC before 2010. Beyond 2010, non-chemotherapeutic agents are increasingly used as the first-line agent for mCRPC [47]. This shift in the choice of agent is most probably related to the better safety profile of the non-chemotherapeutic agents acting on the androgen receptor/signaling pathway. Elderly patients aged 75 years and older also tend to have significantly more high-grade and fatal treatment-related toxicities when treated with docetaxel [48]. There is still no consensus on the sequence to apply the currently available agents for mCRPC treatment as a result of the absence of head-to-head comparisons of these agents in randomized clinical trials (RCTs). Results from large observational studies and systematic reviews of published studies are emerging to define the better sequence of application of the available agents for mCRPC [49, 50]. It is crucial to determine the most effective treatment sequence so that the most effective agent is applied earlier in the therapy sequence since the response to agents applied later in the sequence are generally less remarkable. Safety is another critical factor to be considered in the sequencing of therapy agents so that the most effective and, equally important, the safest agent is applied earlier to preserve and prolong quality life.

A randomized control trial (RCT) is required to define the efficacy and the place of any therapy intervention in medical practice. Results from RCTs evaluating the efficacy, safety, and the place PRLT either with ^{177}Lu-PSMA or ^{225}Ac-PSMA are still being awaited. It is also worth noting that a comparison of results from different RCTs is difficult due to the differences in the patient populations in the different trials. Many insights can be gained from the published retrospective observational studies that have reported the safety and efficacy of ^{225}Ac-PSMA in mCRPC treatment. In the absence of an RCT, a Swimmer plot analysis is a useful pictorial representation of the duration of tumor control in an individual treated with different agents. In the series by Kratochwil and colleagues, using a Swimmer plot analysis, the authors show that ^{225}Ac-PSMA used as a last-line agent performed better or similar to agents applied as the first-, second-, and third-line treatments [31]. This suggests that, perhaps, if applied earlier in the course of the disease, ^{225}Ac-PSMA could have provided a longer duration of disease control than the currently approved agents.

In a study of ^{225}Ac-PSMA therapy in chemotherapy-naïve patients, Sathekge and colleagues reported a PSA decline of 90% or more in 82% of patients and a PSA decline of ≥80% seen in 71% of patients after the first cycle of ^{225}Ac-PSMA administered for mCRPC [51]. In 41% of patients, PSA declined to undetectable levels after two to three cycles of ^{225}Ac-PSMA and remained undetectable for a median of 12 months posttreatment. Tolerable xerostomia was seen in all patients treated, but no patients withdrew from this treatment due to this side effect. No statistically significant decline was seen in the pretreatment versus posttreatment leucocyte count, hemoglobin level, serum creatinine level, or serum albumin level [49]. Docetaxel given in the same setting led to a PSA decline of ≥50% in 45% to 48% of patients with a median duration of PSA response of 7.7 to 8.2 months

[1]. Docetaxel is significantly associated with neutropenia, alopecia, diarrhea, sensory neuropathy, dysgeusia, stomatitis, among other treatment-related toxicities warranting discontinuation of treatment in some patients [1]. Cabazitaxel is another chemotherapeutic agent with a survival benefit in mCRPC in the post-docetaxel setting. Used as a second-line agent in the post-docetaxel setting, cabazitaxel led to a ≥ 50% PSA decline in 39.2% of patients with a median time to PSA progression of 6.4 months [2]. Like docetaxel, cabazitaxel caused significant bone marrow toxicity causing any-grade neutropenia and anemia in more than 90% of patients treated. The severity of side effects led to treatment discontinuation in 18% of patients treated with cabazitaxel [2].

While the evidence from controlled trials in support of the use of ^{225}Ac-PSMA in TAT of mCRPC is being awaited, the available data are already showing good efficacy and tolerability in patients treated in critical clinical situations [28–31, 52]. Here we make a case for the compassionate consideration of the use of ^{225}Ac-PSMA in chemotherapy-naïve patients who may be considered unfit or have refused chemotherapy because of its potential side effects or other consideration, especially if they have previously failed therapy with the novel agents targeting the androgen receptor/signaling pathway (Fig. 26.1). In this setting, ^{225}Ac-PSMA therapy is associated with better PSA response, longer duration of tumor control, better safety profile, and a survival advantage when compared, in an intra-individual fashion or with historical control, against the currently approved life-prolonging agents. While not the subject of discussion in this review, it is worthy to note that similar upfront application ^{177}Lu-PSMA in the chemotherapy-naïve setting is associated with a better response than its application post-taxane chemotherapy [15]. In the work from Bad Berka, Barber and colleagues showed that taxane-naïve patients had significantly better survival with a median PFS and OS of 8.8 months and 27.1 months, respectively, compared with taxane-pretreated patients whose corresponding PFS and OS were 6.0 months and 10.7 months, respectively [15].

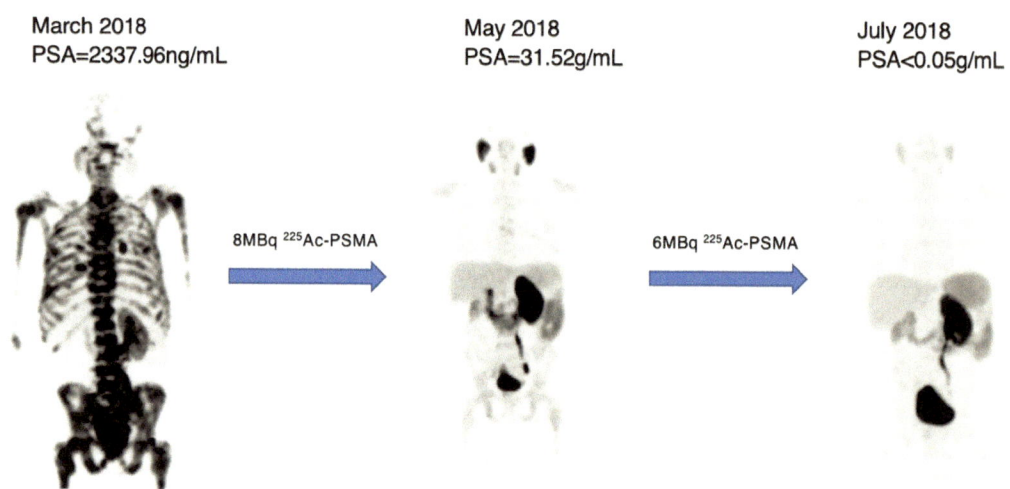

March 2018
PSA=2337.96ng/mL

May 2018
PSA=31.52g/mL

July 2018
PSA<0.05g/mL

8MBq ^{225}Ac-PSMA

6MBq ^{225}Ac-PSMA

Fig. 26.1 A 76-year-old male treated with two cycles of ^{225}Ac-PSMA-617 therapy in March and May 2018. He is known with a large cystic mass in the right kidney. His treatment history included androgen-deprivation therapy and radiotherapy to the spine. He had a remarkable response to ^{225}Ac-PSMA-617 and his serum PSA has remained undetectable to date

26.6 Conclusion and Future Perspectives

In recent times, many agents with the ability to prolong life are now available for routine clinical application in the treatment of men with mCRPC. This widespread availability of treatment options has not translated to consistent more prolonged survival in all climes. More agents, including immunotherapies, drugs targeting oncogenic and genomic pathways, and radionuclide therapies, are being evaluated for their efficacy and safety in mCRPC. Even with the available agents, the sequence to apply drug treatment for the most effective response and most prolonged survival is still a subject of research. TAT with ^{225}Ac-PSMA has shown excellent PSA response, clinical symptom control, and tolerable side effects. It is believed that this excellent performance may be confirmed in controlled trials soon. The understanding of tumor biology is broadening, especially in the late-stage disease where genomic instability and mutations in multiple DNA repair genes are prevalent and drive resistance to therapy. This broadening understanding is providing insight that may guide the future application of combination therapies to attack multiple cancer targets reasonably and safely for effective therapy of mCRPC. ^{225}Ac-PSMA, currently applied as a last-line agent, holds much promise to get a front-line application in the future owing to its excellent efficacy that compares with currently approved agents and its tolerability. Efforts must continue to address salivary gland toxicity. This may be in the form of ligand modification to improve specificity for tumor target, reduce administered activity in combination therapy with other effective agents, or effective pharmacologic salivary gland protection.

Special Paragraph for Prof Rich Baum
Dear Rich and Julitta,

Rich, you are one of the greatest leaders of Nuclear Medicine, I admire and appreciate your achievements and the time you have invested with regards to promoting targeted radionuclide imaging and therapy. To me you have always been a big brother, friend and mentor. I am grateful you are an encouragement, inspiration, and motivation. Julitta and you have always shown me the WARMTH and kindness. I thank you so kindly for making me part of the memorable "Festschrift in Honor of Prof. Baum."

Big Hugs!!!

Mike

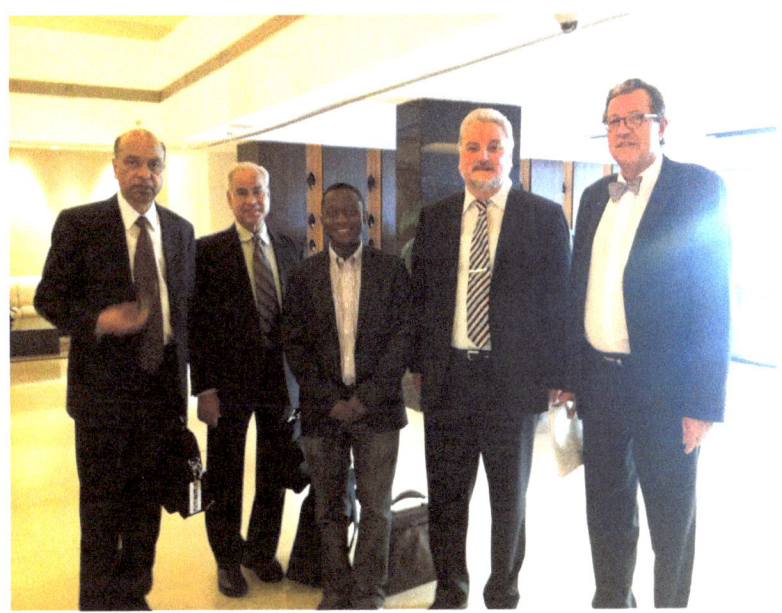

Conflict of Interest All authors declare that they have no conflict of interest.

References

1. Tannock IF, de Wit R, Berry WR, Horti J, Pluzanska A, Chi KN, et al. Docetaxel plus prednisone or mitoxantrone plus prednisone for advanced prostate cancer. N Engl J Med. 2004;351:1502–12.
2. de Bono JS, Oudard S, Ozguroglu M, Hansen S, Machiels JP, Krocak I, et al. Prednisone plus cabazitaxel or mitoxantrone for metastatic castration-resistant prostate cancer progressing after docetaxel treatment: a randomized open-label trial. Lancet. 2010;376:1147–54.
3. de Bono JS, Logothetis CJ, Molina A, Fizazi K, North S, Chu L, Chi KN, et al. Abiraterone and increased survival in metastatic prostate cancer. N Engl J Med. 2011;364:1995–2005.
4. Scher HI, Fizazi K, Saad F, Taplin ME, Sternberg CN, Miller K, et al. Increased survival with enzalutamide in prostate cancer after chemotherapy. N Engl J Med. 2012;367:1187–97.
5. Kantoff PW, Higano CS, Shore ND, Berger ER, Small EJ, Penson DF, et al. Sipuleucel-T immunotherapy for castration-resistant prostate cancer. N Engl J Med. 2010;363:411–22.
6. Parker C, Nilsson S, Heinrich D, Helle SI, O'Sullivan JM, Fosså SD, et al. Alpha emitter radium-223 and survival in metastatic prostate cancer. N Engl J Med. 2013;369:213–23.
7. Culp MB, Soerjomataram I, Efstathiou JA, Bray F, Jemal A. Recent global patterns in prostate cancer incidence and mortality rates. Eur Urol. 2020;77:38–52.
8. Lawal IO, Bruchertseifer F, Vorster M, Morgenstern A, Sathekge MM. Prostate-specific membrane antigen-targeted endoradiotherapy in metastatic prostate cancer. Curr Opin Urol. 2020;30:98–105.
9. Fendler WP, Rahbar K, Hermann K, Kratochwil C, Eiber M. ^{177}Lu-PSMA radioligand therapy for prostate cancer. J Nucl Med. 2017;58:1196–200.
10. Ahmadzadehfar H, Aryana K, Pirayesh E, Farzanehfar S, Assadi M, Fallahi B, et al. The Iranian Society of Nuclear Medicine practical guideline on radioligand therapy in metastatic castration-resistant prostate cancer using ^{177}Lu-PSMA. Iran J Nucl Med. 2018;26:2–8.
11. Kratochwil C, Fendler WP, Eiber M, Baum R, Bozkurt MF, Czernin J, et al. EANM procedure guidelines for radionuclide therapy with ^{177}Lu-labelled PSMA-ligands (^{177}Lu-PSMA-RLT). Eur J Nucl Med Mol Imaging. 2019;46:2536–44.
12. Vorster M, Warwick J, Lawal IO, du Toit P, Vangu M, Nyakale NE, et al. South African guidelines for receptor radioligand therapy (RLT) with Lu-177-PSMA in prostate cancer. S Afr J Surg. 2019;57:45–51.
13. Rahbar K, Ahmadzadehfar H, Kratochwil C, Haberkorn U, Schäfers M, Essler M, et al. German multicenter study investigating ^{177}Lu-PSMA-617 radioligand therapy in advanced prostate cancer patients. J Nucl Med. 2017;58:85–9.
14. Fanti S, Minozzi S, Antoch G, Banks I, Briganti A, Carrio I, et al. Consensus on molecular imaging and theranostics in prostate cancer. Lancet Oncol. 2018;19:e696–708.
15. Barber TW, Singh A, Kulkarni HR, Niepsch K, Bilah B, Baum RP. Clinical outcomes of ^{177}Lu-PSMA radio-

ligand therapy in earlier and later phases of metastatic castration-resistant prostate cancer grouped by previous taxane chemotherapy. J Nucl Med. 2019;60:955–62.

16. Zhang J, Kulkarni HR, Singh A, Schuchardt C, Niepsch K, Langbein T, et al. ^{177}Lu-PSMA-617 radioligand therapy in metastatic castration-resistant prostate cancer patients with a single functioning kidney. J Nucl Med. 2019;60:1579–86.

17. von Eyben FE, Singh A, Zhang J, Nipsch K, Meyrick D, Lenzo N, et al. ^{177}Lu-PSMA radioligand of predominant lymph node metastatic prostate cancer. Oncotarget. 2019;10:2451–61.

18. Yordanova A, Linden P, Hauser S, Meisenheimer M, Kürpig S, Feldmann G, et al. Outcome and safety of rechallenge [177Lu]Lu-PSMA-617 in patients with metastatic prostate cancer. Eur J Nucl Med Imaging. 2019;46:1073–80.

19. Hofman MS, Violet J, Hicks RJ, Ferdinandus J, Thang SP, Akhurst T, et al. [177Lu]-PSMA-617 radionuclide treatment in patients with metastatic castration-resistant prostate cancer (LuPSMA trial): a single-Centre, single-arm, phase 2 study. Lancet Oncol. 2018;19:825–33.

20. Yadav MP, Ballal S, Dwivedi SN, Bal C. Radioligand therapy with ^{177}Lu-PSMA for metastatic castration-resistant prostate cancer: a systematic review and meta-analysis. AJR. 2019;213:1–11.

21. Lawal I, Vorster M, Boshomane T, Ololade K, Ebenhan T, Sathekge M. Metastatic prostate carcinoma presenting as a superscan on ^{68}Ga-PSMA PET/CT. Clin Nucl Med. 2015;40:755–6.

22. Kratochwil C, Haberkorn U, Giesel FL. [225]Ac-PSMA-617 for therapy of prostate cancer. Semin Nucl Med. 2020;50:133–40.

23. Hindié E, Zanotti-Fregonara P, Quinto MA, Morgat C, Champion C. Dose deposits from ^{90}Y, ^{177}Lu, ^{111}In, and [161]Tb in micrometastases of various sizes: implications for radiopharmaceutical therapy. J Nucl Med. 2016;57:759–64.

24. Morgenstern A, Apostolidis C, Kratochwil C, Sathekge M, Krolicki L, Bruchertseifer F. An overview of targeted alpha therapy with [225]Actinium and [213]Bismuth. Curr Radiopharm. 2018;11:200–8.

25. Sgouros G. Dosimetry, radiobiology and synthetic lethality: radiopharmaceutical therapy (RPT) with alpha-particle-emitters. Semin Nucl Med. 2020;50:124–32.

26. Azorín-Vega E, Rojas-Calderón E, Ferro-Flores G, Aranda-Lara L, Jiménez-Mancilla N, Nava-Cabrera MA. Assessment of the radiation absorbed dose produced by ^{177}Lu-iPSMA, [225]Ac-iPSMA and [223]RaCl$_2$ to prostate cancer cell nuclei in a bone microenvironment model. Appl Radiat Isot. 2019;146:66–71.

27. Liu H, Rajasekaran AK, Moy P, Xia Y, Kim S, Navarro V, et al. Constitutive and antibody-induced internalization of prostate-specific membrane antigen. Cancer Res. 1998;58:4055–60.

28. Kratochwil C, Bruchertseifer F, Giesel FL, Weis M, Verburg FA, Mottaghy F, et al. [225]Ac-PSMA-617 for PSMA-targeted α-radiation therapy of metastatic castration-resistant prostate cancer. J Nucl Med. 2016;57:1941–4.

29. Kratochwil C, Bruchertseifer F, Rathke H, Bronzel M, Apostolidis C, Weichert W, et al. Targeted α-radiation therapy of metastatic castration-resistant prostate cancer with [225]Ac-PSMA-617: dosimetry estimate and empirical dose finding. J Nucl Med. 2017;58:1624–31.

30. Kratochwil C, Giesel FL, Stefanova M, Benešová M, Bronzel M, Afshar-Oromieh A, et al. PSMA-targeted radionuclide therapy of metastatic castration-resistant prostate cancer with ^{177}Lu-labeled PSMA-617. J Nucl Med. 2016;57:1170–6.

31. Kratochwil C, Bruchertseifer F, Rathke H, Hohenfellner M, Giesel FL, Haberkorn U, et al. Targeted α-radiation therapy of metastatic castration-resistant prostate cancer with [225]Ac-PSMA-617: swimmer-plot analysis suggests efficacy regarding duration of tumor control. J Nucl Med. 2018;59:759–802.

32. Sathekge M, Bruchertseifer F, Vorster M, Lawal IO, Knoesen O, Mahapane J, et al. Predictors of overall and disease-free survival in metastatic castration-resistant prostate cancer patients receiving [225]Ac-PSMA-617 radioligand therapy. J Nucl Med. 2020;61:62–9.

33. Kratochwil C, Giesel FL, Heussel CP, Kazdal D, Endris V, NNientiedt C, et al. Patients resistant against PSMA-targeting alpha-radiation therapy often harbor mutations in DNA-repair associated genes. J Nucl Med. 2019;10:683.

34. Velho PI, Qazi F, Hassan S, Carducci MA, Denmeade SR, Markowski MC, et al. Efficacy of Radium-223 in bone-metastatic castration-resistant prostate cancer with and without homologous repair gene defects. Eur Urol. 2019;76:170–6.

35. Falck J, Mailand N, Syljuåsen RG, Bartek J, Lukas J. The ATM-Chk2-Cdc25A checkpoint guards against radioresistant DNA synthesis. Nature. 2001;410:842–7.

36. Paschalis A, Sheehan B, Riisnaes R, Rodrigues DN, Gurel B, Bertan C, et al. Prostate-specific membrane antigen heterogeneity and DNA repair defects in prostate cancer. Eur Urol. 2019;76:469–78.

37. Hofman MS, Emmett L. Tumour heterogeneity and resistance to therapy in prostate cancer: a fundamental limitation to prostate-specific membrane antigen theranostics or a key strength. Eur Urol. 2019;76:479–81.

38. Emmet L, Crumbaker M, Ho B, Willowson K, Eu P, Ratnayake L, et al. Results of a prospective phase 2 pilot trial of ^{177}Lu-PSMA-617 therapy for metastatic castration-resistant prostate cancer including imaging predictors of treatment response and pattern of progression. Clin Genitourin Cancer. 2019;17:15–22.

39. Thang SP, Violet J, Sandhu S, Iravani A, Akhurst T, Kong G, et al. Poor outcome for patients with metastatic castration-resistant prostate cancer with low prostate-specific membrane antigen (PSMA) expression deemed ineligible for ^{177}Lu-labelled PSMA radioligand therapy. Eur Urol Oncol. 2019;2:670–6.

40. Kilnoshita Y, Kuratsukuri K, Landas S, Imaida K, Rovito PM Jr, Haas GP. Expression of prostate-specific membrane antigen in normal and malignant human tissues. World J Surg. 2006;30:628–36.

41. Rupp NJ, Umbricht CA, Pizzuto DA, Lenggenhager D, Töpfer A, Müller J, et al. First clinicopathologic evidence of a non-PSMA-related uptake mechanism for ^{68}Ga-PSMA-11 in salivary glands. J Nucl Med. 2019;60:1270–6.

42. Langbein T, Chaussé G, Baum RP. Salivary gland toxicity of PSMA radioligand therapy: relevance and preventive strategies. J Nucl Med. 2018;59:1172–3.

43. van Kalmthout LWM, Lam MGEH, de Kaizer B, Krijger GC, Ververs TFT, de Roos R, et al. Impact of external cooling with icepacks on ^{68}Ga-PSMA uptake in salivary glands. EJNMMI Res. 2018;8:56.

44. Yilmaz B, Nisli S, Ergul N, Gursu RU, Acikgoz OA, Çermik TF. Effect of external colling on Lu-177 PSMA uptake for parotid glands. J Nucl Med. 2019;60:1388.

45. Baum RP, Langbein T, Singh A, Shahinfar M, Schuchardt C, Volk GF, et al. Injection of botulinum toxin for preventing salivary gland toxicity after PSMA radioligand therapy: an empirical proof of a promising concept. Nucl Med Mol Imaging. 2018;52:80–1.

46. Rathke H, Kratochwil C, Hohenberger R, Giesel FL, Bruchertseifer F, Flechsig P, et al. Initial clinical experience performing sialendoscopy for salivary gland protection in patients undergoing [225]Ac-PSMA-617 RLT. Eur J Nucl Med Mol Imaging. 2019;46:139–47.

47. Halwani AS, Rasmussen KM, Patil V, Li CC, Yong CM, Burningham Z, et al. Real-world practice patterns in veterans with metastatic castration-resistant prostate cancer. Urol Oncol. 2020;38:1.e1–1.e10.

48. Abdel-Rahman O. Efficacy and toxicity outcomes of elderly castrate-resistant prostate cancer patients treated with docetaxel—a pooled analysis of 3 randomized studies. Urol Oncol. 2020;38(4):210–5.

49. Caffo O, Wissing M, Bianchini D, Bergman A, Thomsen FB, Schmid S, et al. Survival outcomes from a cumulative analysis of worldwide observational studies on sequential use of new agents in metastatic castration-resistant prostate cancer. Clin Genitourin Cancer. 2020;18:69–76.

50. Maines F, Caffo O, Veccia A, Trentin C, Tortora G, Galligioni E, et al. Sequencing new agents after docetaxel in patients with metastatic castration-resistant prostate cancer. Crit Rev Oncol Hematol. 2015;96:498–506.

51. Sathekge M, Bruchertseifer F, Knoesen O, Reyneke F, Lawal I, Lengana T, et al. [225]Ac-PSMA-617 in chemotherapy-naïve patients with advanced prostate cancer: a pilot study. Eur J Nucl Med Mol Imaging. 2019;46:129–38.

52. Sathekge MM, Bruchertseifer F, Lawal IO, Vorster M, Knoesen O, Lengana T, et al. Treatment of brain metastases of castration-resistant prostate cancer with [225]Ac-PSMA-617. Eur J Nucl Med Mol Imaging. 2019;46:1756–7.

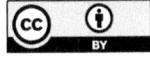

Sola Dosis Facit Venenum: Dosimetry for Molecular Radiotherapy in Bad Berka

Christiane Schuchardt

27.1 Introduction

The story of dosimetry for molecular radiotherapy at the Zentralklinik Bad Berka starts in 2004. At the department of nuclear medicine, Professor Dr. R. P. Baum already performed peptide receptor radionuclide therapy (PRRT) using Y-90 labeled DOTATATE since 1999. In August 2004, the first PRRT using Lu-177 DOTATATE was performed. It was the very first Lu-177 therapy and also the very first dosimetric study.

This first patient was a 41-year old woman, which presented with a sphenoidal meningioma that affected the right optical nerve. The initial diagnosis was in December 2003; after surgery, the MRI still detected residual tumor and she had increasing right-sided defect of field of view. Due to the progressive visual field defect on the right side, the ophthalmologist gave a prognosis of rapidly progressive blindness of the right eye within the next few months. The patient reported increasing visual disturbances and feeling of pressure behind the right eye as well as intermittent headaches.

Before therapy, in order to confirm the SSTR expression of the meningioma, at this time a Tc-99 m EDDA Hynic Toc scintigraphy as well as SPECT was performed. In addition, Ga-68 DOTA-NOC PET/CT was acquired. All imaging studies proved the high SSTR expression of the meningioma (Fig. 27.1).

Because of the high SSTR expression, the patient received 5300 MBq of Lu-177 DOTATATE. After the administration, serial planar whole body scans were performed to measure the time-dependent biodistribution of the radiopharmaceutical (Fig. 27.2).

Based on these uptakes, mean absorbed organ and tumor doses were estimated for the first time. The whole body dose was 0.05 Gy/GBq, the renal mean absorbed dose was about 1 Gy/GBq, and the dose to the meningioma was approximately 7 Gy/GBq or 35 Gy. In addition, the effective half-life of the compound in organs and tumor was also calculated, the longest half-life of 78 h was found in the kidneys and a shorter half-life of 38 h for the tumor.

Three months after this first cycle, the patient was treated again. Since then, just restaging was done and until now the patient is doing fine, she is free of any complaints and her visual field has improved over time.

This success story was the starting shot for dosimetry in molecular radiotherapy in Bad Berka.

C. Schuchardt (✉)
Department for Nuclear Medicine, Zentralklinik Bad Berka GmbH, Bad Berka, Germany
e-mail: christiane.schuchardt@zentralklinik.de

V. Prasad (ed.), *Beyond Becquerel and Biology to Precision Radiomolecular Oncology: Festschrift in Honor of Richard P. Baum*, https://doi.org/10.1007/978-3-031-33533-4_27

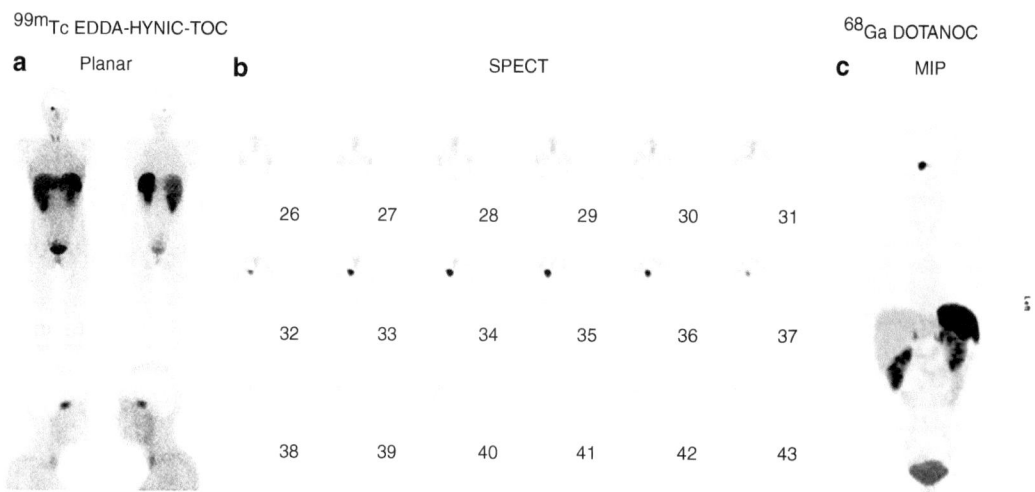

Fig. 27.1 First Lu-177 PRRT patient in Bad Berka before therapy: (**a**) Tc-99 m EDDA Hynic Toc scintigraphy; (**b**) SPECT; (**c**) Ga-68 DOTANOC MIP

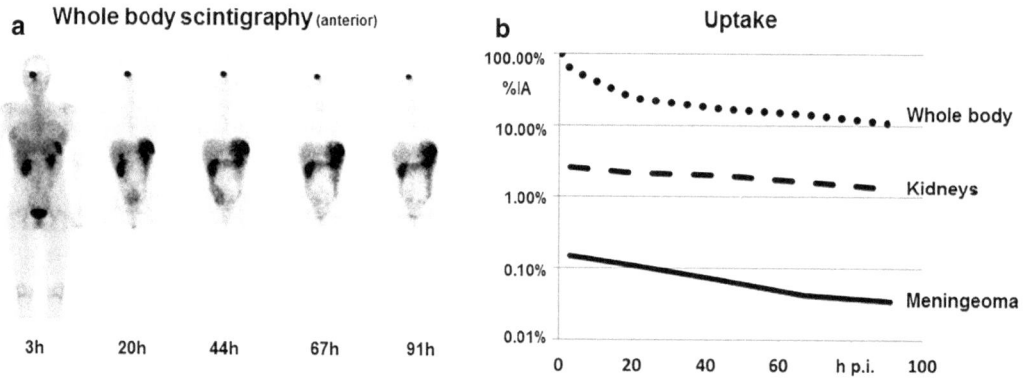

Fig. 27.2 First Lu-177 PRRT patient in Bad Berka: (**a**) first PRRT anterior whole-body scintigraphy; (**b**) corresponding time-activity curves

27.2   Bad Berka Dose Protocol

Dosimetry in Bad Berka was always carried out using an in-house developed dose protocol, the so-called Bad Berka dose protocol (BBDP), which is constantly being further improved.

The BBDP is a so-called hybrid method combining planar and SPECT imaging for dose estimation. The dose estimation requires an accurate determination of the time-dependent activity curve of the organs and tumors to be analyzed. Thus, most important is the correct evaluation of the distribution and the kinetics of the administered radiopharmaceutical [1, 2]. We developed a

practically convenient procedure by adapting the calculation model to our particular conditions. The main objective was to create a method which is practicable in daily clinical routine and to make dosimetry available for all patients. The dosimetric approach is based on the MIRD scheme, and mean absorbed doses are estimated using the OLINDA 2.0 software [3–6]. The workflow of the BBDP is shown in Fig. 27.3.

At least five serial planar whole-body scintigraphies and one regional SPECT/CT were acquired per patient. For planar whole-body (WB) imaging, the following gamma camera settings were implemented: MEDISO spirit DH-V

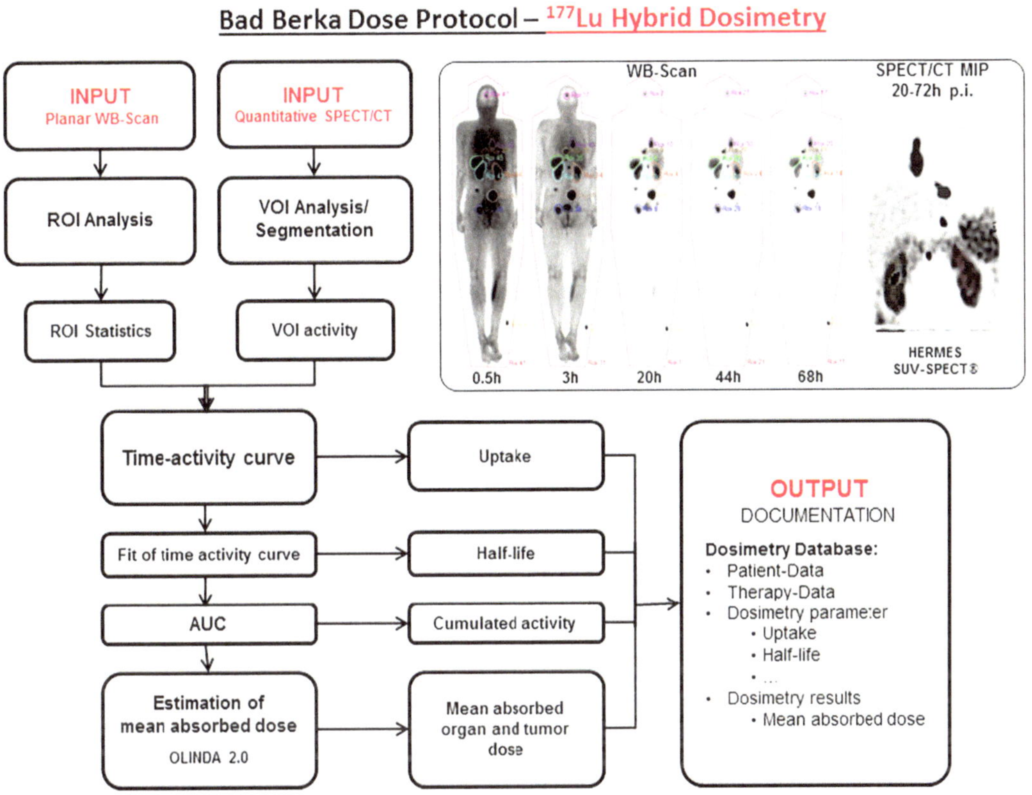

Bad Berka Dose Protocol – ^{177}Lu Hybrid Dosimetry

Fig. 27.3 Workflow Bad Berka Dose Protocol

dual-headed gamma camera (Medical Imaging Systems, Budapest, Hungary), MEGP collimator, 15% energy window, peak at 208 keV, scan speed 15 cm/min. WB scintigraphies were acquired at following time points post injection (p.i.): from 0.5 h p.i. (immediately after administration of therapeutic activity and before bladder voiding) up to 68 h p.i.. Additionally, post-therapy imaging using SPECT/CT of kidneys and/or tumor-involving regions of the body was performed at 24, 48, or 72 h p.i. using a Siemens Symbia T camera system (Siemens Healthcare GmbH, Erlangen, Germany) and the following settings: MELP collimator, peak at 113 keV and 208 keV (15% energy windows and 20% upper and lower scatter window), 128×128 matrix, 32 projections with 30 s per step, body contour.

Since the patients were not allowed to empty the bladder before the first scan, the total body counts acquired immediately after the injection were defined to be 100% of the administered activity. Total body counts on the subsequent scans were expressed as fractions of injected activity (%IA). Regions of interest (ROI) were drawn manually over the source regions over the acquired scintigraphy images, which were then analyzed using the software of the HERMES system (Hermes Medical Solutions, Stockholm, Sweden). Source regions were defined as organs and metastases showing significant specific uptake, which could be clearly delineated on each post-therapy scan. ROIs were always drawn by a physicist in collaboration with a nuclear medicine physician, who selected the suitable lesions for dosimetry (i.e., lesions with the highest uptake in the respective organ). The biodistribution and kinetics of whole body and source organs were determined based on this ROI analysis. The SPECT/CT scans were reconstructed and quantified using the HERMES SUV SPECT software (HERMES Medical Solutions, Stockholm, Sweden). After segmentation, the SPECT activity of source regions was used to scale the time-activity curves obtained from planar imaging. In the next step, these time-activity curves were fitted to mono- or bi-exponential functions in order to calculate effective half-lives and the time-integrated activity coefficient. Mean absorbed organ and tumor doses were finally estimated using OLINDA 2.0. The ICRP 89 adult model and the spheres model were used for normal organs and tumor lesions, respectively (both included in OLINDA 2.0). Volumes of normal organs and tumor lesions were obtained by the latest CT of the patient in order to adopt the model to individual organ and tumor volumes. Organs showing tumor involvement were excluded from dosimetric evaluation.

27.3 Dosimetry in Daily Clinical Routine

The BBDP is a hybrid method which is used in daily clinical routine, with some advantages but also disadvantages. Planar dosimetry represents whole body dosimetry including all organs and metastases, but it is limited by organ superimposition and inaccurate attenuation and scatter correction. Hybrid dosimetry on the other side is using 3D imaging with improved accuracy, but the segmentation is challenging and depending on the number of SPECT/CTs or the field of view, hybrid dosimetry cannot characterize whole body biodistribution. Thus, there are some limitations of the dose estimation:

- Physical/technical:
  - Number of time points.
  - Availability of late scan.
  - Quantification and volumetric analysis.
  - Dose estimation based on models (OLINDA).
- Medical:
  - Patient's condition.
- Time effort for:
  - Patient.
  - Technologist.
  - Physician.
  - Physicist.

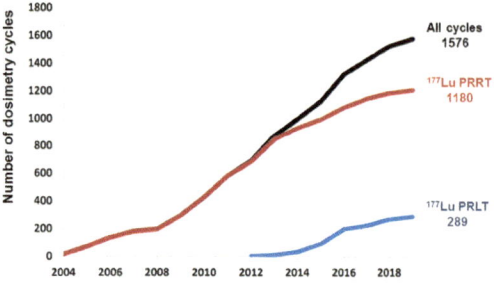

Fig. 27.4 Number of dosimetry cycles performed in Bad Berka for PRRT and PRLT

Consequently, dosimetry is still a dose estimation, an approximation of the mean absorbed dose. The challenge for the clinical use is to find an optimal practical method to enable individual dosimetry for each patient and each therapy cycle (e.g., in comparison to external radiation therapy). The solution is a compromise between the theoretical model and daily circumstances by adapting the MIRD scheme to the special conditions at the department. The BBDP represents the optimal dosimetry procedure for the clinical routine at the nuclear medicine ward of the Zentralklinik Bad Berka.

Until December 2019, dosimetry was performed using the BBDP for 1180 Lu-177 PRRT cycles, and another 289 for Lu-177 PRLT; in total, dosimetry was analyzed for more than 1500 therapy cycles. Figure 27.4 shows the number of dosimetry studies over time as well as the number of studies using different (commonly used) tracers. In the following, some particular examples for the use of dosimetry and the role of dosimetry results will be given.

27.4 Dosimetry for PRRT

Already in 2007 we published first results of dosimetry in PRRT. The comparison of Lu-177 DOTATATE and Lu-177 DOTANOC revealed a higher uptake of DOTANOC for whole body and normal tissue as well as a higher tumor uptake for DOTATATE. The resulting mean absorbed kidney and spleen doses were comparable for both ligands, and the mean absorbed tumor doses tended to be higher for DOTATATE. Based on these dosimetry results, we showed that DOTATATE has characteristics which are more favorable for PRRT of patients with neuroendocrine tumors [7].

In another large patient cohort, we compared DOTATATE, HA-DOTATATE and DOTATOC. We found the lowest renal uptake as well as the lowest renal absorbed dose for DOTATOC. These examples emphasize how dosimetry can help to evaluate the therapy and to find the optimal peptide for PRRT (Fig. 27.5).

A high interpatient variability was found for all dosimetry results. This is not unexpected since heterogeneous groups of patients, having varying receptor densities and tumor burden, were analyzed. In addition, the results showed a high intra-patient variability in the undergoing several cycles of therapy with different peptides. The dosimetry results stored in the database also give the possibility to analyze several therapy cycles of a single patient.

Figure 27.6 shows serial whole body scintigraphies of a patient which presented with a NEN of the pancreas and hepatic, lymph node as well as bone metastases. He received multiple cycles of PRRT over time; the first three cycles were

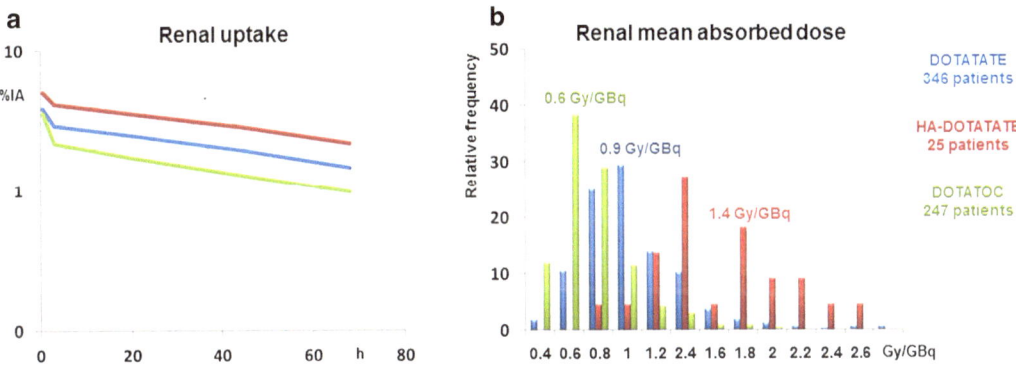

Fig. 27.5 Comparison of renal dosimetry in PRRT using different peptides: (**a**) renal uptake; (**b**) renal mean absorbed dose

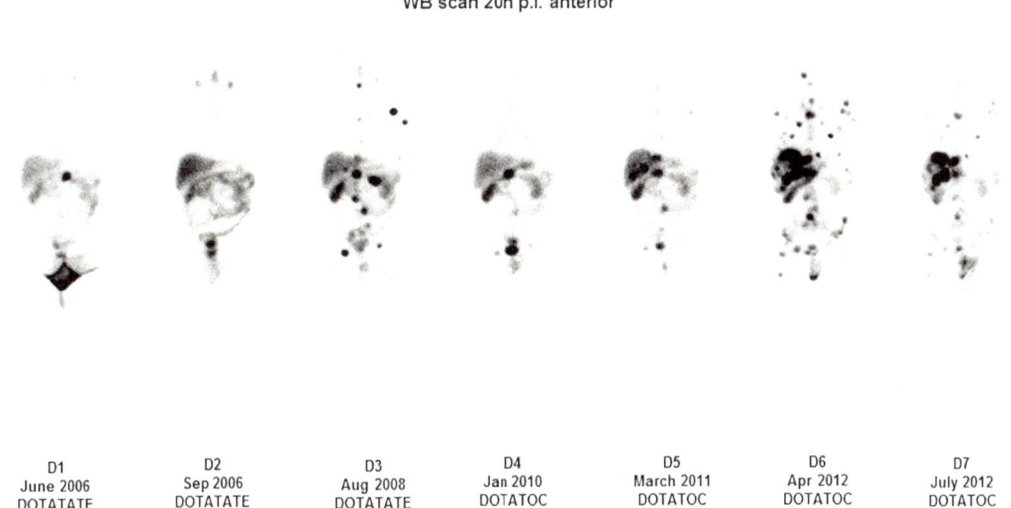

Fig. 27.6 Anterior whole body scintigraphy of serial PRRT cycles over a long period of time in the same patient

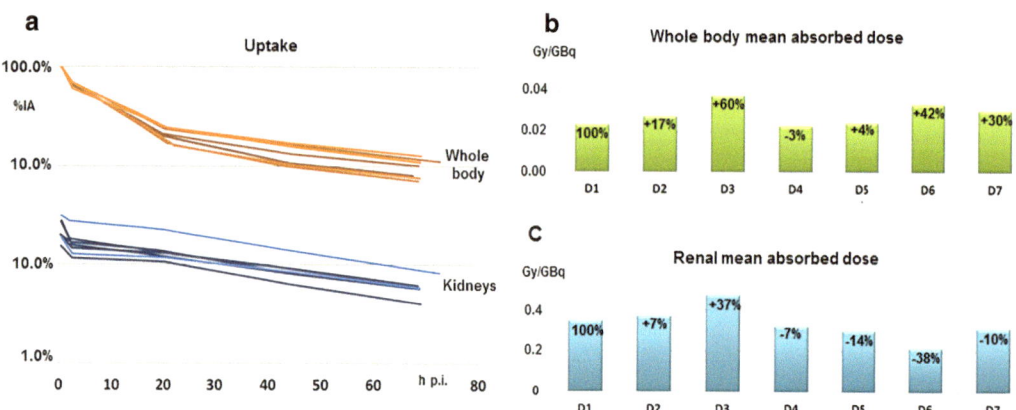

Fig. 27.7 Intra-patient variability of multiple PRRT cycles in the same patient: (**a**) whole body and renal uptake; (**b**) whole body mean absorbed dose; (**c**) renal mean absorbed dose

done using DOTATATE followed by four cycles of DOTATOC. Dosimetry results are shown in Fig. 27.7.

The whole body uptake as well as the renal uptake shows some differences between the dosimetry cycles. Also the resulting mean absorbed doses show some variation over time. If the first whole body dose is considered to be 100%, the whole body dose of consecutive therapies varies from −3 to 60%. The same is true for the renal absorbed dose. Interestingly, the renal doses were less from the fourth therapy on. This could be due to the changing tumor burden, or other therapies in between. The patient received DOTATOC in these cases, so these results could also indicate a lower renal dose when DOTATOC is used.

27.5 PRRT Antagonists

Since over two decades, somatostatin receptor (SSTR) agonists are being used for molecular imaging of SSTR-expressing tumors. Clinical studies with SSTR antagonist-based PET/CT have shown a higher tumor detection rate in SSTR expressing tumors than PET/CT applying the SSTR agonist [8–10]. Consequently, we used dosimetry in order to compare the kinetics and absorbed doses in patients undergoing peptide

receptor radionuclide therapy (PRRT) using the Lu-177 labeled antagonist DOTA-LM3.

Analyzed were biodistribution, effective half-life and mean absorbed organ and tumor doses. Very intense uptake in the tumor lesions as well as significant uptake in the kidneys, spleen and liver was observed in all patients. A rapid clearance of tracer from whole body was also found, whereas the longest effective half-life was obtained for metastases. The dosimetry of Lu-177 antagonists revealed relatively high absorbed tumor and organ doses, where the spleen had the highest absorbed dose of the analyzed normal organs. Additionally, tumor lesions were grouped in bone and liver metastases. A higher uptake, longer effective half-life and higher mean absorbed doses were found for liver metastases compared to bone metastases.

In accordance with imaging studies, we found higher tumor uptake, longer effective half-life and higher mean absorbed organ and tumor doses for the antagonist compared to the agonist DOTATOC (Fig. 27.8).

These first results showed a high accumulation of the antagonist DOTA-LM3 in metastases. Despite the also high mean absorbed organ doses, we concluded that PRRT using DOTA-LM3 appears to be promising, as significantly high tumor doses are achieved.

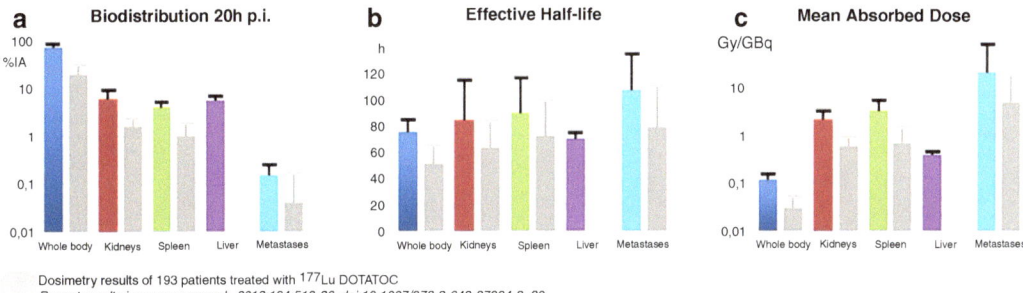

Dosimetry results of 193 patients treated with ^{177}Lu DOTATOC
Recent results in cancer research. 2013;194:519-36. doi:10.1007/978-3-642-27994-2_30

Fig. 27.8 PRRT dosimetry comparison using DOTATOC versus DOTA-LM3: (**a**) biodistribution; (**b**) effective half-life; (**c**) mean absorbed dose

27.6 Dosimetry for PSMA Radioligand Therapy

Besides dosimetry for PRRT, dosimetry for PSMA radioligand therapy (PRLT) is very valuable. The most frequently applied ligands at our center are PSMA I&T (since April 2013) and PSMA-617 [11, 12].

Of particular interest is the variation of dosimetry parameters in correlation with the serum PSA level, as shown by Fig. 27.9. In this study, 19 patients were included. The percentage differences of the tumor and renal absorbed dose during the second PRLT cycle compared to the first one were analyzed. 63% of the patients showed a decrease of absorbed tumor dose and increased renal dose at the second therapy cycle. Additionally these patients also had a lower PSA level after two PRLT cycles. These results indicate a correlation of tumor response and change in PSA level.

An inter-cycle variation in the absorbed tumor and kidney doses was found, which correlates with the change in PSA after PRLT. A decrease in serum PSA, indicative of therapy response in tumors, is therefore associated with a decrease in the absorbed tumor dose during subsequent PRLT cycle and vice versa. A decrease in tumor burden results in an increase in the absorbed renal dose in the next therapy cycle. We concluded finally that the administration of a higher amount of radioactivity in the first cycle seems to be reasonable, since the tumor doses tend to decrease in the subsequent cycles due to therapy response. The results of this study show the direct influence of dosimetry on clinical decision-making and prove the importance of dosimetry in radionuclide therapy.

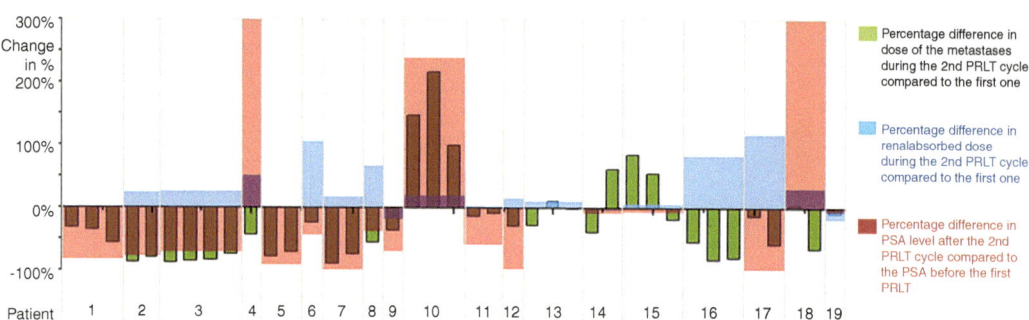

Fig. 27.9 Correlation of dosimetry results and change in PSA

27.7 Conclusions

What is the "best dosimetry?" Historically, in radionuclide therapy, a standardized amount of a radionuclide is administered, neglecting patient size, tumor burden, disease progression and intralesional heterogeneity. External beam radiotherapy on the other hand is highly individualized to maximize the dose to target whilst minimizing radiation dose delivered to normal tissues.

Treatment planning is to deliver what is believed to be the dose of radiation to target to attempt to effect local control and to limit the radiation exposure of dose-limiting organs. There might be some limits, for example, imaging modalities, patient conditions, time effort. However, the following compromise situation may succeed: Start a course with a dose based on the experience of physicians and physicists and acquire necessary data to individualize subsequent treatments – even though intraindividual differences between consecutive therapy cycles are well known.

In summary, we hope that the importance of dosimetry could be pointed out. Using protocols like the BBDP makes it practicable in daily clinical routine within acceptable time and affordable effort. Dosimetry helps to identify optimal ligands, for PRRT as well as for PSMA RLT. It helps to plan the individual treatment. Additionally, dosimetry is important for the evaluation of the therapy: concerning response, benefit and toxicity. Beside PRRT and PRLT, the BBDP can be used to do dose estimations for all

kinds of different tracer, labelled with Lu-177 or even labelled with other nuclides [13–15].

The title of this article is: "Sola Dosis Facit Venenum," which means that the dose makes the poison. Consequently, if one wants to do therapy in nuclear medicine, dosimetry is mandatory. Dosimetry adds a lot of important information to clinical and medical facts in order to find the optimal therapeutic path for each individual patient. But a nuclear medicine department also needs one important prerequisite: the physician who believes in dosimetry. This cannot be taken for granted; sometimes, it is a challenge to make the physician believe in physics, even in nuclear medicine where physics is the base of "practically everything."

Professor Dr. R. P. Baum is such a physician, he always believed in dosimetry results and supported the team all the time. He always encouraged to stay tuned, to use the latest methods to provide the important dosimetry results – always with the aim of finding the best possible therapy for the individual patient.

The author wants to thank Prof Baum for this encouragement and steady support during all the years in Bad Berka. It was an eventful time and a great collaboration between medicine and physics.

References

1. Stabin MG, Siegel JA. Physical models and dose factors for use in internal dose assessment. Health Phys. 2003;85(3):294–310.

2. Sgouros G. Dosimetry of internal emitters. J Nucl Med. 2005;46(1):18S–27S.

3. Siegel JA, Thomas SR, Stubbs JB, Stabin MG, Hays MT, Koral KF, et al. MIRD pamphlet no. 16: Techniques for quantitative radiopharmaceutical biodistribution data acquisition and analysis for use in human radiation dose estimates. J Nucl Med. 1999;40(2):37S–61S.

4. Bolch WE, Eckerman KF, Sgouros G, Thomas SR. MIRD pamphlet No. 21: a generalized schema for radiopharmaceutical dosimetry—standardization of nomenclature. J Nucl Med. 2009;50(3):477–84.

5. Stabin MG, Sparks RB, Crowe E. OLINDA/EXM: the second-generation personal computer software for internal dose assessment in nuclear medicine. J Nucl Med. 2005;46(6):1023–7.

6. Stabin MG, Siegel JA. RADAR dose estimate report: a compendium of radiopharmaceutical dose estimates based on OLINDA/EXM version 2.0. J Nucl Med. 2018;59(1):154–60.

7. Wehrmann C, Senftleben S, Zachert C, Muller D, Baum RP. Results of individual patient dosimetry in peptide receptor radionuclide therapy with 177Lu DOTA-TATE and 177Lu DOTA-NOC. Cancer Biother Radiopharm. 2007;22(3):406–16.

8. Fani M, Nicolas GP, Wild D. Somatostatin receptor antagonists for imaging and therapy. J Nucl Med. 2017;58(Suppl 2):186783.

9. Wild D, Fani M, Fischer R, Del Pozzo L, Kaul F, Krebs S, et al. Comparison of somatostatin receptor agonist and antagonist for peptide receptor radionuclide therapy: a pilot study. J Nucl Med. 2014;55(8):1248–52.

10. Bodei L, Weber WA. Somatostatin receptor imaging of neuroendocrine tumors: from agonists to antagonists. J Nucl Med. 2018;59(6):907–8.

11. Kulkarni HR, Singh A, Schuchardt C, Niepsch K, Sayeg M, Leshch Y, et al. PSMA-based Radioligand therapy for metastatic castration-resistant prostate cancer: the Bad Berka experience since 2013. J Nucl Med. 2016;57(Suppl 3):170167.

12. Baum RP, Kulkarni HR, Schuchardt C, Singh A, Wirtz M, Wiessalla S, et al. Lutetium-177 PSMA Radioligand therapy of metastatic castration-resistant prostate cancer: safety and efficacy. J Nucl Med. 2016;21(115):168443.

13. Baum RP, Prasad V, Muller D, Schuchardt C, Orlova A, Wennborg A, et al. Molecular imaging of HER2-expressing malignant tumors in breast cancer patients using synthetic 111In- or 68Ga-labeled affibody molecules. J Nucl Med. 2010;51(6):892–7.

14. Baum RP, Kluge A, Gildehaus FJ, Bronzel M, Schmidt K, Schuchardt C, et al. Systemic Endoradiotherapy with carrier-added 4-[(131)I]Iodo-L-phenylalanine: clinical proof-of-principle in refractory glioma. Nucl Med Mol Imaging. 2011;45(4):299–307.

15. Baum RP, Singh A, Schuchardt C, Kulkarni HR, Klette I, Wiessalla S, et al. (177)Lu-3BP-227 for neurotensin receptor 1-targeted therapy of metastatic pancreatic adenocarcinoma—first clinical results. J Nucl Med. 2017;12(117):193847.

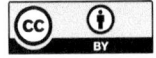

On the Use of ^{203}Pb Imaging to Inform ^{212}Pb Dosimetry for $^{203/212}$Pb Image-Guided Alpha-Particle Therapy for Cancer

28

Stephen Graves, Mengshi Li, Dongyoul Lee, and Michael K. Schultz

28.1 Introduction

Emerging evidence suggests that receptor-targeted radionuclide therapy for cancer has the potential to be transformative for cancer patient care [1–15]. Alpha-particle radionuclide therapy (α-RT), in particular, is receiving considerable attention given the potential advantages of α-RT relative to (beta) β-RT. [1, 3, 5, 6, 16] Of these advantages (relative to β-emitters), higher linear-energy transfer (LET) (100 keV/μm) and resulting increases in primary and secondary ionizations along a relatively short path length in tissue is considered a primary advantage [3, 5, 11, 12, 15, 17]. The major underlying reason for this is that high LET radiation deposition over this short path length results in an increase in double-strand DNA breaks, which is thought to improve cytotoxicity via an improved relative biological effectiveness (RBE) when compared to β-RT. [18–21, 5, 16, 18–36] Of the radionuclides under investigation for α-RT, ^{225}Ac, ^{211}At, ^{212}Pb, ^{212}Bi, and ^{213}Bi have generated considerable enthusiasm [5, 16–36]. Of these, the only available elementally identical radionuclide pair for image-guided radionuclide therapy for cancer is ^{203}Pb/^{212}Pb, where gamma-emitting radionuclide ^{203}Pb can be used for single photon emission computed tomography (SPECT) and ^{212}Pb represents a potentially ideal radionuclide for specific classes of radiopharmaceuticals for delivering alpha particles to cancer cells.

Generator-produced ^{212}Pb ($t_{1/2}$ = 10.6 h; 100% β decay to alpha emitters ^{212}Bi and ^{212}Po) is rec-

S. Graves
Department of Radiology, University of Iowa, Iowa City, IA, USA

Department of Radiation Oncology, University of Iowa, Iowa City, IA, USA

Department of Biomedical Engineering, University of Iowa, Iowa City, IA, USA
e-mail: stephen-graves@uiowa.edu

M. Li · D. Lee
Perspective Therapeutics, Inc., Coralville, IA, USA

M. K. Schultz (✉)
Department of Radiology, University of Iowa, Iowa City, IA, USA

Department of Radiation Oncology, University of Iowa, Iowa City, IA, USA

Perspective Therapeutics, Inc., Coralville, IA, USA

Department of Pediatrics, University of Iowa, Iowa City, IA, USA

Department of Chemistry, University of Iowa, Iowa City, IA, USA
e-mail: michael-schultz@uiowa.edu

V. Prasad (ed.), *Beyond Becquerel and Biology to Precision Radiomolecular Oncology: Festschrift in Honor of Richard P. Baum*, https://doi.org/10.1007/978-3-031-33533-4_28

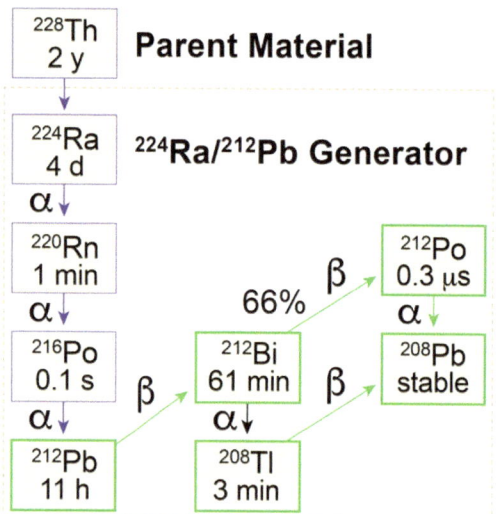

Fig. 28.1 Decay series for the production and use of ^{212}Pb for image-guided radionuclide therapy for cancer

ognized as a promising radionuclide for receptor-targeted α-RT (Fig. 28.1) [10, 33, 37–39]. However, α-decay cannot be used directly for molecular imaging. Therefore, a surrogate imaging radionuclide is required to perform complementary diagnostic imaging. The primary rationale for use of an elementally matched pair of radionuclides for this application is highlighted by recent comparisons of tumor and normal organ uptake of ^{68}Ga- and ^{90}Y-labeled small peptides in which measurable differences in pharmacokinetics were observed in in vivo biodistribution studies in mice [40]. Thus, for ^{212}Pb α-RT, the cyclotron-produced gamma(γ)-emitting radionuclide ^{203}Pb can be used as an elementally identical imaging surrogate [10, 33, 37, 38]. To wit, it can be expected that isotopes of the same element will have identical chemical and biochemical behaviors, adding confidence to predictions of ^{212}Pb α-RT outcomes using ^{203}Pb SPECT and SPECT/CT. However, in this context, uncertainties arise in these assumptions given the relationship between α-RT and imaging that must be considered in evaluation of ^{203}Pb SPECT. Stability of the ^{212}Pb-ligand complex and the potential for biological redistribution of daughter progeny gives rise to a potentially significant uncertainty in the use of ^{203}Pb SPECT

for ^{212}Pb α-RT dosimetry. Here, we discuss factors relating to the introduction of these isotopes for image-guided radionuclide therapy for cancer.

28.2 ^{203}Pb SPECT/CT Imaging in Advance of ^{212}Pb α-RT

One of the potential advantages of ^{212}Pb-based alpha-emitting radiopharmaceuticals is the potential for using quantitative imaging by single photon emission computed tomography (SPECT) and computed tomography (CT) with ^{203}Pb-based surrogates to perform patient-specific dosimetry prior to therapy. It is anticipated that this could be most beneficial early in development process of new radiopharmaceuticals, such as in the preclinical setting and in early clinical trials (e.g., where organ doses can be monitored to develop understanding of the potential for other organ toxicities). SPECT imaging utilizes parallel hole collimation or pinhole collimation to obtain two-dimensional projections of the activity distribution within a patient. From these projected images and density information from CT imaging, a quantitative three-dimensional distribution of the radioactivity can be generated. Each quantitative image describes the activity distribution at a particular point in time, so multiple imaging time points are typically required to characterize the spatiotemporal characteristics of the radiopharmaceutical following administration.

Patient-specific pharmacokinetic data obtained through quantitation can be used to develop understanding by performing retrospective calculations regarding the absorbed dose to tumors and normal tissues. Dosimetry can enable patient-specific treatment optimization by delivering the maximum possible radiation dose to tumors without exceeding normal organ dose limits, which has the potential to improve the overall safety and efficacy of radiopharmaceutical therapies [41, 42]. Without dosimetric guidance, dose to normal tissues has been reported to vary by up to a factor of 5 per administered activity [43]. Based on these findings and observations, a dosimetrically informed therapy planning paradigm may be advantageous vs a "fixed activity" treatment strategy.

In some cases, dosimetry can be performed by administering a relatively low amount of the therapeutic radiopharmaceutical prior to treatment. This has been extensively demonstrated in the setting of radioiodine treatment for thyroid cancer—and this approach is now also the standard practice prior to treatment with iodine-131 labeled metaiodoguanidine (^{131}I-MIBG) for pheochromocytoma or paraganglioma [44, 45]. In other cases, a surrogate radiopharmaceutical is used to predict the biodistribution and pharmacokinetics of the therapeutic radiopharmaceutical. Use of ^{99m}Tc-labeled macroaggregated albumin (^{99m}Tc-MAA) to predict the distribution of ^{90}Y-microspheres is a prominent example, although it is known that the biodistribution of these two radiopharmaceuticals is somewhat dissimilar [46]. In the case of fractionated delivery of radiopharmaceutical therapy (routinely performed with ^{177}Lu-DOTATATE; 7.4 GBq per fraction for a total of 29.6 GBq), dosimetry can be performed directly following each treatment via SPECT CT imaging and medical physics analysis. This retrospective dosimetry approach allows for modification of subsequent administrations to target a specific cumulative dose. In all cases, it is important to note that the dose per administered activity can vary within a given subject based on differing metabolic states at the time of administration, or due to radiation-induced changes in patient physiology over the course of treatment. These observations suggest that a pretreatment dosimetric assessment repeated prior to each therapeutic fraction may be optimal.

In the case of image-guided radionuclide therapy using ^{212}Pb, an elementally identical gamma-emitting radionuclide (i.e., ^{203}Pb) can be employed for patient dosimetry. Practical considerations for quantitative SPECT imaging with ^{203}Pb are likely to parallel methods that have been developed for SPECT/CT following therapy with ^{177}Lu-based agents [47, 48].

Specific considerations include the collimator selection, the number of SPECT projections, the camera orbit trajectory, scatter window selection, dead time correction, attenuation correction, collimator detector response modeling, number of iterative updates during the reconstruction, and partial volume correction. One notable difference compared with methods developed for ^{177}Lu is that a high-energy collimator will likely be needed for use with ^{203}Pb due to the higher energy (279 keV vs 208 keV). In addition, it is possible that the size and makeup of scintillator crystals of the SPECT system may impact the efficiency of detection due the higher energy of the ^{203}Pb emission. A representative small animal image of ^{203}Pb-DOTATOC demonstrates the potential for ^{203}Pb-based SPECT CT (Fig. 28.2).

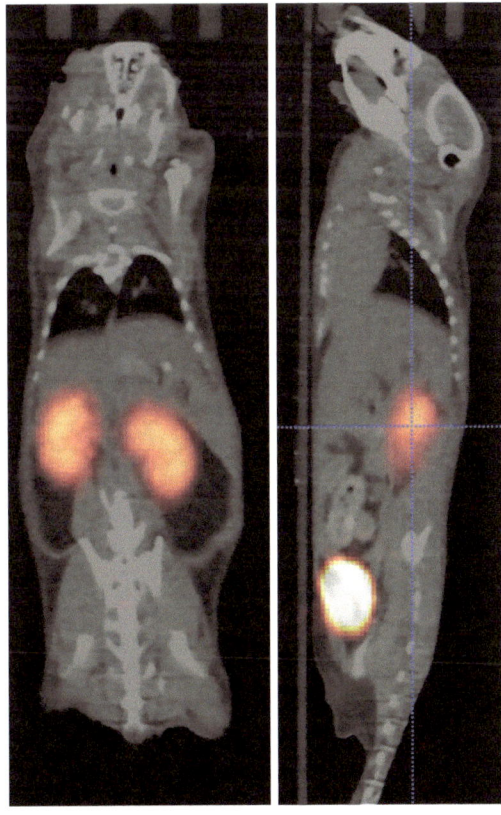

Fig. 28.2 ^{203}Pb-DOTATOC SPECT/CT in healthy ICR mice (HE pinhole collimator; Siemens Inveon)

28.3 Prediction of ^{212}Pb Dosimetry Based on ^{203}Pb Imaging

An elementally identical imaging surrogate (i.e., ^{203}Pb as a surrogate for ^{212}Pb) is potentially advantageous because the chemistry (and biochemistry) of nuclides of the same element are the same. However, potential uncertainties arise in the approach due to the subsequent nuclear transformations that generate ^{212}Pb radionuclide progeny in the ^{212}Pb decay series (Fig. 28.1). This scenario is common to other radiometals currently employed and under investigation for receptor-targeted alpha-particle therapy, including ^{225}Ac and ^{227}Th. A key distinguishing physical characteristic of these two radionuclides (i.e., difference from ^{212}Pb) is that their primary decay is directly by alpha-particle emission, while the ^{212}Pb nuclear transformation to radionuclide progeny ^{212}Bi occurs by beta-particle emission. This is important because the alpha-particle energy of the ^{225}Ac and ^{227}Th decay is undoubtedly sufficient to break the chemical bonds of the chelator-radiometal coupling of the daughter nuclei (i.e., ^{225}Ac–^{221}Fr and ^{227}Th–^{223}Ra). This phenomenon creates an immediate separation of the entire decay-series progeny from the site of the parent radionuclide (i.e., the chelator-ligand complex) that cannot be overcome. This phenomenon is potentially lessened in the case of ^{212}Pb, because the recoil energy imparted to the transforming nucleus is relatively small compared to alpha-particle-induced recoil energy [49]. Nonetheless, a critical parameter in assessing the uncertainty of modeling ^{212}Pb-based radionuclide therapy using ^{203}Pb imaging surrogates is an understanding of the potential for migration of ^{212}Pb decay series radionuclides from the site of ^{212}Pb decay. Within this context, the half-lives of ^{212}Po ($t_{1/2}$ 300 psec.) and ^{208}Tl ($t_{1/2}$ 3 min.) are sufficiently short such that understanding of the potential for ^{212}Bi to migrate from the site of ^{212}Pb decay is considered sufficient information to inform the uncertainty in using ^{203}Pb as a model for predicting ^{212}Pb alpha-particle dosimetry.

Within this context, one key parameter that remains in question is the kinetic stability of ^{212}Bi generated by the decay of ^{212}Pb within the chelator moieties employed for binding the radionuclides to the receptor-targeted ligands employed for delivering radiation to the tumor microenvironment. Extensive studies of the potential for differences in biodistribution of ^{212}Pb and ^{212}Bi (using the various chelator-ligand combinations for ^{212}Pb chelation and tumor delivery) have not been reported. The limited studies that have been reported explored the kinetic stability of ^{212}Bi generated by ^{212}Pb in the in vitro or in vivo setting. One study examined ^{203}Pb(II) and ^{206}Bi(III) chelate stability using a tetracarboxy chemical form of the chelator DOTA with no peptide ligand attached. This investigation showed that the chemical exchange of both Pb and Bi complexes with DOTA occur rather slowly in aqueous solution at physiologically relevant pH (pH 4–10). However, this study revealed that in the case of this tetra-carboxy DOTA derivative (free chelator without a peptide attached), approximately 30% of ^{212}Pb beta decays can result in the release of daughter ^{212}Bi from the chelator coupling, representing a potentially significant uncertainty that could be introduced with respect to pretreatment dosimetry that employs a ^{203}Pb-labeled agent as a surrogate for ^{212}Pb [50–52]. Further studies are required to develop a more detailed understanding of the chelator coupling with ^{212}Bi created by ^{212}Pb decay and it is anticipated that the stability of the ^{212}Pb-chelator complexes will be chelator-specific. An examination of this type for specific chelator-modified peptide conjugates will be needed to develop a more empirical understanding for individual radiopharmaceuticals.

A majority of energy released during the ^{212}Pb decay chain arises via alpha emissions of ^{212}Bi ($t_{1/2}$ 61 min) and that of the short-lived ^{212}Bi daughter, ^{212}Po ($t_{1/2}$: 0.3 μs). The radioactive half-life of ^{212}Bi may be long enough to redistribute within the body according to its own pharmacokinetics depending on the tissue type—and depending on whether the bismuth atom is released within a cell or in the extracellular environment. Reported pharmacokinetic data provides some information regarding the biological fate of radioactive bismuth ions in humans. As is the case for numerous other elements, the International Commission on Radiological Protection (ICRP) has created a pharmacokinetic model for bismuth based on human data from accidental or intentional exposures to radiobismuth [53]. This model is reproduced in Fig. 28.3 with transfer rate constants specified in Table 28.1. Most forms of bismuth (those prone to ionic dissociation) clear rapidly from the blood with significant accumulation in the kidneys and liver. With consideration given toward bismuth released within tumors, activity that is released into extracellular fluid (represented by the rapid turnover compartment in Fig. 28.3) will clear quickly ($k = 66$ d^{-1}) into the plasma, and subsequently into the liver ($k = 30$ d^{-1}) and renal structures ($k = 36$ d^{-1}). For this reason, dose to tumors may be overestimated by ^{203}Pb imaging, and dose to other normal tissues may be underestimated. The potential for new chelator technologies to be introduced that protect the integrity of the daughter-chelator coupling post-decay of ^{212}Pb has the potential to mitigate this uncertainty and more research in this area is needed.

In order to estimate the degree of systematic error from ^{203}Pb-based predictions of ^{212}Pb biodistribution, the pharmacokinetic model described by Fig. 28.3 and Table 28.1 was implemented in a MatLab script. Bismuth ions were assumed to be generated in various subcompartments (soft tissue, kidneys, liver, blood), and the fate of ions at the time of radioactive decay were tallied. Organ-specific time activity curves for the case where ions are released within the tumor extracellular compartment is shown in Fig. 28.4. Transfer of activity from the extracellular soft tissue space to the plasma occurs rapidly, followed by localization in the kidneys and liver within approximately 1 h. Integration of these time activity curves reveals that 50% of released bismuth ions would decay prior to leaving the soft tissue compartment, while the blood, liver, and kidneys receive 8%, 13%, and 15% of decays, respectively. In the case of bismuth released while the radiopharmaceutical is in the blood, only 10% of ^{212}Bi decays occur prior to clearance from the blood, while the liver, kidneys, and other soft tissues receive 17%, 19% and 37% of decays, respectively. Other combinations of "source" and "target" organs are listed in Table 28.2. Data generated from this pharmacokinetic modeling, combined with information regarding the fraction of ^{212}Bi daughters that are released from a particular chelator, allows for improved accuracy when extrapolating from ^{203}Pb imaging.

Fig. 28.3 Pharmacokinetic model of bismuth in the body, reproduced with permission from ICRP 137 [53]

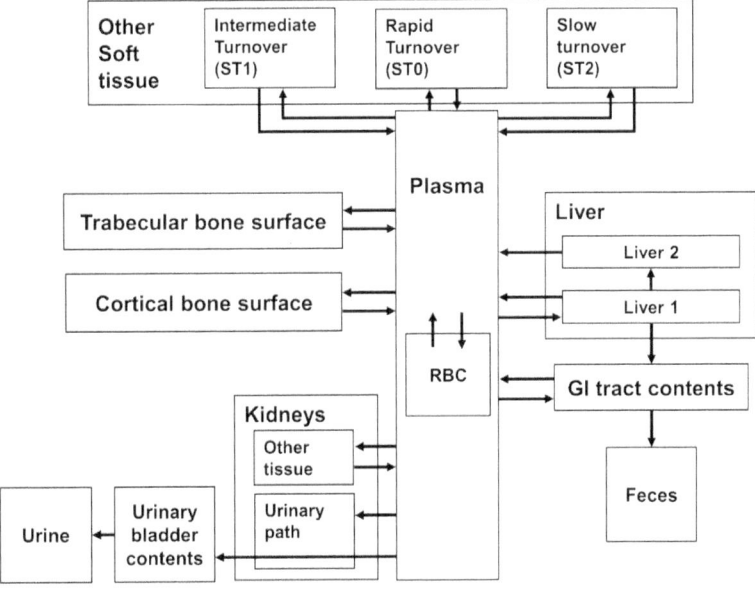

Table 28.1 Transfer coefficients for bismuth pharmacokinetic model. Reproduced with permission from ICRP 137 [53]

From	To	Transfer coefficient (d⁻¹)
Plasma	Urinary bladder contents	20
Plasma	Right colon contents	4
Plasma	RBC	0.5
Plasma	ST0	300
Plasma	ST1	4.2
Plasma	ST2	1.3
Plasma	Liver 1	30
Plasma	Urinary path (kidneys)	30
Plasma	Other kidney tissue	5
Plasma	Cortical bone surface	2.5
Plasma	Trabecular bone surface	2.5
RBC	Plasma	0.173
ST0	Plasma	66
ST1	Plasma	0.0347
ST2	Plasma	0.00116
Liver 1	Small intestine contents	0.208
Liver 1	Liver 2	0.139
Liver 2	Plasma	0.0693
Urinary path (kidneys)	Urinary bladder contents	0.693
Other kidney tissues	Plasma	0.139
Cortical bone surface	Plasma	0.0347
Trabecular bone surface	Plasma	0.0347

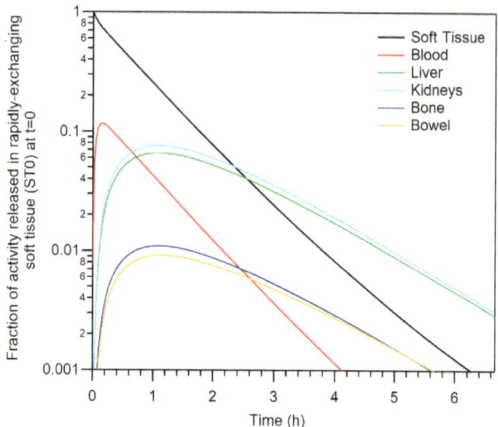

Fig. 28.4 Time-activity curves following a release of free ^{212}Bi within the extracellular soft tissue space, such as what would be observed with non-internalized tumor uptake of a radiopharmaceutical

If the fraction of bismuth ions released (f) is known, a generalized formalism can be devised to account for this redistribution effect by correcting ^{203}Pb-derived time-integrated activities:

$$\bar{A}(r_i) = (1-f)\bar{A}_{raw}(r_i) + f\sum_{r_S}\bar{A}_{raw}(r_s)\psi(r_i \leftarrow r_s)$$

In this formalism, $\bar{A}_{raw}(r_i)$ is the time-integrated activity for a given organ (r_i) without correcting for the redistribution effect, and $A(r_i)$

is the corrected time-integrated activity for that organ. The fractional transfer of time-integrated activity from a given source organ (r_s) to the organ of interest (r_i) is represented by the product of f and $\psi(r_i \leftarrow r_s)$ (Table 28.2), where $\psi(r_i \leftarrow r_s)$ describes the probability of a given bismuth ion decaying in r_i when it was released from r_s. More sophisticated microdosimetric correction factors could potentially be developed if sub-organ pharmacokinetic models were utilized in a similar fashion to what has been described here. Once $A(r_i)$ is determined for each tissue type, patient-specific dosimetry can proceed according to MIRD methods [54]. It is worth noting that within this formalism the release of activity within tumors should be treated separately from other soft tissues in the body, and that the additive correction—$\sum_{r_S}\bar{A}_{raw}(r_s)\psi(r_i \leftarrow r_s)$—should distribute time-integrated activity uniformly over all soft tissues, including tumors. Also notable is that this methodology could potentially be extended to ^{225}Ac-based radiopharmaceuticals to estimate dose due to redistribution of daughters (^{211}Fr, ^{207}At, ^{213}Bi). In this way, a more detailed understanding of the potential off-target dosimetry can be obtained that can be used for more precise image-guided radionuclide therapy treatment planning.

Table 28.2 Fraction of energy deposited in normal structures as a function of where ^{212}Bi is released. When ^{212}Bi is released in liver, kidneys, and intracellular soft tissue compartments (ST1, ST2), the biological redistribution of ^{212}Bi is negligible prior to decay. Consideration should be given to ^{212}Bi that is released in the extracellular soft-tissue compartment (ST0) as well as ^{212}Bi that is released in the blood plasma

Source compartment	Fraction of energy deposited from free ^{212}Bi						
	Blood	Soft tissue	Liver	Kidneys	Bone	Bowel	Urine
Plasma	0.096	0.372	0.168	0.191	0.028	0.025	0.120
Rapid turnover tissue (ST0)	0.077	0.497	0.134	0.153	0.023	0.020	0.096
Intermediate turnover tissue (ST1)	0.000	0.999	0.000	0.000	0.000	0.000	0.000
Slow turnover tissue (ST2)	0.000	1.000	0.000	0.000	0.000	0.000	0.000
Liver 1	0.000	0.000	0.988	0.000	0.000	0.012	0.000
Liver 2	0.000	0.002	0.996	0.001	0.000	0.000	0.000
Urinary path, kidney	0.000	0.000	0.000	0.960	0.000	0.000	0.040
Other kidney tissue	0.001	0.003	0.001	0.993	0.000	0.000	0.001
Bone	0.000	0.001	0.000	0.000	0.998	0.000	0.000

28.4   Summary and Future Directions

Alpha-emitting radiopharmaceutical therapy shows promise for improving the therapeutic efficacy of existing and future targeting ligands by limiting off-target irradiation and by preempting many cell survival mechanisms (e.g., DNA repair, hypoxia). In addition to the potency of alpha radiation, dosimetry-guided therapies have been shown to be potentially safer and more effective than RPT administration under a fixed-activity paradigm. Among the candidates of alpha-emitting radioisotopes, ^{212}Pb shows promise for use under a theranostic paradigm, whereby ^{203}Pb can be used for dosimetry and treatment planning.

In this chapter, we have presented an approach for accurately estimating the dosimetry of ^{212}Pb-based radiopharmaceuticals using ^{203}Pb as a surrogate. Moving forward, it will be necessary to establish more precisely the uncertainties arising under this paradigm and to experimentally validate the model used to predict the redistribution of ^{212}Bi following the decay of ^{212}Pb. One way to approach this problem would be to perform comparative biodistribution studies, whereby a ^{212}Pb-bearing compound is administered to a mouse that is sacrificed at specified time points postinjection. Tissue samples would be acquired promptly, and quantitative gamma spectrometry could be performed to differentiate between the location of ^{212}Pb and ^{212}Bi (unsupported vs supported) (and progeny) in the body. The gamma emission energies of ^{212}Pb (E_γ: 239 keV, 43.6%), ^{212}Bi (E_γ: 727 keV, 6.7%), ^{212}Po (E_γ: 570 keV, 2%), and ^{208}Tl (E_γ: 583 keV, 85%) are sufficiently distinct and abundant as to enable quantitative energy-peak spectroscopic measurements by sodium iodide solid scintillation detectors and by high-purity germanium detector. The challenging aspects of this experiment are (1) minimizing the time between animal sacrifice and spectroscopic measurements, and (2) appropriately modeling the decay of unsupported ^{212}Bi, and ingrowth of ^{212}Bi in tissues where ^{212}Pb is present. Careful uncertainty analysis will be required when considering the alteration of redistribution dosimetric modeling parameters.

Experiments are also needed to elucidate the toxicity of bioconjugated and free ^{212}Bi in tissues of interest, normalized to tissue mean dose. It has been shown that microdosimetric factors, such as what organ sub-structure the radioactivity resides in, can substantially alter organ-level toxicity [55]. Therefore, on a per-radiopharmaceutical basis, it may be important to consider the differential distribution of free ^{212}Bi ions and radiopharmaceutical-bound activity.

Research productivity in the field of αRPT is growing rapidly, as evidenced by the ~ten-fold increase in publications per year over the last

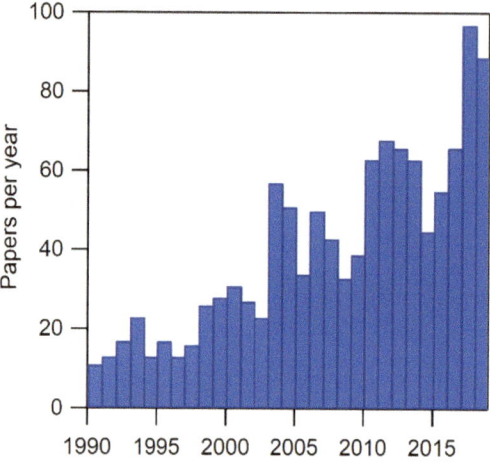

Fig. 28.5 PubMed results by year for the search terms ^{212}Pb, ^{225}Ac, ^{212}Bi, ^{213}Bi, ^{211}At, and ^{227}Th

30 years (Fig. 28.5). Human therapy studies have shown promising preliminary results, and the field of αRPT is benefiting from the development of new and innovative beta-emitting radiopharmaceutical therapies. We foresee continued growth in research productivity in this area, as well as improved patient care standards as technologies progress. Lead-212 is likely to play a key role in the progress toward personalized αRPT.

References

1. Bartlett M. From the inside out: radionuclide radiation therapy. Australas Phys Eng Sci Med. 2016;39(2):357–9. https://doi.org/10.1007/s13246-016-0455-9.
2. Hardiansyah D, Guo W, Kletting P, Mottaghy FM, Glatting G. Time-integrated activity coefficient estimation for radionuclide therapy using PET and a pharmacokinetic model: a simulation study on the effect of sampling schedule and noise. Med Phys. 2016;43(9):5145. https://doi.org/10.1118/1.4961012.
3. Iagaru AH, Mittra E, Colletti PM, Jadvar H. Bone-targeted imaging and radionuclide therapy in prostate cancer. J Nucl Med. 2016;57(Suppl 3):19S–24S. https://doi.org/10.2967/jnumed.115.170746. PubMed PMID: 27694165; PMCID: PMC5093914.
4. Jin ZH, Furukawa T, Degardin M, Sugyo A, Tsuji AB, Yamasaki T, Kawamura K, Fujibayashi Y, Zhang MR, Boturyn D, Dumy P, Saga T. alphaV-beta3 integrin-targeted radionuclide therapy with 64Cu-cyclam-RAFT-c(-RGDfK-)4. Mol Cancer Ther. 2016;15(9):2076–85. https://doi.org/10.1158/1535-7163.MCT-16-0040.
5. Kratochwil C, Giesel FL, Stefanova M, Benesova M, Bronzel M, Afshar-Oromieh A, Mier W, Eder M, Kopka K, Haberkorn U. PSMA-targeted radionuclide therapy of metastatic castration-resistant prostate cancer with 177Lu-labeled PSMA-617. J Nucl Med. 2016;57(8):1170–6. https://doi.org/10.2967/jnumed.115.171397.
6. Kwekkeboom DJ, Krenning EP. Peptide receptor radionuclide therapy in the treatment of neuroendocrine tumors. Hematol Oncol Clin North Am. 2016;30(1):179–91. https://doi.org/10.1016/j.hoc.2015.09.009.
7. Li W, Liu Z, Li C, Li N, Fang L, Chang J, Tan J. Radionuclide therapy using (1)(3)(1)I-labeled anti-epidermal growth factor receptor-targeted nanoparticles suppresses cancer cell growth caused by EGFR overexpression. J Cancer Res Clin Oncol. 2016;142(3):619–32. https://doi.org/10.1007/s00432-015-2067-2.
8. Lo Russo G, Pusceddu S, Prinzi N, Imbimbo M, Proto C, Signorelli D, Vitali M, Ganzinelli M, Maccauro M, Buzzoni R, Seregni E, de Braud F, Garassino MC. Peptide receptor radionuclide therapy: focus on bronchial neuroendocrine tumors. Tumour Biol. 2016;37:12991. https://doi.org/10.1007/s13277-016-5258-9.
9. Nonnekens J, van Kranenburg M, Beerens CE, Suker M, Doukas M, van Eijck CH, de Jong M, van Gent DC. Potentiation of peptide receptor radionuclide therapy by the PARP inhibitor olaparib. Theranostics. 2016;6(11):1821–32. https://doi.org/10.7150/thno.15311. PubMed PMID: 27570553; PMCID: PMC4997239.
10. Norain A, Dadachova E. Targeted radionuclide therapy of melanoma. Semin Nucl Med. 2016;46(3):250–9. https://doi.org/10.1053/j.semnuclmed.2015.12.005.
11. Otte A. Neuroendocrine tumors: peptide receptors radionuclide therapy (PRRT). Hell J Nucl Med. 2016;19(2):182. https://doi.org/10.1967/s0024499100378.
12. Takahashi A, Miwa K, Sasaki M, Baba S. A Monte Carlo study on (223)Ra imaging for unsealed radionuclide therapy. Med Phys. 2016;43(6):2965–74. https://doi.org/10.1118/1.4948682.
13. Weber WA, Morris MJ. Molecular imaging and targeted radionuclide therapy of prostate cancer. J Nucl Med. 2016;57(Suppl 3):3S–5S. https://doi.org/10.2967/jnumed.116.175497.
14. Werner RA, Lapa C, Ilhan H, Higuchi T, Buck AK, Lehner S, Bartenstein P, Bengel F, Schatka I, Muegge DO, Papp L, Zsoter N, Grosse-Ophoff T, Essler M, Bundschuh RA. Survival prediction in patients undergoing radionuclide therapy based on intratumoral somatostatin-receptor heterogeneity. Oncotarget. 2016;8:7039. https://doi.org/10.18632/oncotarget.12402.
15. Zukotynski K, Jadvar H, Capala J, Fahey F. Targeted radionuclide therapy: practical applications and future prospects. Biomark Cancer. 2016;8(Suppl 2):35–8.

https://doi.org/10.4137/BIC.S31804. PubMed PMID: 27226737; PMCID: PMC4874742.

16. Kratochwil C, Bruchertseifer F, Giesel FL, Weis M, Verburg FA, Mottaghy F, Kopka K, Apostolidis C, Haberkorn U, Morgenstern A. 225Ac-PSMA-617 for PSMA targeting alpha-radiation therapy of patients with metastatic castration-resistant prostate cancer. J Nucl Med. 2016. Epub 2016/07/09.;57:1941. https://doi.org/10.2967/jnumed.116.178673.

17. Wild D, Frischknecht M, Zhang H, Morgenstern A, Bruchertseifer F, Boisclair J, Provencher-Bolliger A, Reubi JC, Maecke HR. Alpha- versus beta-particle radiopeptide therapy in a human prostate cancer model (213Bi-DOTA-PESIN and 213Bi-AMBA versus 177Lu-DOTA-PESIN). Cancer Res. 2011;71(3):1009–18. https://doi.org/10.1158/0008-5472.CAN-10-1186.

18. Hobbs RF, Howell RW, Song H, Baechler S, Sgouros G. Redefining relative biological effectiveness in the context of the EQDX formalism: implications for alpha-particle emitter therapy. Radiat Res. 2014;181(1):90–8. https://doi.org/10.1667/RR13483.1. PubMed PMID: 24502376; PMCID: PMC3984880.

19. Sgouros G. Alpha-particles for targeted therapy. Adv Drug Deliv Rev. 2008;60(12):1402–6. https://doi.org/10.1016/j.addr.2008.04.007.

20. Sgouros G, Hobbs RF, Song H. Modelling and dosimetry for alpha-particle therapy. Curr Radiopharm. 2011;4(3):261–5. PubMed PMID: 22201712; PMCID: PMC4332831.

21. Sgouros G, Roeske JC, McDevitt MR, Palm S, Allen BJ, Fisher DR, Brill AB, Song H, Howell RW, Akabani G, Bolch WE, Brill AB, Fisher DR, Howell RW, Meredith RF, Sgouros G, Wessels BW, Zanzonico PB. MIRD pamphlet No. 22 (abridged): radiobiology and dosimetry of alpha-particle emitters for targeted radionuclide therapy. J Nucl Med. 2010;51(2):311–28 . Epub 2010/01/19. https://doi.org/10.2967/jnumed.108.058651.

22. Akabani G, Kennel SJ, Zalutsky MR. Microdosimetric analysis of alpha-particle-emitting targeted radiotherapeutics using histological images. J Nucl Med. 2003;44(5):792–805.

23. Behr TM, Behe M, Jungclas H, Jungclas H, Becker W, Sgouros G. Higher relative biological efficiency of alpha-particles: in vitro veritas, in vitro vanitas? Eur J Nucl Med. 2001;28(9):1435–6.

24. Behr TM, Behe M, Stabin MG, Wehrmann E, Apostolidis C, Molinet R, Strutz F, Fayyazi A, Wieland E, Gratz S, Koch L, Goldenberg DM, Becker W. High-linear energy transfer (LET) alpha versus low-LET beta emitters in radioimmunotherapy of solid tumors: therapeutic efficacy and dose-limiting toxicity of 213Bi- versus 90Y-labeled CO17-1A Fab' fragments in a human colonic cancer model. Cancer Res. 1999;59(11):2635–43.

25. Elgqvist J, Frost S, Pouget JP, Albertsson P. The potential and hurdles of targeted alpha therapy—clinical trials and beyond. Front Oncol. 2014;3:324.

https://doi.org/10.3389/fonc.2013.00324. PubMed PMID: 24459634; PMCID: PMC3890691.

26. Hauck ML, Larsen RH, Welsh PC, Zalutsky MR. Cytotoxicity of alpha-particle-emitting astatine-211-labelled antibody in tumour spheroids: no effect of hyperthermia. Br J Cancer. 1998;77(5):753–9. PubMed PMID: 9514054; PMCID: PMC2149964

27. Humm JL, Chin LM. A model of cell inactivation by alpha-particle internal emitters. Radiat Res. 1993;134(2):143–50.

28. Jurcic JG, Larson SM, Sgouros G, McDevitt MR, Finn RD, Divgi CR, Ballangrud AM, Hamacher KA, Ma D, Humm JL, Brechbiel MW, Molinet R, Scheinberg DA. Targeted alpha particle immunotherapy for myeloid leukemia. Blood. 2002;100(4):1233–9.

29. Kim YS, Brechbiel MW. An overview of targeted alpha therapy. Tumour Biol. 2012;33(3):573–90. https://doi.org/10.1007/s13277-011-0286-y.

30. Kratochwil C, Giesel FL, Bruchertseifer F, Mier W, Apostolidis C, Boll R, Murphy K, Haberkorn U, Morgenstern A. (2)(1)(3)bi-DOTATOC receptor-targeted alpha-radionuclide therapy induces remission in neuroendocrine tumours refractory to beta radiation: a first-in-human experience. Eur J Nucl Med Mol Imaging. 2014;41(11):2106–19. https://doi.org/10.1007/s00259-014-2857-9. PubMed PMID: 25070685; PMCID: PMC4525192.

31. Macklis RM, Kinsey BM, Kassis AI, Ferrara JL, Atcher RW, Hines JJ, Coleman CN, Adelstein SJ, Burakoff SJ. Radioimmunotherapy with alpha-particle-emitting immunoconjugates. Science (New York, NY). 1988;240(4855):1024–6. Epub 1988/05/20.

32. McDevitt MR, Sgouros G, Finn RD, Humm JL, Jurcic JG, Larson SM, Scheinberg DA. Radioimmunotherapy with alpha-emitting nuclides. Eur J Nucl Med. 1998;25(9):1341–51.

33. Miao Y, Hylarides M, Fisher DR, Shelton T, Moore H, Wester DW, Fritzberg AR, Winkelmann CT, Hoffman T, Quinn TP. Melanoma therapy via peptide-targeted {alpha}-radiation. Clin Cancer Res. 2005;11(15):5616–21. Epub 2005/08/03. https://doi.org/10.1158/1078-0432.ccr-05-0619.

34. Sgouros G, Song H. Cancer stem cell targeting using the alpha-particle emitter, 213Bi: mathematical modeling and feasibility analysis. Cancer Biother Radiopharm. 2008;23(1):74–81. https://doi.org/10.1089/cbr.2007.0408. PubMed PMID: 18298331; PMCID: PMC2977973.

35. Wadas TJ, Pandya DN, Solingapuram Sai KK, Mintz A. Molecular targeted alpha-particle therapy for oncologic applications. AJR Am J Roentgenol. 2014;203(2):253–60. https://doi.org/10.2214/AJR.14.12554. PubMed PMID: 25055256; PMCID: PMC4490786.

36. Zalutsky MR. Targeted alpha-particle therapy of microscopic disease: providing a further rationale for clinical investigation. J Nucl Med. 2006;47(8):1238–40.

37. Miao Y, Figueroa SD, Fisher DR, Moore HA, Testa RF, Hoffman TJ, Quinn TP. 203Pb-labeled alpha-melanocyte-stimulating hormone peptide as an imaging probe for melanoma detection. J Nucl Med. 2008;49(5):823–9. Epub 2008/04/17. https://doi.org/10.2967/jnumed.107.048553.

38. Miao Y, Quinn TP. Peptide-targeted radionuclide therapy for melanoma. Critical Rev Oncol. 2008;67(3):213–28. Epub 2008/04/05. https://doi.org/10.1016/j.critrevonc.2008.02.006.

39. Martin ME, Sue O'Dorisio M, Leverich WM, Kloepping KC, Walsh SA, Schultz MK. "click"-cyclized (68)Ga-labeled peptides for molecular imaging and therapy: synthesis and preliminary in vitro and in vivo evaluation in a melanoma model system. Recent Results Cancer Res. 2013;194:149–75. https://doi.org/10.1007/978-3-642-27994-2_9.   PubMed PMID: 22918759; PMCID: PMC3799893.

40. Fani M, Maecke HR. Radiopharmaceutical development of radiolabelled peptides. Eur J Nucl Med Mol Imaging. 2012;39(Suppl 1):S11–30. Epub 2012/03/06. https://doi.org/10.1007/s00259-011-2001-z.

41. Strigari L, Konijnenberg M, Chiesa C, Bardies M, Du Y, Gleisner KS, Lassmann M, Flux G. The evidence base for the use of internal dosimetry in the clinical practice of molecular radiotherapy. Eur J Nucl Med Mol Imaging. 2014;41(10):1976–88.

42. Garske-Román U, Sandström M, Baron KF, Lundin L, Hellman P, Welin S, Johansson S, Khan T, Lundqvist H, Eriksson B. Prospective observational study of 177 Lu-DOTA-octreotate therapy in 200 patients with advanced metastasized neuroendocrine tumours (NETs): feasibility and impact of a dosimetry-guided study protocol on outcome and toxicity. Eur J Nucl Med Mol Imaging. 2018;45(6):970–88.

43. Menda Y, Madsen MT, O'Dorisio TM, Sunderland JJ, Watkins GL, Dillon JS, Mott SL, Schultz MK, Zamba GK, Bushnell DL. 90Y-DOTATOC dosimetry–based personalized peptide receptor radionuclide therapy. J Nucl Med. 2018;59(11):1692–8.

44. Pryma DA, Chin BB, Noto RB, Dillon JS, Perkins S, Solnes L, Kostakoglu L, Serafini AN, Pampaloni MH, Jensen J. Efficacy and safety of high-specific-activity 131I-MIBG therapy in patients with advanced pheochromocytoma or paraganglioma. J Nucl Med. 2019;60(5):623–30.

45. Lassmann M, Reiners C, Luster M. Dosimetry and thyroid cancer: the individual dosage of radioiodine. Endocr Relat Cancer. 2010;17(3):R161–R72.

46. Kim SP, Cohalan C, Kopek N, Enger SA. A guide to 90Y radioembolization and its dosimetry. Phys Med. 2019;68:132–45.

47. Dewaraja YK, Frey EC, Sgouros G, Brill AB, Roberson P, Zanzonico PB, Ljungberg M. MIRD pamphlet no. 23: quantitative SPECT for patient-specific 3-dimensional dosimetry in internal radionuclide therapy. J Nucl Med. 2012;53(8):1310–25.

48. Ljungberg M, Celler A, Konijnenberg MW, Eckerman KF, Dewaraja YK, Sjögreen-Gleisner K. MIRD pamphlet no. 26: joint EANM/MIRD guidelines for quantitative 177Lu SPECT applied for dosimetry of radiopharmaceutical therapy. J Nucl Med. 2016;57(1):151–62.

49. Azure MT, Archer RD, Sastry KS, Rao DV, Howell RW. Biological effect of lead-212 localized in the nucleus of mammalian cells: role of recoil energy in the radiotoxicity of internal alpha-particle emitters. Radiat Res. 1994;140(2):276–83. Epub 1994/11/01. PubMed PMID: 7938477; PMCID: PMC3321059.

50. Gansow OA, Wu C, Goldenberg D. Advanced methods for radiolabeling monoclonal antibodies with therapeutic radionuclides. In: Cancer therapy with radiolabeled antibodies. Boca Raton, FL: CRC; 1995. p. 63–76.

51. Gansow O, Brechbiel M, Pippin C, McMurry T, Lambrecht R, Colcher D, Schlom J, Roselli M, Strand M, Huneke R. Lead and bismuth complexes of functionalized dtpa ligands and of the polyazacycloalkane-n-acetic acid dota-utility for radioimmunoimaging and radioimmunotherapy. Antib Immunoconjug Radiopharm. 1991;4(4):413–25.

52. Mirzadeh S, Kumar K, Gansow OA. The chemical fate of 212Bi-DOTA formed by β-decay of 212Pb (DOTA) 2. Radiochim Acta. 1993;60(1):1–10.

53. Paquet F, Bailey M, Leggett RW, Lipsztein J, Marsh J, Fell T, Smith T, Nosske D, Eckerman KF, Berkovski V. ICRP publication 137: occupational intakes of radionuclides: part 3. Ann ICRP. 2017;46(3–4):1–486.

54. Wessels BW, Konijnenberg MW, Dale RG, Breitz HB, Cremonesi M, Meredith RF, Green AJ, Bouchet LG, Brill AB, Bolch WE. MIRD pamphlet No. 20: the effect of model assumptions on kidney dosimetry and response—implications for radionuclide therapy. J Nucl Med. 2008;49(11):1884–99.

55. Hobbs RF, Song H, Huso DL, Sundel MH, Sgouros G. A nephron-based model of the kidneys for macro-to-micro α-particle dosimetry. Phys Med Biol. 2012;57(13):4403.

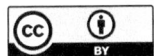

Radioiodine-Labeled Meta-Iodobenzylguanidine for Imaging and Treatment of Pheochromocytoma/ Paraganglioma and Neuroblastoma

29

Manfred Fischer and Matthias Schmidt

29.1 Introduction

The main topic of the International Symposium – Theranostics/Precision Oncology at Bad Berka/ Germany, 12–14th December 2019 was "Looking Back and Moving Forward" (Fig. 29.1).

Colleagues, already being specialists in radiology, starting specialization in nuclear medicine, were asked in 1973 (M.F.):"Why are you doing that, nuclear medicine is a dying specialty because of the development of computed tomography and high-sophisticated ultrasound?"Following the statement of the British physiologist Ernest Starling (1866-1927), "The physiology of today is the medicine of tomorrow," I was convinced that nuclear medicine would have a future as long as we would perform functional diagnostic and targeted therapeutic procedures. Manfred Fischer (MF) met Richard P. Baum in two special moments of his career. The very first time,

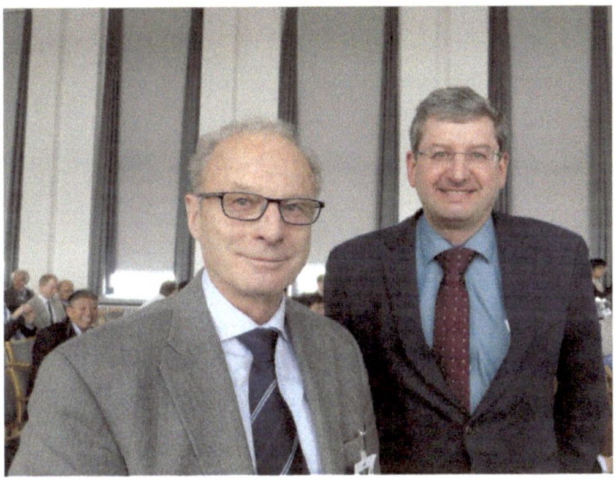

Fig 29.1 Manfred Fischer (left) and Matthias Schmidt (right) at the International Symposium on the Occasion of the 20th Anniversary of Molecular Radiotherapy at Zentralklinik Bad Berka and Inauguration of the ICPO Foundation, December 12-14, 2019 | Zentralklinik Bad Berka

M. Fischer
Institute of Radiology, Nuclear Medicine and
Radiation Therapy, Kassel, Germany

M. Schmidt (✉)
Oberarzt, Arzt für Nuklearmedizin, FEBNM,
Universität zu Köln, Medizinische Fakultät und
Uniklinik Köln, Klinik und Poliklinik für
Nuklearmedizin, Köln, Germany
e-mail: matthias.schmidt@uk-koeln.de

when Richard Baum had to pass an exam to become specialist in nuclear medicine, I was one of the two examiners. After he answered (nearly) all our questions correctly, we decided after a brief confidential discussion that he was ready to become a specialist in nuclear medicine. Some years later, he asked me if I could perform a treatment of a peritoneal carcinomatosis of an ovarian cancer in my department in Kassel/Germany, because he did not have isolation beds for radionuclide therapy in his university hospital in Frankfurt at that time. This

V. Prasad (ed.), *Beyond Becquerel and Biology to Precision Radiomolecular Oncology: Festschrift in Honor of Richard P. Baum*, https://doi.org/10.1007/978-3-031-33533-4_29

was the first treatment with the radiolabeled monoclonal antibody in ovarian cancer in Germany.

In June 2010, Matthias Schmidt (MS) had the opportunity to spend a week with Prof. Baum in Bad Berka to learn about peptide receptor radionuclide therapy which had not yet been introduced at the department of nuclear medicine, University Hospital of Cologne. It is almost impossible to describe how inspiring it was to be with Prof. Richard Baum in his department. MS had known him from excellent talks before, but how Prof. Baum talks to patients was an outstanding experience. It is a very special combination of outstanding patient care, extraordinary enthusiasm for nuclear medicine, precision oncology and deep knowledge that makes him a very special colleague. He openly allowed to spread his knowledge. In 2011, MS attended the "1st World Congress on Ga-68 and Peptide Receptor Radionuclide Therapy (PRRNT) THERANOSTICS – On the Way to Personalized Medicine" with Prof. Baum being the congress president. It was most impressive how many colleagues from continents even as far away as Australia came to the rather remote location of Bad Berka, being in close proximity to Weimar – a location that stands for outstanding cultural and intellectual achievements. This event as well as the present congress in 2019 were highly enjoyable days combining outstanding presentations with an social evening event allowing to meet very interesting people from all over the world in person (Fig. 29.2).

Another regular opportunity to meet Prof. Baum are the "Hamburger Nuclear Medicine Days," a 3-day educational program once a year with MS being the scientific coordinator since 2013. Prof. Baum holds his very special Friday morning lecture about positron emission tomography and radionuclide therapies. Every year, Prof. Richard Baum presents vividly the most up-to-date information making his lectures an outstanding experience for about 30 doctors most of them being in their advanced years of specialization. For me, these times are a pleasure to experience his energy, his profound knowledge and his visionary ideas.

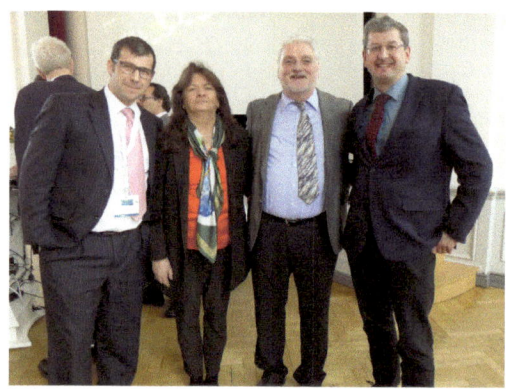

Fig 29.2 Michael Kreissl (left), Richard Baum with his wife (middle), and Matthias Schmidt (left) at the International Symposium on the Occasion of the 20th Anniversary of Molecular Radiotherapy at Zentralklinik Bad Berka and Inauguration of the ICPO Foundation, December 12-14, 2019 | Zentralklinik Bad Berka

"Molecular imaging: probes used to visualize, characterize, and measure biological processes in living systems. Both endogenous molecules and exogenous probes can be molecular agents" (SNM molecular center 2007). These probes may also be used for therapeutic procedures.

The World Health Organization (WHO) published in 2017 a new classification of tumors of endocrine organs [1]. In chap. 5, a new definition and description of tumors of the adrenal medulla and extra-adrenal paraganglia is given, including pheochromocytoma, extra-adrenal paraganglioma, neuroblastic tumors of the adrenal gland (neuroblastoma), composite pheochromocytoma, and composite paraganglioma. One characteristic clinical feature of all of them is an excessive synthesis of catecholamines.

In 1967, first time adrenal medullary hormone epinephrine and its precursors were radiolabeled with ^{14}C [2]. In the following decade, several groups studied mainly radiolabeled dopamine and its analogues. The first radioiodinated compound developed by the same group, was the bretylium analogue p-RIBA (III), showing a high affinity to the adrenal medulla [3]. Within 2 years, Donald M Wieland and coworkers developed by changing the chemical structure ^{131}ortho-iodobenzyldimethyl-2-hydroxyethyl ammonium. In tissue distribution studies with dogs, high tracer uptake was observed in the adrenal medulla [4]. Labeling meta- (or para-) iodobenzylguanidine with ^{125}I, these tracers showed a significantly higher concentration in adrenomedullary tissue with a long retention in the chromaffin storage granules. Meta-iodobenzylguanidine as a derivative of guanethidine acts as an analogue of noradrenalin and can be used for anatomico-functional imaging and treatment. It enters the sympathetic cells via the norepinephrine transporters and is stored in the intracellular secretory granules and/or cytoplasm. The authors recommended to use these tracers for scintigraphic imaging of the adrenal medulla, pheochromocytomas, and neuroblastomas [5] (Fig. 29.3) (Chem structures).

29.1.1 Pheochromocytoma/Paraganglioma

29.1.1.1 Manfred Fischer

WH Beierwaltes published an article [6] and mentioned the evaluation of the use of ^{131}I-mIBG for treating medullary hyperplasia. From diagnostic scans, his group suggested that similar to radioiodine therapy of thyroid cancer, a radiation dose to pheochromocytoma metastases of about 5000 rad/100 mCi of ^{131}I-mIBG may be reached. Using this approach, we started to treat three female patients (two of them 16 years., one of 73 years. of age) suffering from metastatic pheochromocytoma between July 1982 and May 1983, administering single dose of 2.4 upto 5 GBq (cummulative activities between 5 and 9.2 GBq) [7].

As in diagnostic scintigraphies, ^{131}I-mIBG uptake in pheochromocytomas may vary in a wide range from false negative to true positive. An overall sensitivity in diagnostic scans of 87.4% (range 78.4–94.3%) and specificity of 98.9–100% was observed in true positive pheochromocytomas [8]. This variability seems to be independent from the specific activity of the tracer. The same is evident, comparing tracer uptake versus plasma und intratumoral noradrenaline levels [9]. In a small group of other neuroendocrine tumors like medullary thyroid cancer, ganglioneuroma, neuroectodermal tumor, neurofibromatosis, oat cell carcinoma, and melanoma ($n = 36$) 25 were false negative in the ^{131}I-mIBG scintigraphy. In two patients with carcinoid and one with medullary thyroid cancer, following true positive diagnostic ^{131}I-mIBG scintigraphy, ^{131}I-mIBG therapy was performed with no change in disease in two patients and progressive disease in one patient. In 43 cases of pheochromocytoma or functional paraganglioma in children or adolescents (≤18 years) (24 m, 19 f) a positive

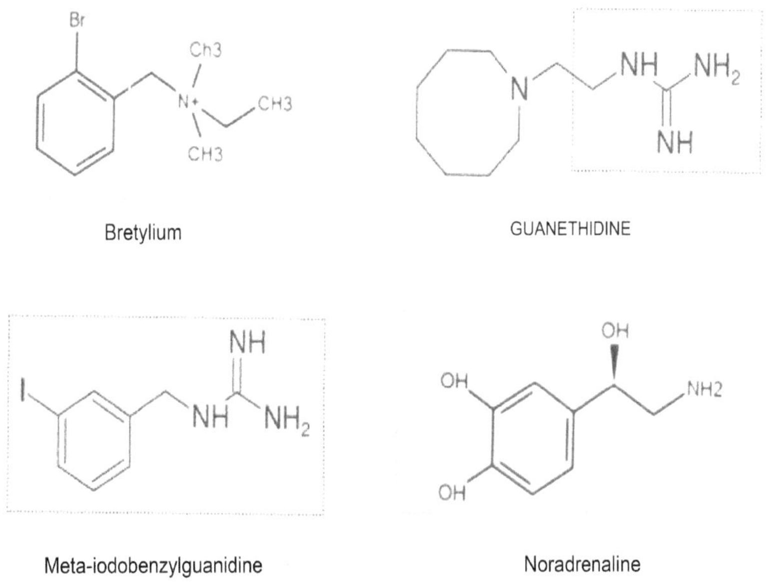

Fig. 29.3 Chemical structure of Bretylium, Guanethidine, meta-iodobenzylguanidine, and Noradrenaline

Bretylium

GUANETHIDINE

Meta-iodobenzylguanidine

Noradrenaline

[131]I-mIBG scintigraphy was observed in 36 patients (84%) whereas false negative results were observed in 12%. The false negative rate in computed tomography was higher (20%). Thirteen of 24 (54%) unifocal tumors, which were considered to be benign, proved to be multifocal and/or malignant. Only 15 tumors in this group were staged as malignant at the time of primary diagnosis. Ultimately 26 (60%) proved to have malignant tumors, confirmed by local recur-

rence or distant metastases upto 26 years after initial surgery. Therefore lifelong follow-up with effective diagnostic procedures like ^{123}I-MIBG seems to be mandatory [10].

In 1991, we summarized the results of 13 patients with malignant pheochromocytoma and one female patient with an intra-adrenal probably benign pheochromocytoma (Fig. 29.4). The first patient treated in our center got two times a sequential ^{131}I-mIBG therapy (cummulative

Fig. 29.4 ^{131}I-mIBG accumulation in an intra-adrenal pheochromocytoma

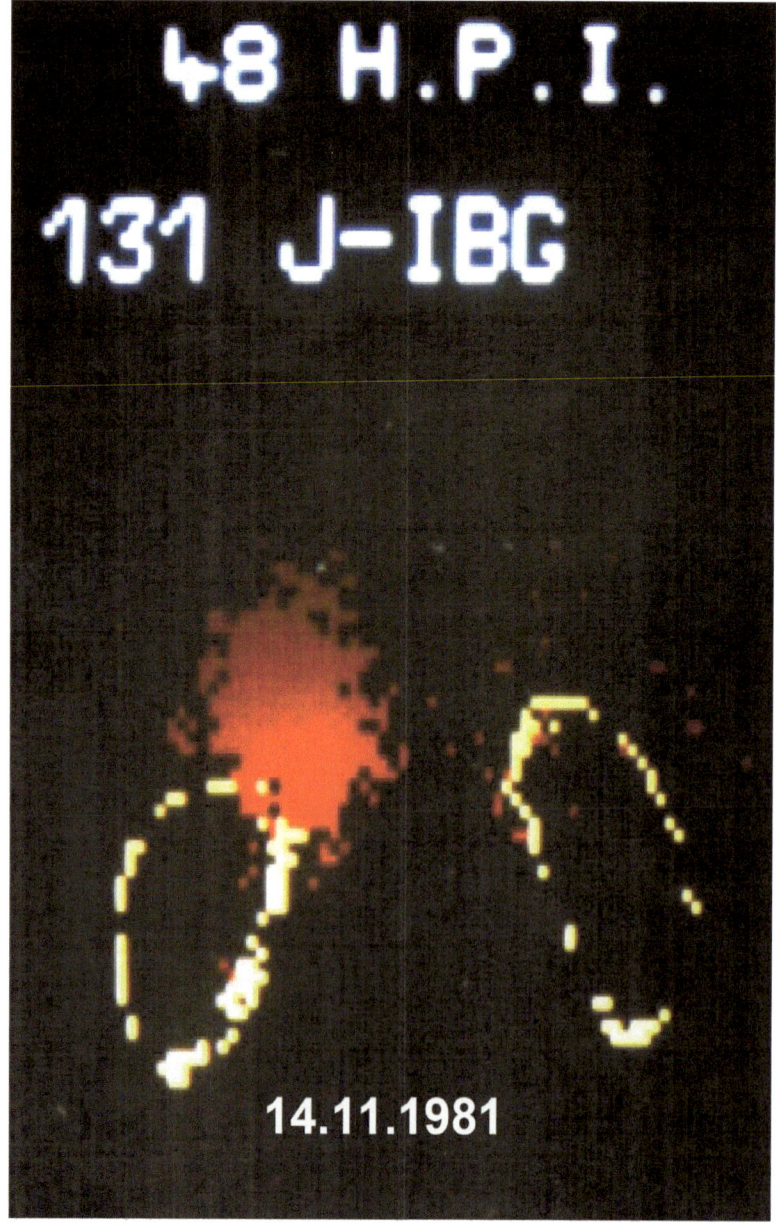

activity 50 GBq) with an ineffective chemotherapy in between. After a follow-up of about 10 years, she finally died from her progressive tumor. In a young boy (13 years at start of ^{131}I-mIBG therapy) with inoperable lymph node metastasis of a malignant pheochromocytoma, invading the liver, the tumor encapsulated totally after four courses of ^{131}I-mIBG treatment (cum.

Activity 20.4 GBq) (Fig. 29.5). Surgical complete removal of the primary tumor and lymph node metastasis was possible. This patient now is father of a boy, who was diagnosed by MRI suffering from a bilateral adrenal tumor about 30 years later. Lab tests showed elevated catecholamines. By ^{123}I-MIBG whole body scan and PET/CT (Fig. 29.6) the bilateral neuroendocrine

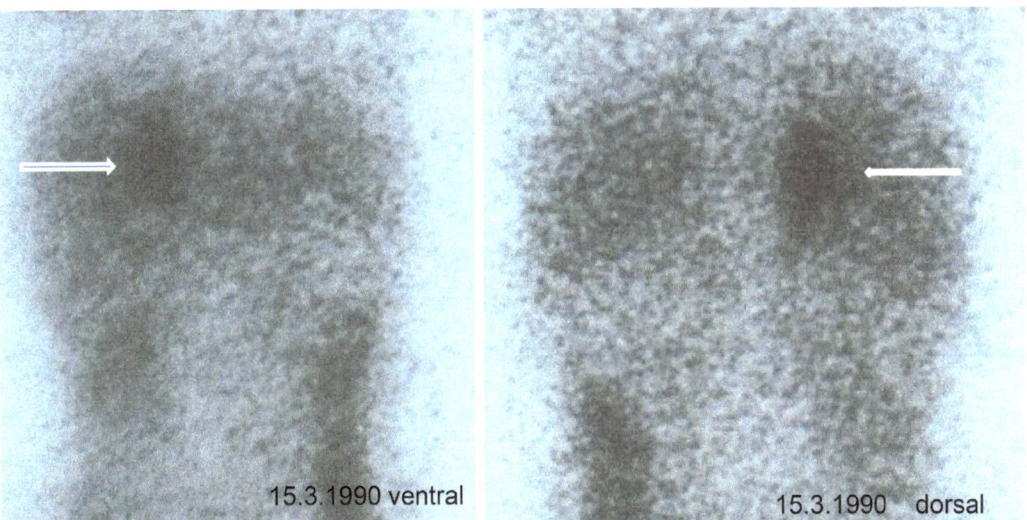

Fig. 29.5 N.D. (14yrs.), post-therpeutic scan: metastatic pheo.; lymph node metastasis infiltrating the liver. 3 cycles with a cum. activity of 18.5 GBq ^{131}I-mIBG

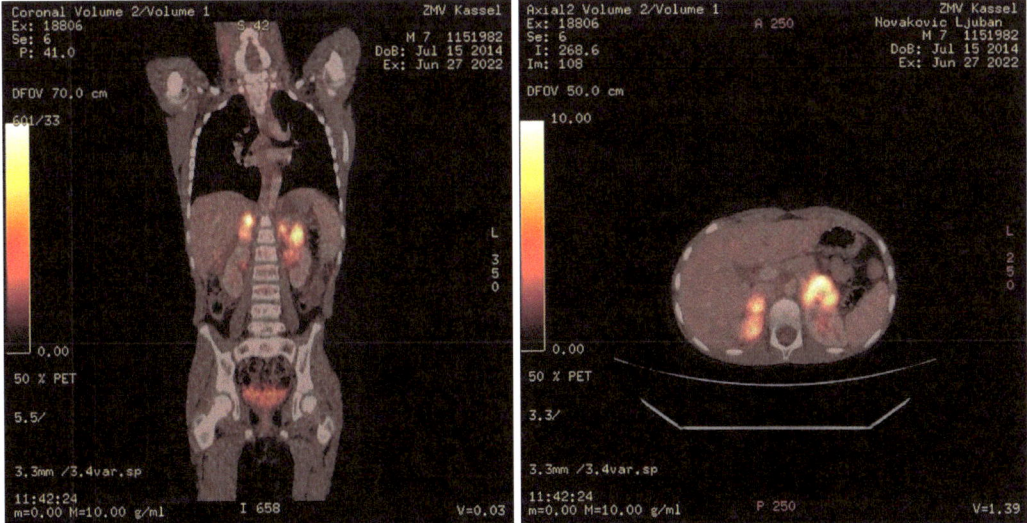

Fig. 29.6 ^{68}Ga-DOTATOC PET/CT of the 8 years old boy with a bilateral familial pheochromocytoma. The left tumor shows a lobulated structure with partly inhomogeneous intensive tracer uptake; the right gland shows an irregular structure with intensive tracer uptake. No extra-adrenal tracer uptake was shown in the pre-surgery whole-body scan (With courtesy of Dr. S. Ortega-Lawerenz)

tumor was confirmed without showing extra-adrenal tracer uptake, excluding metastatic disease. The son was transferred from Serbia to the same hospital, where we treated his father already. By surgery the tumor tissue was removed totally. During the follow-up period of nearly 2 year the patient is symptom-free. ^{131}I.MIBG therapy was not needed. One should keep in mind the "rule of 10" in this rare neuroendocrine disease with an incidence of 2–8 per million per year in the USA: in 1/10 patients the pheochromocytoma is bilateral, in 1/10 malignant, in 1/10 extra-adrenal and in 1/10 familial [11]. In this family, one can find three of them. The father suffered from a malignant, the son from a bilateral tumor and the disease is familial. The activity administered in patients we treated because of malignant disease ranged from 15 to 42.7 GBq. The mean follow-up time was 30.2 months (range 9–97 months). In one patient with malignant pheochromocytoma and a soft tissue metastasis in the mouth in one of five of the therapeutic courses the total activity was administered via an intra-arterial catheter into the arteria carotis externa. Tumor uptake and intratumoral residence time of the activity in this local metastasis was not significantly different from intravenous activity administration (Fig. 29.7). The clinical symptoms improved in all patients. Four of the patients died in the follow-up time [12].

Probably in all studies, mentioned above, low-specific-activity ^{131}I-mIBG (LSA-^{131}I-mIBG) was used for treatment of these patients. The disadvantage of this compound is a very high amount of unlabeled MIBG, competing for norepinephrine transporter binding sites and disrupting the norepinephrine-reuptake mechanism negatively. In an open, single-arm multicenter trial, 49 patients with pheochromocytoma and 19 patients with paraganglioma were treated with a very high-specific-activity ^{131}I-mIBG(HAS-^{131}I-mIBG) between 2009 and 2014. Thirty-three (49%) of all treated patients had a response regarding hypertension control with a reduction of at least 50% of hypertensive medication. Even 59 (92%) patients had an objective tumor response (partial response $n = 15$; stable disease

$n = 44$). The median overall survival (OS) was 37 months (range 31–49 months) and 5-years OS 36%. These data suggest a broad tumor effect of HAS-^{131}I-mIBG. The number of severe adverse events in the long-term follow-up was comparable with those in earlier trials using LSA-^{131}I-mIBG two secondary malignancies (1 acute myeloid and 1 acute lymphocytic leukemia). Hematologic adverse events under HSA-^{131}I-mIBG therapy were higher than under LSA-^{131}I-mIBG [13].

In some of our patients, we observed decreasing tracer uptake following repeated ^{131}I-mIBG treatment courses (Fig. 29.8). Using ^{111}In-Octreotide scintigraphy in these patients, they might show positive tracer uptake. In those patients, we went on using unlabeled Somatostatin® for further treatment to improve or stabilize clinical symptoms.

MIBG sensitivity drops down in metastatic pheochromocytomas and paragangliomas to even <50% of paragangliomas with germline mutations with succinate dehydrogenase subunits. Most of these lesions strongly express somatostatin receptors [14]. Five somatostatin receptor subtypes are known. The overexpression of these subtypes may be different in benign or malignant pheochromocytomas. The majority (about 90%) of pheochromocytomas and paragangliomas overexpress somatostatin subtype 3 and/or 2A. Subtype 2A is overexpressed mainly in extra-adrenal pheochromocytomas [15]. Comparing the detection rate per lesion of pheochromocytoma and paraganglioma by different imaging procedures, PET studies using ^{68}Ga-DOTA-SST were significantly better than other PET-tracer studies and $^{123/131}$I-MIBG scintigraphy, especially in tumors overexpressing SSTR2, whereas ^{68}Ga-DOTATOC binds more to SSTR2 and SSRT5, ^{68}Ga-DOTANOC shows a high affinity to all SSTRs except SSTR1 [16].

Since several years, radiotagged somatostatin receptor agonists are developed for diagnostic and therapeutic procedures in patients suffering from such neuroendocrine tumors [17], which express somatostatin receptors. More recently for therapy β-emitters like ^{90}Y or ^{177}Lu are used for

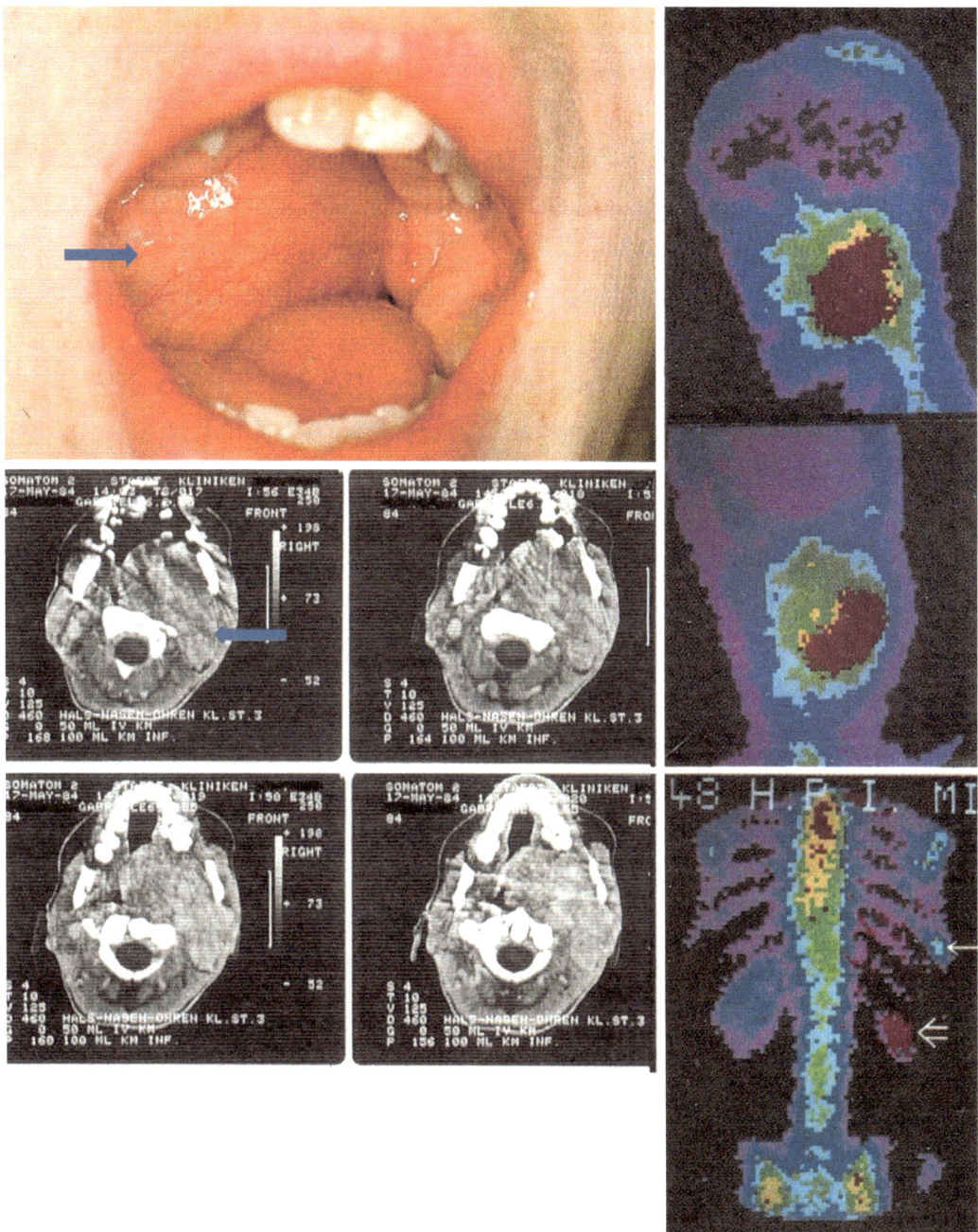

Fig. 29.7 Female pat. with malignant pheo: primary left adrenal gland, soft tissue metastasis right neck with compression in the mouth (blue arrow), bone mets

labeling either DOTATOC or DOTATATE. In a prospective observational trial in 200 patients with advanced neuroendocrine tumors, dosimetry of kidneys and bone marrow was performed to evaluate the impact on efficacy and outcome after treatment with ^{177}Lu-DOTA-octreotate. Most patients were suffering from advanced small intestine or pancreatic NET, only three from paraganglioma and one from a pheochromocytoma. Complete remission was reached in 1

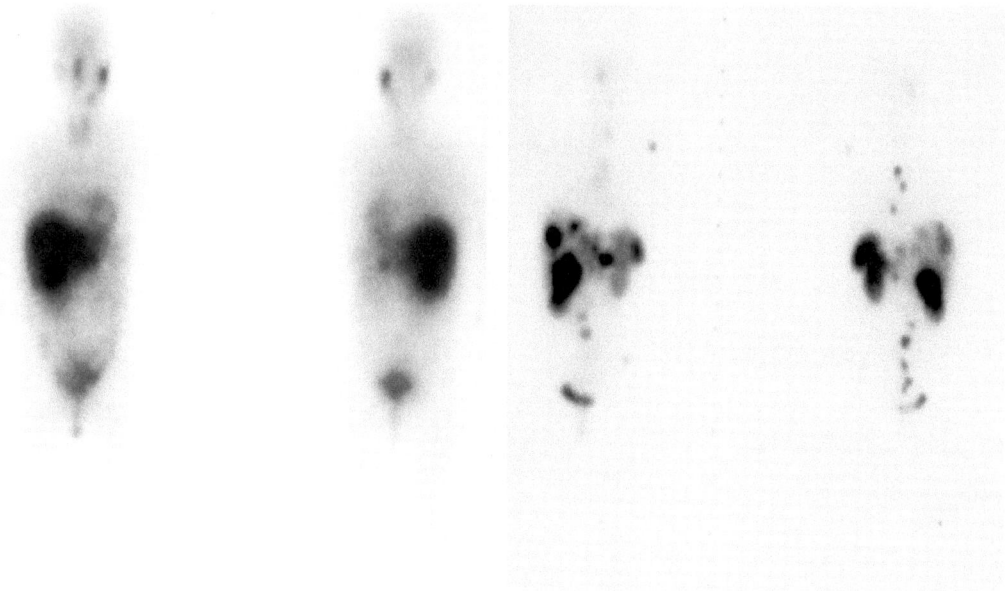

Fig 29.8 Malignant pheochromocytoma after 3 cycles with ^{131}I-mIBG with negative 123-I MIBG scintigraphy (left), but positive [111]In Octreotide scintigraphy. (right). Pat. was then treated with Sandostatin®

patient (0.5%), partial response in 47 (23.5%) and stable disease in 135 (67.5%) patients. The overall survival was 54 months in those who reached an absorbed dose in kidneys of 23 Gy in multiple treatment cycles, 25 months in those with lower absorbed doses. Toxicity was very similar to those observed in ^{131}I-mIBG therapy, resulting in acute leukemia (1.5%) and chronic leukemia (0.5%) of all patients in long-term observation [18]. Puranik and coworkers published results about more inoperable head and neck paragangliomas treated with ^{90}Y and or ^{177}Lu DOTATATE. Five patients were treated two times, one received three, and four others four courses. Mean follow-up time was 2.1 years (range 0.5–7 years). None of the patients developed new lesions, four of them showed partial response, five stable disease [19].

During the annual meeting of the European Association of Nuclear Medicine 2019 in Barcelona, the group of R.P. Baum presented a poster about a new somatostatin receptor antagonist for NET therapy [20]. For therapy, this NOGADA-LM3 was labeled with [177]Lu. In diagnostic scans with 68Ga NOGADA-LM3, high uptake in the tumors was observed, also fast

whole-body clearance. In comparison with post-therapeutic scans with 68Ga DOTATATE, more metastases were observed because of a better tumor-to-background ratio (Fig. 29.9). Because of these promising aspects, further clinical studies are needed.

29.1.2 Neuroblastoma

29.1.2.1 Matthias Schmidt
Neuroblastoma is the most common extracranial pediatric solid tumor, first recognized in 1910 by Dr. James Homer Wright Homer Wright [21]. Neuroblastoma commonly presents in children younger than 2 years of age, with 90% being younger than 5 years of age. There is marked variability in clinical behavior ranging from spontaneous regression or differentiation into benign tumors to rapid and progressive disease with fatal outcome. One subgroup, high-risk neuroblastoma, is difficult to treat and requires multimodal therapy (Table 29.1).

Current treatment for high-risk neuroblastoma patients consists of induction chemotherapy followed by a consolidation therapy including

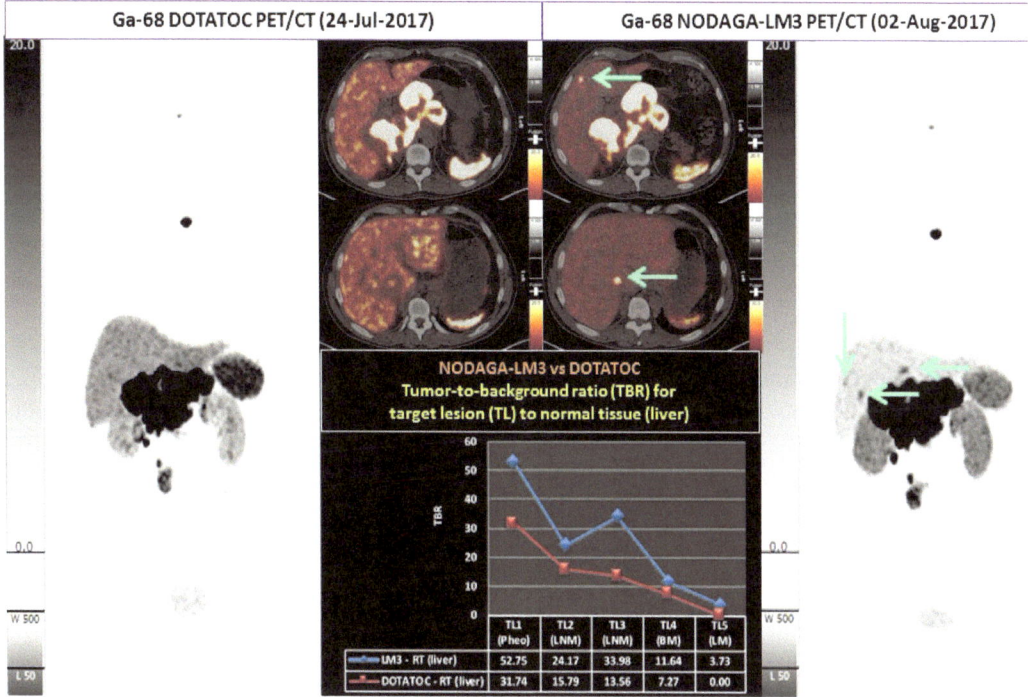

Fig. 29.9 Malignant pheochromocytoma: higher tumor-to-normal liver ratio on Ga-68 NOGADA-LM3 PCT/CT compared to Ga-68 DOTATOC PET/CT allows detection of 3 additional liver metastases (blue arrows). (Courtesy Prof. Dr. RP. Baum)

Table 29.1 Stage according to the International Neuroblastoma Risk Group (INRG) stages [22]

Stage	Description
L1	Localized tumor not involving vital structures as defined by the list of imaging-defined risk factors and confined to one body part
L2	Loco-regional tumor with presence of one more image-defined risk factors
M	Distant metastatic disease (except stage MS)
MS	Metastatic disease in children younger than 18 months with metastases confined to skin, liver, and/or bone marrow

autologous stem cell transplantation. Surgery for the primary tumor and/or metastases and external radiation therapy are additional therapeutic modalities. Despite aggressive treatment regimens, high-risk neuroblastoma continues to have a devastating mortality rate of more than 40% and 5-year overall survival of patients with stage IV neuroblastoma only 30–50% [23]. ^{131}I-mIBG therapy is one treatment option [24–26]

29.2 ^{131}I-mIBG for Initial Therapy

First-line ^{131}I-mIBG therapy was developed in The Netherlands [27]. In 1991, Hoefnagel and coworkers recommended the use of ^{131}I-mIBG therapy in advanced neuroblastoma as a first-line treatment just after diagnosis. They stated that children's better general condition prior to following surgery and/or chemotherapy might be more unaffected, and shrinkage of the primary tumor would be advantageous for a surgical resection [28]. Kraal et al. analyzed response rates of ^{131}I-mIBG therapy in patients with newly diagnosed high-risk neuroblastoma. In one study, the objective response rate (ORR) was 73% after surgery; the median overall survival was 15 months (95% confidence interval (CI) 7 to 23); 5-year overall survival was 14.6%; median event-free survival was 10 months (95% CI 7 to 13); and 5-year event-free survival was 12.2%. In the other study, the ORR was 56% after myeloablative therapy and autologous stem cell transplantation; 10-year overall survival was 6.25%; and event-free survival was not reported. With regard to short-term adverse effects, one study showed a prevalence of 2% (95% CI 0% to 13%; best-case scenario) for death due to myelosuppression. After the first cycle of ^{131}I-mIBG therapy in one study, platelet toxicity occurred in 38% (95% CI 18% to 61%), neutrophil toxicity in 50% (95% CI 28% to 72%), and hemoglobin toxicity in 69% (95% CI 44% to 86%); after the second cycle this was 60% (95% CI 36% to 80%) for platelets and neutrophils and 53% (95% CI 30% to 75%) for hemoglobin. In one study, the prevalence of hepatic toxicity during or within 4 weeks after last the ^{131}I-mIBG treatment was 0% (95% CI 0% to 9%; best-case scenario). Neither study reported cardiovascular toxicity and sialadenitis. There were no secondary malignancies observed (0%, 95% CI 0% to 9%), but only five children survived more than 4 years [29].

29.3 ^{131}I-mIBG in Stage III or IV Neuroblastoma

[131]I-mIBG therapy in high-risk neuroblastoma patients started in 1984 [25], and these early studies focused on feasibility and toxicity. There is a lack of prospective randomized controlled trials about ^{131}I-mIBG therapy in neuroblastoma patients. Data are mostly taken from retrospective series. Seven studies with a total of 151 patients reported on highly variable ^{131}I-mIBG activities per treatment cycle 2.59–16.65 GBq (70–450 mCi) and on a response rate (complete or mostly partial response) of 17–66%. Phase I/II studies used ^{131}I-mIBG in progressive, refractory or relapsed high-risk neuroblastoma. In 1998, Matthay et al. reported on the treatment of 30 patients with escalating doses from 96.2–673.4 MBq/kg. None of the patients treated with 444 MBq/kg (12 mCi/kg) or less experienced prolonged neutropenia and therefore did not require autologous stem cell rescue. In contrast, two of five patients treated with 555 MBq/kg (15 mCi/kg) and four of nine patients treated with 666 MBq/kg (18 mCi/kg) required stem cell rescue. The maximum tolerated dose for patients without stem cell support was 444 MBq/kg (12 mCi/kg) being nowadays a usually used activity. The objective response rate was 37%, with most of the responses observed in patients receiving 444 MBq/kg (12 mCi/kg) or higher ^{131}I-mIBG. Median survival time following ^{131}I-mIBG therapy was 6 months [30]. Summarizing the results of 25 studies, Wilson et al. reported about an objective tumor response ranging from 0% to 75%, mean 32% [24, 26]. In Germany, ^{131}I-mIBG is given at the end of induction chemotherapy in case of persistent mIBG-avid disease before autologous stem cell transplantation [31].

29.4 ^{131}I-mIBG after Induction Chemotherapy

In the German NB85 trial, 47 high-risk neuroblastoma patients without complete response after induction chemotherapy were treated with a mean activity of 330 MBq (8.9 mCi) ^{131}I-mIBG/kg resulted in a response rate of 46.8%. In the German NB2004 study (End of study 31.12.2016), ^{131}I-mIBG therapy was scheduled in patients with non-progressing I-123-mIBG positive tumor tissue at the end of induction therapy. The effect of ^{131}I-mIBG therapy was analyzed retrospectively in 111 high-risk neuroblastoma patients: Forty patients received ^{131}I-mIBG therapy using a median activity of 444 MBq ()/kg body weight. By univariate analysis, patients who underwent ^{131}I-mIBG therapy had a better 3-year event-free survival (3-y-EFS 46 ± 8%) and 3-year overall survival (3-y-OS 58 ± 9%) than 71 patients without ^{131}I-mIBG therapy (3-y-EFS 19 ± 5%, $p = 0.003$; 3-y-OS 43 ± 6%, $p = 0.037$). However, subgroup analysis of 66 patients who underwent high-dose chemotherapy with autologous stem cell transplantation (ASCT) during treatment found a very similar outcome with ^{131}I-mIBG (3-y-EFS 49 ± 9%, 3-y-OS 59 ± 10%) and without ^{131}I-mIBG therapy (3-y-EFS 33 ± 9%, $p = 0.171$; 3-y-OS 59 ± 9%, $p = 0.285$) due to the dominating effect of ASCT. By multivariate anal-

I-123-mIBG
Mar 2017

7,0 GBq I-131-mIBG
Apr 2017

I-123-mIBG
Jun 2017

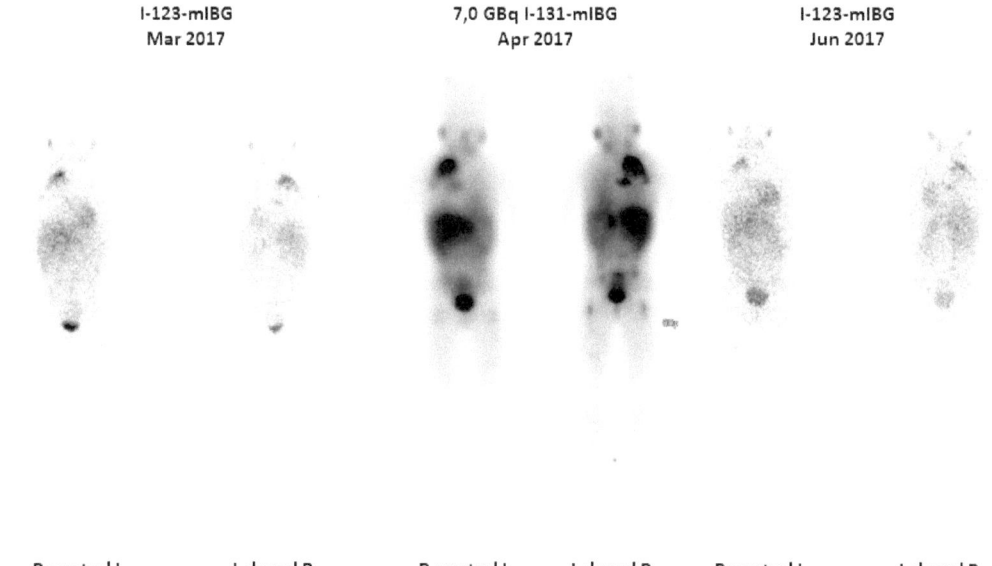

R ventral L   L dorsal R   R ventral L   L dorsal R   R ventral L   L dorsal R

Fig. 29.10 Four year old male child with neuroblastoma IV with primary tumor in the right thoracic apex with infiltration of neuroforamina C7-Th4 and multiple skeletal lesions in the skull, ribs and vertebrae, pelvis and fem- ora. Post-therapy ^{131}I-mIBG WBS shows more extensive skeletal disease. Subsequent ^{123}I-mIBG WBS demon- strates a decrease in number of lesions and intensity of uptake in the primary tumor and skeletal lesions

ysis, ^{131}I-mIBG therapy had no independent impact on EFS ($p = 0.494$) and OS ($p = 0.891$). Only ASCT, external beam radiation therapy and MYCN amplification were important for EFS and OS. Thus, an independent advantage of ^{131}I-mIBG therapy could not be proven in this ret- rospective analysis. Several problems have been addressed with this study: ^{131}I-mIBG therapy was delivered in multiple hospitals with highly vari- able activities of ^{131}I-mIBG (median activity 0.45 GBq (12 mCi), range: 0.14–1.46 GBq (3.8– 39.5 mCi) / kg body weight). Results were influ- enced by local decisions as only 40 patients from 111 potentially eligible patients with ^{123}I-mIBG- positive residual disease at the end of induction chemotherapy actually received ^{131}I-mIBG ther- apy. As the patient numbers would allow detec- tion of a difference between ^{131}I-mIBG therapy and no ^{131}I-mIBG therapy exceeding 20%, a smaller difference between these treatment options seemed likely from a clinical perspective, but was impossible to detect. As this study was based on the retrospective evaluation of the German NB97 trial, no dosimetric data were available. The pattern and intensity of ^{123}I-mIBG

uptake were not analyzed with regard to treat- ment selection and outcome. In this group of heavily pretreated children, mIBG uptake was highly variable [31]. Fig. 29.10 is an example for treatment response after ^{131}I-mIBG therapy in a 4-year-old male child with neuroblastoma IV being initially treated with chemotherapy accord- ing to NB-2004 trial protocol HR including 7.0 GBq of ^{131}I-mIBG at the end of the induction chemotherapy before autologous stem cell transplantation.

29.5   Side Effects of ^{131}I-mIBG Therapy

The most important and usually intermediate complication of ^{131}I-mIBG therapy is related to hematotoxicity due to bone marrow irradiation. Neutropenia and thrombocytopenia are the most likely side effects and can be effectively over- come in combination with autologous stem cell transplantation. Matthay et al. demonstrated in a phase I trial that 30% of patients receiving ≥555 MBq (15 mCi)/kg of ^{131}I-mIBG had prolonged and significant myelosuppression which could be abrogated with infusion of autologous hematopoietic stem cells. Hematological toxicity is more noticeable in patients with bone marrow metastases and patients who received higher whole-body radiation doses. Hematopoietic cell transplantation was required in about one-third of patients treated with 666 MBq (18 mCi)/kg ^{131}I-mIBG. In contrast, all patients treated with less than 444 MBq (12 mCi)/kg of ^{131}I-mIBG did not need hematopoietic cell transplantation.

Early complications include nausea and vomiting in 10–20% of patients. Sialadenitis is seen with a relatively high frequency, while permanent xerostomia is rare. Modak et al. reported on transient sialadenitis in nine neuroblastoma patients who had received 444–666 MBq (12–18 mCi)/kg of ^{131}I-mIBG. Five patients had bilateral parotid swelling, two patients with associated buccal discomfort within 24 h of injection which subsided within 48 h. Grade 3 or 4 serum amylase elevation was documented in 8/8 patients tested [median 1336; range: 576–8830 U/L] which normalized [25–125 U/L] within 4–14 [median 5.5] days. Serum lipase remained normal. Patients did not develop subsequent dry mouth or dysphagia.

Blood pressure-related adverse advents are rare: antihypertensive drugs were required in 2.8% of 218 ^{131}I-mIBG administrations.

Veno-occlusive liver disease (VOLD) is an important early complication in patients who received ^{131}I-mIBG therapy followed by myeloablative chemotherapy and hematopoietic cell transplantation. The new approaches to neuroblastoma therapy (NANT) consortium reported that 6 of 22 patients had VOLDs after the therapies and an apparently high rate of VOLD was seen in the patients with a low glomerular filtration rate. In contrast, no VOLD was seen in patients receiving double infusions of high-dose ^{131}I-mIBG without chemotherapy. A decreased clearance of the chemotherapeutic agents was considered a major cause of VOLD.

Late complications include persistent hematotoxicity and thyroid dysfunction. Van Santen et al. reported about the development of a TSH ≥4.5 mU/L in 16 (64%) out of 25 neuroblastoma patients treated with ^{131}I-mIBG and concluded that occurrence of thyroid dysfunction after treatment with ^{131}I-mIBG for neuroblastoma is high, in spite of potassium iodide prophylaxis requiring close thyroid follow-up. In addition, they reported on an improved thyroid blockade with thyroxine, methimazole and potassium iodide with 19 / 23 patients (86%) of patients having a normal thyroid function after a mean follow-up of 19 months. Clement et al. reported on long-term efficacy of thyroid prophylaxis. Defining thyroid dysfunction as a plasma TSH > 5.0 mU/L or the use of levothyroxine thyroid disorders was seen in 12/24 patients available for long-term evaluation with a mean follow-up of 9.0 years after ^{131}I-mIBG treatment demonstrating the significant risk of thyroid damage. Thus, the incidence of thyroid disorders was high and increases with advancing time. No deleterious effects of ^{131}I-mIBG therapy on the parathyroid glands were found. As hypothyroidism can be easily treated, this side effect is usually not considered as serious.

Other less likely complications include fatigue secondary to anemia, sterility, and amenorrhea but these side effects are usually an effect of the combination with other therapies such as chemotherapy. Clement et al. published two patients with ovarian insufficiency after treatment with ^{131}I-mIBG therapy. Hepatic, adrenal, or cardiac dysfunction have rarely been reported.

Secondary malignancies have been reported with an incidence of less than 5%. In a report from Italy, two leukemia, one angiomatoid fibrous histiocytoma, one schwannoma, and one rhabdomyosarcoma occurred in 119 patients with neuroblastoma after ^{131}I-mIBG therapy. The University of California group from San Francisco described that leukemia was observed in 3 of 95 patients with refractory neuroblastoma at 7, 11, and 12 months after ^{131}I-mIBG therapy. It was difficult to clarify the main factors of the secondary malignancies, because all patients received several intensive therapies including chemotherapy and ^{131}I-mIBG therapy. Papillary thyroid carcinomas have been reported in two of nine patients with thyroid nodules [32].

29.6 Radiation Exposure/Dosimetry

Heterogeneity in ^{131}I-mIBG uptake, tumor characteristics, and radiation resistance, as well as limitations of the current equipment and methods make correlation of dosimetry with response a continuing challenge [33]. Tumor dosimetry is an extensive topic on which progress has been achieved [34–37]. The main problem is that acquisition of serial whole body imaging in children is usually not possible. Usually, empirical treatment activities are usually chosen, and posttherapeutic wholebody and SPECT examinations are performed. Without stem cell support, the maximum allowable bone marrow absorbed dose consists of 2 Gy for adults and 2.5 Gy for children. If stem cell rescue is available, higher bone marrow doses are possible. In a series of 16 neuroblastoma patients in whom serial imaging after ^{131}I-mIBG was possible, typical whole-body absorbed doses were found in the region of 2 Gy (range: 1.0–2.9 Gy) whereas tumor absorbed doses in turn covered a span between 10 and 60 Gy using a therapeutic activity of 444 MBq/kg body weight [37].

In sum, ^{131}I-mIBG therapy is a long-standing established treatment modality. Upfront ^{131}I-mIBG therapy was mainly used in the Netherlands. ^{131}I-mIBG in case of residual mIBG-avid disease at the end of induction chemotherapy was included in the German protocol. ^{131}I-mIBG therapy was used in case of relapse in international studies. Due to the rarity of the disease, data are limited and there is only little innovation so far. The optimal timing of ^{131}I-MIBG therapy within the multidisciplinary therapy in not yet defined [38]. A new therapeutical aspect may be the use of [211]At metaastatobenzylguanidine, causing less hematotoxicity, shown in animal experiments [39].

With the recent establishment of new therapies, it may be possible to develop more effective therapeutic strategies in high-risk neuroblastoma patients. Few data are available on the effectiveness of PRRT [40]. A British trial was set up to evaluate how effective ^{177}Lu-DOTATATE is in children with high-risk relapsed or refractory neuroblastoma and determine the safety and adverse events of the treatment experienced by patients on the study (Eudra-CT-Nr. 2012-000510-10, https://www.clinicaltrialsregister.eu/ctr-search/trial/2012-000510-10/results).

It may be concluded as stated by Kayano D and Kinuya S still in 2018 "MIBG therapy indicate their efficacy, especially in patients with advanced neuroblastoma and pheochromocytoma/paragangliomas [41].

References

1. Lloyd RV, Osamura RY, Klöppel G, Rodai J, editors. WHO classification of tumours of endocrine organs. Lyon: International Agency for Research on Cancer; 2017.
2. Morales JO, Beierwaltes WH, Counsell RE, et al. The concentration of radioactivity from labeled epinephrine and its precursors in the dog adrenal medulla. J Nucl Med. 1967;8:800–9.
3. Korn N, Buswink A, Yu T, et al. A radioiodinated bretyllium analog as a potential agent for scanning the adrenal medulla. J Nucl Med. 1977;18:87–9.
4. Wieland DM, Swanson DP, Brown LE, Beierwaltes WH. Imaging the adrenal medulla with an I-131-labeled antiadrenergic agent. J Nucl Med. 1979;20:155–8.
5. Wieland DM, Wu J-I, Brown LE, et al. Radiolabled adrenergic neuron-blocking agents: adrenomedullary imaging with ^{131}I-iodobenzylguanidine. J Nucl Med. 1980;21:349–53.
6. Beierwaltes WH. New horizons for therapeutic nuclear medicine in 1981. J Nucl Med. 1981;22:549–54.
7. Fischer M, Winterberg B, Müller-Rensing R, et al. Nuklearmedizinische Therapie des Phäochromozytoms. Nuc Compact. 1983;14:172–6.
8. Shapiro B, Copp JE, Sisson JC, et al. Iodine-131 metaiodobenzylguanidine for the location of suspected pheochromocytoma: experience in 400 cases. J Nucl Med. 1985;26:576–85.
9. Fischer M, Vetter W, Winterberg B, et al. Scintigraphic localization of phaeochromocytomas. Clin Endocrinol. 1984;20:1–7.
10. Khafagi FA, Shapiro B, Fischer M, et al. Phaeochromocytoma and funtioning paraganglioma in childhood and adolescence: role of iodine 131 metaiodobenzylguanidine. Eur J Nucl Med. 1991;18:191–8.
11. Conzo G, Pasquali D, Colantuoni V, et al. Current concepts of pheochromocytoma. Intern J Surg. 2014;12:469–74.

12. Fischer M. Therapy of pheochromocytoma with [131I] metaiodobenzylguanidine. J Nucl Biol Med. 1991;35:292–4.
13. Pryma DA, Chin BB, Noto RB, et al. Efficacy and safety of high-specific-activity 131I-MIBG therapy in patients with advanced pheochromocytoma or paraganlioma. J Nucl Med. 2019;60:623–30.
14. Mak IYF, Hayes AR, Khoo B, Grossman A. Peptide receptor radionuclide therapy as a novel treatment for metastatic and invasive phaeochromocytoma and paraganglioma. Neuroendocrinology. 2019;109:287–98.
15. Mundschenk J, Unger N, Schulz S, et al. Somatostatin receptor subtypes in human pheochromocytoma: subcellular expression pattern and functional relevance for octreotide scintigraphy. J Clin Endocrinol Metab. 2003;88:5150–7.
16. Han S, Suh CH, Woo S, et al. Performance of 68Ga-DOTA-conjugated somatostatin receptor-targeting PET in detection of pheochromocytomas and paraganlioma: a systematic review and metaanalysis. J Nucl Med. 2019;60:369–76.
17. Bodei L, Zaknun JJ, Mueller-Brand J, et al. The joint IAEA, EANM, and SNMMI practical guidance on peptide receptor radionuclide therapy (PRRNT) in neuroendocrine tumours. Eur J Nucl Med Mol Imaging. 2013;40:800–16.
18. Garske-Román U, Sandström M, Baron K-F, et al. Prospective observational study of 177Lu-DOTA-octreotate therapy in 200 patients with advanced metastasized neuroendocrine tumours (NETs): feasibility and impact of a dosimetry-guided study protocol on outcome and toxicity. Eur J Nuc Med Mol Imaging. 2018;45:970–88.
19. Puranik AD, Kulkarni HR, Singh A, Baum RP. Peptide receptor radionuclide therapy with 90Y/177Lu-labeled peptides for inoperable head and neck paragangliomas (glomus tumours). Eur J Nucl Med Mol Imaging. 2015;42:1223–30.
20. Schuchardt C, Wiessalla S, Kulkarni HR et al. Peptide radio receptor therapy with SSTR antagonists: biokinetics and dosimetry of Lu-177 DOTA-LM3. EANM Annual Meeting. 2019. Abstr.
21. Wright JH. Neurocytoma or neuroblastoma. A kind of tumor not generally recognized. J Exp Med. 1910;12:556–61.
22. Monclair T, Brodeur GM, Ambros PF, et al. The international neuroblastoma risk group (INRG) staging system: an INRG task force report. J Clin Oncol. 2009;27:298–303.
23. Schmidt M, Hero B, Simon T. I-131-mIBG therapy in neuroblastoma: established role and prospective applications. Clin Transl Imaging. 2016;4:87–101.
24. Wilson JS, Gains JE, Moroz V, Wheatley K, Gaze MN. A systematic review of 131I-meta iodobenzylguanidine molecular radiotherapy for neuroblastoma. Eur J Cancer. 2014a;50(4):801–15.
25. Treuner J, Feine U, Niethammer D, et al. Scintigraphic imaging of neuroblastoma with [131-I] iodobenzylguanidine. Lancet. 1984;1:333–4.
26. Wilson JS, Gains JE, Moroz V, Wheatley K, Gaze MN. A systematic review of 131I-meta iodobenzylguanidine molecular radiotherapy for neuroblastoma. Eur J Cancer. 2014b;50:801–15.
27. De Kraker J, Hoefnagel KA, Verschuur AC, van Eck B, van Santen HM, Caron HN. Iodine-131-metaiodobenzylguanidine as initial induction therapy in stage 4 neuroblastoma patients over 1 year of age. Eur J Cancer. 2008;44:551–6.
28. Hoefnagel CA, deKraker J, et al. Preoperative [131I] metaiodobenzylguanidine therapy of neuroblastoma at diagnosis. J Nucl Biol Med. 1919;35:248–51.
29. Kraal KC, van Dalen EC, Tytgat GA, Van Eck-Smit BL. Iodine-131-meta-iodobenzyl-guanidine therapy for patients with newly diagnosed high-risk neuroblastoma. Cochrane Database Syst Rev. 2017;4:CD010349.
30. Matthay KK, DeSantes K, Hasegawa B, Huberty J, Hattner RS, Ablin A, et al. Phase I dose escalation of 131I-metaiodobenzylguanidine with autologous bone marrow support in refractory neuroblastoma. J Clin Oncol. 1998;16:229–36.
31. Schmidt M, Simon T, Hero B, Eschner W, Dietlein M, Sudbrock F, et al. Is there a benefit of 131 I-MIBG therapy in the treatment of children with stage 4 neuroblastoma? A retrospective evaluation of the German neuroblastoma trial NB97 and implications for the German neuroblastoma trial NB2004. Nuklearmedizin. 2006;45:145–51.
32. Bleeker G, Schoot RA, Caron HN, de Kraker J, Hoefnagel CA, van Eck BL, Tytgat GA. Toxicity of upfront 131I-metaiodobenzylguanidine (131I-MIBG) therapy in newly diagnosed neuroblastoma patients: a retrospective analysis. Eur J Nucl Med Mol Imaging. 2013;40:1711–7.
33. Taggart D, Dubois S, Matthay KK. Radiolabeled metaiodobenzylguanidine for imaging and therapy of neuroblastoma. Q J Nucl Med Mol Imaging. 2008;52:403–18.
34. Buckley SE, Chittenden SJ, Saran FH, Meller ST, Flux GD. Whole-body dosimetry for individualized treatment planning of 131I-MIBG radionuclide therapy for neuroblastoma. J Nucl Med. 2009;50:1518–24.
35. Buckley SE, Saran FH, Gaze MN, Chittenden S, Partridge M, Lancaster D, et al. Dosimetry for fractionated (131)I-mIBG therapies in patients with primary resistant high-risk neuroblastoma: preliminary results. Cancer Biother Radiopharm. 2007;22:105–12.
36. Lassmann M, Chiesa C, Flux G, Bardiès M. EANM dosimetry committee guidance document: good practice of clinical dosimetry reporting. Eur J Nucl Med Mol Imaging. 2011;38:192–200.

37. Sudbrock F, Schmidt M, Simon T, Eschner W, Berthold F, Schicha H. Dosimetry for ^{131}I-MIBG therapies in metastatic neuroblastoma, phaeochromocytoma and paraganglioma. Eur J Nucl Med Mol Imaging. 2010;37:1279–90.

38. Kraal, Timmermann, et al. Peripheral stem cell apheresis is feasible post [131]Iodine. Metaiodobenzylguinidine-therapy in high-risk neuroblastoma, but results in delayed platelet reconstitution. Clin Cancer Res. 2019;25:1012.

39. Agrawal A, Rangarajan V, et al. MIBG (metaiodobenzylguanidine) theranostics in pediatric and adult malignancies. Brit J Radiol. 2018;91:20180103.

40. Schmidt M, Baum RP, Simon T, Howman-Giles R. Therapeutic nuclear medicine in pediatric malignancy. Q J Nucl Med Mol Imaging. 2010;54:411–28.

41. Kayano D, Kinuya S. Current consensus on I-131 MIBG therapy. Nucl Med Mol Imaging. 2018;52:254–65.

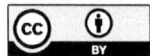

Ajit S. Shinto

30.1 Aim

The aim of this investigator-led study is to introduce a real-world experience of how a mentor could change the course of one's life.

30.2 Materials and Methods

Would definitely not survive a thorough scientific appraisal, but evidence was painstakingly reminisced, collated, distilled, and transcribed.

30.3 Results

Results were some wonderful experiences which had the power to challenge, stimulate, and empower one's heart and mind to the limitless possibilities if the intent is true and consuming.

30.4 Conclusion

It is a life worth having lived, if you touch the lives of many, have inspired someone to be better, to be the leader that is also a ladder for others to climb higher, to be a dreamer who recognizes the potential of other's dreams and lends them the hand that gives them a gentle support to move ahead continuously.

This might be considered incongruous in such a learned text, but what I do have is a story. And like all stories, I hope it catches your attention, makes you a part of the journey, think a bit and take parts of it for your own life and give it the suitable conclusion that each mind is uniquely capable of conjuring.

We hosted the first ever nuclear medicine congress of the southern chapter of the Society of Nuclear Medicine, India, in Coimbatore in September 2013, where the late Dr Ajit Padhy and his team from World Association of Radiopharmaceutical and Molecular Therapy (WARMTH) helped us set up the Re 188 therapeutic program during the Congress. However, it was also a very saddening affair that he succumbed to a massive heart attack after reaching home in Singapore the day after the Congress. In his memory, I was asked to present the data on Re 188 Lipiodol therapy for liver cancer at the World Congress in Cancun in 2014. I entered the hall and it was packed to the hilt with an international audience, and my eyes immediately rested on the moderators of the session upfront on the stage. It was the talk before mine, and I realized that one of the moderators, this huge bearded giant of a man was expounding and professing with such an impact, that I stood in awe. I was nervous to

A. S. Shinto (✉)
Department of Nuclear Medicine, Theranostics
Center of Excellence, Apollo Proton Cancer Centre,
Chennai, Tamil Nadu, India
e-mail: drajit_shinto@apollohospitals.com

© The Author(s) 2024
V. Prasad (ed.), *Beyond Becquerel and Biology to Precision Radiomolecular Oncology: Festschrift in Honor of Richard P. Baum*, https://doi.org/10.1007/978-3-031-33533-4_30

begin with, as it was my first presentation at an international stage and the work I was presenting was all of 7 months vintage. Anyway, I walked up as serenely as possible and delivered for the next 25 minutes our initial single center experience of treating liver cancers with this new product. I had no idea how this project would be received and looked up as I finished to a silent audience. And then out of nowhere came a thunderous voice on the mike from the very same moderator with a – THAT'S OUSTANDING DATA, please give him a huge round of applause. That was my very first interaction with Prof. Richard Baum and it had already made such a deep impact on me. What it taught me was to be supportive and encouraging of the work that is being done by your colleague, however junior or inexperienced he or she may be. To nurture when it need not be done is a gift.

During the same Congress, I was called for a special meeting with the executive committee of WARMTH, wherein I was asked to summarize the Rhenium project and the potential challenges as well as way forward. Prof. Baum was the then president of WARMTH, and after listening to the synopsis and discussing with the other senior members, decreed that I should be the Chairman of a new task force to propagate Rhenium therapies across the globe on behalf of the Late Dr. Padhy and as a legacy of WARMTH. Indeed, it was such a great boost to my confidence, and it really felt like there was a strong wind under my sail taking me in a new direction. In retrospect, I was astonished by his ability to delegate a project on behalf of an international organization to a newcomer and a relative stranger such as I. It spoke volumes of his ability to trust and motivate and to constantly keep moving forward with a vision that would inspire others around him.

After reaching back to India, with so many thoughts whirling in my brain as to how to take this project forward, I learnt with alarm that the only commercial supplier of the Re 188 generator had stopped its production and distribution due to nonviability of the product and that I do not have the main item, that is, Re 188 to continue this project. I really did not know what to do and that is when I decided to write to Prof. Baum to ask him if he could help in any way. EANM

meeting that year was in Gothenburg, and on behalf of me, he organized a round table meeting with the major isotope suppliers of the world and asked me to present my case. In essence, what he had done was to leverage his standing in the professional NM community and to lean on industry personally to try and help me to do what was effectively not going to benefit him in any way. So, mainly due to his persuasiveness and weight behind me, we got one of the companies to agree to actually give on a regular basis a subsidized WARMTH generator with a built-in fee for academic and research development. To those of us who have battled the industry on multiple fronts, you would understand how difficult it would be to convince a business entity to support a commercially nonviable product. It inspired me to think – of what good is your clout and influence, if you cannot use it to develop something or help someone out and to do so with no personal gain, not expecting anything in return.

One of the key areas lacking with the propagation of the Re 188 project was the general lack of awareness of the product. To address this challenge, I envisaged the first world Rhenium Congress in 2015 with an idea to bring all the stakeholders, industry, reactor companies, pharmacy, dosimetry specialists,clinicians, and researchers working with Re 188 from around the globe together to Coimbatore, a tier 2 city in South India; which again was a stupendous step forward and was never imagined on such a large or an international scale. Of course my main inspiration was Prof. Baum who had conceptualized and organized the First World Gallium Congress in 2011, which was very successful. When I reached out to him for support as the incumbent president of WARMTH, he immediately warmed up to the idea and was enthusiastic with his suggestions. Not only was he prompt in responding to calls of help, but he also went out of his way to get us the major funding for the Congress, called up favors owed from his colleagues to help get me support and even flew down on his own expense as well as sponsored researchers who could not afford to come down due to financial constraints. Learning point: No idea is your own, go out on a limb to help someone who wants to do something new or useful when you can and always propagate knowledge. We had delegates and faculties from over 35 countries who flew in on their own expense to attend this novel meeting. In fact, when many of them applied for their visa to India to attend the meeting and said they wanted to go to Coimbatore, the officials of the Indian embassy had very less idea of where this city was or why would anyone from say Colombia or Russia go there.

I remember wanting to ask his support on multiple things during a meeting in South Africa wherein, he was to leave early and the only time that we had left was actually the bus ride to the conference venue. I had my pen and paper as it was a short ride and I did not want to forget something. I said I wanted to host the second Rhenium Congress and also wanted to combine it with some other international agency such as IAEA, SRS, ISCORN, WTA, WARMTH or SNMI. Typical of Richard, he said great, let us do this with all of them .The 2017 Congress had all of the above agencies supporting us and it was due to the indefatigable effort from him personally many a time that made it possible. For me, it was amazing how he would take the time out, to discuss and encourage and not just promise, but to actually act on that discussion and enable its fruition. He was unfazed by enormity, the bigger the better.

I was ecstatic that Prof Baum had landed in Coimbatore for the Rhenium Congress, and I visited him on the same day in his hotel room to check on him as well as to invite him for a private dinner. He politely refused to come out that evening saying he had to prepare for his lectures that he was due to give the next day and he also said that he never uses the same presentation twice. He always believed that you should respect the audience and the platform and put in your best when up there. Indeed it was an inspiration for me, that how much ever you grow, always do your job to the best of your ability and never take a podium or the ability to educate and influence other minds for granted. Due diligence matters.

During many an interaction with my clinical colleagues who had trained with him or were working with him, when asked what is the secret of his success; the answer consistently revolved around three things. Hard work (he came most days in the wee hours of the morning 3–5 am), a great clinician (an attribute which many of us NM physicians are distancing ourselves from), and ability to believe in yourself and take that risk, provided you have the patient's good as your endpoint. I have kept these guiding mantras in my pursuit of success in the professional arena, and still have a long way to go.

His ability to remember even the most elusive and what you would consider the most minute or inconsequential detail has always amazed me, and in part, I feel it is because of his inherent curiosity. I remember many a times, even across the dinner plate, when he hears something new, he would always ask it to be sent to him so that he could read it and understand better. He would take great pride in pronouncing words and names the exact correct way and would remember fondly the details of a particular wine at a dinner or even the entertainment on an evening way back in time. The abiding lesson learnt was that the tiny details matter and it embellishes the ability to live life to the fullest.

It was after great difficulty that I had convinced a journal to come out with an entire issue based on Re 188, covering all relevant topics from bench to clinical and research avenues. However, the stumbling block was to find financial support for this issue. It took a 2 min call for help to Dr. Baum, who asked me to go ahead and decided to fund it himself. Not only did he do that, he handed over the money personally to me when he saw me next, in a cover marked with the current euro exchange rate and was exact to the last cent. If in a position to give, give freely and easily, do not make the recipient ask many times and most importantly do not give like it does not mean anything to you – be accountable even when you are beneficent.

In all my series of conversations with him, the one thing that I always admired was his ability to cut through the molasses and reach to the core of the person. He had a way of knowing who would stand up to their pitch, who could walk the talk and pick the winning horse or even the one that would not give up. He always respected the hustle, knowing that opportunities are everywhere and the person who did the hard yards to reach wherever they were now, needed to be respected.

Some enduring images are of professor with the traditional white "veshti" and a cigar in his mouth at the Rhenium Congress, to shouting out: "someone give this German a beer," to pulling me aside to a restaurant in the lunch break of a conference saying "I can't be eating these box lunches anymore if I have a choice." Make things count, a meal, an evening to cherish, a ready quip, a hearty laugh, a good beer, and time well spent: celebrate the small things.

Some of the small things the Re 188 taskforce has achieved over the past few years that need to be celebrated have been summarized. We have been able to stabilize the Re 188 generator availability and also convince agencies to produce commercially available cold kits for labeling in a cost-effective manner. Multipronged training has

been imparted to multiple centers in different countries to use this technology, conducted two world congresses, had editorials and journal issues dedicated to Re 188, sparked bench chemistry and dosimetric research in various universities across the globe and even have ongoing collaborative multicentric trials.

With support from so many unbelievable people that I have met in my journey with Re 188, the chief among them being key members of WARMTH and Prof Baum, I continue to walk feeling stronger with every step; maybe that is what happens when you journey with Hercules.

Conflict of Interest/Financial Disclosure None.

Financial Support and Conflict of Interest Nil

Reference

1. Experience-based medicine.

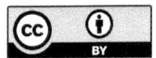

CXCR4 Theranostics: A Potential Game Changer in Solid Tumors and Hematological Malignancies

31

Singh Baljinder, Watts Ankit,
Amit Singh Shekhawat, Singh Ashwin,
Pankaj Malhotra, Abdul Waheed, Kaur Harneet,
Rani Nisha, Renu Madan, Sunil Arora,
B. D. Radotra, Vikas Prasad, Hans J. Wester,
and Digambar Behera

31.1 Background

A knowledge of receptor expression on the tumor is the key for therapy directed at these receptors and traditionally has been obtained by assay of biopsy material. Advances in molecular cancer biology have demonstrated that many of these

S. Baljinder (✉) · W. Ankit · A. S. Shekhawat
S. Ashwin · A. Waheed · K. Harneet · R. Nisha
Department of Nuclear Medicine, PGIMER,
Chandigarh, India

P. Malhotra
Internal Medicine, PGIMER, Chandigarh, India

R. Madan
Radiotherapy, PGIMER, Chandigarh, India

S. Arora
Immunopathology, PGIMER, Chandigarh, India

B. D. Radotra
Histapathology, PGIMER, Chandigarh, India

V. Prasad
Division of Nuclear Medicine, Mallinckrodt Institute
of Radiology, Washington University in Saint Louis,
St. Louis, MO, USA
e-mail: pvikas@wustl.edu

H. J. Wester
Pharmaceutical Radiochemistry, Technical University
of Munich, Munich, Germany

D. Behera
Pulmonary Medicine, PGIMER, Chandigarh, India

tumor targets are receptors and have been reported as earliest targets for cancer diagnosis as well as therapy, with notable success in the effective treatment in few cancers [1]. One such important class of molecules/targets is a class of chemokine receptors, and the human chemokine system includes more than 50 chemokines and 20 chemokine receptors [2]. These receptors play an important role in cancer progression in terms of tumor growth, senescence, angiogenesis, epithelial-mesenchymal transition, metastasis, and evading the host immune system [3]. Among these chemokine receptors, CXCR4 is the most widely expressed receptor on malignant tumors, and its role in tumor biology has been studied extensively [4]. The chemokine CXCL12 is the sole ligand of CXCR4 and the majority of research focusing on the role of CXCR4 in cancer relates to this chemokine/chemokine-receptor pair [5, 6]. Upregulation of CXCR4 has been reported in at least 23 different epithelial, mesenchymal, and hematopoietic cancers [7, 8]. CXCR4 overexpression in tumor tissues has also been correlated with tumor aggressiveness, increased risk of metastasis, and a higher probability of recurrence [9].

It has been reported that an increased CXCR4 receptor density is often associated with metastatic disease which in turn leads to a poor prog-

V. Prasad (ed.), *Beyond Becquerel and Biology to Precision Radiomolecular Oncology: Festschrift in Honor of Richard P. Baum*, https://doi.org/10.1007/978-3-031-33533-4_31

nosis [10]. Tumor receptor imaging offers a complementary role not only in providing a non-invasive evidence of tumor receptor expression but also in the evaluation of the entire tumor burden and characterization of the tumor hetero-geneity. Therefore, noninvasive imaging using high-throughput PET probes targeting CXCR4 receptors may yield important diagnostic and prognostic information pertinent to the disease process [11]. Plerixafor (AMD-3100), an immu-nostimulant is a peptide that has been approved by Food and Drug Administration (FDA, USA) as a CXCR4-targeted therapy for hematopoietic stem cell mobilization in AML (Acute Myeloid Leukemia) and non-Hodgkin's Lymphoma (NHL) patients [12]. Several CXCR4-specific PET (^{64}Cu; ^{68}Ga) tracers (AMD-3100; Trade Name—Plerixafor) have been developed but were restricted to preclinical applications [13]. However, the only PET tracer that has undergone the transition to clinical applications is ^{68}Ga-labeled Pentixafor. This PET tracer (devel-oped by a German group) was developed after certain modifications (without changing the physiochemical properties in the motif (Plerixafor—the parent compound)) allowing chemical binding with the metal chelator (DOTA) for achieving effective coupling with ^{68}Ga [14]. These authors in their extensive animal and pre-liminary human studies have shown that the tracer localizes in the CXCR4-expressing tumors (lymphoma) with high target to nontarget ratios [15]. Further, these authors have shown that ^{68}Ga-Pentixafor offers favorable dosimetry exhibiting whole-body radiation exposure of 2.3 mSv to patients which is almost one-third of that received from a conventional ^{18}F-FDG PET scan [16].

The use of Gallium-68 (half-life $t_{1/2} = 68$ min; positron emission intensity—87%) is on the rise [17]. Several favorable properties of this radionu-clide include superior image quality compared to SPECT radionuclides (e.g., indium-111) and the potential for an on-demand production via gen-erator technologies that provide reliable and high-purity ^{68}Ga in sufficient quantities for rou-tine radiopharmaceutical production without the need for expensive cyclotron operations [18, 19].

Generator technologies for ^{68}Ga production, chemistry of gallium, and emerging applications for ^{68}Ga radiopharmaceuticals have been reviewed in detail [18, 20]. These physicochemi-cal properties provide a strong basis for develop-ing specific ^{68}Ga-labeled probes for molecular imaging in various human cancers including solid tumors and hematological malignancies [15, 21–23].

The central role of CXCR4 in cancer patho-genesis and metastasis is proven beyond doubt; however, no in vivo method suitable for whole-body CXCR4 disease quantification has been described till late. This unmet clinical need or the scientific question has been addressed and 68Ga-Pentixafor having high affinity for CXCR4 receptors have been developed. They synthesized and developed ^{68}Ga-Pentixafor which is a CXCR4 targeting high-affinity nuclear probe and have evaluated the radiotracer in small-cell lung can-cer models [22]. Further, proof of concept (POC) studies with ^{68}Ga-Pentixafor in lymphoma-xenografted animal models and in first human hematological malignancies are highly encourag-ing [23, 24]. And human dosimetry studies dem-onstrated excellent pharmacokinetics and low radiation burden to patients [16]. In expanding clinical applications of this novel tracer, it has been shown both in preclinical and clinical stud-ies that the tracer provides a high contrast image in comparison to ^{18}F-FDG PET in advanced stage multiple myeloma patients [23]. The other diag-nostic applications of ^{68}Ga-Pentixafor in glioma and some other cancers known to have higher degrees of CXCR4 expression are also emerging. We will discuss in this chapter the CXCR4 ther-anostics in lung cancer, multiple myeloma, and glioma.

31.2 CXCR4-Targeted PET Imaging in Lung Cancer

Lung cancer is one of the most common (after breast cancer) malignancies globally and within India amongst males alone as well as in the com-bined male and female population [25, 26]. Lung cancer (LC) alone causes higher number of deaths than that caused by the combination of the other four (breast, colon, pancreas, and prostate) common malignancies [25]. Both epidemiological data and molecular understanding of the disease pathophysiology has shown that LC is associated with cigarette smoking and occupational/environmental factors [26–29]. Approximately, 80% of the LC cases are of the non-small cell lung cancer (NSCLC) and frequently present with advanced disease at initial diagnosis (stages IIIB and IV) where the traditional treatment options like chemotherapy and radiation therapy are aimed at disease and symptom control rather than at achieving a cure [27, 28].

The diagnostic workup of suspected lung cancer depends upon the type, that is, NSCLC or small-cell lung cancer (SCLC), the size and site of the primary lung cancer. This approach involves accurate tissue diagnosis (histopathology and advanced immune-histochemical analysis), staging, and functional evaluation by radiological imaging techniques with high sensitivity and specificity. Amongst, over 150 factors, the tumor stage which guides the therapeutic options (surgery/radiation therapy/chemotherapy) is considered as the most significant prognostic indicator in LC patients [30–33]. Despite significant advances in diagnostic, staging, and surgical techniques as well as availability of newer targeted (both chemo/radio) therapies, the death rate from lung carcinoma has remained high [34, 35].

Hybrid ^{18}F-FDG PET/CT imaging remains the mainstay of the diagnostic workup of patients with lung cancer [36]. This imaging technique scores high over the conventional radiological techniques for example, computed tomography (CT) and magnetic resonance imaging (MRI) in terms of both sensitivity and specificity [37]. Although ^{18}F-FDG/PET imaging has proven its utility in monitoring response to appropriate therapies at early time intervals, yet this technique has fewer limitations. These include its inability to differentiate inflammatory/infectious pathologies from tumor recurrence/relapse, and the high background FDG uptake interferes with the detection of metastatic lesions in the brain [38,

39]. On the other hand, ^{18}F-FLT, a marker of cell proliferation has high specificity for solid tumors. However, this imaging technique has inherent problem of lower uptake thereby poor image contrast, not making it an ideal PET tracer especially for response assessment [40, 41].

Philips et al. reported that distant metastases from NSCLC require a CXCL12 chemotactic gradient [42]. Furthermore, they found CXCL12 levels to be significantly higher in metastatic organs than that in the primary tumors. Likewise, SCLC preferentially metastasizes to the marrow, which has high constitutive CXCL12 expression [43]. The signaling via CXCR4 on SCLC cells induces activation and signaling of tumor-associated integrins that apparently play an important role in tumor progression [44]. A positive correlation between CXCR4 expression and clinical outcome in lung cancer has been reported. In a very interesting study by Spano et al. [45], it was observed that the patients having CXCR4-positive nuclear staining demonstrated confinement of CXCR4 presence in the nucleus and is associated with better patients' survival than those having the receptor expression on the cytoplasmic membrane with absent nuclear staining.

In a recent study, Vag et al. reported their first experience on the use of ^{68}Ga-Pentixafor PET imaging, targeting CXCR4 receptors in solid tumors [21]. These authors concluded that the detectability of solid cancers was found to be lower for ^{68}Ga-Pentixafor than for ^{18}F-FDG PET. However, this study included a small and heterogeneous cohort of 21 patients out of which only two were of NSCLC. The highest SUV_{max} of 10.9 was observed in a NSCLC patient followed by pancreatic cancer (6.2), HCC (5.0), and breast cancer (3.3). On the other hand, highest SUV_{max} of 13.8 was noted in the cervical metastases of the patient with cancer of unknown primary (CUP). In another study, Lapa et al. [22] studied the feasibility of CXCR4-directed ^{68}Ga-Pentixafor PET/CT imaging in ten patients of small-cell lung carcinoma (SCLC) and compared results with ^{18}F-FDG PET/CT or ^{68}Ga-DOTA-TOC PET/CT. These authors concluded that noninvasive imaging of CXCR4 expression in SCLC is feasible and ^{68}Ga-Pentixafor as a novel PET tracer might serve as a readout for confirming the CXCR expression which might serve as a prerequisite for potential CXCR4-directed radio-chemotherapies.

In a preliminary study [46], we have shown that ^{68}Ga-Pentixafor PET/CT demonstrated higher CXCR4 density in SCLC compared to NSCLC and had superior performance in detection of brain metastases which is a known limitation of ^{18}F-FDG PET imaging. We expanded our initial cohort to image 100 lung cancer patients with ^{68}Ga-Pentixafor PET/CT. We found that the SUV_{max} values on ^{68}Ga-pentixafor PET/CT were 6.14 ± 2.14 and 8.0 ± 1.9 in squamous ($n = 60$) and adenocarcinoma ($n = 20$) variants of the NSCLC, respectively. The corresponding values were highest in SCLC (n = 20; SUV_{max} 10.30 ± 5.0). Similarly, the CXCR4 quantitative values expressed as Mean Fluorescence Index (MFI) for in vivo measure of CXCR4 receptor density were 136.0 ± 80; 288 ± 121, and 348 ± 99 in squamous, adenocarcinoma, and SCLC respectively. These findings highlight that the uptake of the tracer increased as a function of the receptor density which in turn supports the specific binding of the tracer to CXCR4 receptors (Fig. 31.1). A representative IHC-stained slide showing CXCR4+ SCLC patient and a control (CXCR4-negative) slide is shown in Fig. 31.2. We have reported that 68Ga-Pentixafor PET/CT targets CXCR4 receptors non-invasively and its uptake varies as a function of CXCR4 receptors' density in different lung cancer subtypes [47]. This imaging

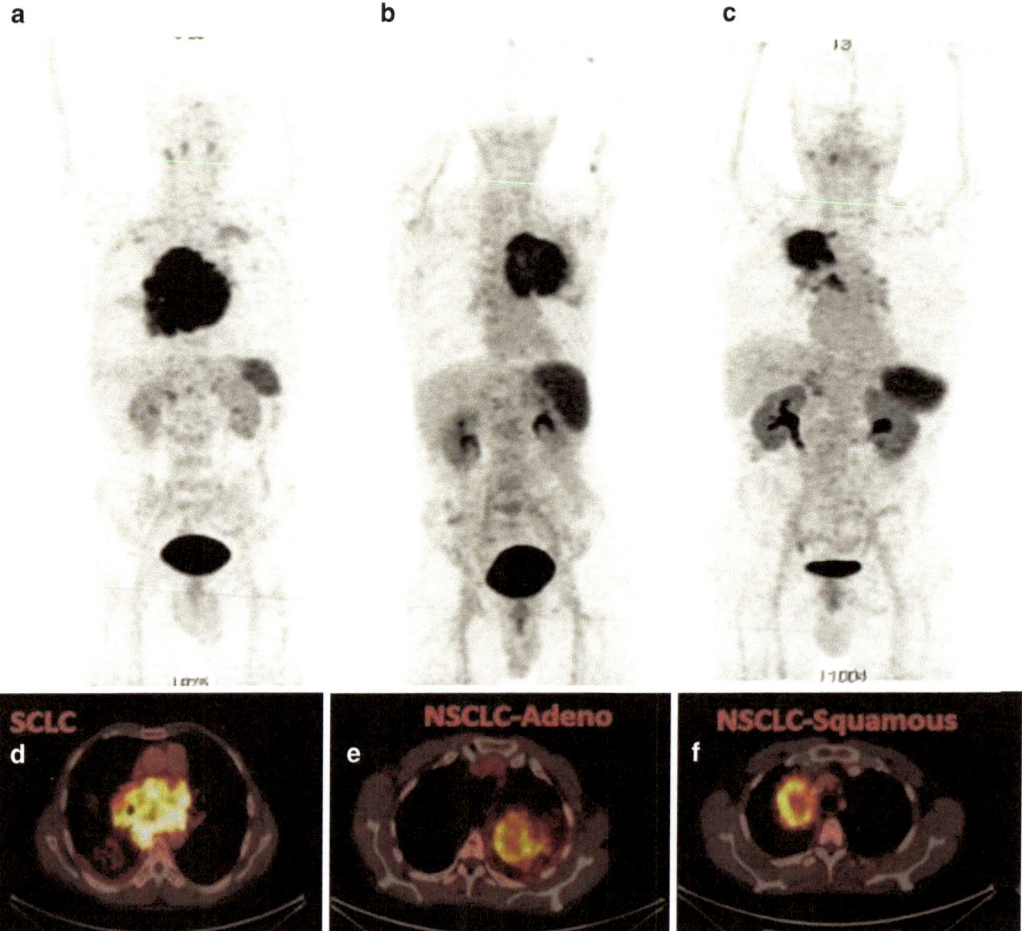

Fig. 31.1 68Ga-Pentixafor PET/CT images in a SCLC patient (**a, d**), NSCLC adenocarcinoma (**b, e**) and NSCLC-squamous (**c, f**) showing SUV_{max} values of 13.2, 10.0, and 7.2 and MFI of 413, 208, and 99.0, respectively

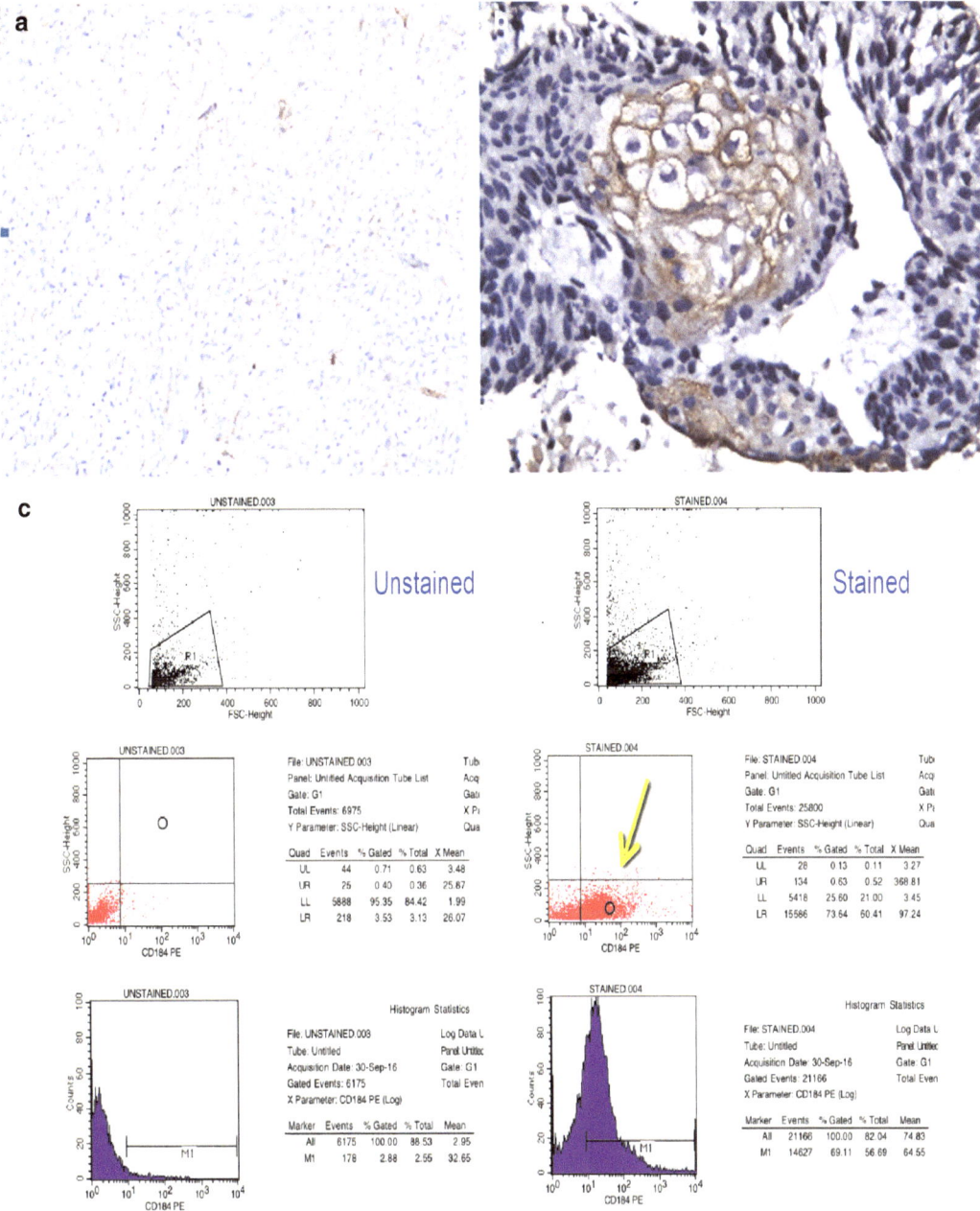

Fig. 31.2 Immuohistochemistry (IHC) analysis showing no stained cells in a control slide (**a**) and slide demonstrating stained CXCR4+ tumor cells (**b**) and quantitative FACS analysis (**c**) showing fractions of unstained and stained cells (CXCR4+ tumor cells) in a SCLC patient

technique can thus be used for lung cancer disease assessment and for patient selection for appropriate CXCR inhibitor therapies and, especially, α/β-targeted radionuclide therapies. Further, this novel PET tracer has the potential of becoming a powerful tool for monitoring therapy response to CXCR4 inhibitors and also for the development of emerging alpha/beta-targeted therapies in advanced stage lung carcinoma.

31.3 CXCR4-Targeted PET Imaging in Multiple Myeloma

Multiple myeloma (MM) is characterized by the clonal proliferation of malignant plasma cells and accounts for 1.0% of all the cancers and 10.0% of all the hematological malignancies [48, 49]. MM patients often present with skeletal and renal involvement and immunodeficiency [50]. Despite significant advances in treatment for MM, most patients will eventually go into relapse or become refractory to the chemotherapeutic interventions [51]. Therefore, the prognosis for MM patients remains poor and the 5-year survival rate is around 45.0% [52]. This underscores the need to properly understand the tumor biology and find new targets for diagnosis and treatment of MM [53]. ^{18}F-FDG PET has a proven role in the diagnosis, staging, response assessment, and management of MM [54, 55]. However, ^{18}F-FDG PET has its own limitations, as a significant decrease in the SUV_{max} value (versus the baseline value) on the post-therapy follow-up has been reported to be not correlating with the progression-free survival [56].

The clinical utility of ^{68}Ga-Pentixafor PET/CT imaging for in vivo imaging of CXCR4 whole-body disease burden has been reported in few recent studies. ^{68}Ga-Pentixafor as a novel PET tracer having high affinity for CXCR4 has been shown to be superior or equal to ^{18}F-FDG for the detection of myeloma lesions [57–59]. Herrmann et al. [23] in their first preliminary clinical experience reported that after disease mapping with ^{68}Ga-Pentixafor PET/CT, CXCR4-targeted radiotherapy with Pentixather appears to be a promising novel treatment option in combination with cytotoxic chemotherapy and autologous stem cell transplantation, especially for patients with advanced multiple myeloma. Therefore, ^{68}Ga-Pentixafor/^{177}Lu/^{90}Y-Pentixather is emerg-

ing as a potential theranostics' pair for treatment of CXCR4-targeting therapies when other available treatment options in advanced stage MM patients have failed.

Our experience [59] with ^{68}Ga-Pentixafor PET/CT in MM at PGIMER, Chandigarh, India, showed a higher lesion detection rate with ^{68}Ga-Pentixafor PET compared to ^{18}F-FDG PET (Fig. 31.3). We concluded that the dual tracer imaging may provide additional information on spatial and temporal heterogeneity of MM and may have significance for response evaluation to CXCR4-targeting pharmacologic or endo-radiotherapeutic therapies in CXCR4-positive and FDG-negative disease variants of multiple myeloma. In a recent study [60] in 30 MM patients, ^{68}Ga-Pentixafor PET/CT showed a higher positive disease detection rate than ^{18}F-FDG PET/CT (93.3 vs. 53.3%, $p = 0.005$). They further observed that the bone marrow tracer uptake of ^{68}Ga-Pentixafor correlated positively ($p < 0.05$) with the end organ damage, staging, and laboratory markers of tumor disease burden including serum β2-microglobulin, serum-free light chain, and 24 h urine light chain. They concluded that ^{68}Ga-Pentixafor PET/CT is a promising tracer in the assessment of newly diagnosed MM patients. The application of ^{68}Ga-Pentixafor PET/CT in other hematological malignancies is emerging. In a recent study by Luo et al., the application of ^{68}Ga-Pentixafor PET/CT was expanded in patients with Waldenstrom macroglobulinemia/lymphoplas-macytic lymphoma (WM/LPL) and compared results with ^{18}F-FDG PET/CT [61]. ^{18}F-FDG PET/CT has limitations in the evaluation of WM/LPL which is an indolent B-cell lymphoma and primarily involves the bone marrow. They reported that ^{68}Ga-Pentixafor PET/CT had a higher positive rate for disease detection than ^{18}F-FDG PET/CT (100.0% vs. 58.8%; $p = 0.023$).

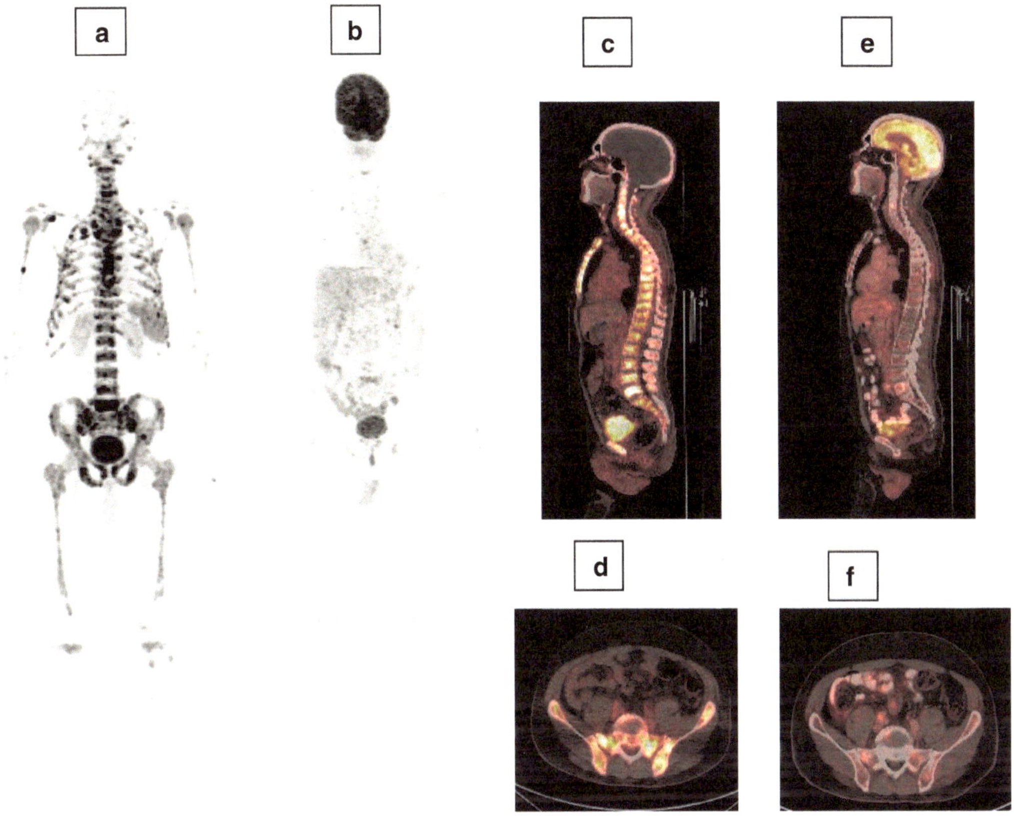

Fig. 31.3 ^{68}Ga-Pentixafor PET/CT in a 60-year-old man with mutiple myeloma and diffuse bony pains. PET/CT images show diffuse and focal tracer uptake in the axial and appendicular skeleton (MIP image **a**), fused PET/CT (trans-axial **c**, sagittal **d**) images show diffuse and focal increased tracer uptake in multiple marrow and lytic skeletal lesions. The corresponding ^{18}F-FDG PET/CT images (**e**, **f**) did not show any abnormal uptake in marrow and anywhere in the skeleton

31.4 CXCR4-Targeted PET Imaging in Glioblastoma Multiforme (GBM)

Gliomas are the most common primary tumors of the central nervous system (CNS) with a reported annual incidence of 20.5/100,000 [62]. Glioblastoma multiforme (GBM) usually have a infiltrative pattern of growth, and surgery is often incomplete, so radiotherapy with or without concurrent chemotherapy has become part of the current treatment regimens to significantly improve the survival in such patients [63]. In the post-surgery/chemoradiation follow-up of glioma, an accurate identification of the disease recurrence and radiation necrosis is important as the treat-ment strategy for recurrence warrants a change in treatment, whereas radiation necrosis will require continuation of the standard treatment [64]. So, there is a need for noninvasive imaging techniques for the accurate differentiation of tumor necrosis from recurrence and for response assessment to chemoradiation [65, 66].

Over the past few decades, different amino acid-based PET tracers, such as ^{18}F-fluoro-ethyl-tyrosine (^{18}F-FET), ^{18}F-fluoro-choline (^{18}F-FCH), and ^{11}C-methionine (^{11}C-MET) have been used in targeting various metabolic and molecular pathways that may add valuable diagnostic information especially in clinically challenging situations to improve diagnosis, detect tumor extent, and to help in therapy planning [67]. Among these tracers, ^{11}C-MET is one of the most extensively investigated PET tracers in the diagnostic workup of glioma. ^{11}C-MET accumulates extensively in proliferating tumors by the mechanism of increased amino acid transport and protein synthesis [68]. Undoubtedly, ^{18}F-FDG PET/CT is not of much use in GBM and all other PET tracers have their own limitations in terms of logistical and cumbersome radiolabeling issues. Therefore, alternative tracers which are easy to synthesize and can be made widely available widely with "ready to label" strategies are needed for the accurate detection and postsurgical/chemoradiation follow-up in GBM.

There has been growing evidence that CXCR4 is overexpressed in GBM and is associated with tumor angiogenesis as well as associated with poor survival outcomes [7–9, 69, 70]. It has also been shown in animal xenograft models that treatment with CXCR4 antagonist significantly inhibits tumorigenicity and tumor growth and proliferation [71]. The latter suggests that CXCR4 may play a crucial role in promoting the growth of gliomas in humans. Therefore, the CXCR4/CXCL12 axis represents a highly relevant molecular target of cancer biology and offers promising new approaches and techniques for targeted cancer therapy [72, 73].

In a recent study [74], ^{68}Ga-Pentixafor PET/CT was used for the detection of primary/recurrent glioma in 15 patients. In this pilot study, the tracer retention was noted in the vast majority of patients, and histological analysis from the tumor areas with high ^{68}Ga-Pentixafor uptake confirmed the CXCR4 expression. On the other hand, regions of the same tumor without apparent tracer uptake showed no or low receptor expression. Further, in this study, head-to-head comparison with ^{18}F-FET PET/CT in 11/15 cases showed similar SUV_{mean} and SUV_{max} values of the two tracers; however, the TBR (target-to-background ratio) for SUV_{mean} and SUV_{max} values were higher for ^{68}Ga-pentixafor by multiples of 37 and 19, thereby resulting in excellent image contrast. It was concluded in this study that ^{68}Ga-Pentixafor PET served as readout for visualization of intracranial CXCR4 expression which might prove as a useful theranostic tool for sensitive noninvasive in vivo quantification of CXCR4 tumor pheno-

typing. The latter may serve as a useful guide for prognostication and selection of patients who might benefit from CXCR4-directed therapies including β/α radionuclide therapies.

We conducted a pilot study [75] at PGIMER, Chandigarh, India, using ^{68}Ga-Pentixafor PET/CT for quantitative imaging of CXCR4 expression in 28 GBM patients having clinical suspicion of recurrent/residual disease. All the patients received radical radiotherapy (54.0–60.0 Gy) after surgery with or without concurrent temozolomide as indicated and underwent ^{68}Ga-Pentixafor PET/CT and conventional ceMRI of the brain. ^{68}Ga-Pentixafor PET/CT findings with focally increased uptake of the radiotracer were interpreted as positive for recurrent/residual disease in 13/14 patients. The mean SUV_{max} value in these patients ($n = 13$) was 5.25 ± 2.07 (range: 2.71–9.69). PET/CT findings were concurrent with MRI findings in all the 14 patients. A representative ^{68}Ga-Pentixafor PET image in a patient (58 yrs., female) with recurrent tumor in central primary GBM disease showing intense uptake of the radiotracer ($SUV_{max} = 7.9$) is presented in Fig. 31.4. The only (1/14) patient who had no focal uptake anywhere in the brain on ^{68}Ga-Pentixafor PET was interpreted as negative

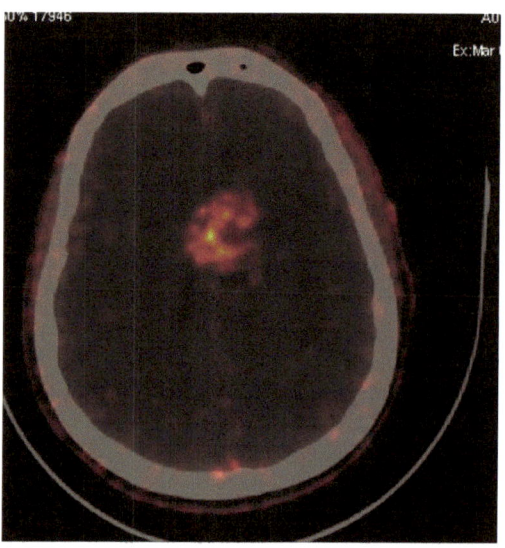

Fig. 31.4 ^{68}Ga-Pentixafor PET/CT in a 58-year-old woman with recurrent centrally located primary GBM (lateral ventricular region) showing intense uptake of the radiotracer ($SUV_{max} = 7.9$) and an excellent tumor to background contrast

for any residual/recurrent disease. The ceMRI finding in this patient was also negative and was reported as gliosis. The results of this preliminary study demonstrated that ^{68}Ga-Pentixafor PET imaging in GBM (known to have high CXCR4 expression) is viewed to open up new theranostics applications (with beta and alpha radionuclides) for long-term survival benefits. However, the diagnostic utility of this tracer needs to be validated in a large cohort of patients through multicentric trials.

31.5 Conclusion

CXCR4 and its ligand CXCL12 are intricately involved in the growth and proliferation of both solid tumors as well as hematologic malignancies. Noninvasive assessment of CXCR4 expression by PET/CT imaging can provide a useful tool in the management of a variety of oncologic conditions, both in terms of diagnostic and theranostic capabilities. Solid malignancies such as lung, breast, brain, prostate, and colorectal cancer and hematologic malignancies such as multiple myeloma, Waldenstrom macroglobulinemia, acute and chronic leukemia, and non-Hodgkin's lymphoma have shown to overexpress CXCR4. Further large and prospectively planned studies can explore the diagnostic performance of ^{68}Ga-Pentixafor PET/CT versus the conventional imaging techniques.

The need of the hour in aggressive malignancies such as glioblastoma multiforme is the development of novel therapies that can prolong survival, improve quality of life, and potentially offer a cure in these patients. Radionuclide therapies, such as intralesional injection of ^{213}Bi-labled substance-P in GBM has shown some promising results [76]. In this context, the increased expression of CXCR4 in GBM has been utilized to develop novel peptide-based theranostics with beta/alpha emitters [77, 78]. This approach may expand our future PRRT armamentarium in GBM healthcare as an alternative to radio-immunotherapy.

References

1. Mankoff DA, Link JM, Linden HM, Sundararajan L, Krohn KA. Tumor receptor imaging. J Nucl Med. 2008;49(4):149S–63S.
2. Sarvaiya PJ, Guo D, Ulasov I, Gabikian P, Lesniak MS. Chemokines in tumor progression and metastasis. Oncotarget. 2013;4(12):2171–85.
3. Furusato B, Mohamed A, Uhlén M, Rhim JS. CXCR4 and cancer. Pathol Int. 2010;60(7):497–505.
4. Zlotnik A, Burkhardt AM, Homey B. Homeostatic chemokine receptors and organ-specific metastasis. Nat Rev Immunol. 2011;11(9):597–606.
5. Bleul CC, Farzan M, Choe H, Parolin C, Clark-Lewis I, Sodroski J, et al. The lymphocyte chemoattractant SDF-1 is a ligand for LESTR/fusin and blocks HIV-1 entry. Nature. 1996;382(6594):829–33.
6. Burger JA, Stewart DJ, Wald O, Peled A. Potential of CXCR4 antagonists for the treatment of metastatic lung cancer. Expert Rev Anticancer Ther. 2011;11(4):621–30.
7. Balkwill FR. The chemokine system and cancer. J Pathol. 2012;226:48–57.
8. Fulton AM. The chemokine receptors CXCR4 and CXCR3 in cancer. Curr Oncol Rep. 2009;11:125–31.
9. Jiang YP, Wu XH, Shi B, Wu WX, Yin GR. Expression of chemokine CXCL12 and its receptor CXCR4 in human epithelial ovarian cancer: an independent prognostic factor for tumor progression. Gynecol Oncol. 2006;103:226–33.
10. Liao WC, Wang HP, Huang HY, Wu MS, Chiang H, Tien YW, et al. CXCR4 expression predicts early liver recurrence and poor survival after resection of pancreatic adenocarcinoma. Clin Transl Gastroenterol. 2012;3:e22.
11. Kuil J, Buckle T, van Leeuwen FW. Imaging agents for the chemokine receptor 4 (CXCR4). Chem Soc Rev. 2012;41:5239–61.
12. Domanska UM, Kruizinga RC, Nagengast WB, Timmer-Bosscha H, Huls G, de Vries EG, et al. A review on CXCR4/CXCL12 axis in oncology: no place to hide. Eur J Cancer. 2013;49(1):219–30.
13. Nguyen QD, Aboagye EO. Imaging the life and death of tumors in living subjects: preclinical PET imaging of proliferation and apoptosis. Integr Biol. 2010;2:483–95.
14. Gourni E, Demmer O, Schottelius M, D'Alessandria C, Schulz S, Dijkgraaf I, et al. PET of CXCR4 expression by a (68)Ga-labeled highly specific targeted contrast agent. J Nucl Med. 2011;52(11):1803–10.
15. Wester HJ, Keller U, Schottelius M, Beer A, Philipp-Abbrederis K, Hoffmann F, et al. Disclosing the CXCR4 expression in lymphoproliferative diseases by targeted molecular imaging. Theranostics. 2015;5(6):618–30.
16. Herrmann K, Lapa C, Wester HJ, Schottelius M, Schiepers C, Eberlein U, et al. Biodistribution and

radiation dosimetry for the chemokine receptor CXCR4-targeting probe 68Ga-Pentixafor. J Nucl Med. 2015;56(3):410–6.

17. Schultz MK, Donahue P, Musgrave NI, Zhernosekov K, Naidoo K, Razbash A, et al. An increasing role for 68Ga-PET imaging: a perspective on the availability of parent 68Ge material for generator manufacturing in an expanding market. Postgrad Med Edu Res. 2013;47(1):26–30.

18. Roesch F. Maturation of a key resource - the germanium-68/gallium-68 generator: development and new insights. Curr Radiopharm. 2012;5(3):202–11.

19. Buchmann I, Henze M, Engelbrecht S, Eisenhut M, Runz A, Schafer M, et al. Comparison of 68Ga-DOTATOC PET and 111In-DTPAOC (Octreoscan) SPECT in patients with neuroendocrine tumours. Eur J Nucl Med Mol Imaging. 2007;34(10):1617–26.

20. Prata MI. Gallium-68: a new trend in PET Radiopharmacy. Curr Radiopharm. 2012;5(2):142–9.

21. Vag T, Gerngross C, Herhaus P, Eiber M, Philipp-Abbrederis K, Graner FP, et al. First experience with chemokine receptor CXCR4-targeted PET imaging of patients with solid cancers. J Nucl Med. 2016;57(5):741–6.

22. Lapa C, Lückerath K, Rudelius M, Schmid JS, Schoene A, Schirbel A, et al. [68Ga]-Pentixafor-PET/CT for imaging of chemokine receptor 4 expression in small cell lung cancer--initial experience. Oncotarget. 2016;7(8):9288–95.

23. Herrmann K, Schottelius M, Lapa C, Osl T, Poschenrieder A, Hänscheid H, et al. First-in-human experience of CXCR4 directed Endoradiotherapy with 177Lu- and 90Y-labeled Pentixather in advanced-stage multiple myeloma with extensive intra and extramedullary disease. J Nucl Med. 2016;57(2):248–51.

24. Demmer O, Gourni E, Schumacher U, Kessler H, Wester HJ. PET imaging of CXCR4 receptors in cancer by a new optimized ligand. Chem Med Chem. 2011;6(10):1789–91.

25. Singh N, Aggarwal AN, Gupta D, Behera D, Jindal SK. Unchanging clinico-epidemiological profile of lung cancer in North India over three decades. Cancer Epidemiol. 2010;34:101–4.

26. Behera D, Balamugesh T. Lung cancer in India. Indian J Chest Dis Allied Sci. 2004;46:269–81.

27. Singh N, Aggarwal AN, Gupta D, Behera D, Jindal SK. Quantified smoking status and non-small cell lung cancer stage at presentation: analysis of a north Indian cohort and a systematic review of literature. J Thorac Dis. 2012;4:474–84.

28. Singh N, Mootha VK, Madan K, Aggarwal AN, Behera D. Tumor cavitation among lung cancer patients receiving first-line chemotherapy at a tertiary care Centre in India: association with histology and overall survival. Med Oncol. 2013;30:602.

29. Jemal A, Siegel R, Xu J, Ward E. Cancer statistics, 2010. CA Cancer J Clin. 2010;60(5):277–300.

30. Pao W, Girard N. New driver mutations in non-small-cell lung cancer. Lancet Oncol. 2011;12(2):175–80.

31. Pao W, Hutchinson KE. Chipping away at the lung cancer genome. Nat Med. 2012;18(3):349–51.

32. Alberg AJ, Ford JG, Samet JM. Epidemiology of lung cancer: ACCP evidence-based clinical practice guidelines. Chest. 2007;132(3 Suppl):29S–55S.

33. Siegel R, Desantis C, Virgo K, Stein K, Mariotto A, Smith T, et al. Cancer treatment and survivorship statistics, 2012. CA Cancer J Clin. 2012;62(4):220–41.

34. Spiro SG, Silvestri GA. One hundred years of lung cancer. Am J Respir Crit Care Med. 2005;172(5):523–9.

35. Barker JM, Silvestri GA. Lung cancer staging. Curr Opin Pulm Med. 2002;8:287–93.

36. Cuaron J, Dunphy M, Rimner A. Role of FDG-PET scans in staging, response assessment, and follow-up care for non-small cell lung cancer. Front Oncol. 2013;2:208.

37. Gupta NC, Graeber GM, Rogers JS, Bishop HA. Comparative efficacy of positron emission tomography with FDG and computed tomographic scanning in preoperative staging of non-small cell lung cancer. Ann Surg. 1999;229:286–91.

38. Weber WA, Avril N, Schwaiger M. Relevance of positron emission tomography (PET) in oncology. Strahlenther Onkol. 1999;175:356–73.

39. Marom EM, McAdams HP, Erasmus JJ, Goodman PC, Culhane DK, Coleman RE, et al. Staging non-small cell lung cancer with whole-body PET. Radiology. 1999;212:803–9.

40. Bhoil A, Singh B, Singh N, Kashyap R, Watts A, Sarika S, et al. Can 3′-deoxy-3′-(18)F-fluorothymidine or 2′-deoxy-2′-(18)F-fluoro-d-glucose PET/CT better assess response after 3-weeks treatment by epidermal growth factor receptor kinase inhibitor, in non-small lung cancer patients? Preliminary results. Hell J Nucl Med. 2014;17(2):90–6.

41. Sohn HJ, Yang YJ, Ryu JS, Oh SJ, Im KC, Moon DH, et al. 18F-Fluorothymidine positron emission tomography before and 7 days after Gefitinib: treatment predicts response in patients with advanced adenocarcinoma of the lung. Clin Cancer Res. 2008;14:7423–9.

42. Phillips RJ, Burdick MD, Lutz M, Belperio JA, Keane MP, Strieter RM. The stromal derived factor-1/CXCL12-CXC chemokine receptor 4 biological axis in non-small cell lung cancer metastases. Am J Respir Crit Care Med. 2003;167(12):1676–86.

43. Hartmann TN, Burger JA, Glodek A, Fujii N, Burger M. CXCR4 chemokine receptor and integrin signaling co-operate in mediating adhesion and chemoresistance in small cell lung cancer (SCLC) cells. Oncogene. 2005;24:4462–47.

44. Sethi T, Rintoul RC, Moore SM, MacKinnon AC, Salter D, Choo C, et al. Extracellular matrix proteins protect small cell lung cancer cells against apoptosis: a mechanism for small cell lung cancer growth and drug resistance in vivo. Nat Med. 1999;5:662–8.

45. Spano J, Andre F, Morat L, Sabatier L, Besse B, Combadiere C, et al. Chemokine receptor CXCR4 and early-stage non-small cell lung cancer: pattern of expression and correlation with outcome. Ann Oncol. 2004;15:613–7.

46. Watts A, Singh B, Basher R, Singh H, Bal A, Kapoor R, et al. 68Ga-Pentixafor PET/CT demonstrating higher CXCR4 density in small cell lung carcinoma than in non-small cell variant. Eur J Nucl Med Mol Imaging. 2017;44(5):909–10.

47. Watts A, Singh B, Singh H, Bal A, Kaur H, Dhanota N, et al. (68Ga)Ga-Pentixafor PET/CT imaging for in vivo CXCR4 receptor mapping in different lung cancer histologic sub-types: correlation with quantitative receptors' density by immunochemistry techniques. Eur J Nucl Med Mol Imaging. 2023;50:1216–27.

48. Raab MS, Podar K, Breitkreutz I, Richardson PG, Anderson KC. Multiple myeloma. Lancet. 2009;374(9686):324–39.

49. Jemal A, Clegg LX, Ward E, Ries LA, Wu X, Jamison PM, et al. Annual report to the nation on the status of cancer, 1975–2001, with a special feature regarding survival. Cancer. 2004;101(1):3–27.

50. Hanrahan CJ, Christensen CR, Crim JR. Current concepts in the evaluation of multiple myeloma with MR imaging and FDG PET/CT. Radiographics. 2010;30(1):127–42.

51. Laubach JP, Mahindra A, Mitsiades CS, Schlossman RL, Munshi NC, Ghobrial IM, et al. The use of novel agents in the treatment of relapsed and refractory multiple myeloma. Leukemia. 2009;23(12):2222–32.

52. Lütje S, de Rooy JW, Croockewit S, Koedam E, Oyen WJ, Raymakers RA. Role of radiography, MRI and FDG-PET/CT in diagnosing, staging and therapeutical evaluation of patients with multiple myeloma. Ann Hematol. 2009;88(12):1161–8.

53. Domanska UM, Kruizinga RC, Nagengast WB, Timmer-Bosscha H, Huls G, de Vries EG, Walenkamp AM. A review on CXCR4/CXCL12 axis in oncology: no place to hide. Eur J Cancer. 2013;49(1):219–30.

54. Bartel TB, Haessler J, Brown TL, Shaughnessy JD, van Rhee F, Anaissie E, et al. F18-fluorodeoxyglucose positron emission tomography in the context of other imaging techniques and prognostic factors in multiple myeloma. Blood. 2009;114(10):2068–76.

55. Dimitrakopoulou-Strauss A, Hoffmann M, Bergner R, Uppenkamp M, Haberkorn U, Strauss LG. Prediction of progression-free survival in patients with multiple myeloma following anthracycline-based chemotherapy based on dynamic FDG-PET. Clin Nucl Med. 2009;34(9):576–84.

56. Bredella MA, Steinbach L, Caputo G, Segall G, Hawkins R. Value of FDG PET in the assessment of patients with multiple myeloma. AJR Am J Roentgenol. 2005;184(4):1199–204.

57. Philipp-Abbrederis K, Herrmann K, Knop S, Schottelius M, Eiber M, Lückerath K, et al. In vivo molecular imaging of chemokine receptor CXCR4 expression in patients with advanced multiple myeloma. EMBO Mol Med. 2015;7(4):477–87.

58. Lapa C, Schreder M, Schirbel A, Samnick S, Kortüm KM, Herrmann K, et al. [68Ga]Pentixafor-PET/CT for imaging of chemokine receptor CXCR4 expression in multiple myeloma - comparison to [18F]FDG and laboratory values. Theranostics. 2017;7(1):205–12.

59. Shekhawat AS, Singh B, Malhotra P, et al. Imaging CXCR4 receptors expression for staging multiple myeloma by using 68Ga-Pentixafor PET/CT: comparison with 18F-FDG PET/CT. Br J Radiol. 2022;95:20211272.

60. Pan Q, Cao X, Luo Y, Li J, Feng J, Li F. Chemokine receptor-4 targeted PET/CT with 68Ga-Pentixafor in assessment of newly diagnosed multiple myeloma: comparison to 18F-FDG PET/CT. Eur J Nucl Med Mol Imaging. 2020;47(3):537–46.

61. Luo Y, Cao X, Pan Q, Li J, Feng J, Li F. 68Ga-Pentixafor PET/CT for imaging of chemokine receptor 4 expression in Waldenström Macroglobulinemia/Lymphoplasmacytic lymphoma: comparison to 18F-FDG PET/CT. J Nucl Med. 2019;60(12):1724–9.

62. Jessen KR. Glial cells. Int J Biochem Cell Biol. 2004;36:1861–7.

63. Ahmed R, Oborski MJ, Hwang M, Lieberman FS, Mountz JM. Malignant gliomas: current perspectives in diagnosis, treatment, and early response assessment using advanced quantitative imaging methods. Cancer Manag Res. 2014;6:149–70.

64. Parvez K, Parvez A, Zadeh G. The diagnosis and treatment of pseudoprogression, radiation necrosis and brain tumor recurrence. Int J Mol Sci. 2014;15:11832–46.

65. Kumar AJ, Leeds NE, Fuller GN, Van Tassel P, Maor MH, Sawaya RE, et al. Malignant gliomas: MR imaging spectrum of radiation therapy- and chemotherapy-induced necrosis of the brain after treatment. Radiology. 2000;217:377–84.

66. Deng SM, Zhang B, Wu YW, Zhang W, Chen YY. Detection of glioma recurrence by 11C-methionine positron emission tomography and dynamic susceptibility contrast-enhanced magnetic resonance imaging: a meta-analysis. Nucl Med Commun. 2013;34:758–66.

67. Huang C, McConathy J. Radiolabeled amino acids for oncologic imaging. J Nucl Med. 2013;54:1007–10.

68. Okubo S, Zhen HN, Kawai N, Nishiyama Y, Haba R, Tamiya T. Correlation of L-methyl-11 C-methionine (MET) uptake with L-type amino acid transporter 1 in human gliomas. J Neuro-Oncol. 2010;99:217–25.

69. Tabouret E, Tchoghandjian A, Denicolai E, Delfino C, Metellus P, Graillon T, et al. Recurrence of glioblastoma after radio-chemotherapy is associated with an angiogenic switch to the CXCL12-CXCR4 pathway. Oncotarget. 2015;6(13):11664–75.

70. Bian XW, Yang SX, Chen JH, Ping YF, Zhou XD, Wang QL, et al. Preferential expression of chemokine receptor CXCR4 by highly malignant human gliomas and its association with poor patient survival. Neurosurgery. 2007;61(3):570–8.

71. Rubin JB, Kung AL, Klein RS, Chan JA, Sun Y, Schmidt K, et al. A small-molecule antagonist of CXCR4 inhibits intracranial growth of primary brain tumors. Proc Natl Acad Sci U S A. 2003;100(23):13513–8.

72. Uy GL, Rettig MP, Motabi IH, McFarland K, Trinkaus KM, Hladnik LM, et al. A phase 1/2 study of chemo-sensitization with the CXCR4 antagonist plerixafor in relapsed or refractory acute myeloid leukemia. Blood. 2012;119:3917–24.

73. Kuhne MR, Mulvey T, Belanger B, Chen S, Pan C, Chong C, et al. BMS-936564/MDX-1338: a fully human anti-CXCR4 antibody induces apoptosis in vitro and shows antitumor activity in vivo in hematologic malignancies. Clin Can Res. 2013;19:357–66.

74. Lapa C, Lückerath K, Kleinlein I, Monoranu CM, Linsenmann T, Kessler AF, et al. (68) Ga-Pentixafor-PET/CT for imaging of chemokine receptor 4 expression in glioblastoma. Theranostics. 2016;6(3):428–34.

75. Watts A, Arora D, Kumar N, Thakur S, Basher R, Radotra B, et al. 68Ga-Pentixafor PET/CT offers high contrast image for the detection of CXCR4 expres-sion in recurrent glioma. J Nucl Med. 2019;60(suppl 1):491.

76. Krolicki L, Bruchertseifer F, Kunikowska J, Koziara H, Królicki B, Jakuciński M, et al. Prolonged survival in secondary glioblastoma following local injection of targeted alpha therapy with ^{213}Bi-substance P analogue. Eur J Nucl Med Mol Imaging. 2018;45(9):1636–44.

77. Schottelius M, Osl T, Poschenrieder A, Hoffmann F, Beykan S, Hänscheid H, et al. [177Lu] -pentixather: comprehensive preclinical characterization of a first CXCR4-directed endoradiotherapeutic agent. Theranostics. 2017;7(9):2350–62.

78. Buck AK, Stolzenburg A, Hänscheid H, Schirbel A, Lückerath K, Schottelius M, Wester HJ, Lapa C. Chemokine receptor—directed imaging and ther-apy. Methods. 2017;130:63–71.

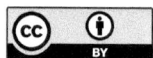

Mathew L. Thakur

32.1 Introduction

Cancer is complex yet commonplace, and the most terrifying disease of mankind. Among men in the USA, prostate cancer (PCa) is particularly lethal, second only to cancers of the lung and bronchus combined [1]. In 2020, more than 30,000 men will succumb to PCa, and more than 240,000 new PCa cases will be identified in the USA alone [1]. PCa affects one in every 6 men who are 60 years or older and affects African-Americans at a rate 2.4 times greater than European-Americans [1].

To treat these patients effectively, clinicians have a large array of options. However, even the novel agents such as abiraterone and enzalutamide offer only a limited survival benefit to the patients. For patients with skeletal metastases, FDA-approved Radium-223 chloride, (Xofigo) enhances the survival for up to 3.6 months. Furthermore Ra-223 chloride targets only osteoblastic lesions and does not provide effective treatment to visceral or nodal metastatic lesions. A continued search for more effective treatment has recently led to the development of a theranostic agent Lutetium-177-PSMA-617 (Lu-177-PSMA-617), although not yet approved by FDA for use in the USA, is being commonly used in

many continents such as Europe, Asia, Australia and South Africa. At the time of this writing, the agent is in clinical trials in the USA. With three or more cycles of Lu-177-PSMA-617 treatments of approximately 7.4 GBq (200 mCi) each, progression-free survival of up to 13.6 months has been reported [2]. The best success of the Lu-177-PSMA-617 treatment consists of >50% PSA decline in 45% of the patients, partial regression in 56%, stable disease in 7% and progressive disease in 3.6% of the patients [2–4]. Progression-free survival for 3.6 months to 13.7 months has also been reported [2–4].

Although the results are encouraging, several weaknesses of Lu-177-PSMA-617 treatment have surfaced. First, PSMA is expressed only on 80% to 85% of PCa which requires patient to be screened, for PSMA expression using Ga-68-PSMA-11 PET scan. Second, extensive uptake of Lu-177-PSMA-617 in salivary glands leaves most patients with mild-to-severe xerostomia to minimize which some investigators have chosen to block the uptake using botulinum toxin (another pre-Lu-177-PSMA-617 treatment procedure). Third, considerable myelocytic toxicity and fatigue have been also reported in patients receiving Lu-177-PSMA-617. Fourth, Lu-177-PSMA-617 has approximately 75% renal excretion in 24 h, exerting radiation risk to renal medulla and bladder wall. Blocking renal uptake with certain amino acids prior to Lu-177-PSMA-617 treatment, a third pretreatment proce-

M. L. Thakur (✉)
Thomas Jefferson University, Philadelphia, PA, USA
e-mail: mathew.thakur@jefferson.edu

V. Prasad (ed.), *Beyond Becquerel and Biology to Precision Radiomolecular Oncology: Festschrift in Honor of Richard P. Baum*, https://doi.org/10.1007/978-3-031-33533-4_32

dure, has been also considered. Fifth, Lu-177 contains approximately 0.1% Lu-177 m as an impurity. Lu-177 m has a half-life of 110 days. The urinary excretion of up to 75% of injected Lu-177 m within 24 h together with the longer lived Lu-177 m creates a waste disposal problem particularly for those patients who are incontinent and wear diapers.

These issues, in addition to the pretreatment procedures, not only add to the treatment cost but are also undesirable to the patients already stressed emotionally and weakened physically. In addition, the PSMA treatment eliminates 15 to 20% of the needy PCa patients who do not express PSMA. Improved agents with similar or better therapeutic effectiveness but without the persistent weaknesses are desirable.

32.2   Our Approach

Our proposed approach to treat PCa, its metastases and recurrence is driven by targeting an endogenous genetic product overexpressed when cells suffer genetic mutations that ignite cancerous transformation. VPAC mediates VIP (vasoactive intestinal peptide) and PACAP (pituitary adenylate cyclase activating peptide) growth hormone function in all types of PCa irrespective of the PCa heterogeneity [5–9].

These characteristic fingerprints, the VPAC cell surface receptors, express themselves at the onset of the malignancy, and may be prior to the elevation of PSA, and well before the cell morphology is altered this forms the basis of histologic diagnosis [5]. However, the expression on malignant cell surface has not yet been investigated for treating PCa and its metastases. Over the past few years, we have developed a small radioactive molecule (Cu-64-TP3805) that has high-affinity (Kd 3.1×10^{-9} M) VPAC receptors expressed in high density on all PCa cells. Our PET imaging studies in humans have shown that Cu-64-TP3805 detects primary PCa, bone metastatic lesions, and malignant lymph nodes with >95% sensitivity [10–19]. Furthermore, the agent has no urinary excretion, has no salivary gland uptake, no bone marrow uptake, and only a small uptake in the renal cortex, not sensitive to radiation damage.

Copper-64 has other radionuclide, a beta-emitting Copper-67, (t½ 2.6 day, γ-185 KeV (40%) and βmax- 580 KeV) which can be easily used to synthesize Cu-67-TP3805 using a well-established procedure in our laboratory and can be used for theranostic applications in PCa patients. Since (1) the tissue range (0.6 mm) and the linear energy transfer for Cu-67 is the same as Lu-177,and since Cu-67-TP3805, will have (2) the same tissue distribution as that of Cu-64-TP-3805 with high uptake both in primary PCa and its metastatic lesions, (3) no urinary excretion, (4) no salivary gland uptake, and (5) since VPAC is expressed in high density on all PCa types, the Cu-67-TP3805 treatment will be readily applicable to all PCa patients without having to perform patient suitability examination or having to deliver any of the antitoxicity, preventive procedures. These virtues of Cu-67-TP3805 for theranostic applications are listed in Table 32.1.

Table 32.1 Theranostic Cu-67-TP3805 at a glance

Characteristics	Lu-177-PSMA	Cu-67-TP3805	Advantages of Cu-67-TP3805
Tissue range	0.6 mm	0.6mm	Same as Lu-177
Receptor expression on PCa type	80%–85%	100%	• No patient screening procedure required • 100% of the PCa patients can be treated
Tissue distribution			
Salivary gland	Yes	No	• No xenograft • No Botulinum Toxin pretreatment required
Renal	Yes (cortex and medulla)	Cortex only	• No renal damage • No amino acid treatment required
Bladder	Yes	No	• Primary PCa lesion can be diagnosed and treated
Metastatic lesions	Yes	Yes	• All distant metastatic lesions can be treated
Cancer stem cells	No	Yes	• Cancer stem cells can be targeted • Minimize recurrence

32.3 VPAC Receptor and Its Expression on PCa

VPAC, a genomic biomarker, belongs to the superfamily of G protein-coupled surface receptors which are expressed in high density (10^4–10^5/cell) on all PCa types cells at the onset of oncogenesis [20–25]. On stroma, normal cells and benign masses VPAC is minimally present (5–10/cell). Since VPAC receptors are expressed on all PCa, for theranostic use of Cu-67-TP3805, patient-qualifying screening studies, like those required with Lu-177-PSMA-617 treatment, will not be necessary.

Reubi and colleagues [6–9] examined more than 600 tumors and their metastases using immunohistochemistry and conclusively reported that VPAC and VPAC2 receptors are overexpressed on a variety of frequently occurring human tumors including those of the breast and prostate. On 100% of the human prostate tumors examined ($n = 35$), VPAC receptors were predominantly overexpressed on PCa tissues and VPAC2 on stroma, to a lesser extent. Although VPAC receptors exist on normal cells, their expression is lower than on malignant cells on which the receptor density is high.

A 28 amino acid peptide VIP has high affinity for VIP receptors and the 27 amino acid peptide PACAP has high affinity for VIP and PACAP1 combined. VPAC receptors are overexpressed on all PCa including metastatic lesions (Figs. 32.1, 32.2, 32.3 and 32.4). High expression of VPAC receptors ($>10^4$/cell) has been observed by others. Both VIP_{28} and $PACAP_{27}$ have high affinity for VPAC (VPAC and VPAC2 receptors) [6–9].

Therefore, we had hypothesized that radiolabeled VIP and PACAP1 or their analogues will provide us with excellent biomolecules for accurate and sensitive detection of human PCa. The probe can also detect metastases, and be used to determine therapeutic effectiveness.

Lu-177-PSMA **Cu-64-TP3805**

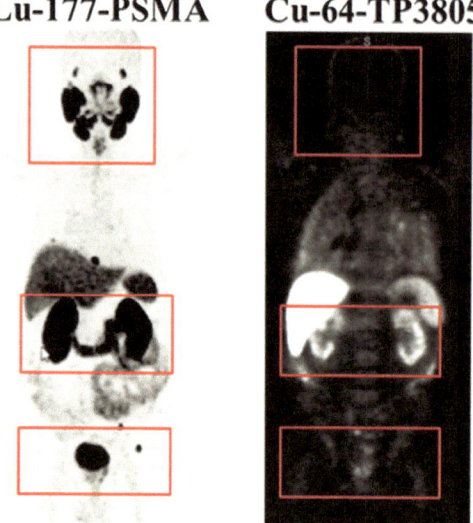

Fig. 32.1 Comparison of tissue distribution of Lu-177-PSMA and Cu-64-TP3805 (targeting VPAC)

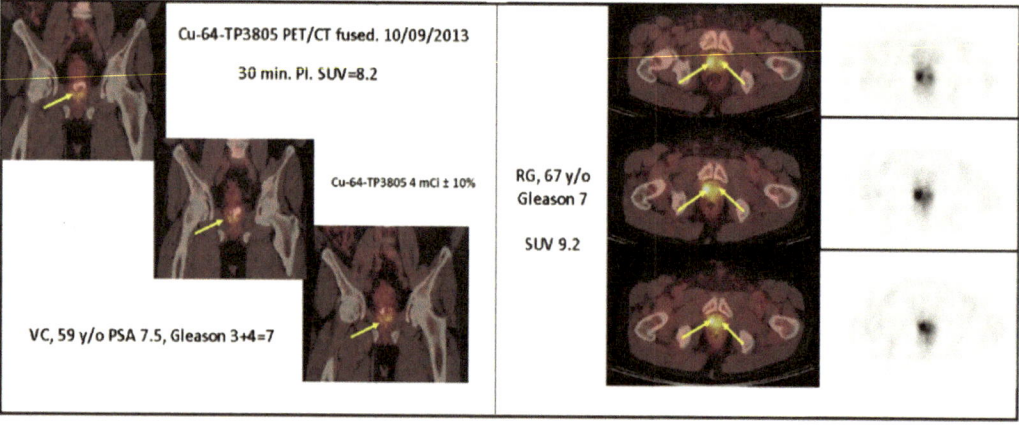

Fig. 32.2 PET images of two PCa patients (Gleason 3+4), 1 h post injection of approximately 4 mCi Cu-64-TP3805. Radical prostatectomy was performed 1 week later. Histology confirmed PCa malignancy

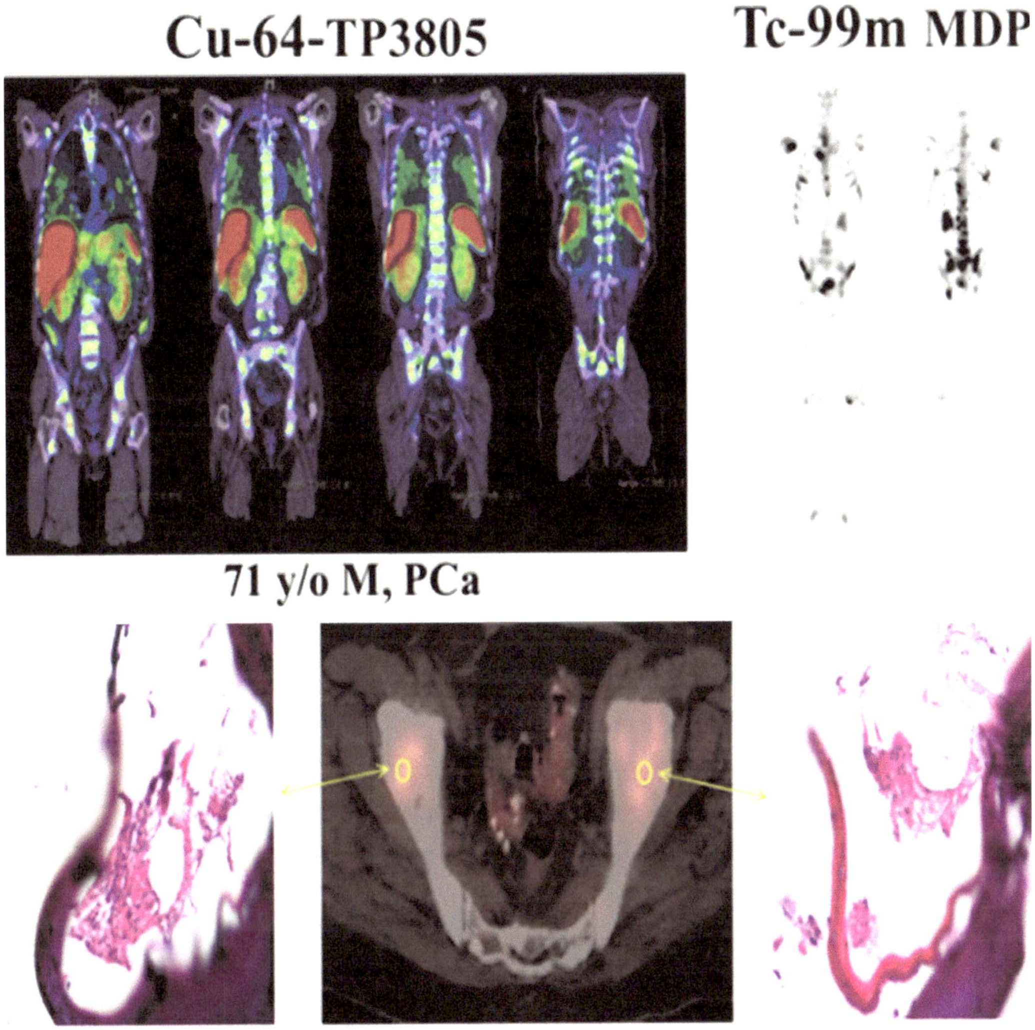

Cu-64-TP3805

Tc-99m MDP

71 y/o M, PCa

Fig. 32.3 A 70 year old male consented to the Cu-64-TP3805 PET imaging. Images showed multiple bone lesions secondary to his PCa. Histological examination of the bone biospy confirmed that the lesions were malignant

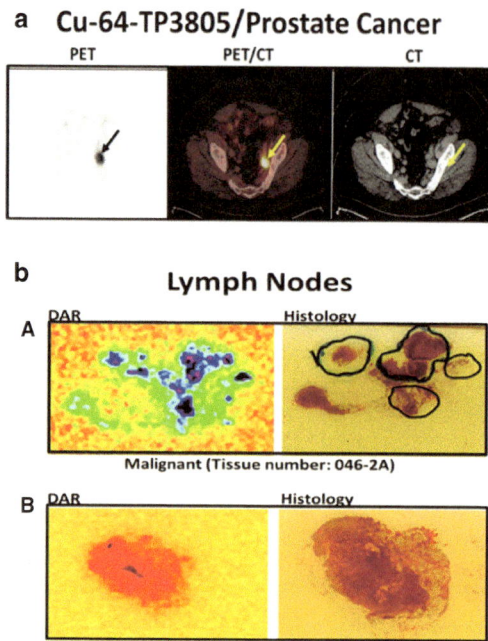

Fig. 32.4 (**a**) Cu-64-TP3805 PET imaging of small lymph node (arrow, SUVmax 7.15) in a 61 y/o PCa patient. (**b**) Digital auto radiography (DAR) of a malignant lymph node (A). Left panel shows Cu-64-TP3805 bound to malignant cells as confirmed by histology (right panel) of the same lymph node. (B) Left panel benign lymph node has no Cu-64-TP3805 uptake. Histology (right panel) shows absence of malignant cells

with I-123 successfully imaged a number of human tumors [31]. Following PACAP homology, these gene receptors are recently named VPAC (for VIP1 and PACAP2 combined) and VPAC2 (for VIP2 and PACAP3 combined). PACAP, a 38-amino acid peptide, isolated from bovine hypothalamus, was named PACAP because it stimulated the accumulation of intracellular and extracellular cAMP in monolayer cultures of rat anterior pituitary cells [20, 32]. PACAP, a neurotransmitter and member of the VIP family, is ten times more potent than VIP in stimulating adenylate cyclase in pituitary cells [32]. PACAP has three gene receptors, PACAP1, 2, and 3. Gottschall et al. [33] isolated 27-amino acid PACAP (PACAP$_{27}$) from bovine hypothalamus and concluded that PACAP$_{38}$ and PACAP$_{27}$ were equally active and derived from a single 176-amino acid precursor. PACAP$_{27}$, like VIP, has an amidated C-terminus and histidine at the N-terminus. Nineteen of the 27 amino acids of PACAP$_{27}$ are homologous. The fact that PACAP$_{27}$ recognizes and has high affinity (Kd = 1.5 nM) for both VIP and PACAP (VPAC) receptors that are overexpressed on PCa cells suggests that PACAP or its bioactive analogue may also be a suitable agent to image PCa [8, 10–17].

32.4 VIP, PACAP, and Their Analogues

VIP is a 28-amino acid peptide initially isolated from porcine intestine [26]. VIP, whose structure is common in humans, pigs and rats, is a hydrophobic, basic peptide that contains three lysine (position 13, 18, 19) and two arginine (position 12, 14) residues. From the essential histidine residue at the N-terminus to the amidated C terminus, all 28 amino acids of VIP are required for high-affinity binding and biological activity [27].

VIP gene receptors (VIP1 and VIP2) have been detected on the cell membrane of normal intestinal [28] and bronchial epithelial cells [21–23] and are overexpressed on various cancer cells, including colonic adenocarcinoma [23, 29], pancreatic carcinoma [30], and cancers of the prostate [6–9]. VIP (Tyr10 and Tyr22) labeled

32.5 Synthesis of N2(S-Benzyl)$_2$ Containing VIP and PACAP

We synthesized one analogue of VIP$_{28}$ (TP3939) and one of PACAP$_{27}$ (TP3805) that are more potent and biologically stable than VIP$_{28}$. Vasoactive intestinal peptide (VIP) bound to a C-terminal diaminodithiol (N$_2$S$_2$) chelator was synthesized on a Wang resin using ABI 341A peptide synthesizer (Applied Biosystems, Inc.) [10, 18]. The analogues were prepared, purified, and characterized by American Peptide Company (Sunnyvale, CA) and named after their molecular weights as TP3805 and TP3939. Although peptides have been conjugated with chelating agents such as DOTA (1, 4, 7, 10-tetraazadocdecane -N, N″, N′, N, −tetra acetic acid), it requires a prepared and pre-purified peptide to which DOTA is to be conjugated. The conjugated product then needs further purification and characterization. Preparation of our analogues is a one-step process that provides efficiency, saves time, and provides a N_2S_2 type of chelating moiety for strong chelation with Cu-64.

Our data show that these Cu-64 probes are highly stable in vivo [11, 12]. Furthermore, the high VIP affinity for receptors on malignant cells and subsequent internalization minimizes its proteolysis and allows cell detection, as we have demonstrated in both mice and humans [10–19, 34]. These analogues have the high IC50 values (4.4 nM and 5.3 nM, respectively) among the many that have been synthesized and evaluated [20, 32].

The rationale for choosing TP3939 analogues was as follows. VIP28 is comprised of three aromatic moieties at Phe6, Tyr10, and Tyr22, a negatively charged site at Asp3 and a lone pair structure at His1. Although all five sites are required for complete binding to receptors with high affinity, substitutions at position 22 of 3-OCH3–4-OH-Phe and Lys12, Nle17, Val26, Thr28-VIP produced the best results, increasing potency by four times (IC50 = 4.4 nM vs. 15 nM) over VIP_{28}. Higher affinity may enhance tumor uptake and improve image quality. Again, our recent preliminary data in humans, obtained using Tc-99 m-TP3654, a VIP analogue are consistent with this hypothesis [34].

32.6 Cu-64-TP3805 and Its Tissue Distribution in Humans

Cu-64-TP3805, designed and extensively validated in our receptors laboratory, has a high affinity (3.1×10^{-9} M) for VPAC receptors [10, 18, 19]. The agent is highly stable in vivo, has no urinary excretion, has no salivary gland uptake, and has renal uptake only in the cortex, resistant to radiation damage (Fig. 1). The hypothesis therefore is that by targeting VPAC receptors will eliminate (a) patient treatment qualifying PET imaging, (b) subsequent xerostomia without botulinum toxin pretreatment, and (c) reduce renal toxicity preventing renal pretreatment.

32.7 Ability of VPAC Target to Image Primary PCa, and Its Metastases in Bone and Lymph Nodes

Following targeting VPAC receptors, and validating our hypothesis in TRAMP (Transgenic Adenocarcinoma of the Mouse Prostate) mice, we have studied 45 patients with primary PCa and metastatic lesions by PET imaging with Cu-64-TP3805 [18]. As confirmed by postsurgical histology, all primary and metastatic lesions were imaged with >95% sensitivity (Figs. 32.2, 32.3 and 32.4). These data support the notion that VPAC is a highly suitable target for theranostic applications of Cu-67-TP3805 for treating PCa and its metastatic lesions.

32.8 Suitability of Cu-67 for Theranostic Application

Copper-67 is a commercially available, 2.6 day half-lived radionuclide that has radiation characteristics similar to that of Lu-177 (Table 32.2), including its β tissue range of 0.6 mm and linear energy transfer (LET). Since Cu-67 has the same chemical properties as that of Cu-64, we can prepare Cu-67-TP3805 using the same well-established procedure in our laboratory. Therefore, Copper-67, available commercially without longer lived radionuclide contamination,

Table 32.2 How does copper-67 compare with Lu-177?

	Cu-67	Lu-177
Half-life	**2.6 days**	6.7 days
Beta tissue range (Range × 90)	**0.6mm**	**0.6mm**
SPECT gamma	**YES (γ-185 KeV β⁻ 580 KeV)**	**YES (γ-208 KeV β⁻ 497 KeV)**
Theranostic PET same element	**YES**	**NO**
Hospitalization required	**NO**	**NO**
Production method	**Accelerator**	Reactor
Example radiopharmaceutical	Sartate™	Lutathera®

can be easily prepared as Cu-67-TP3805 and be effectively used to target VPAC receptors. The attractive radiation characteristics of Cu-67 have already drawn considerable attention leading to clinical trials treating neuroblastoma using SARTATE™ composed of Cu-67-labeled peptide, MeCOSar-Tyr3-octreatate [35] (Table 32.2).

Reflecting on the present, planning for the future and prompted by the highly encouraging results in our laboratory, our quest is to systematically investigate targeting VPAC receptors using beta-emitting Cu-67-TP3805 for theranostic applications of primary and metastatic PCa. In addition to the anticipated high benefit-to-risk ratio of Cu-67-TP3805 as a theranostic, VPAC receptors are expressed on many other oncologic diseases, such as the cancers of the breast, bladder, lung, ovary, and brain [6–9, 13, 17, 36, 37]. It is therefore, reasonable to postulate that Cu-67-TP3805 may serve as a useful theranostic agent to treat many other cancers as well.

Acknowledgments The author thanks Dr. Prof. Richard Baum and his colleagues for their pioneer role and leadership in the establishment the modern theranostic field in general and the PCa theranostic in particular. This book will serve as a compendium of the lifelong scholarly activities and collaborative research of Dr. Prof. Richard Baum in advancing medical science and treatment of oncologic diseases. We salute him and thank him for his decades of friendship.

The author also gratefully acknowledges the contributions of his colleagues in basic, preclinical, and translational clinical investigations in exploring the role of VPAC receptors in oncologic applications and the financial support of NIH (NCI), DOD and Thomas Jefferson University.

References

1. Cancer Facts & Figures 2019. American Cancer Society. 2019. https://www.cancer.org/content/dam/cancer-org/research/cancer-facts-and-statistics/annual-cancer-facts-and-figures/2019/cancer-facts-and-figures-2019.pdf.
2. Baum RP, Kulkarni HR, Schuchardt C, Singh A, Wirtz M, Wiessalla S, Schottelius M, Mueller D, Klette I, Wester H-J. 177Lu-labeled prostate-specific membrane antigen radioligand therapy of metastatic castration-resistant prostate cancer: safety and efficacy. J Nucl Med. 2016;57(7):1006–13. https://doi.org/10.2967/jnumed.115.168443.
3. McBean R, O'Kane B, Parsons R, Wong D. Lu177-PSMA therapy for men with advanced prostate cancer: initial 18 months experience at a single Australian tertiary institution. J Med Imaging Radiat Oncol. 2019;63:538. https://doi.org/10.1111/1754-9485.12891.
4. Turner JH. Recent advances in theranostics and challenges for the future. Br J Radiol. 2018;91(1091):20170893. https://doi.org/10.1259/bjr.20170893; Epub 2018/03/23. PubMed PMID: 29565650; PMCID: PMC6475948.
5. Lelievre VPN, Wasche JA. In: Vaudry HAA, editor. The biological significance of PACAP and PACAP receptors in human tumors: from cell lines to cancers. Springer Publishing Co.; 2003.
6. Reubi JC. In vitro identification of vasoactive intestinal peptide receptors in human tumors: implications for tumor imaging. J Nucl Med. 1995;36(10):1846–53.
7. Reubi JC, Laderach U, Waser B, Gebbers JO, Robberecht P, Laissue JA. Vasoactive intestinal peptide/pituitary adenylate cyclase-activating peptide receptor subtypes in human tumors and their tissues of origin. Cancer Res. 2000;60(11):3105–12.
8. Reubi JC. In vitro evaluation of VIP/PACAP receptors in healthy and diseased human tissues. Clinical implications. Ann N Y Acad Sci. 2000;921:1–25.
9. Reubi JC. Neuropeptide receptors in health and disease: the molecular basis for in vivo imaging. J Nucl Med. 1995;36(10):1825–35.
10. Thakur ML, Aruva MR, Gariepy J, Acton P, Rattan S, Prasad S, Wickstrom E, Alavi A. PET imaging of oncogene overexpression using 64Cu-vasoactive intestinal peptide (VIP) analog: comparison with 99mTc-VIP analog. J Nucl Med. 2004;45:1381–9.
11. Zhang KAM, Shanthly N, Cardi CA, Rattan S, Patel C, Kim C, McCue PA, Wickstrom E, Thakur ML. PET imaging of VPAC1 expression in experimental and spontaneous prostate cancer. J Nucl Med. 2008;49(1):112–21. https://doi.org/10.2967/jnumed.107.043703; PMCID: PMC5850935.
12. Zhang K, Aruva MR, Shanthly N, Cardi CA, Patel CA, Rattan S, Cesarone G, Wickstrom E, Thakur ML. Vasoactive intestinal peptide (VIP) and pituitary adenylate cyclase activating peptide (PACAP) receptor specific peptide analogues for PET imaging of breast cancer: in vitro/in vivo evaluation. Regul Pept. 2007;144(1–3):91–100. https://doi.org/10.1016/j.regpep.2007.06.008; PubMed PMID: 17727979; PMCID: PMC2587158.
13. Leylon FPJJS, et al. VIP 1 receptors are present in breast cancer biopsy specimens. Am Assoc Cancer Res. 1998;38:117.
14. Pallela VR, Thakur ML, Chakder S, Rattan S. 99mTc-labeled vasoactive intestinal peptide receptor agonist: functional studies. J Nucl Med. 1999;40(2):352–60; Epub 1999/02/20.
15. Kolan HRPV, Thakur ML. Technetium-99m labeled vasoactive intestinal peptide, (VIP): preparation and preliminary evaluation. J Label Compd Radiopharm.

1997;40(11):721–811.   https://doi.org/10.1002/jlcr.2580401101.

16. Rao PS, Thakur ML, Pallela V, Patti R, Reddy K, Li H, Sharma S, Pham HL, Diggles L, Minami C, Marcus CS. 99mTc labeled VIP analog: evaluation for imaging colorectal cancer. Nucl Med Biol. 2001;28(4):445–50.

17. Thakur ML. Genomic biomarkers for molecular imaging: predicting the future. Semin Nucl Med. 2009;39(4):236–46.   https://doi.org/10.1053/j.semnuclmed.2009.03.006; PubMed PMID: 19497401; PMCID: PMC2731478.

18. Tripathi SKTE, Gomella L, Kim S, McCue P, Intenzo C, Birbe R, Gandhe A, Kumar P, Thakur M. VPAC1 targeted (64)cu-TP3805 positron emission tomography imaging of prostate cancer: preliminary evaluation in man. Urology. 2016;88:111–8. https://doi.org/10.1016/j.urology.2015.10.012;   PMCID: PMC4788593.

19. Trabulsi EJ, Tripathi SK, Gomella L, Solomides C, Wickstrom E, Thakur ML. Development of a voided urine assay for detecting prostate cancer noninvasively: a pilot study. BJU Int. 2017;119(6):885–95. https://doi.org/10.1111/bju.13775; Epub 2017/01/12. PubMed PMID: 28075510; PMCID: PMC5444967.

20. Bolin DR, Cottrell J, Garippa R, Michalewsky J, Rinaldi N, Simko B, O'Donnell M. Structure-activity studies on the vasoactive intestinal peptide pharmacophore. 1. Analogs of tyrosine. Int J Pept Protein Res. 1995;46(3–4):279–89. https://doi.org/10.1111/j.1399-3011.1995.tb00599.x; Epub 1995/09/01.

21. Paul S, Said SI. Characterization of receptors for vasoactive intestinal peptide solubilized from the lung. J Biol Chem. 1987;262(1):158–62; Epub 1987/01/05.

22. Moody TW. Peptides and growth factors in non-small cell lung cancer. Peptides. 1996;17(3):545–55. https://doi.org/10.1016/0196-9781(95)02148-5; Epub 1996/01/01.

23. Couvineau A, Laburthe M. The human vasoactive intestinal peptide receptor: molecular identification by covalent cross-linking in colonic epithelium. J Clin Endocrinol Metab. 1985;61(1):50–5. https://doi.org/10.1210/jcem-61-1-50; Epub 1985/07/01.

24. Sreedharan SP, Robichon A, Peterson KE, Goetzl EJ. Cloning and expression of the human vasoactive intestinal peptide receptor. Proc Natl Acad Sci U S A. 1991;88(11):4986–90.   https://doi.org/10.1073/pnas.88.11.4986; Epub 1991/06/01. PubMed PMID: 1675791; PMCID: PMC51792.

25. Zia H, Leyton J, Loecho T, Moody TW. PACAP receptors are present on breast cancer cell lines. Am Assoc Cancer Res. 1997;38:117.

26. Said SI, Mutt V. Polypeptide with broad biological activity: isolation from small intestine. Science. 1970;169(3951):1217–8.

27. Chakder S, Rattan S. The entire vasoactive intestinal polypeptide molecule is required for the activation of the vasoactive intestinal polypeptide receptor: functional and binding studies on opossum internal anal sphincter smooth muscle. J Pharmacol Exp Ther. 1993;266(1):392–9.

28. Blum AM, Mathew R, Cook GA, Metwali A, Felman R, Weinstock JV. Murine mucosal T cells have VIP receptors functionally distinct from those on intestinal epithelial cells. J Neuroimmunol. 1992;39(1–2):101–8.   https://doi.org/10.1016/0165-5728(92)90179-o; Epub 1992/07/01.

29. el Battari A, Martin JM, Luis J, Pouzol O, Secchi J, Marvaldi J, Pichon J. Solubilization of the active vasoactive intestinal peptide receptor from human colonic adenocarcinoma cells. J Biol Chem. 1988;263(33):17685–9; Epub 1988/11/25.

30. Le Meuth V, Farjaudon N, Bawab W, Chastre E, Rosselin G, Guilloteau P, Gespach C. Characterization of binding sites for VIP-related peptides and activation of adenylate cyclase in developing pancreas. Am J Phys. 1991;260(2 Pt 1):G265–74. https://doi.org/10.1152/ajpgi.1991.260.2.G265;   Epub 1991/02/01.

31. Virgolini I, Raderer M, Kurtaran A, Angelberger P, Banyai S, Yang Q, Li S, Banyai M, Pidlich J, Niederle B, Scheithauer W, Valent P. Vasoactive intestinal peptide-receptor imaging for the localization of intestinal adenocarcinomas and endocrine tumors. N Engl J Med. 1994;331(17):1116–21. https://doi.org/10.1056/NEJM199410273311703.

32. Bolin DR, Cottrell J, Garippa R, Rinaldi N, Senda R, Simko B, O'Donnell M. Comparison of cyclic and linear analogs of vasoactive intestinal peptide. Drug Des Discov. 1996;13(3–4):107–14; Epub 1996/04/01.

33. Gottschall PE, Tatsuno I, Miyata A, Arimura A. Characterization and distribution of binding sites for the hypothalamic peptide, pituitary adenylate cyclase-activating polypeptide. Endocrinology. 1990;127(1):272–7.   https://doi.org/10.1210/endo-127-1-272; Epub 1990/07/01.

34. Thakur ML, Zhang K, Berger A, Cavanaugh B, Kim S, Channappa C, Frangos AJ, Wickstrom E, Intenzo CM. VPAC1 receptors for imaging breast cancer: a feasibility study. J Nucl Med. 2013;54(7):1019–25. https://doi.org/10.2967/jnumed.112.114876; PubMed PMID: 23651947; PMCID: PMC5506835.

35. 67Cu-SARTATE™ peptide receptor radionuclide therapy administered to pediatric patients with high-risk neuroblastoma. Clarity Pharmaceuticals Ltd. https://clinicaltrials.gov/ct2/show/NCT04023331.

36. Gespach C, Bawab W, de Cremoux P, Calvo F. Pharmacology, molecular identification and functional characteristics of vasoactive intestinal peptide receptors in human breast cancer cells. Cancer Res. 1988;48(18):5079–83. Epub 1988/09/15

37. Moody TW, et al. VIP: a VIP agonist for localizing breast cancer tumors. Peptides. 1998;19:585–92.

J. Harvey Turner

What evidence is required to establish that 68Ga/177Lu-PSMA radioligand theranostic management of advanced metastatic prostate cancer provides meaningful clinical benefit in terms of prolonged overall survival (OS) and enhanced quality of life (QOL)?

How might it be unequivocally demonstrated that this radionuclide molecular-targeted approach represents a significant, affordable, available improvement in clinical outcome over that achievable with current standard of care, such that it becomes adopted into mainstream clinical oncology practice worldwide?

Where do we start?

If we were to choose 2018 as our point of departure, we would see a *tabula rasa* of oncologist ignorance, and even denial, of the existence of precision radionuclide targeted diagnosis and therapy of prostate cancer. The comprehensive, authoritative, state-of-the-art review on recent accomplishments and future challenges in management of metastatic prostate cancer, published in the *New England Journal of Medicine* in 2018 [1] failed to mention either 68Ga-PSMA PET-CT diagnosis or 177Lu-PSMA beta therapy, let alone 225Ac-PSMA alpha therapy. Viewed from a North American perspective, theranostic radionuclide precision oncology does not exist for the

quarter million patients with metastatic prostate cancer diagnosed per annum in the USA by superseded CT methodology and 99mTc-MDP bone scans [2].

The first report of 68Ga-PSMA –PET localization of human tumors in prostate cancer patients was published in 2013 [3]. The potential for theranostics was quickly appreciated in Europe and Australia where, over the next 5 years, 68Ga-PSMA-PET replaced CT, and was shown to be superior to MR, in those centers offering this imaging modality [4]. A multicenter German study reported change in intended management in 39% of patients after 68Ga-PSMA-PET-CT [5]. A prospective multicenter Australian study of patients presenting with newly diagnosed, or recurrent, prostate cancer, demonstrated alteration of planned treatment in over half the patients [6]. Both these theranostic management studies were published in 2018, in the American scientific literature.

Most recently, a review of the German national experience showed even greater impact of 68Ga-PSMA-PET-CT on prostate cancer management, occasioning change of intended treatment in two-thirds of patients [7]. It was remarked that 68Ga-PSMA-PET-CT had been incorporated into the German guideline and, more significantly, into the prostate cancer management guideline of the European Association of Urology. Meanwhile, whilst an American-German coauthored paper reported the major

J. H. Turner (✉)
The University of Western Australia,
Murdoch, Australia
e-mail: Harvey.Turner@health.wa.gov.au

© The Author(s) 2024
V. Prasad (ed.), *Beyond Becquerel and Biology to Precision Radiomolecular Oncology: Festschrift in Honor of Richard P. Baum*, https://doi.org/10.1007/978-3-031-33533-4_33

impact of 68Ga-PSMA-PET-CT on salvage radiotherapy planning [8], the accompanying, more skeptical, editorial perspective, by a past president of the Society of Nuclear Medicine was entitled "Transformational Change in Prostate Cancer Management?" [9].

The "Appropriate Use Criteria for Imaging Evaluation of Biochemical Recurrence of Prostate Cancer After Definitive Primary Treatment" published April 2020 in the *Journal of Nuclear Medicine* merely remarks that "the new class of PSMA-targeted PET radiotracers has generated considerable interest and are [sic] discussed briefly, although these agents are currently not approved for routine clinical use in the United States" [10]. The American Society of Clinical Oncology (ASCO) Guideline for optimum imaging strategies for advanced prostate cancer e-published January 2020 in *Journal of Clinical Oncology* stated "a number of studies have reported on the major impact of PSMA PET imaging on management of patients with prostate cancer, although the potential influence on outcome will need additional investigations" [11]. A 2020 UK review of management of de novo metastatic prostate cancer cited eight diverse definitive studies, none of which made reference to 68Ga-PSMA PET/CT [12]. Significantly, the reviewers remarked that currently no international consensus has been reached on the definition of oligometastatic disease. They did, however, acknowledge that the advent of improved imaging of metastatic disease, such as 68Ga-PSMA, is likely to positively affect the survival outcomes achieved with metastasis-directed therapy [12].

The definitive prospective randomized multicenter phase 3 study of 68Ga-PSMA PET/CT imaging commenced in 2017, in Australia [13]. The results in 302 men with newly diagnosed prostate cancer provide compelling evidence that PSMA PET/CT has better accuracy, with consequent change in management, fewer equivocal results, and lower radiation exposure compared with current standard-of-care imaging with CT and bone scanning [14]. Accuracy of 68Ga-PSMA PET/CT was 27% greater than for conventional imaging (92% vs. 65%). Comparison of sensitivity (85% vs. 38%) and specificity (98% vs. 91%) also demonstrated significant advantage of 68Ga-PSMA PET/CT over CT and bone scanning. The authors conclude that PSMA PET/CT is better than, and can replace, conventional imaging with CT and bone scan for staging men with high-risk prostate cancer before surgery or radiotherapy with curative intent, and they recommended that existing guidelines should be reviewed [14].

It is to be hoped that this well-designed Australian multicenter RCT will persuade oncologists, urologists, and radiologists worldwide to adopt the essential imaging component of the theranostic paradigm. 68Ga-PSMA-PET-CT is the mandated prerequisite for eligibility for 177Lu-PSMA, or 225Ac-PSMA therapy, as encapsulated in Professor Richard Baum's maxim: "we see what we treat, and we treat what we see." It is likely, however, that this truth will become self-evident only when the actual efficiency of 177Lu-PSMA radioligand therapy is irrefutably demonstrated.

So, how do we obtain such unassailable evidence?

Academic centers throughout Germany have been applying theranostic management of metastatic castrate-resistant prostate cancer (mCRPC) with 68Ga/177Lu-PSMA since 2013 [15, 16]. Hundreds of patients have been treated on compassionate patient usage protocols, and several retrospective reports of encouraging responses have been published [16–18]. In particular, OS was significantly longer in patients who were chemotherapy-naïve [19]. However, the protocols were diverse, patient populations were heterogeneous, and surrogate endpoints varied. The resulting "evidence" of efficacy was not deemed worthy of acceptance by the oncologist community, which demands rigorous prospective clinical trials on agreed protocols, with uniform patient eligibility criteria and predefined endpoints. Notwithstanding the absence of formal oncologist approbation, the manifestly favorable clinical outcomes of 177Lu-PSMA-RLT of mCRPC, achieved with minimal toxicity, have resulted in hundreds of patients requesting treatment with these theranostic agents, which are not currently approved in any regulatory jurisdiction in the world.

The European Association of Nuclear Medicine (EANM) has taken the unprecedented step of preparing a guideline for this unapproved radionuclide therapy, which they acknowledge can be offered individually on the basis of compassionate patient use and in accordance with the best actual knowledge [20]. The ethical basis of the EANM guideline is stated to be: "In line with the declaration of Helsinki, it is considered ethically justified (and a legally recognized necessity of excuse) to apply a well-reasoned but unapproved intervention compared with withholding such a promising treatment from patients due to formal regulatory or administrative issues." The guideline is intended to provide a base for the harmonization of PSMA-radioligand therapy protocols, wherein the EANM "strongly advocates the development of PSMA-radioligand therapy within the context of adequately powered multicenter clinical trials with appropriate endpoints."

What form should such clinical trials take, in order to establish efficiency in the global population of prostate cancer patients?

A 2020 review of five key studies of metastasis-directed therapy in men with oligometastatic prostate cancer failed to mention 177Lu/225Ac-PSMA radioligand therapy [12]. It was remarked that large-cohort randomized controlled trials (RCTs) exploring the effects of metastasis-directed therapies would help to establish the potential OS benefits of this approach and possibly overcome the prohibitive financial barrier currently preventing the use of such approaches beyond the clinical trial setting by facilitating insurance coverage and reimbursement [12].

RCTs have been the acknowledged gold standard for evaluation of the efficacy of novel anticancer agents over the past 50 years. However, with the advent of precision oncology, such as radionuclide molecular-targeted therapy of prostate cancer, major flaws have been exposed in RCT methodology [21]. The demonstration of efficacy, in terms of a statistically significant advantage in respect of arbitrary surrogate endpoints in a highly selected patient population, often does not translate to improved survival and QOL in the real world of clinical practice. In fact, most of the novel anticancer agents approved after RCT over the past decade failed to achieve a clinically meaningful benefit on the ASCO and the European Society of Medical Oncology (ESMO) scales which measure efficiency of drugs in terms of substantial improvement of OS and QOL, and which also show cost-benefit [22].

The magnitude of the increasing incidence and mortality of prostate cancer throughout the world render meeting the unmet need for a proven remedy an urgent imperative. RCTs, quite apart from their expense, and highly selected patient population, take years to come to fruition, during which time the affected population-at-large is denied access to the agent being tested.

In addition, those patients allocated to the control arm of a RCT are also denied, what is postulated to be, the most effective treatment. For example, 250 of the mCRPC patients assigned to standard-of-care control arm in the VISION RCT (NCT03511664) of 177Lu-PSMA-617-RLT will not be able to receive the active treatment given to the 500 patients on the study arm [23]. The ethical rationale for this deprivation of 177Lu-PSMA-617 in the control cohort is said to be the existence of equipoise, as carefully explained to each RCT participant in the process of obtaining informed consent: "Investigators must impart a clear understanding that 177Lu-PSMA-617 has not, to date, shown any survival advantage or any other metric of clinical benefit over the standard of care." However, in an earlier prospective study; the pre-VISION Study, using the same eligibility criteria, the same treatment protocol, and the same endpoints, the same authors reported favorable surrogate endpoints: best PSA response (>50% decline) in more than half the treated patients (53.7%), and median PFS 49.2 months, and conclude: "Therefore it seems reasonable to prefer the 7.5GBq [VISION] regimen in most patients" [24].

Nonetheless, the major ethical objection to any RCT is that the research subject is treated as a means to an end of demonstrating the statistically significant efficacy of the agent, rather than the clinical benefit of the patient on study. The patient treated on a research study has a moral right to be treated as an end in themselves, which is denied them in the design of RCTs.

How can we preserve the beneficent doctor-patient relationship and provide what is believed to be the best management of advanced prostate cancer, yet, at the same time, obtain the required evidence of efficiency which would be acceptable to oncologists, urologists, and regulatory authorities throughout the world?

ASCO has released a policy statement asserting the importance of phase 1 clinical trials as a treatment modality with potential clinical benefit for patients with advanced stage malignancies [25]. Similarly, the US FDA also acknowledges that a primary aim of phase 1 trials is to gain early evidence of effectiveness [26]. This official recognition of early phase trials offering potential individual clinical benefit to all participants raises another ethical problem for subsequent RCTs. If drug access in phase 1 studies is considered therapeutic, how can investigators downstream of successful phase 1 trials ethically deprive half their human research subjects of study product in the RCT? Furthermore, drug regulator policies may restrict drug access, or limit commercial claims of efficacy based upon phase 1/2 trials, until validated by later restrictive RCT which confines availability to a highly select few.

The first prospective proof-of-concept phase 2 clinical trial of 177Lu-PSMA-617 in mCRPC was a single center Australian study (ANZ CTR 12615000912583), which demonstrated efficacy in 30 patients with advanced disease progressing after chemotherapy [27]. The treatment protocol was individualized within the parameters later enumerated in the EANM procedure guideline [20]. This seminal study demonstrates the practicality of personalizing 177Lu-PSMA treatment cycles to address the individual needs of the patient at the discretion of their treating physician. This real-world applicable study achieved rapid and substantial improvement in QOL and surrogate markers of response, without any sig-

nificant toxicity. The authors concluded that this evidence supports the need for RCTs to further assess efficacy compared with current standard of care. However, whilst RCT may establish efficacy in a selected cohort of patients, it cannot provide the critical evaluation of efficiency in the global population of patients with advanced prostate cancer, nor can it address the practical problems of availability, affordability, and accessibility throughout the world [21].

The real issue of timely access to novel cancer therapies is not one of regulatory delay, but rather of archaic, overly restrictive, non-pragmatic RCT designs with limited distribution of investigation sites. RWE can help hasten the approval process and provide both access and strong evidence of meaningful gains in QOL and OS in large representative patient populations [28].

The important concept proven by the pathfinding prospective phase 2 study of 177Lu-PSMA-617 in mCRPC [27] is the capacity to individualize patient treatment within a harmonized protocol to obtain clinically meaningful scientific data which are credible and generalizable. Thus we now have a template for the translation of 177Lu-PSMA-RLT to real-world management of mCRPC on a harmonized protocol standardized to the EANM guideline.

Appropriate logistics exist in at least 50 countries where 68Ga/177Lu-PSMA theranostics is currently practiced on compassionate usage programs. The World Association for Radiopharmaceutical and Molecular Therapy (WARMTH) is coordinating an international prospective audit of patients receiving 177Lu-PSMA treatment under locally authorized individual patient access programs throughout the world and will collect, collate, and analyze real-world data (RWD) from patients treated on a harmonized protocol standardized on the EANM guideline. This multicenter international study: National Investigators Global Harmonization Theranostics CAncer of Prostate (NIGHTCAP) Study has very simple endpoints, comprising OS and QOL [29]. Assessment of QOL is by patient-reported outcome (PRO), which is language-independent and based upon patient selection of images on a standard 5-point emoji scale app on their smart phone [30].

Clinical access to 68Ga/177Lu-PSMA is provided through local compassionate patient usage programs, under existing national regulatory agency approvals, and all therapy and follow-up is at the discretion of the treating physician. This individualized molecular targeted theranostic management, within the harmonized EANM protocol guideline, does not require serial imaging or laboratory investigations to define surrogate response, given that the NIGHTCAP Study endpoints are limited to those which are of fundamental concern to the mCRPC patient: QOL and OS [29]. The COVID pandemic precluded performance of the NIGHTCAP Study but the design principles remain valid for real-world evidence of effectiveness.

Inevitably, novel evolving modifications will improve future outcomes of treatment of mCRPC. These potential developments may include incorporation of combination chemotherapy, such as cabazitaxel with 177Lu-PSMA in the ongoing TheraP Study [27], or sequential beta and alpha radionuclide therapy with 177Lu-PSMA and 225Ac-PSMA in tandem approaches [31, 32]. As soon as these novel combination therapies, which might also include chemo-immunotherapies, are shown to be safe and efficacious, they can be seamlessly incorporated into a modified harmonized adaptive NIGHTCAP Study protocol in real time as they become available. This rapid response and real-time flexibility contrasts with the rigid, locked-in protocol design, and inherent obsolescence of RCTs.

Thus, every patient on the NIGHTCAP Study would have received cutting-edge optimized theranostic management which is deemed to be most appropriate for them by their own personal physician, according to the most up-to-date real-time RWD. This ethically and scientifically sound approach to clinical outcome research is encapsulated in the ASCO Presidential Address of 2019 "Caring for every patient, learning from every patient" [33]. In the NIGHTCAP Study design, nothing be lost in translation into real-world evidence of efficiency of 177Lu-PSMA radioligand therapy of metastatic prostate cancer in routine oncology clinical practice throughout the world.

References

1. Sartor O, de Bono JS. Metastatic prostate cancer. N Engl J Med. 2018;378:645–57.
2. Bray F, Ferlay J, Soerjomataram I, et al. Global cancer statistics 2018: GLOBOCAN. Estimates of incidence and mortality worldwide for 36 cancers in 185 countries. CA Cancer J Clin. 2018;394:17–31. https://doi.org/10.3322/caac.21492.
3. Afshar-Oromich A, Malcher A, Eder M, et al. PET imaging with a [68Ga] gallium-labelled PSMA ligand for the diagnosis of prostate cancer: biodistribution in humans and first evaluation of tumour lesions. Eur J Nucl Med Mol Imaging. 2013;40:486–95.
4. Lenzo NP, Meyrick D, Turner JH. Review of gallium-68 PSMA PET/CT imaging in the management of prostate cancer. Diagnostics. 2018;8:16. https://doi.org/10.3390/diagnostics8010016.
5. Afaq A, Alahmed S, Chen S-H, et al. Impact of 68Ga-prostate-specific membrane antigen PET/CT on prostate cancer management. J Nucl Med. 2018;59:89–92. https://doi.org/10.2967/jnumed.117.192625.
6. Roach PJ, Francis R, Emmett L, et al. The impact of 68Ga-PSMA PET/CT on management intent in prostate cancer: results of an Australian prospective multicentre study. J Nucl Med. 2018;59:82–8. https://doi.org/10.2967/jnumed.117.197160.
7. Schmidt-Hegemann N-S, Eze C, Li M, et al. Impact of 68Ga-PSMA PET/CT on the radiotherapeutic approach to prostate cancer in comparison to CT: a retrospective analysis. J Nucl Med. 2019;60:963–70. https://doi.org/10.2967/jnumed.118.220855.
8. Calais J, Czernin J, Cao M, et al. 68Ga-PSMA-11 PET/CT mapping of prostate cancer biochemical recurrence after radical prostatectomy in 270 patients with a PSA level of less than 1.0ng/mL: impact on salvage radiotherapy planning. J Nucl Med. 2018;59:230–7. https://doi.org/10.2967/jnumed.117.201749.
9. Jadvar H, Ballas LK. Transformational change in prostate cancer management? J Nucl Med. 2018;59:228–9.
10. Jadvar H, Ballas LK, Choyke PL, et al. Appropriate use criteria for imaging evaluation of biochemical recurrence of prostate cancer after definitive primary treatment. J Nucl Med. 2020;61:552–62. https://doi.org/10.2967/jnumed.119.240929.
11. Trabulsi EJ, Rumble RB, Jadvar H, et al. Optimum imaging strategies for advanced prostate cancer: ASCO guideline. J Clin Oncol. 2020;38:1963. https://doi.org/10.1200/jco.19.02757.
12. Connor MJ, Shah TT, Horan G, et al. Cytoreductive treatment strategies for de novo metastatic prostate cancer. Nat Rev Clin Oncol. 2020;17:168. https://doi.org/10.1038/s41571-019-0284-3[13].
13. Hofman MS, Murphy DG, Williams SG, et al. A prospective randomised multicentre study of the impact of gallium-68 prostate specific membrane antigen (PSMA) PET/CTimaging for staging high-risk prostate cancer prior to curative-intent surgery or radiotherapy (proPSMA study): clinical trial protocol. BJU Int. 2018;122:783–93.

14. Hofman MS, Lawrentschuk N, Francis RJ, et al. Prostate-specific membrane antigen PET-CT in patients with high-risk prostate cancer before curative-intent surgery or radiotherapy (proPSMA): a prospective, randomised, multicentre study. Lancet. 2020;395:1208–16. https://doi.org/10.1016/S0140-6736(20)30314-7.

15. Weineisen M, Schottelius M, Simecek J, et al. 68Ga- and 177Lu-labeled PSMA I&T: optimization of a PSMA-targeted theranostic concept and first proof-of-concept human studies. J Nucl Med. 2015;56:1169–79. https://doi.org/10.2967/jnumed.115.158550.

16. Kulkarni HR, Singh A, Schuchardt C, et al. PSMA-based radioligand therapy for metastatic castration-resistant prostate cancer: the bad berka experience since 2013. J Nucl Med. 2016;57:97S–104S. https://doi.org/10.2967/jnumed.115.170167.

17. Kulkarni HR, Singh A, Langbein T, et al. Theranostics of prostate cancer: from molecular imaging to precision molecular radiotherapy targeting the prostate-specific membrane antigen. Br J Radiol. 2018;91:20180308. https://doi.org/10.1259/bjr.20180308.

18. Rahbar K, Ahmadzadehfar H, Kratochwil C, et al. German multicentre study investigating 177Lu-PSMA-617 radioligand therapy in advanced prostate cancer patients. J Nucl Med. 2017;58:85–90. https://doi.org/10.2967/jnumed.116.183194.

19. Ahmadzadehfar H, Rahbar K, Baum RP, et al. Prior therapies as prognostic factors of overall survival in metastatic castration-resistant prostate cancer patients treated with [177Lu]Lu-PSMA-617. A WARMTH multicentre study (the 617 trial). Eur J Nucl Med Mol Imaging. 2020;48:113. https://doi.org/10.1007/s00259-020-04797-9.

20. Kratochwil C, Fendler PW, Eiber M, et al. EANM procedure guidelines for radionuclide therapy with 177Lu-labelled PSMA-ligands (177Lu-PSMA-RLT). Eur J Nucl Med Mol Imaging. 2019;46:2536–44. https://doi.org/10.1007/s00259-019-04485-3.

21. Turner JH. Theranostic outcomes in clinical practice of oncology: what, so what, now what? What's more. Cancer Biother Radiopharm. 2019;34:135–40. https://doi.org/10.1089/cbr.2019.29006.jht(2019).

22. Das M. Many FDA-approved cancer drugs might lack clinical benefit. Lancet Oncol. 2018;19:e82. https://doi.org/10.1016/S1470-2045(17)30954-3.

23. Rahbar K, Bodei L, Morris MJ. Is the vision of radioligand therapy for prostate cancer becoming a real- ity? An overview of the phase 3 VISION trial and its importance for the future of theranostics. J Nucl Med. 2019;60:1504–6.

24. Seifert R, Kessel K, Schlack K, et al. Radioligand therapy using [(177)Lu]Lu-PSMA-617 in mCRPC: a pre-VISION single-center analysis. Eur J Nucl Med Mol Imaging. 2020;47:2106. https://doi.org/10.1007/s00259-020-04703-3.

25. Weber JS, Levit LA, Adamson PC, et al. American Society of Clinical Oncology policy statement update: the critical role of phase 1 trials in cancer research and treatment. J Clin Oncol. 2015;33:278–84. https://doi.org/10.1200/jco.2014.58.2635.

26. Burris HA III. Correcting the ASCO position on phase 1 clinical trials in cancer. Nat Rev Clin Oncol. 2020;17:125. https://doi.org/10.1038/s41571-019-0311-4(2020).

27. Hofman MS, Violet J, Hicks RJ, et al. [(177)Lu]-PSMA-617 radionuclide treatment in patients with metastatic castration-resistant prostate cancer (LuPSMA trial): a single-centre, single-arm, phase 2 study. Lancet Oncol. 2018;19:825–3.

28. Raphael MJ, Gyawali B, Booth CM. Real-world evidence and regulatory drug approval. Nat Rev Clin Oncol. 2020;17:271–2.

29. Turner JH. Real-world evidence of clinical outcomes in precision radionuclide oncology: the NIGHTCAP study of 177Lu-PSMA in metastatic prostate cancer. Curr Pharm Des. 2020;26:1–5. https://doi.org/10.2174/1381612826666200312141347.

30. Thompson CA, Novotny PJ, Bartz A, et al. Development of a novel emoji scale to measure patient-reported outcomes in cancer patients. J Clin Oncol. 2018;36(7 suppl):174. https://doi.org/10.1200/jco.2018.36.7suppl.174.

31. Khreish F, Ebert N, Ries M, et al. 225Ac-PSMA-617/177Lu-PSMA-617 tandem therapy of metastatic castration-resistant prostate cancer: pilot experience. Eur J Nucl Med Mol Imaging. 2020;47:721–8. https://doi.org/10.1007/s00259-019-04612-0.

32. Kulkarni HR, Zhang J, Singh A, et al. Tandem PSMA radioligand therapy using ac-225 and Lu-177 in advanced prostate cancer: safety and efficacy. Eur J Nucl Med Mol Imaging. 2019;46:S236–S7.

33. Bertagnolli MM. 2019 ASCO presidential address: caring for every patient, learning from every patient. J Clin Oncol. 2019;2019(37):2301–5. https://doi.org/10.1200/jco.19.01584.

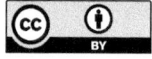

Uptake of ^{68}Ga-DOTATATE and ^{68}Ga-DOTATOC in Primary Neuroendocrine Tumors, Metastases, and Normal Liver Tissue: Is There a Significant Difference?

34

Mila V. Todorović-Tirnanić, Cees J. A. van Echteld,
Milan M. Gajić, and Richard P. Baum

34.1 Introduction

Although they have historically been considered as rare tumors, recent data suggest that neuroendocrine tumors (NETs) are more common than might be expected [1, 2]. Reported annual age-adjusted incidence is 5.25/100,000 [3]. NETs may arise anywhere in the human body, but the most common location of the primary lesion is the gastroenteropancreatic (GEP) tract, followed by the lungs. GEP NETs originate from the diffuse endocrine system of the gastrointestinal tract and pancreas [4]. A wide spectrum of biologically active peptides can be produced by NET cells (e.g., serotonin, gastrin, glucagon, and insulin) which are stored in vesicles, whose proteins (chromogranin A and synaptophysin) are common markers of GEP NETs [5].

The majority of GEP NETs (primaries and metastases) express somatostatin receptors, five distinct subtypes (sstr 1 to 5) of which have been identified, all of them binding native somatostatin. Somatostatin (sst) is a small, cyclic neuropeptide formed of 14 or 28 amino acids, both originating from the same preprotein, and is present in neurons and endocrine cells. It inhibits the secretion of a wide range of hormones. Its antiproliferative action controls cell growth with the potential for therapeutic application. Somatostatin actions are mediated by transmembrane domain G-protein-coupled receptors, and multiple subtypes of these receptors frequently coexist in the same cell [6, 7].

Naturally occurring sst has a very low metabolic stability *in vivo* with a half-life of less than 2 min. Therefore, more stable synthetic sst analogues have been developed [7, 8] which for *in vivo* diagnostic purposes have been labeled with gamma emitters: first with I-123 [9] and subsequently with In-111 [10], Tc-99 m [11–13], Ga-67 [14], and with positron emitters: C-11 [15], F-18 [16, 17], Ga-68 [14], Cu-64 [18], Sc-44 [19], and Tb-152 [20].

M. V. Todorović-Tirnanić
Faculty of Medicine, University of Belgrade, Belgrade, Serbia

Center of Nuclear Medicine, Clinical Center of Serbia, Belgrade, Serbia

C. J. A. van Echteld (✉)
ABX-CRO Advanced Pharmaceutical Services, Forschungsgesellschaft mbH, Dresden, Germany
e-mail: cees.van.echteld@abx-cro.com

M. M. Gajić
Faculty of Medicine, Institute of Medical Statistics and Informatics, University of Belgrade, Belgrade, Serbia

R. P. Baum
Theranostics Center for Molecular Radiotherapy and Molecular Imaging, Zentralklinik Bad Berka, Bad Berka, Germany

© The Author(s) 2024
V. Prasad (ed.), *Beyond Becquerel and Biology to Precision Radiomolecular Oncology: Festschrift in Honor of Richard P. Baum*, https://doi.org/10.1007/978-3-031-33533-4_34

^{68}Ga-DOTATOC and ^{68}Ga-DOTATATE (Fig. 34.1) are the most established somatostatin receptor PET tracers and both have been recently approved in USA and Europe. Both radiopharmaceuticals enabled higher lesion detection rate than conventional ^{111}In-DTPA-octreotide SPECT scintigraphy [21, 22], and changed the clinical management in most patients with negative or inconclusive findings on ^{111}In-DTPA-octreotide scintigraphy [22]. Furthermore, dosimetric data showed the effective dose of ^{111}In-DTPA-octreotide to be approximately three to five times higher than for the ^{68}Ga-labeled somatostatin analogs [23].

In GEP NET sstr 2 is overexpressed most abundantly, followed by sstr 1 and 5, rarely sstr 3 and 4 [24]. Higher presence of sstr 3 is revealed in pancreatic NET (incidence up to 71%) [25], compared with non-pancreatic NET. In vitro, it

has been shown that ^{68}Ga-DOTATATE binds to sstr 2, with an approximately tenfold higher affinity than ^{68}Ga-DOTATOC. On the other hand, ^{68}Ga-DOTATOC binds also to sstr 5 with significantly lesser affinity than to sstr 2, but with five-fold higher affinity compared to ^{68}Ga-DOTATATE [26]. However, for various radionuclides, such an affinity difference between DOTATOC and DOTATATE could not be confirmed in humans. To clarify this discrepancy, Poeppel et al. [27] have conducted a study on 40 NET patients undergoing both ^{68}Ga-DOTATATE and ^{68}Ga-DOTATOC PET/CT. They also performed a separate subgroup analysis of 27 GEP-NET patients [28]. Both these studies showed a small but significantly higher number of lesions detected by ^{68}Ga-DOTATOC and unexpectedly higher SUVmax in both primary tumors and metastases, but not in kidneys. Hence, a

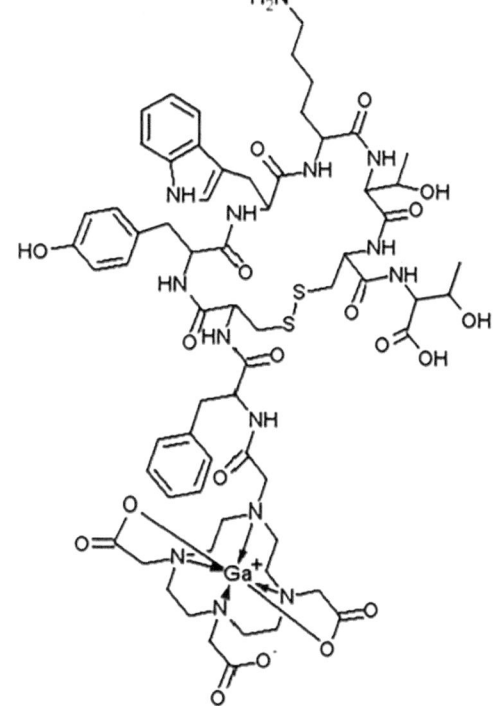

^{68}Ga-DOTATOC   **[68]Ga-DOTATATE**

Fig. 34.1 Structural formulas of ^{68}Ga-DOTATOC and ^{68}Ga-DOTATATE, where TOC and TATE stand, respectively, for D-Phe-Cys-Tyr-D-Trp-Lys-Thr-Cys-Thr(OH) and D-Phe-Cys-Tyr-D-Trp-Lys-Thr-Cys-Thr. Difference in structure is highlighted with blue square [29]

significantly higher kidney-to-tumor ratio for ^{68}Ga-DOTATOC was reported. The authors conclude that the approximately tenfold higher in vitro affinity of ^{68}Ga-DOTATATE for sstr 2 is not clinically relevant. Yet, in another study on 10 NET patients undergoing both ^{68}Ga-DOTATATE and ^{68}Ga-DOTATOC PET/CT, Velikyan et al. [29] state a preference for ^{68}Ga-DOTATATE because of healthy organ distribution and excretion, although their conclusion is not fully supported by their data and their tumor-to-healthy organ ratios for liver, kidney, and spleen were all in favor of ^{68}Ga-DOTATOC. Therefore, the aim of this study was to resolve this discrepancy by comparing in another group of GEP NET patients the in vivo distribution of the two radiopharmaceuticals in the same patients by determining their SUVmax values in primary tumors, metastases, and in normal liver.

34.2 Methods

Thirty eight histologically confirmed well-differentiated GEP NET patients with clinically, biochemically, and morphologically stable disease (selected from 800 NET patients), 19 female and 19 male (mean age 61.8 ± 12.1 years; age range 24–79 years) were submitted to first a ^{68}Ga-DOTATATE and subsequently a ^{68}Ga-DOTATOC PET/CT study on two consecutive visits as part of a usual workup, with 197 days (117–311 days range) in between. Well-differentiated GEP NET primary tumors included: 1 duodenal, 18 pancreatic, 2 cecal, 12 ileal, 3 jejunal, 1 mesenteric, and 1 GEP NET in appendix.

Patients had either not been on octreotide therapy or had octreotide therapy suspended for 6 weeks prior to ^{68}Ga-DOTATOC/^{68}Ga-DOTATATE PET/CT. Labeling and quality control of the radiopharmaceuticals were performed according to methods described previously [30]. ^{68}Ga-DOTATOC and ^{68}Ga-DOTATATE were prepared in the radiopharmacy of the Zentralklinik Bad Berka under GMP conditions and used in patients in agreement with specific German regulations for the use of in-house prepared radio-pharmaceuticals and in accordance with regulations of the Federal Office for Radiation Protection (Bundesamt für Strahlenschutz). Patients were given 1.5 L of water-equivalent oral contrast dispersion Gastrografin 1 h before the start of acquisition. To increase renal washout and decrease radiation exposure to the urinary bladder, 20 mg of furosemide was given i.v. after injection of ^{68}Ga-DOTATOC/^{68}Ga-DOTATATE.

All patients were examined on a dual-modality PET/CT scanner (Biograph duo; Siemens Medical Solutions). On average, acquisition started 87 min after injection of 123 ± 9 MBq of ^{68}Ga-DOTATATE, and 90 min after injection of 119 ± 8 MBq of ^{68}Ga-DOTATOC, each with a peptide mass dose of 12 μg.

First, a topogram was acquired. The patients were given 100 mL of intravenous contrast (by an automated injection pump), followed by computed tomography (CT) scanning in the craniocaudal direction with 30 s delay after injection, and PET scanning in the caudocranial direction. After scatter and attenuation correction, PET emission data were reconstructed using an attenuation-weighted ordered-subsets maximization expectation approach with two iterations and eight subsets on 128 × 128 matrices and with a 5 mm Gaussian post-reconstruction filtering.

The PET/CT images were assessed using E.soft (syngo-based nuclear medicine software). In each of 76 patient PET/CT studies (38 PET/CT studies for each radiopharmaceutical), regions of interest (ROIs) were outlined in normal liver tissue, in the primary tumor as well as in all liver, lymph node, soft tissue, and bone metastases on PET/CT fusion images. For the liver ROI, the normal tissue of the liver was chosen with care as not to include possible metastases, present in the liver tissue of some GEP NET patients. The ROIs positioned were verified in all three planes (transversal, coronal, and sagittal).

SUVmax for all outlined ROIs in both studies (^{68}Ga-DOTATATE and ^{68}Ga-DOTATOC) were determined and mean SUVmax values for ^{68}Ga-DOTATATE and ^{68}Ga-DOTATOC in normal liver tissue, primary tumors, and metastases (in liver, lymph nodes, soft tissues, and bones) were calculated and compared.

Statistical analysis was performed using a General Linear Model for Repeated Measures procedure. Radiopharmaceutical had two variables, and the type of tissue had six variables (primary GEP NET, metastases in the liver, soft tissue, lymph nodes, bones, and normal liver tissue). Sidak's test enabled comparison between accumulation of both radiopharmaceuticals (SUVmax values) in primary tumor, in metastases in liver, lymph nodes, bones, soft tissues, and in normal liver tissue.

34.3 Results

The intravenous injections of ^{68}Ga-DOTATATE and ^{68}Ga-DOTATOC were well tolerated. No local or systemic side effects were evident during the time of observation (up to 180 min post injection). Examples of data reconstruction and image analysis are displayed in Fig. 34.2a for ^{68}Ga-DOTATATE and in Fig. 34.2b for ^{68}Ga-DOTATOC.

On 76 PET/CT studies (38 ^{68}Ga-DOTATATE and 38 ^{68}Ga-DOTATOC in 38 GEP NET patients), 548 regions of interest (36 over primary tumors, 196 over liver metastases, 134 over lymph nodes metastases, 86 over bone metastases, 34 over soft tissue metastases, 62 over normal liver tissue) were outlined and SUVmax values were determined and compared (Table 34.1).

For both ^{68}Ga-DOTATATE and ^{68}Ga-DOTATOC, the highest SUVmax values were measured in primaries, followed by liver-, soft tissue- and lymph node-metastases. Of all metastases, bone metastases had the lowest SUVmax for both radiopharmaceuticals (Fig. 34.3). Almost identical values for ^{68}Ga-DOTATATE and ^{68}Ga-DOTATOC SUVmax were registered in normal liver tissue.

^{68}Ga-DOTATOC had higher SUVmax values (mean SUVmax = 15.10) compared to ^{68}Ga-DOTATATE (mean SUVmax = 12.67) in all measured tumor tissues (the difference was statistically highly significant: $F = 27.174$; $p < 0.001$) (Tables 34.1 and 34.2). The significance of the differences between ^{68}Ga-DOTATOC and ^{68}Ga-DOTATATE accumulation (SUVmax values) in primary GEP NET tumors (Sidak's test results), in metastases in the liver, lymph nodes, bones, and soft tissues, and in normal liver tissue are displayed in Table 34.2.

Comparison of radiopharmaceutical uptake (SUVmax) in different tumor tissues, as well as in tumor tissue and normal liver tissue, where a significant difference was found (for both ^{68}Ga-DOTATATE and ^{68}Ga-DOTATOC), is shown in Table 34.3. Highly significant difference was registered in primary tumor, in liver metastases, and in lymph node metastases. Significant difference was registered in bone metastases. Notwithstanding these highly significant differences in SUV max values, considerable variability in the preferred tracer uptake was still observed, as shown in Table 34.4. No significant difference existed in soft tissue metastases (higher values were obtained for ^{68}Ga-DOTATOC compared to ^{68}Ga-DOTATATE, but without statistically significant difference), and in normal liver tissue.

Fig. 34.2 (a) Maximum intensity projection, transversal, sagittal and frontal (coronal) fused PET/CT images obtained with ^{68}Ga-DOTATATE in the same patient with pancreatic corpus and tail NET displayed. A ROI around a metastasis in S5/6 of the liver is outlined on all fused images. SUVmax = 21.5. (b) Maximum intensity projec-tion, transversal, sagittal, and frontal (coronal) fused PET/CT images obtained with ^{68}Ga-DOTATOC in a patient with pancreatic corpus and tail NET displayed. A ROI around a metastasis in S5/6 of the liver is outlined on all fused images. SUVmax = 26.0

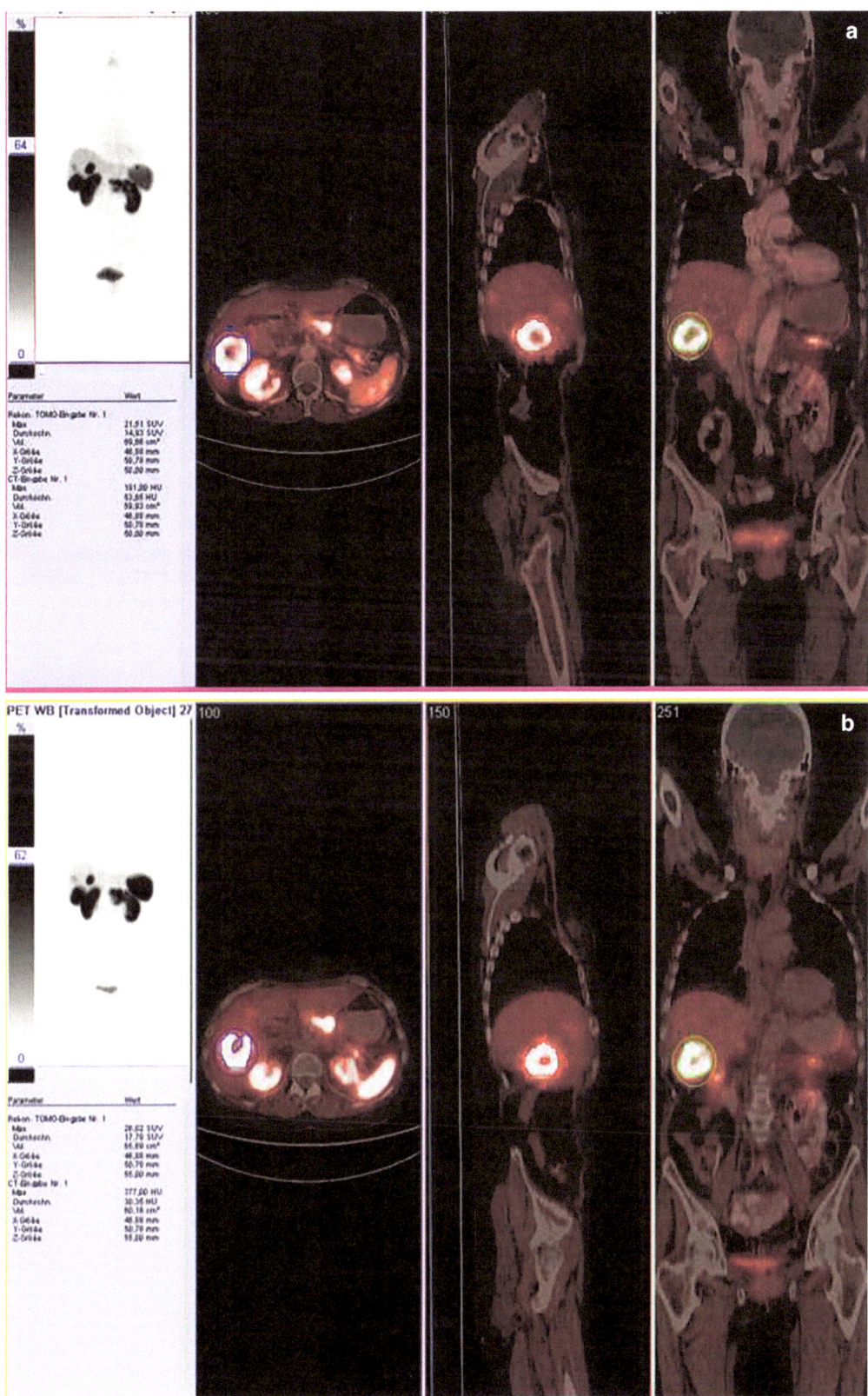

Table 34.1 Results of SUVmax measurements in ⁶⁸Ga-DOTATATE and ⁶⁸Ga-DOTATOC PET/CT studies on 38 GEP NET patients with stable disease

Radiopharmaceutical	Tissue	SUVmax value		
		Mean	SD	Number
⁶⁸Ga-DOTATATE	Primary tumor	20.39	13.68	18
	Metastasis in the liver	15.41	9.43	98
	Lymph node metastasis	11.96	9.52	67
	Bone metastasis	7.48	5.72	43
	Soft tissue metastasis	15.30	16.37	17
	All lesions	12.67	10.45	243
	Normal liver	6.82	1.66	31
⁶⁸Ga-DOTATOC	Primary tumor	24.23	20.11	18
	Metastasis in the liver	17.86	11.36	98
	Lymph node metastasis	15.20	13.32	67
	Bone metastasis	9.87	7.98	43
	Soft tissue metastasis	17.32	18.77	17
	All lesions	15.10	13,27	243
	Normal liver	6.89	1.82	31

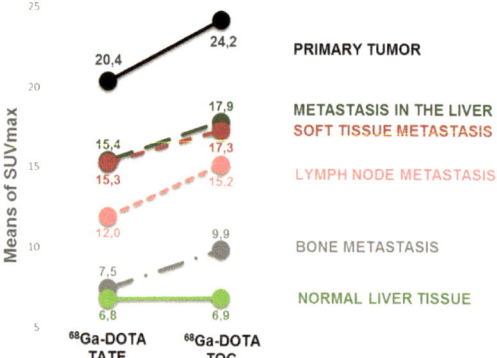

Fig. 34.3 Comparison between mean SUVmax values of ⁶⁸Ga-DOTATATE and ⁶⁸Ga-DOTATOC in the normal liver, primary tumor and its metastases (in the liver, lymph nodes, soft tissues, and bones)

Table 34.2 Significance of the difference between ⁶⁸Ga-DOTATOC and ⁶⁸Ga-DOTATATE accumulation (SUVmax values) in primary GEP NET tumors, in metastases in the liver, lymph nodes, bones and soft tissues, and in normal liver tissue

Tissue	Mean difference in SUVmax values (⁶⁸Ga-DOTATOC SUVmax—⁶⁸Ga-DOTATATE SUVmax)	Statistical significance(p) (pairwise comparison; adjustment for multiple comparisons: Sidak)
Primary tumor	3.839	0.008
Metastasis in the liver	2.449	0.000
Lymph node metastasis	3.239	0.000
Bone metastasis	2.386	0.011
Soft tissue metastasis	2.018	0.173
All lesions	2.430	0.000
Normal liver	0.071	0.948

Table 34.3 Comparison of radiopharmaceutical uptake (SUVmax) in different tumor tissues, as well as in tumor tissue and normal liver tissue, where a significant difference was found

Radiopharmaceutical uptake comparisons	^{68}Ga-DOTATATE SUVmaxdifference			^{68}Ga-DOTATOC SUVmaxdifference		
	Mean	Statistical significance		Mean	Statistical significance	
		p			p	
Primary tumor vs. bone metastases	12.92	0.000	High	14.37	0.001	High
Primary tumor vs. normal liver tissue	13.57	0.000	High	17.34	0.000	High
Primary tumor vs. lymph node metastases	8.43	0.012	Significant	9.03	0.079	No
Liver vs. bone metastases	7.94	0.000	High	8.00	0.006	High
Liver metastases vs. normal liver tissue	8.59	0.000	High	10.97	0.000	High
Soft tissue vs. normal liver tissue	8.48	0.044	Significant	10.42	0.069	No
Lymph node metastases vs. normal liver tissue	5.14	0.167	No	8.31	0.027	Significant

Table 34.4 Frequency of higher SUVmax for ^{68}Ga-DOTATATE and ^{68}Ga-DOTATOC in 243 GEP NET lesions

Tissue	Higher SUVmax		Equal SUVmax	Lesion number
	^{68}Ga-DOTATATE	^{68}Ga-DOTATOC		
Primary net	7	10	1	18
Hepatic mets	35	62	1	98
Lymph node mets	17	48	2	67
Bone mets	9	34	0	43
Soft tissue mets	5	11	1	17
All	73	165	5	243

34.4 Discussion

In vivo molecular imaging by somatostatin analogue-based PET/CT has become the gold standard in clinical practice for diagnostics of GEP NET [31, 32]. These peptides exhibit fast pharmacokinetics, fast target localization, fast blood clearance, and fast renal excretion [33]. Scanning time is short and radiation dose is low [33]. Additional qualities are high sensitivity, high resolution, high detection rate, high image contrast, and the possibility of accurate quantification [33].

In this study, we have demonstrated a significantly higher accumulation of ^{68}Ga-DOTATOC compared to ^{68}Ga-DOTATATE, not only in primary tumors, but also in metastases (hepatic, lymph node and bone). In soft tissue metastases, ^{68}Ga-DOTATOC SUVmax tended to be higher too, but the difference was not statistically significant. The results from this study are very similar to the results obtained by Poeppel et al. [27, 28], who also found significantly higher SUV max for ^{68}Ga-DOTATOC compared to ^{68}Ga-DOTATATE, although actual SUVmax values for different lesion types show differences between both studies, which may be explained by individual variations in receptor densities. Nevertheless, for ^{68}Ga-DOTATOC, Poeppel et al. [28] reported the highest SUVmax for primary tumors, followed in decreasing order by metastases in liver, lymph nodes and bone, which is identical to the order found in this study. For ^{68}Ga-DOTATATE, a similar sequence was observed in this study, albeit with lower SUVmax values than for ^{68}Ga-DOTATOC, whereas Poeppel et al. reported a marginally higher SUVmax in liver metastases than in primary tumors for ^{68}Ga-DOTATATE. However, it needs to be emphasized that the difference in SUVmax between primary tumors and hepatic metastases in the present study was not significant, whereas this was not tested by Poeppel et al.

Explanations for the different SUVmax values of ^{68}Ga-DOTATOC and ^{68}Ga-DOTATATE [27, 29] have been sought in the different in vitro affinity profiles for the various sst receptor subtypes of these ligands [6, 7]. ^{68}Ga-DOTATATE has the highest in vitro affinity for sstr 2 (IC50 = 0.20 ± 0.04 nM/L), even higher than natural somatostatin-28 (IC50 = 2.7 ± 0.3 nM/L). Affinity of ^{68}Ga-DOTATOC for sstr 2 (IC50 = 2.5 ± 0.5 nM/L) is similar to natural somatostatin-28, but tenfold lower than the affinity of ^{68}Ga-DOTATATE. However, ^{68}Ga-DOTATOC has 39% higher affinity for sstr 3 (IC50 = 613 ± 140 nM/L) and fivefold higher for sstr 5 (IC50 = 73 ± 21 nM/L) compared to DOTATATE (IC= > 1000 nM/L for sstr 3 and IC50 = 377 ± 18 nM/L for sstr 5) [26, 34]. However, at the peptide mass dose used in this study, the highest tracer plasma concentration that can be reached is in the low nanomolar, if not the subnanomolar, range. At this concentration, the only appreciable binding that may be expected for both tracers is with sstr 2 and any binding to other sst receptor subtypes will be very minor or negligible, even when the protein mass of the different receptor subtypes would be comparable. Predicted binding will be even less when taking into account that only a very small fraction of the peptide is actually radiolabeled and that the in vitro affinity of the unlabeled tracers is lower than for the ^{68}Ga-labeled tracers [26].

These latter considerations would certainly correspond with the significant correlation of membranous sstr 2 expression as determined by immunohistochemistry and ^{68}Ga-DOTATOC PET/CT SUVmax in patients with NETs [35]. Interestingly, Kaemmerer et al. demonstrated highly significant correlations between the SUVmax in ^{68}Ga-DOTANOC PET/CT scans and immunoreactive scores of both sstr 2A and sstr 5 of NET patients [36]. Importantly, Wild et al. have reported for ^{68}Ga-DOTANOC an sstr 2 IC50 = 1.9 ± 0.4 nM/L and an sstr 5 IC50 = 7.2 ± 1.6 nM/L, both values in the low nanomolar range [37]. However, even if for ^{68}Ga-DOTATOC and ^{68}Ga-DOTATATE only binding to sstr 2 plays a role, the higher SUVmax of ^{68}Ga-DOTATOC is in remarkable contrast with the reported >10 times higher in vitro affinity of ^{68}Ga-DOTATATE for sstr 2. As Poeppel et al. concluded, this >10 times higher in vitro affinity of ^{68}Ga-DOTATATE did not prove to be clinically relevant. The affinity profiles for the various somatostatin receptor subtypes have been established in vitro in transfected cell cultures. The in vivo affinity for these somatostatin receptor subtypes expressed in their native environment may be further determined by, for instance, allosteric modulation and/or receptor clustering, which may impact the various ligand affinities differently. In this respect, it is highly interesting to note that in transfected cells expressing both sstr 2 and sstr 5, substantial heterodimerization was observed depending on the type of sst-agonist. The sstr 2/sstr 5 heterodimerization resulted in augmented receptor recycling and an approximate tenfold increase in efficiency for G-protein-coupling and MAPK activation [38, 39]. Unfortunately, the effects of DOTATOC and DOTATATE on formation of sstr homo- and heterodimers and their functional consequences are unknown.

In therapeutic applications with higher plasma concentrations of somatostatin analogues, binding to sstr subtypes with lower affinities may become more relevant. The most commonly expressed subtypes in GEP NETs are known to be sstr 2A and sstr 5. The expression of sstr 2 and sstr 5 has a prognostic role as reported by Corleto et al. [40]. They observed a significantly better survival rate in patients with well-differentiated endocrine carcinomas expressing sstr 2, sstr 5 and Ki-67 < 2%, treated with somatostatin analogues, compared to those with sstr 2 and sstr 5 negative tumors and Ki-67 ≥ 2% ($p < 0.038$). Five years survival rates were 91% vs. 43%, respectively. The positive prognostic role of expression of sstr 2 and sstr 5 is possibly related to the high affinity that the available somatostatin analogs display for these two specific sstr subtypes [40]. Interestingly, when going from well-differentiated endocrine tumors to poorly differentiated endocrine carcinomas, the densi-

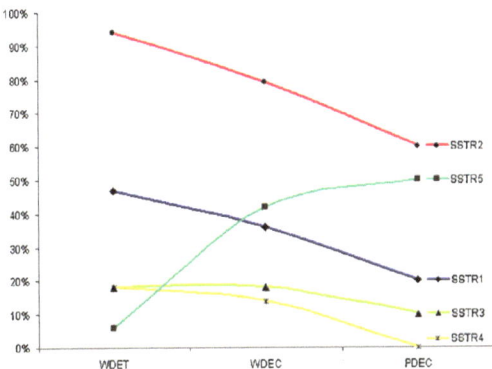

Fig. 34.4 Percentage of GEP-NETs with sstr 1–5 expression according to WHO classification. *WDET* well-differentiated endocrine tumor, *WDEC* well-differentiated endocrine carcinoma, *PDEC* poorly differentiated endocrine carcinoma. (Adapted with permission from [25], copyright Elsevier)

ties of sstr 1, sstr 2, sstr 3, and sstr 4 all decrease, but the density of sstr 5 shows a substantial increase [25] (Fig. 34.4).

We could not register differences in uptake between the two radiopharmaceuticals in normal liver tissue, which had significantly lower SUVmax values than primaries and liver- and lymph node metastases. In a previous publication [41], we have compared in vivo uptake of ⁶⁸Ga-DOTATOC in liver and prostate (being threefold lower in the prostate) with in vitro sstr 2 expression (being sixfold greater in prostate) [42]. Higher liver uptake of ⁶⁸Ga-DOTATOC than expected on the basis of sstr 2 expression has been related to normal peptide metabolism in the liver [42, 43]. Our result of almost identical uptake of ⁶⁸Ga-DOTATOC and ⁶⁸Ga-DOTATATE in normal liver tissue supports this explanation. ⁶⁸Ga-DOTATOC SUVmax values for renal parenchyma at 1 h, 2 h, and 3 h and for liver at 1 h and 2 h were found to be lower than ⁶⁸Ga-DOTATATE SUVmax values [29], while the tumor-to-kidney ratio has been reported to be higher than that of ⁶⁸Ga-DOTATATE [29, 44]. Added to the higher ⁶⁸Ga-DOTATOC SUVmax values for primary tumors and metastases, this would make ⁶⁸Ga-DOTATOC, the preferred peptide for somatostatin receptor imaging. However, we have also

shown considerable variability in preferred peptide uptake, suggesting that for therapy planning somatostatin receptor imaging with both peptides would be optimal, ideally with the same peptide amount as planned for therapy. Unfortunately, although ¹⁷⁷Lu is currently the most widely used radionuclide for peptide receptor radionuclide therapy in NET patients, the affinity profiles of ¹⁷⁷Lu-DOTATOC and ¹⁷⁷Lu-DOTATATE for the various sstr have not been published to date.

34.4.1 Potential Limitations

For each patient, the first somatostatin receptor imaging reported in this study was performed with ⁶⁸Ga-DOTATATE, the second with ⁶⁸Ga-DOTATOC. However, as already mentioned, we have only selected patients, with clinically, biochemically, and morphologically stable disease on both occasions.

Partial volume effect in this study, described for lesions whose diameter is smaller than two or three times the scanner resolution [45], had no influence on the results, since both radiopharmaceuticals were compared under the same conditions in the same patients, in the same primaries and in the same metastases.

34.5 Conclusions

On average, ⁶⁸Ga-DOTATOC shows significantly higher uptake in GEP-NET primary tumors and metastases than ⁶⁸Ga-DOTATATE. However, we have also observed considerable variability in preferred peptide uptake. Optimal therapy planning would therefore require somatostatin receptor imaging with both these peptides.

Conflict of Interest Mila V. Todorović-Tirnanić, Cees J.A. van Echteld, Milan M. Gajić, and Richard P. Baum declare that they have no conflict of interest. Mila V. Todorović-Tirnanić was International Atomic Energy Agency (IAEA, TC Project SRB/6/005) fellow from February to April 2010 at the Department of Nuclear Medicine and Centre for PET/CT, Zentralklinik Bad Berka, when this work was done.

Ethical Approval The institutional review board of Zentralklinik Bad Berka has approved this retrospective study.

Informed Consent Informed consent was obtained from all patients in accordance with German regulations concerning administration of radiolabeled substances to humans and documentation of the data in a database for future studies.

References

1. Ambrosini V, Campana D, Tomassetti P, Fanti S. 68Ga-labelled peptides for diagnosis of gastroenteropancreatic NET. Eur J Nucl Med Mol Imaging. 2012;39(Suppl 1):S52–60.

2. Yao JC, Hassan M, Phan A, Dagohoy C, Leary C, Mares JE, Abdalla EK, Fleming JB, Vauthey JN, Rashid A, Evans DB. One hundred years after "carcinoid": epidemiology of and prognostic factors for neuroendocrine tumors in 35,825 cases in the United States. J Clin Oncol. 2008;26:3063–72.

3. Modlin IM, Kidd M, Latich I, Zikusoka MN, Shapiro MD. Current status of gastrointestinal carcinoids. Gastroenterology. 2005;128:1717–51.

4. Modlin IM, Lye KD, Kidd M. A 5-decade analysis of 13,715 carcinoid tumors. Cancer. 2003;97:934–59.

5. Wiedenmann B, John M, Ahnert-Hilger G, Riecken EO. Molecular and cell biological aspects of neuroendocrine tumors of the gastroenteropancreatic system. J Mol Med (Berl). 1998;76:637–47.

6. Reubi JC. Peptide receptor expression in GEP-NET. Virchows Arch. 2007;451(Issue 1 Supplement):47–50.

7. Reubi JC, Waser B. Concomitant expression of several peptide receptors in neuroendocrine tumors: molecular basis for in vivo multireceptor targeting. Eur J Nucl Med Mol Imaging. 2003;30:781–93.

8. Bombardieri E, Maccauro M, De Deckere E, Savelli G, Chiti A. Nuclear medicine imaging of neuroendocrine tumors. Ann Oncol. 2001;12(suppl2):S51–61.

9. Krenning EP, Kwekkeboom DJ, Bakker WH, Breeman WA, Kooij PP, Oei HY, van Hagen M, Postema PT, de Jong M, Reubi JC, et al. Somatostatin receptor scintigraphy with [111In-DTPA-D-Phe1]- and [123I-Tyr3]-octreotide: the rotterdam experience with more than 1000 patients. Eur J Nucl Med. 1993;20:716–31.

10. de Jong M, Bakker WH, Krenning EP, Breeman WA, van der Pluijm ME, Bernard BF, Visser TJ, Jermann E, Béhé M, Powell P, Mäcke HR. Yttrium-90 and indium-111 labelling, receptor binding and biodistribution of [DOTA0,d-Phe1,Tyr3]octreotide, a promising somatostatin analogue for radionuclide therapy. Eur J Nucl Med. 1997;24:368–71.

11. Decristoforo C, Mather SJ, Cholewinski W, Donnemiller E, Riccabona G, Moncayo R. 99mTc-EDDA/HYNIC-TOC: a new 99mTc-labelled

12. Maina T, Nock B, Nikolopoulou A, Sotiriou P, Loudos G, Maintas D, Cordopatis P, Chiotellis E. [99mTc]Demotate, a new 99mTc-based [Tyr3]octreotate analogue for the detection of somatostatin receptor-positive tumours: synthesis and preclinical results. Eur J Nucl Med Mol Imaging. 2002;29:742–53.

13. Storch D, Béhé M, Walter MA, Chen J, Powell P, Mikolajczak R, Mäcke HR. Evaluation of [99mTc/EDDA/HYNIC0]octreotide derivatives compared with [111In-DOTA0,Tyr3, Thr8]octreotide and [111In-DTPA0]octreotide: does tumor or pancreas uptake correlate with the rate of internalization? J Nucl Med. 2005;46:1561–9.

14. Smith-Jones PM, Stolz B, Bruns C, Albert R, Reist HW, Fridrich R, Mäcke HR. Gallium-67/gallium-68-[DFO]-octreotide—a potential radiopharmaceutical for PET imaging of somatostatin receptor-positive tumors: synthesis and radiolabeling in vitro and preliminary in vivo studies. J Nucl Med. 1994;35:317–25.

15. Henriksen G, Schottelius M, Poethko T, Hauser A, Wolf I, Schwaiger M, Wester HJ. Proof of principle for the use of 11C-labelled peptides in tumour diagnosis with PET. Eur J Nucl Med Mol Imaging. 2004;31:1653–7.

16. Hofmann M, Maecke H, Börner R, Weckesser E, Schöffski P, Oei L, Schumacher J, Henze M, Heppeler A, Meyer J, Knapp H. Biokinetics and imaging with the somatostatin receptor PET radioligand (68)Ga-DOTATOC: preliminary data. Eur J Nucl Med. 2001;28:1751–7.

17. Wester HJ, Schottelius M, Scheidhauer K, Meisetschläger G, Herz M, Rau FC, Reubi JC, Schwaiger M. PET imaging of somatostatin receptors: design, synthesis and preclinical evaluation of a novel 18F-labelled, carbohydrated analogue of octreotide. Eur J Nucl Med Mol Imaging. 2003;30:117–22.

18. Sprague JE, Peng Y, Sun X, Weisman GR, Wong EH, Achilefu S, Anderson CJ. Preparation and biological evaluation of copper-64-labeled tyr3-octreotate using a cross-bridged macrocyclic chelator. Clin Cancer Res. 2004;10:8674–82.

19. Singh A, van der Meulen NP, Müller C, Klette I, Kulkarni HR, Türler A, Schibli R, Baum RP. First-in-human PET/CT imaging of metastatic neuroendocrine neoplasms with cyclotron-produced 44Sc-DOTATOC: a proof-of-concept study. Cancer Biother Radiopharm. 2017;32:124–32.

20. Baum RP, Singh A, Benešová M, Vermeulen C, Gnesin S, Köster U, Johnston K, Müller D, Senftleben S, Kulkarni HR, Türler A, Schibli R, Prior JO, van der Meulen NP, Müller C. Clinical evaluation of the radiolanthanide terbium-152: first-in-human PET/CT with 152Tb-DOTATOC. Dalton Trans. 2017;46:14638–46.

21. Gabriel M, Decristoforo C, Kendler D, Dobrozemsky G, Heute D, Uprimny C, Kovacs P, Von Guggenberg E, Bale R, Virgolini IJ. 68Ga-DOTA-Tyr3-octreotide

PET in neuroendocrine tumors: comparison with somatostatin receptor scintigraphy and CT. J Nucl Med. 2007;48:508–18.

22. Srirajaskanthan R, Kayani I, Quigley AM, Soh J, Caplin ME, Bomanji J. The role of 68Ga-DOTATATE PET in patients with neuroendocrine tumors and negative or equivocal findings on 111In-DTPA-octreotide scintigraphy. J Nucl Med. 2010;51:875–82.

23. Walker RC, Smith GT, Liu E, Moore B, Clanton J, Stabin M. Measured human dosimetry of 68Ga-DOTATATE. J Nucl Med. 2013;54:855–60.

24. Reubi JC. Peptide receptors as molecular targets for cancer diagnosis and therapy. Endocr Rev. 2003;24:389–427.

25. Zamora V, Cabanne A, Salanova R, Bestani C, Domenichini E, Marmissolle F, Giacomi N, O'Connor J, Méndez G, Roca E, Argentum Working Group. Immunohistochemical expression of somatostatin receptors in digestive endocrine tumours. Dig Liver Dis. 2010;42:220–5.

26. Reubi JC, Schar JC, Waser B, Wenger S, Heppeler A, Schmitt JS, et al. Affinity profiles for human somatostatin receptor subtypes SST1-SST5 of somatostatin radiotracers selected for scintigraphic and radiotherapeutic use. Eur J Nucl Med. 2000;27:273–82.

27. Poeppel TD, Binse I, Petersenn S, Lahner H, Schott M, Antoch G, Brandau W, Bockisch A, Boy C. 68Ga-DOTATOC versus 68Ga-DOTATATE PET/CT in functional imaging of neuroendocrine tumors. J Nucl Med. 2011;52:1864–70.

28. Poeppel TD, Binse I, Petersenn S, Lahner H, Schott M, Antoch G, Brandau W, Bockisch A, Boy C. Differential uptake of 68Ga-DOTATOC and 68Ga-DOTATATE in PET/CT of gastroenteropancreatic neuroendocrine tumors. Recent Results Cancer Res. 2013;194:353–71.

29. Velikyan I, Sundin A, Sörensen J, Lubberink M, Sandström M, Garske-Román U, Lundqvist H, Granberg D, Eriksson B. Quantitative and qualitative intrapatient comparison of 68Ga-DOTATOC and 68Ga-DOTATATE: net uptake rate for accurate quantification. J Nucl Med. 2014;55:204–10.

30. Zhernosekov KP, Filosofov DV, Baum RP, Aschoff P, Bihl H, Razbash AA, Jahn M, Jennewein M, Rösch F. Processing of generator-produced 68Ga for medical application. J Nucl Med. 2007;48:1741–8.

31. Kaemmerer D, Athelogou M, Lupp A, Lenhardt I, Schulz S, Peter L, Hommann M, Prasad V, Binnig G, Baum RP. Somatostatin receptor immunohistochemistry in neuroendocrine tumors: comparison between manual and automated evaluation. Int J Clin Exp Pathol. 2014;7:4971–80.

32. Treglia G, Castaldi P, Rindi G, Giordano A, Rufini V. Diagnostic performance of gallium-68 somatostatin receptor PET and PET/CT in patients with thoracic and gastroenteropancreatic neuroendocrine tumours: a meta-analysis. Endocrine. 2012;42:80–7.

33. Naji M, Al-Nahhas A. 68Ga-labelled peptides in the management of neuroectodermaltumours. Eur J Nucl Med Mol Imaging. 2012;39(suppl.1):S61–7.

34. Antunes P, Ginj M, Yhang H, et al. Are radiogallium-labelled DOTA-conjugated somatostatin analogues superior to those labeled with other radiometals? Eur J Nucl Med Mol Imaging. 2007;34:982–93.

35. Miederer M, Seidl S, Buck A, Scheidhauer K, Wester HJ, Schwaiger M, et al. Correlation of immunohistopathological expression of somatostatin receptor 2 with standardised uptake values in 68Ga-DOTATOC PET/CT. Eur J Nucl Med Mol Imaging. 2009;36:48–52.

36. Kaemmerer D, Peter L, Lupp A, Schulz S, Sänger J, Prasad V, Kulkarni H, Haugvik SP, Hommann M, Baum RP. Molecular imaging with 68Ga-SSTR PET/CT and correlation to immunohistochemistry of somatostatin receptors in neuroendocrine tumors. Eur J Nucl Med Mol Imaging. 2011;38:1659–68.

37. Wild D, Mäcke HR, Waser B, Reubi JC, Ginj M, Rasch H, Müller-Brand J, Hofmann M. 68Ga-DOTANOC: a first compound for PET imaging with high affinity for somatostatin receptor subtypes 2 and 5. Eur J Nucl Med Mol Imaging. 2005;32:724.

38. Grant M, Alturaihi H, Jaquet P, Collier B, Kumar U. Cell growth inhibition and functioning of human somatostatin receptor type 2 are modulated by receptor heterodimerization. Mol Endocrinol. 2008;22:2278–92.

39. Kumar U. G-protein coupled receptors dimerization: diversity in somatostatin receptors subtypes. J Pharmacogenom Pharmacoproteomics. 2013;4:120.

40. Corleto VD, Falconi M, Panzuto F, Milione M, De Luca O, Perri P, Cannizzaro R, Bordi C, Pederzoli P, Scarpa A, DelleFave G. Somatostatin receptor subtypes 2 and 5 are associated with better survival in well-differentiated endocrine carcinomas. Neuroendocrinology. 2009;89:223–30.

41. Todorović-Tirnanić MV, Gajić MM, Obradović VB, Baum RP. Gallium-68 DOTATOC PET/CT in vivo characterization of somatostatin receptor expression in the prostate. Cancer Biother Radiopharm. 2014;29:108–15.

42. Boy C, Heusner TA, Poeppel TD, et al. 68Ga-DOTATOC PET/CT and somatostatin receptor (sst1-sst5) expression in normal human tissue: correlation of sst2 mRNA and SUVmax. Eur J Nucl Med Mol Imaging. 2011;38:1224–36.

43. Prasad V, Baum RP. Biodistribution of Ga-68 labeled somatostatin analogue DOTA-NOC in patients with neuroendocrine tumours: characterisation of uptake in normal organs and tumour lesions. Q J Nucl Med Mol Imaging. 2010;54:61–7.

44. Schuchardt C, Kulkarni HR, Prasad V, Zachert C, Müller D, Baum RP. The Bad Berka dose protocol: comparative results of dosimetry in pepide receptor radionuclide therapy using ^{177}Lu-DOTATATE, ^{177}Lu-DOTANOC, and ^{177}Lu-DOTATOC. Recent Results Cancer Res. 2013;194:519–36.

45. Soret M, Bacharach SL, Buvat I. Partial-volume effect in PET tumor imaging. J Nucl Med. 2007;48:932–45.

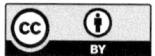

Damian Wild

35.1 Introduction

Somatostatin receptor (SST) scintigraphy for imaging and somatostatin analogues for treatment have been used for the management of patients for more than 20 years. In the last 20 years, important developments have improved the management of patients with neuroendocrine tumours (NETs) or neuroendocrine neoplasias (NENs): (1) introduction of peptide receptor radionuclide therapy (PRRT) with radiolabelled SST agonists such as ^{90}Y- or ^{177}Lu-DOTA-TOC and ^{177}Lu-DOTA-TATE [1], (2) invention of SST PET/CT with radiolabelled SST agonists, such as ^{68}Ga-DOTA-TOC, ^{68}Ga-DOTA-TATE and ^{68}Ga-DOTA-NOC which allows most sensitive staging and restaging of NETs as well as the identification of those patients who will benefit from PRRT (theranostic approach) [2], (3) evaluation of PRRT in a randomized, controlled phase III trial with an intervention arm (^{177}Lu-DOTA-TATE plus somatostatin analogue octreotide LAR), and a control arm (high-dose octreotide LAR) showing the superiority of PRRT in comparison to the treatment with somatostatin analogues [3], (4) discovery that PRRT with

α-emitters is likely to perform better than with β-emitters in certain conditions [4], (5) last, but not least, introduction of SST antagonists, which seem to recognize more bindings sites on SST-expressing cancer cells and show favourable pharmacokinetics and better tumour visualization than agonists despite of very poor internalisation rates [5, 6].

Current preclinical and clinical developments of radiolabelled SST antagonists for theranostics (imaging and therapy) and their clinical potential, not only in NETs but also on other tumours are discussed here.

35.2 Part I. Preclinical Development of SST Antagonists for Theranostics

More than 20 years ago, Bass et al. found that the inversion of chirality at position 1 and 2 of the octapeptide (octreotide family) converted an agonist into a potent antagonist [7]. Afterwards, structure activity relationship studies done by Hocart et al. revealed different potent antagonists [8] which were used as lead structures by Jean Rivier (Salk Institute for Biologic Studies, La Jolla, CA), Jean Claude Reubi (University of Bern, Switzerland), and Helmut R. Mäcke (University Hospital Basel, Switzerland) for the collaborative development of SST antagonists for labelling with radiometals [5, 9].

D. Wild (✉)
Division of Nuclear Medicine, University Hospital Basel, Basel, Switzerland
e-mail: Damian.Wild@usb.ch

© The Author(s) 2024

V. Prasad (ed.), *Beyond Becquerel and Biology to Precision Radiomolecular Oncology: Festschrift in Honor of Richard P. Baum*, https://doi.org/10.1007/978-3-031-33533-4_35

The first radiolabelled SST antagonists were labelled with Indium-111 (^{111}In) via the DOTA (1,4,7,10-tetraazacyclododecan-1,4,7,10-tetraacetic acid) chelator and were based on the somatostatin receptor subtype 2 (SST2)-specific antagonist BASS (p-NO$_2$-Phe-cyclo(D-Cys-Tyr-D-Trp-Lys-Thr-Cys)D-Tyr-NH$_2$) (Table 35.1), developed by Bass et al. [7], and the SST3-specific antagonist SST3-ODN-8, developed by Reubi et al. [10]. Comparison of these new SST selective antagonists (^{111}In-DOTA-BASS and ^{111}In-DOTA-SST3-ODN-8) with highly potent SST agonists (^{111}In-DTPA-TATE which is SST2 specific and ^{111}In-DOTA-NOC which has affinity for SST3, in addition to SST2 and SST5) showed somewhat unexpected results in mice bearing human SST2- and SST3-expressing xenografts:

1. Tumour uptake was more than 1.5-fold higher with the antagonist, despite of the lower receptor affinity [5].
2. Tumour uptake was longer lasting with the antagonist, despite the lack of tumour cell internalisation [5, 11].

An important finding of these first studies was that radiolabelled SST antagonists recognized a larger number of binding sites in vitro than radiolabelled SST agonists [5].

Table 35.1 Affinities of metallated somatostatin analogues (IC$_{50}$ in nM)

Metallated somatostatin analogue	Chemical structure	Affinity					Clinical development
		SST1	SST2	SST3	SST4	SST5	
Agonist							
In-DTPA-octreotide[a]	^{111}In-DTPA-D-Phe-cyclo (Cys-Phe-D-Trp-Lys-Thr-Cys)Thr(ol)	>10'000	22 ± 3.6	182 ± 13	>1000	237 ± 52	EMA approved
Ga-DOTA-TOC[a]	^{68}Ga-DOTA-D-Phe-cyclo (Cys-thy-D-Trp-Lys-Thr-Cys)Thr(ol)	>10'000	2.5 ± 0.5	613 ± 140	>1'000	73 ± 21	Prospective phase II
Ga-DOTA-TATE[a]	^{68}Ga-DOTA-D-Phe-cyclo (Cys-Tyr-D-Trp-Lys-Thr-Cys)Thr	>10'000	0.2 ± 0.04	>1'000	300 ± 140	377 ± 18	EMA approved
Lu-DOTA-TATE[b]	^{177}Lu-DOTA-D-Phe-cyclo (Cys-Tyr-D-Trp-Lys-Thr-Cys)Thr	>10'000	2.0 ± 0.8	162 ± 16	>1'000	>1'000	EMA approved
Ga-DOTA-NOC[c]	^{68}Ga-DOTA-D-Phe-cyclo (Cys-1-Nal-D-Trp-Lys-Thr-Cys)Thr(ol)	>10'000	1.9 ± 0.4	40 ± 5.8	260 ± 74	7.2 ± 1.6	Prospective phase II
Antagonist							
In-DOTA-BASS[d]	^{111}In-DOTA-p-NO$_2$-Phe--cyclo (D-Cys.Tyr-D-Trp-Lys-Thr-Cys) D-Tyr-NH$_2$	>1'000	9.4 ± 0.4	>1'000	380 ± 57	>1'000	Preliminary clinical data
Ga-NODAGA-JR10[e]	^{68}Ga-NODAGA-p-NO$_2$-Phe-cyclo[D-Cys-Tyr-D-Aph(Cbm)-Lys-Thr-Cys]-D-Tyr-NH$_2$	>1'000	6.5 ± 0.5	>1'000	>1'000	>1'000	No clinical data
Ga-DOTA-JR11[e] (Ga-OPS201)	^{68}Ga-DOTA-p-cl-Phe--cyclo[D-Cys-Aph(hor)-D-Aph(Cbm)-Lys-Thr-Cys]-D-Tyr-NH$_2$	>1'000	29 ± 2.7	>1'000	>1'000	>1'000	Prospective theranostic
Ga-NODAGA-JR11[e] (Ga-OPS202)	^{68}Ga-NODAGA-p-cl-Phe--cyclo[D-Cys-Aph(hor)-D-Aph(Cbm)-Lys-Thr-Cys)-D-Tyr-NH$_2$	>1'000	1.2 ± 0.2	>1'000	>1'000	>1'000	Prospective phase I/II

(continued)

Table 35.1 (continued)

Metallated somatostatin analogue	Chemical structure	Affinity					Clinical development
		SST1	SST2	SST3	SST4	SST5	
Lu-DOTA-JR11[e] (Lu-OPS201)	^{177}Lu-DOTA-p-cl-Phe--cyclo[D-Cys-Aph(hor)-D-Aph(Cbm)-Lys-Thr-Cys]-D-Tyr-NH$_2$	>1'000	0.7 ± 0.2	>1'000	>1'000	>1'000	Prospective phase I/II
Ga-NODAGA-LM3[e]	^{68}Ga-NODAGA-p-cl-Phe--cyclo[D-Cys-Tyr-D-Aph(Cbm)-Lys-Thr-Cys]-D-Tyr-NH$_2$	>1'000	1.3 ± 0.3	>1'000	>1'000	>1'000	Prospective phase II
Ga-DOTA-LM3[e]	^{68}Ga-DOTA-p-cl-Phe--cyclo[D-Cys-Tyr-D-Aph(Cbm)-Lys-Thr-Cys]-D-Tyr-NH$_2$	>1'000	12.5 ± 4.3	>1'000	>1'000	>1'000	Prospective phase II

All data are mean ± SED, except Lu-DOTATATE data, which are mean ± SD (laboratory that generated Lu-DOTA-TATE data was different from laboratory that generated the rest of the data). *1-Nal* 1-naphtyl-alanine, *Aph(Hor)* 4-amino-L-hydroorotyl-phenylalanine, *D-Aph(Cbm)* D-4-amino-carbamoyl-phenylalanine, *EMA* European Medicines Agency

[a] Data are from Reubi et al. [15]
[b] Data are from Schottelius et al. [16]
[c] Data are from Wild et al. [17]
[d] Data are from Ginj et al. [5]
[e] Data are from Fani et al. [13]

35.2.1 Second Generation of Radiolabelled SST Antagonists

The same collaborative group (Jean Rivier, Jean Claude Reubi and Helmut R. Mäcke) designed the second generation of SST antagonists with improved SST2 affinities for labelling with the positron emitter Gallium-68 (^{68}Ga) for PET/CT imaging as well as β^--emitters (^{177}Lu and ^{90}Y) for therapy: this included different SST2 specific antagonists such as JR10 (p-NO$_2$-Phe-cyclo-D--Tyr-NH$_2$), JR11 (Cpa-cyclo-D-Tyr-NH$_2$), and LM3 (p-Cl-Phe-cyclo[D-Cys-Tyr-D-Aph(Cbm)-Lys-Thr-Cys]D-Tyr-NH$_2$) [9, 12, 13], in combination with two chelators, namely, DOTA and NODAGA (1,4,7-triazacyclononane,1-glutaric acid-4,7-acetic acid), (Table 35.1).

Biodistribution and affinity studies with ^{68}Ga-labelled DOTA- and NODAGA-SST2 antagonists indicated that the chelate made the difference as ^{68}Ga-NODAGA conjugates improved the affinity to SST2 and increased the SST2-specific tumour uptake [13, 14]. Furthermore, the Ga(III)-DOTA-SST2 antagonists had a lower affinity for SST2 than the respective Y(III)-DOTA-, Lu(III)-DOTA-, or In(III)-DOTA-SSTR2 antagonists (Table 35.1), [13]. For the understanding of the potential of radiolabelled SST2 antagonists, the comparison with high-affinity SST2 agonists is crucial. For example, ^{68}Ga-DOTA-JR11 and ^{68}Ga-NODAGA-JR11, having a lower affinity for SST2 (~145-fold and ~ six-fold) than ^{68}Ga-DOTA-TATE (Table 35.1), demonstrated in vivo tumour uptake that was 1.3-fold and 1.7-fold higher in a preclinical head-to-head comparison [13].

SST2 antagonists indicated not only superior biodistribution and tumour uptake in combination with ^{68}Ga for PET/CT imaging but also with β^--emitters for a therapeutic approach. For example, a head-to-head comparison of 10 pmol ^{177}Lu-DOTA-JR11 and 10 pmol ^{177}Lu-DOTA-TATE showed significantly higher tumour uptake for ^{177}Lu-DOTA-JR11 (11.7 ± 2.15% injected

activity per gram) than for ^{177}Lu-DOTA-TATE (3.66 ± 0.54% injected activity per gram) at 72 h after injection resulting in a 2.6 times higher tumour radiation dose [14]. Importantly, also tumour-to-background dose ratios (kidney, bone marrow, spleen, and liver) were higher with ^{177}Lu-DOTA-JR11 than with ^{177}Lu-DOTA-TATE. The tumour-to-background dose ratio could be further enhanced by increasing the amount of ^{177}Lu-DOTA-JR11 from 10 pmol to 200 pmol (e.g., tumour-to-liver dose ratios were 20.9 with 10 pmol peptide mass and 44.9 with 200 pmol peptide mass) [14]. Comparison of ^{177}Lu-DOTA-JR11 and ^{177}Lu-DOTA-TATE in a mice xenograft study indicated a higher median survival rate (71 vs. 61 day) and a longer delay in tumour growth (26 ± 7 vs. 18 ± 5 day) in ^{177}Lu-DOTA-JR11 treated mice [18]. Similar results are found by Albrecht et al. comparing ^{177}Lu-DOTA-JR11 with ^{177}Lu-DOTA-TOC [19]. Despite the fact that 88 ± 1% of the SST2 antagonist remained on the surface of the tumour cells, ^{177}Lu-DOTA-JR11 showed several time higher tumour uptake and caused at least 60% more DNA double-strand breaks than ^{177}Lu-DOTA-TATE [18]. Head-to-head comparison of ^{90}Y-DOTA-JR11 and ^{177}Lu-DOTA-JR11 revealed a lower therapeutic index of ^{90}Y-DOTA-JR11 with a ~ 20% lower tumour-to-kidney uptake ratio and a > 4 times higher effective dose in treated mice [14]. Furthermore, ^{111}In-DOTA-JR11 cannot be used as a surrogate of ^{90}Y-DOTA-JR11 for imaging and dosimetry studies because of differences in their pharmacokinetics and affinity for SST2 [13, 14].

Based on the affinity profile and preclinical in vivo studies [9, 12, 13] the following radiotracers were advancing into patients:

1. ^{68}Ga-NODAGA-JR11 and ^{68}Ga-NODAGA-LM3 for PET/CT imaging.
2. ^{177}Lu-DOTA-JR11 for therapy with its theranostic companion ^{68}Ga-DOTA-JR11 and ^{68}Ga-NODAGA-JR11.
3. ^{177}Lu-DOTA-LM3 for therapy with its theranostic companion ^{68}Ga-NODAGA-LM3 and and ^{68}Ga-DOTA-LM3.

Table 35.2 SST2 binding in different human tumours

Tumour	Respective in vitro autoradiography study: SSTR antagonist/SSTR agonist	Samples (n)	Antagonist-to-agonist ratio
Non-Hodgkin lymphoma	^{125}I-JR11/^{125}I-Tyr[3]-octreotide[a]	15	14.0
	^{177}Lu-DOTA-BASS/^{177}Lu-DOTA-TATE[b]	12	4.8
Renal cell carcinoma	^{125}I-JR11/^{125}I-Tyr[3]-octreotide[a]	12	10.9
	^{177}Lu-DOTA-BASS/^{177}Lu-DOTA-TATE[b]	10	5.1
Breast cancer	^{125}I-JR11/^{125}I-Tyr[3]-octreotide[a]	13	7.9
	^{177}Lu-DOTA-BASS/^{177}Lu-DOTA-TATE[b]	7	11.4
Pheochromocytoma	^{125}I-JR11/^{125}I-Tyr[3]-octreotide[a]	5	17.6
	^{177}Lu-DOTA-BASS/^{177}Lu-DOTA-TATE[b]	10	12.3
Ileal NET	^{125}I-JR11/^{125}I-Tyr[3]-octreotide[a]	4	3.8
	^{177}Lu-DOTA-BASS/^{177}Lu-DOTA-TATE[b]	9	4.2
Medullary thyroid cancer	^{125}I-JR11/^{125}I-Tyr[3]-octreotide[a]	5	21.8
Small cell lung cancer	^{125}I-JR11/^{125}I-Tyr[3]-octreotide[a]	4	4.5
Paraganglioma	^{125}I-JR11/^{125}I-Tyr[3]-octreotide[a]	2	15.6
Lung NET	^{125}I-JR11/^{125}I-Tyr[3]-octreotide[a]	1	6.4

[a] Data are from Reubi et al. [20]
[b] Data are from Cescato et al. [21]

35.3 Part II. Novel Indications for Theranostics with SST Antagonists

The binding capacity of radiolabelled SST antagonists and agonists were compared in human tissue samples from nine different tumours using in vitro autoradiography with the following SST antagonist/agonist pair: ^{125}I-JR11/^{125}I-Tyr[3]-octreotide [20] and ^{177}Lu-DOTA-BASS/^{177}Lu-DOTA-TATE [21], (Table 35.2). The SST2 binding affinities (IC_{50}) of the SST antagonist/agonist pair were similar [20, 21]. Importantly, in all cases, the radiolabelled SST antagonist bound to more SST2 sites in all tumours with an uptake that was 3.8 to 21.8 times higher than with the agonist (Table 35.2). Of particular interest is the fact that tumours other than gastroenteropancreatic neuroendocrine tumours (GEP-NETs) and lung NETs have the potential to become targets for radiolabelled SST2 antagonists despite of the relatively low SST2 expression, for example: non-Hodgkin lymphomas, renal cell carcinoma, breast cancer, pheochromocytoma, paraganglioma, medullary thyroid cancer, small cell lung cancer and paraganglioma.

35.4 Part III. Clinical Development of SST Antagonists

Based on these promising in vitro human tumour data as well as in vivo animal data transition into clinic was started with the most promising diagnostic and therapeutic SST2 antagonists.

35.4.1 Studies with Diagnostic SST Antagonists

First clinical evidence that imaging with SST2 antagonists may be superior to agonists was published in 2011 [6]. In this prospective study, ^{111}In-DOTA-BASS total body scintigraphy and SPECT/CT was compared with the U.S. Food and Drug Administration-approved radiotracer ^{111}In-DTPA-octreotide (OctreoScan, Mallinckrodt) and contrast-enhanced CT studies in the same five patients with NETs or thyroid cancer. The affinity profile of ^{111}In-DOTA-BASS and ^{111}In-DTPA-octreotide are in the same range (Table 35.1). A lesion-based analyses revealed a higher tumour detection rate with ^{111}In-DOTA-BASS (25/28 lesions) than with ^{111}In-DTPA-octreotide (17/28 lesions).

Based on affinity studies and preclinical results, the second generation of SST2 antagonist ^{68}Ga-NODAGA-JR11 = ^{68}Ga-OPS202 (Table 35.1) was selected for PET/CT imaging studies. Nicolas et al. performed a single-center, prospective phase I/II study with 12 GEP-NET patients comparing PET/CT with two microdoses of ^{68}Ga-NODAGA-JR11 and one microdose of the potent SSTR2 agonist ^{68}Ga-DOTA-TOC (ClinicalTrials.gov identifier: NCT02162446). The amount and activity of 15/50 µg and 150 MBq ^{68}Ga-NODAGA-JR11 was well tolerated and showed favourable dosimetry results and imaging properties with best tumour contrast between 1 and 2 h after injection [22]. Lesion-based comparison with ^{68}Ga-DOTA-TOC PET/CT showed a significantly higher sensitivity for ^{68}Ga-NODAGA-JR11 PET/CT: 93.7% (95% CI: 85.3–97.6%) vs. 59.2% (95% CI: 36.3–79.1%) [23]. In this study, diagnostic efficacy measures were compared against contrast-enhanced CT or MRI as the standard for comparison.

Several studies were performed with ^{68}Ga-DOTA-JR11 despite its 24 times lower affinity for SST2 compared to ^{68}Ga-NODAGA-JR11 (Table 35.1) [24–26]. Zhu et al. compared prospectively ^{68}Ga-DOTA-JR11 and ^{68}Ga-DOTA-TATE PET/CT in the same patients with NETs [25]. As in the study of Nicolas et al. they detected significantly more liver lesions with the SST2 antagonist (552 vs. 365), but at the same time significantly less bone lesions (158 vs. 388), compared to ^{68}Ga-DOTA-TATE. Importantly, ^{68}Ga-DOTA-JR11 showed a lower tumour uptake than the SST2 agonist ^{68}Ga-DOTA-TATE. This is in contrast to the study of Nicolas et al. who prospectively compared ^{68}Ga-NODAGA-JR11 and ^{68}Ga-DOTA-TOC PET/CT in the same patients [23]. Zhu et al. identified two reasons for this finding: (1) ^{68}Ga-DOTA-JR11 has a much lower affinity for SST2 than ^{68}Ga-NODAGA-JR11 (Table 35.1), (2) the study design may cause a bias as ^{68}Ga-DOTA-TATE PET/CT was always performed 24 h ahead of ^{68}Ga-DOTA-JR11 PET/CT. This can cause a saturation/internalisation of

SST2 [27]. The different comparator—[68]Ga-DOTA-TATE instead of ^{68}Ga-DOTA-TOC—is unlikely a confounder explaining the different findings as ^{68}Ga-DOTA-TOC showed higher tumour uptake than ^{68}Ga-DOTA-TATE in a previous study [28].

^{68}Ga-NODAGA-LM3 is another antagonist with similar SST2 affinity as ^{68}Ga-NODAGA-JR11 (Table 35.1). So far, there were only abstracts available with a brief summary of results from two retrospective compassionate use studies with ^{68}Ga-NODAGA-LM3 PET/CT. The first study showed in 40 patients with GEP-NET, lung NET, paraganglioma/pheochromocytoma etc. that PET/CT imaging with ^{68}Ga-NODAGA-LM3 is feasible [29]. The other study compared ^{68}Ga-NODAGA-LM3 and ^{68}Ga-DOTA-TOC PET/CT in ten paraganglioma patients. ^{68}Ga-NODAGA-LM3 PET/CT detected many more lesions (243 vs. 177) including many more bone lesions (190 vs. 143) than ^{68}Ga-DOTA-TOC PET/CT [30].

35.4.2 Studies with Therapeutic SST Antagonists

Based on affinity studies and preclinical results, the second generation of SST2 antagonist ^{177}Lu-DOTA-JR11 = ^{177}Lu-OPS201 (Table 35.1) was selected for a therapeutic first-in-human study: In a single-centre, prospective proof-of-principle study (phase 0 study), tumour and organ doses of ^{177}Lu-DOTA-JR11 and ^{177}Lu-DOTA-TATE were compared in the same four patients with advanced, metastatic neuroendocrine neoplasia (NEN), grade 1–3 [31]. The most relevant findings were a 3.5-fold higher median tumour dose as well as >two-fold higher tumour-to-kidney dose ratios with ^{177}Lu-DOTA-JR11 compared to ^{177}Lu-DOTA-TATE, tumour doses of up to 487 Gy and moderate adverse events with one grade 3 thrombocytopenia after treatment with three cycles (total 15.2 GBq) of ^{177}Lu-DOTA-JR11. Reidy-Lagunes et al., however, described grade 4

Table 35.3 Summary of study results with therapeutic SST antagonists

Radiotracer, identifier No.	Study design, study protocol	Subjects	Best objective response (RECIST 1.1)	1-year PFS	Thrombocytopenia, neutropenia, (CTCAE grade 3/4)
^{177}Lu-DOTA-JR11[a], NCT02609737	Single Centre, phase I, 1–2 cycles (5.0–15 GBq)	20 NETs	45%	~75%	20%, 15%
^{177}Lu-DOTA-JR11[b], NCT02592707	Multicentre, phase I/II interims analysis, 3 cycles (~13 GBq)	35 NETs	30%	90%	14%, 6%
^{177}Lu-DOTA-LM3[c]	Single Centre compassionate use, 1–4 cycles	51 NENs	36%	NA	6% NA

[a]Data are from Reidy-Lagunes et al. [32]
[b]Data are from Nicolas et al. [33]
[c]Data are from Zhang et al. [34]

hematotoxicity (leukopenia, neutropenia, and thrombocytopenia) in four of the first seven patients with NETs treated with two cycles of ^{177}Lu-DOTA-JR11 (total activity between 10.5 and 14.7 GBq) [32]. Hence, their single-centre phase I study was suspended, and the protocol modified to limit the cumulative absorbed bone marrow dose. The most important results of the whole study are summarized in Table 35.3. ^{177}Lu-DOTA-JR11 (^{177}Lu-OPS201) is currently evaluated in a phase I/II multicentre study (ClinicalTrials.gov identifier: NCT02162446) and its "sister" compound ^{177}Lu-DOTA-LM3 is evaluated in a single-centre compassionate use study. So far, there were only abstracts available with a brief summary of results from both studies [33, 34]. Table 35.3 shows the most important findings of those studies.

35.5 Part IV. Current and Future Developments

The high potential and promising results of diagnostic and therapeutic radiolabelled SST antagonists have attracted several research groups to further evaluate radiolabelled SST antagonists. Table 35.4 shows an overview of such studies that are listed within ClinicalTrials.gov. The results of these studies are expected to be published in the near future.

The antagonist approach has huge potential to offer new and better theranostic procedures for patients. Here is an overview about possible future developments to achieve this ambition:

1. There are other tumours than GEP-NETs that show high potential for theranostic applications with SST antagonists, for example, non-Hodgkin lymphoma, renal cell carcinoma, breast cancer, pheochromocytoma, paraganglioma, medullary thyroid cancer, small cell lung cancer, lung NET, and other neoplasms with SST2 expression, including tumours with low levels of SST2 expression.

2. Optimizing the SST antagonist approach which includes the reduction of bone marrow toxicity by using alternative radionuclides, for example, α-emitters and β$^-$-emitters with suitable characteristics such as long half-lives, short range, etc.

3. Using other receptor systems for the antagonist approach, for example, gastrin-releasing peptide receptor and cholecystokinin receptor subtype 2.

Last, but not least randomized phase II/III studies evaluating radiolabelled NODAGA-JR11/DOTA-JR11, radiolabelled NODAGA-LM3/DOTA-LM3 or other promising radiolabelled SST antagonists are needed in larger-scale multi-

Table 35.4 Overview about current registered studies

Identifier No.	Radiotracer	Study design, study aim	Enrolled subjects	Status
NCT03220217	^{68}Ga-NODAGA-JR11 (^{68}Ga-OPS202)	Multicentre, randomized, dose-confirmation, phase II study	27 GEP-NET	Completed
NCT04491851	^{68}Ga-NODAGA-LM3 vs. ^{68}Ga-DOTA-LM3 ^{68}Ga-NODAGA-LM3 vs. ^{68}Ga-NODAGA-JR11	Single-Centre, randomized phase II study	30 NET	Unknown status
NCT02592707	^{177}Lu-DOTA-JR11 (^{177}Lu-OPS201)	Multicentre, open-label phase I/II study to evaluate safety, peptide dose and preliminary efficacy	40 GEP-NET, lung NET, pheochromocytoma, paraganglioma	Terminated
NCT03773133	Theranostic pair ^{68}Ga-OPS202 and ^{177}Lu-OPS201	Multicentre, open-label phase I/II study to evaluate safety and preliminary efficacy	9 SCLC or (HR+)/(HER2-) breast cancer	Terminated

centre trials as a theranostic approach in patients with GEP-NETs or other tumours with SST2 expression.

35.6 Conclusion

Until recently it was thought that internalisation of the radiotracer was mandatory for diagnostic and therapeutic SST targeting. Ginj et al. proposed 15 years ago that radiolabelled SST antagonists are superior to SST agonists despite the lack of internalisation [5]. Recently it has been shown that ^{68}Ga-NODAGA-JR11 and ^{68}Ga-NODAGA-LM3 PET/CT revealed the best clinical results among all tested SST antagonists and are clearly superior compared to PET/CT with the potent SST2 agonist ^{68}Ga-DOTA-TOC. PRRT with ^{177}Lu-DOTA-JR11 and ^{177}Lu-DOTA-LM3 is very effective with a high objective response rate (30–45%) and an excellent 1-year PFS of 90% despite of using treatment protocols with low activities (< 15 GBq) given in one to three cycles. The dose limiting organ is the bone marrow, at least for ^{177}Lu-DOTA-JR11. These results warrants larger-scale randomized phase II/III trials in patients

with GEP-NETs and tumours that have not yet been in the focus for SST targeting. Current evidence from preclinical work, binding capacity studies with different human tumour samples and clinical studies support the shift towards SST antagonists.

Acknowledgements I would like to acknowledge Melpomeni Fani, University Hospital Basel, who critically read the chapter and Richard P. Baum, Curanosticum Wiesbaden Frankfurt, who provided me with results of his ^{68}Ga-NODAGA-LM3 and ^{177}Lu-DOTA-LM3 studies.

Disclosure The author of this chapter is a consultant for Ipsen Pharma SAS. There is no other potential conflict of interest which is relevant to this chapter.

References

1. Ambrosini V, Fani M, Fanti S, Forrer F, Maecke HR. Radiopeptide imaging and therapy in Europe. J Nucl Med. 2011;52(Suppl 2):42S–55S.
2. Baumann T, Rottenburger C, Nicolas G, Wild D. Gastroenteropancreatic neuroendocrine tumours (GEP-NET)—imaging and staging. Best Pract Res Clin Endocrinol Metab. 2016;30(1):45–57.

3. Strosberg J, El-Haddad G, Wolin E, Hendifar A, Yao J, Chasen B, et al. Phase 3 trial of (177)Lu-Dotatate for midgut neuroendocrine tumors. N Engl J Med. 2017;376(2):125–35.

4. Kratochwil C, Giesel FL, Bruchertseifer F, Mier W, Apostolidis C, Boll R, et al. (2)(1)(3)bi-DOTATOC receptor-targeted alpha-radionuclide therapy induces remission in neuroendocrine tumours refractory to beta radiation: a first-in-human experience. Eur J Nucl Med Mol Imaging. 2014;41(11):2106–19.

5. Ginj M, Zhang H, Waser B, Cescato R, Wild D, Wang X, et al. Radiolabeled somatostatin receptor antagonists are preferable to agonists for in vivo peptide receptor targeting of tumors. Proc Natl Acad Sci U S A. 2006;103(44):16436–41.

6. Wild D, Fani M, Behe M, Brink I, Rivier JE, Reubi JC, et al. First clinical evidence that imaging with somatostatin receptor antagonists is feasible. J Nucl Med. 2011;52(9):1412–7.

7. Bass RT, Buckwalter BL, Patel BP, Pausch MH, Price LA, Strnad J, et al. Identification and characterization of novel somatostatin antagonists. Mol Pharmacol. 1996;50(4):709–15.

8. Hocart SJ, Jain R, Murphy WA, Taylor JE, Coy DH. Highly potent cyclic disulfide antagonists of somatostatin. J Med Chem. 1999;42(11):1863–71.

9. Cescato R, Erchegyi J, Waser B, Piccand V, Maecke HR, Rivier JE, et al. Design and in vitro characterization of highly sst2-selective somatostatin antagonists suitable for radiotargeting. J Med Chem. 2008;51(13):4030–7.

10. Reubi JC, Schaer JC, Wenger S, Hoeger C, Erchegyi J, Waser B, et al. SST3-selective potent peptidic somatostatin receptor antagonists. Proc Natl Acad Sci U S A. 2000;97(25):13973–8.

11. Wang X, Fani M, Schulz S, Rivier J, Reubi JC, Maecke HR. Comprehensive evaluation of a somatostatin-based radiolabelled antagonist for diagnostic imaging and radionuclide therapy. Eur J Nucl Med Mol Imaging. 2012;39(12):1876–85.

12. Fani M, Del Pozzo L, Abiraj K, Mansi R, Tamma ML, Cescato R, et al. PET of somatostatin receptor-positive tumors using 64Cu- and 68Ga-somatostatin antagonists: the chelate makes the difference. J Nucl Med. 2011;52(7):1110–8.

13. Fani M, Braun F, Waser B, Beetschen K, Cescato R, Erchegyi J, et al. Unexpected sensitivity of sst2 antagonists to N-terminal radiometal modifications. J Nucl Med. 2012;53(9):1481–9.

14. Nicolas GP, Mansi R, McDougall L, Kaufmann J, Bouterfa H, Wild D, et al. Biodistribution, pharmacokinetics, and dosimetry of (177)Lu-, (90)Y-, and (111) in-labeled somatostatin receptor antagonist OPS201 in comparison to the agonist (177)Lu-DOTATATE: the mass effect. J Nucl Med. 2017;58(9):1435–41.

15. Reubi JC, Schar JC, Waser B, Wenger S, Heppeler A, Schmitt JS, et al. Affinity profiles for human somatostatin receptor subtypes SST1-SST5 of somatostatin radiotracers selected for scintigraphic and radiotherapeutic use. Eur J Nucl Med. 2000;27(3):273–82.

16. Schottelius M, Simecek J, Hoffmann F, Willibald M, Schwaiger M, Wester HJ. Twins in spirit—episode I: comparative preclinical evaluation of [(68)Ga] DOTATATE and [(68)Ga]HA-DOTATATE. EJNMMI Res. 2015;5:22.

17. Wild D, Macke HR, Waser B, Reubi JC, Ginj M, Rasch H, et al. 68Ga-DOTANOC: a first compound for PET imaging with high affinity for somatostatin receptor subtypes 2 and 5. Eur J Nucl Med Mol Imaging. 2005;32(6):724.

18. Dalm SU, Nonnekens J, Doeswijk GN, de Blois E, van Gent DC, Konijnenberg MW, et al. Comparison of the therapeutic response to treatment with a 177Lu-labeled somatostatin receptor agonist and antagonist in preclinical models. J Nucl Med. 2016;57(2):260–5.

19. Albrecht J, Exner S, Groetzinger C, Prasad S, Konietschke F, Beindorff N, et al. Multimodal imaging of two-cycle PRRT with (177)Lu-DOTA-JR11 and (177)Lu-DOTATOC in an orthotopic neuroendocrine xenograft tumor mouse model. J Nucl Med. 2020;62:393.

20. Reubi JC, Waser B, Macke H, Rivier J. Highly increased 125I-JR11 antagonist binding in vitro reveals novel indications for sst2 targeting in human cancers. J Nucl Med. 2017;58(2):300–6.

21. Cescato R, Waser B, Fani M, Reubi JC. Evaluation of 177Lu-DOTA-sst2 antagonist versus 177Lu-DOTA-sst2 agonist binding in human cancers in vitro. J Nucl Med. 2011;52(12):1886–90.

22. Nicolas GP, Beykan S, Bouterfa H, Kaufmann J, Bauman A, Lassmann M, et al. Safety, biodistribution, and radiation dosimetry of (68)Ga-OPS202 in patients with gastroenteropancreatic neuroendocrine tumors: a prospective phase I imaging study. J Nucl Med. 2018;59(6):909–14.

23. Nicolas GP, Schreiter N, Kaul F, Uiters J, Bouterfa H, Kaufmann J, et al. Sensitivity comparison of (68) Ga-OPS202 and (68)Ga-DOTATOC PET/CT in patients with gastroenteropancreatic neuroendocrine tumors: a prospective phase II imaging study. J Nucl Med. 2018;59(6):915–21.

24. Krebs S, Pandit-Taskar N, Reidy D, Beattie BJ, Lyashchenko SK, Lewis JS, et al. Biodistribution and radiation dose estimates for (68)Ga-DOTA-JR11 in patients with metastatic neuroendocrine tumors. Eur J Nucl Med Mol Imaging. 2019;46(3):677–85.

25. Zhu W, Cheng Y, Wang X, Yao S, Bai C, Zhao H, et al. Head-to-head comparison of (68)Ga-DOTA-JR11 and (68)Ga-DOTATATE PET/CT in patients with metastatic, well-differentiated neuroendocrine tumors: a prospective study. J Nucl Med. 2020;61(6):897–903.

26. Krebs S, O'Donoghue JA, Biegel E, Beattie BJ, Reidy D, Lyashchenko SK, et al. Comparison of (68)Ga-DOTA-JR11 PET/CT with dosimetric (177) Lu-satoreotide tetraxetan ((177)Lu-DOTA-JR11) SPECT/CT in patients with metastatic neuroendocrine tumors undergoing peptide receptor radionuclide therapy. Eur J Nucl Med Mol Imaging. 2020;47(13):3047–57.

27. Reubi JC, Waser B, Cescato R, Gloor B, Stettler C, Christ E. Internalized somatostatin receptor subtype 2 in neuroendocrine tumors of octreotide-treated patients. J Clin Endocrinol Metab. 2010;95(5):2343–50.

28. Poeppel TD, Binse I, Petersenn S, Lahner H, Schott M, Antoch G, et al. 68Ga-DOTATOC versus 68Ga-DOTATATE PET/CT in functional imaging of neuroendocrine tumors. J Nucl Med. 2011;52(12):1864–70.

29. Singh A, Kulkarni H, Langbein T, Mueller D, Senftleben S, Fani M, et al. PET/CT imaging of somatostatin receptor expressing solid tumors with the novel somatostatin receptor antagonist 68Ga-NODAGA-LM3. J Nucl Med. 2018;59(supplement 1):42.

30. Singh A, Zhang J, Kulkarni H, Langbein T, Baum R. First-in-human study of a novel somatostatin receptor antagonist 68Ga-NODAGA-LM3 for molecular imaging of paraganglioma patients. J Nucl Med. 2019;60(supplement 1):339.

31. Wild D, Fani M, Fischer R, Del Pozzo L, Kaul F, Krebs S, et al. Comparison of somatostatin receptor agonist and antagonist for peptide receptor radionuclide therapy: a pilot study. J Nucl Med. 2014;55(8):1248–52.

32. Reidy-Lagunes D, Pandit-Taskar N, O'Donoghue JA, Krebs S, Staton KD, Lyashchenko SK, et al. Phase I trial of well-differentiated neuroendocrine tumors (NETs) with radiolabeled somatostatin antagonist (177)Lu-Satoreotide Tetraxetan. Clin Cancer Res. 2019;25(23):6939–47.

33. Nicolas GP, Ansquer C, Lenzo NP, McEwan S, Wild D, Hicks RJ. An international open-label study on safety and efficacy of 177Lu-satoreotide tetraxetan in somatostatin receptor positive neuroendocrine tumours (NETs): an interim analysis. Ann Oncol. 2020;31(supplement 4):S771.

34. Zhang J, Singh A, Schuchardt C, Macke H, Mueller D, Kulkarni H, et al. First-in-human study of a novel SSTR antagonist177Lu-DOTA-LM3 for peptide receptor radionuclide therapy in patients with advanced metastatic NENs and low SSTR agonist binging. J Nucl Med. 2020;61(supplement 1):414.

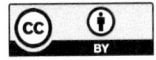

Molecular In Vitro and In Vivo Diagnostics as the Impartible Basis of Multimodal Therapy Approaches in Precision Oncology

Ralph M. Wirtz

In 2000, more than two decades ago, genome-wide gene expression profiling became available and thereafter led to the dissection of cancer biology across almost all entities [1–3]. First, the molecular portraits based on RNA expression profiling (termed "heat maps") were used in breast cancer to identify luminal, ERBB2-positive, and basal tumors. Interestingly, these subtypes not only elucidated the underlying biology but also directly suggested targeted treatment intervention with luminal tumors being hormone-dependent, ERBB2-positive tumors exposing the transmembrane receptor Her-2/neu and basal tumors lacking homogenous expression of typical targeted treatment options, with the latter being termed "triple negative" later on. Interestingly, genome-wide mutation analysis later on revealed that the luminal subtype, while bearing most mutations (such as PIK3CA) exhibited lowest immunogenicity and frequently absence of tumor-infiltrating lymphocytes. In contrast, the basal subtype turned out to have lowest rate of classical oncogens, but was dominated by loss-of-function mutation of p53 [4], while almost half of basal tumors being infiltrated by large amounts of immune cells. This led to the assumption that hormone regulation affects immune cell recognition and three biological axes (hormone, immune, and proliferation axis) were built up for breast cancer as being the coordinates of the biological universe of breast cancer [5, 6]. The therapeutic implication of these fundamental insights were further explored and validated the distinct sensitivity towards antihormonal treatment, ERBB2 targeting, and chemotherapy. Interestingly, the hormone-insensitive, highly proliferating basal and ERBB2-positive tumors with higher amounts of immune cell infiltrates did respond best to neoadjuvant treatment with superior outcome [7]. As one consequence, the concept arose to develop RNA-based vaccination concepts in the post-neoadjuvant situation of triple negative breast cancer not responding to neoadjuvant chemotherapy by targeting individual neo-epitope patterns [8], which has been investigated in the subsequent "Merit" trial with positive proof of concept [9]. In line with this, the first approval of checkpoint therapy treatment in breast cancer happened in the triple negative breast cancer subtype [10].

Almost 10 years after their first description in 2000, the molecular subtypes of breast cancer became integral part for patient stratification in breast cancer by semiquantitative recapitulation using conventional immune histochemistry methods [11] or by molecular methods using standard PCR methods to quantify key targets after RNA extraction from routinely fixed tissues using the in vitro diagnostic "MammaTyper®" test system [12–14].

R. M. Wirtz (✉)
Stratifyer Molecular Pathology GmbH,
Köln, Germany
e-mail: ralph.wirtz@stratifyer.de

V. Prasad (ed.), *Beyond Becquerel and Biology to Precision Radiomolecular Oncology: Festschrift in Honor of Richard P. Baum*, https://doi.org/10.1007/978-3-031-33533-4_36

As a next step, this new IVD technology was validated in other disease entities in which molecular subtyping initially identified in breast cancer just started to be recognized as being potentially hormone-driven such as ovarian cancer [15, 16], lung cancer, [17, 18] and bladder cancer [19–21].

Importantly the quantitative determination or the main drug targets in breast cancer, that is, estrogen receptor (= ESR1, gene name) and the receptor-tyrosine kinase HER-2/neu (= ERBB2; gene name) revealed that only high mRNA over-expression of the targets is associated with addiction to the target and respective response and efficacy to the treatment. As one example in the NSABP B14 breast cancer trial comparing 5-year tamoxifen vs. placebo in ER-positive tumors by IHC, only tumors with high ESR1 mRNA expression did benefit from the antihormonal treatment, while immunohistochemical staining failed to be predictive [22]. Moreover, the large NSABP P1 prevention trial validated that the benefit of Tamoxifen treatment was restricted to the prevention of very high ESR1 mRNA expression [21]. Similarly, for ERBB2 targeting by the two antibodies Tratuzumab and Pertuzumab within the neoadjuvant TRYPHAENA trial, a large translational program revealed that ERBB2 over-expression remained to be the only marker for patient selection of anti-ERBB2 treatments and therapy benefit prediction [23]. Apparently molecular in vitro diagnostics in breast cancer teaches us that it is the quantitation of the treatment target which is of utmost importance for therapy guidance and precision of treatment efficacy prediction.

Moreover, this directly leads to one of the hallmarks of in vivo diagnostics/theranostics, which presumes that uptake of radioactive ligands is strongly correlated to receptor density on the surface tissue. We therefore evaluated whether the surface expression of SSTR2 receptors as determined by semiquantitative IHC and fully quantitative PCR methods in vitro might be related to the uptake of SSTR2 ligands (DOTA-TOC, DOTA-NOC and DOTA-TATE) in patients suffering neuroendocrine pancreatic tumors [24]. It turned out that conventional IHC methods by

immune reactivity score (IRS) only trended to predict uptake as determined by positive correlation with SUV mean ($c = 0.39$ $p = 0.11$). In contrast quantitative, molecular assessment of SSTR2 mRNA expression by PCR correlated very strongly with SUV mean ($c = 0.85$ $p < 0.001$) and equally well as SUV max itself did correlate with SUV mean ($c = 0.90$ $p < 0.001$). This demonstrates as proof-of-principle that target assessment by molecular in vitro and in vivo methods being quantitative by nature do perfectly fit for patient selection for imaging and potentially subsequent radionuclide treatment approaches.

However, tumor response to radionuclide treatments does not only dependent on total uptake, but also on tumor biological aspects such as intrinsic and neoplastic DNA repair capacity, proliferation status, hormone dependence, and tumor microenvironment. Precision oncology approaches have to take these complex interactions into account to improve completeness of therapy responses and thereby support long-term survival. As one example, the biology of the Prostate-Specific Membrane Antigen (PSMA) in prostate cancer might serve as being one of the most advanced radionuclide therapies. PSMA is a transmembrane glycoprotein, whose expression on prostate epithelium is of functional importance for cell migration and chromosome stability [25] and inversely regulated by androgens with increased activity found in tumor cells that become androgen-independent [26]. Superior efficacy of radioligand PSMA treatment (177Lu-PSMA-617) compared to standard of care in castration-resistant, metastatic prostate cancer previously treated with at least one androgen-receptor-pathway inhibitor and one or two taxane regimens and who had PSMA-positive gallium-68 (68Ga)-labeled PSMA-11 positron-emission tomographic-computed tomographic scans has been demonstrated [27]. Median overall survival reached 15.3 month for PSMA-targeted therapy versus 11.3 months for standard of care (Hazard ratio 0.62 $p < 0.0001$). Systematic review emphasizes clinical benefit for this radioligand therapy with 46% of patients achieving a reduction in PSA values >50% (and 75% had a decrease in PSA levels posttreatment) and an overall clinical benefit rate of 75.5% (37.2% of patients with PR and 38.3% SD) [28]. However, despite clear superiority over standard treatment, this study shows that singular radionuclide treatment still has limited efficacy in metastatic prostate cancer, as most patients progress and die of the disease. Molecular tissue analysis of repair genes such as BRCA1, BRCA2, ATM, CHEK2 may be one causal role for resistance or response to PSMA targeting with loss DNA-damage "recognition and signaling" genes resulting in resistance and loss of DNA-damage "repair" (such as BRCA2) being associated with increased radiosensitivity [29]. Interestingly, such "BRCAness" might be induced by PARP inhibition as has been shown in model systems [30]. Moreover, hormone receptors and signaling pathways (PTEN, AKT, PI3K, CDK1) contribute to development of resistance towards PARP inhibition [31], while PARP2 interacts with AR signaling, which in turn regulates PSMA expression. The multitude of functional interaction demonstrates that there is need of precise dissection of gene alteration, target quantitation and pathway pattern analytics in vitro to allow precise, multimodal approaches and adjusted therapy sequences, which combine radionuclide therapies with antihormonal, immune/vaccination therapies and simultaneous multitargeting by upcoming Antibody-Drug Conjugates (ADC). However, these therapeutic, multimodal approaches should in turn be monitored by molecular means again combining in vitro and in vivo approaches based on molecular assessment of tissue, urine, and blood diagnostics and pre- versus post-treatment imaging. Ultimately, these approaches shall not only be designed to govern direct tumor cell killing, but rather provoke systemic, longer lasting immune effects, that allow long-term survival. Most recently, we could show that long-term survival in metastatic NSCLC treated with first-line pembrolizumab monotherapy could be predicted after first cycle by quantitation of dynamic changes of immune cell mRNA signatures from peripheral blood pre- versus post-treatment [32]. Such approaches provide new early outcome indicators and may therefore be helpful to accelerate adopted preci-

sion oncology strategies and underline the importance of inducing immune responses in the advanced treatment settings. In summary, molecular research in the past decades pave the way for fundamentally new insights and treatment approaches with combined molecular in vitro and in vivo diagnostics emerging as the impartible basis of upcoming, multimodal therapy approaches in precision oncology.

References

1. Sorlie T, et al. Gene expression patterns of breast carcinomas distinguish tumor subclasses with clinical implications. Proc Natl Acad Sci U S A. 2001;98:10869–74.
2. Perou CM, et al. Molecular portraits of human breast tumours. Nature. 2000;406:747–52.
3. Sorlie T. Molecular portraits of breast cancer: tumor subtypes as distinct disease entities. Eur J Cancer. 2004;40:2667–75.
4. The cancer genome atlas research network (TCGA). Comprehensive molecular portraits of human breast tumors. Nature. 2012;490(61):61–70.
5. Schmidt M, Böhm D, von Törne C, et al. The humoral immune system has a key prognostic impact in node-negative breast cancer. Cancer Res. 2008;68(13):5405–13.
6. Schmidt M, Hengstler JG, von Törne C, et al. Coordinates in the universe of node-negative breast cancer revisited. Cancer Res. 2009;69(7):2695–8.
7. Denkert C, Loibl S, Noske A, et al. Tumor-associated lymphocytes as an independent predictor of response to neoadjuvant chemotherapy in breast cancer. J Clin Oncol. 2010;28(1):105–13.
8. Wirtz RM, Sahin U. 3rd generation gene signatures—genome wide sequencing and subtype specific characteristics. Annual Meeting of the german society of gynecology. 2013.
9. Schmidt M, et al. T-cell responses induced by an individualized neoantigen specific immune therapy in post (neo)adjuvant patients with triple negative breast cancer. ESMO. 2020;31:S276.
10. Schmid P, et al. Atezolizumab and nab-paclitaxel in advanced triple-negative breast cancer. N Engl J Med. 2018;379(22):2108–21.
11. Goldhirsch A, et al. Strategies for subtypes—dealing with the diversity of breast cancer: highlights of the St Gallen international expert consensus on the primary therapy of early breast cancer 2011. Ann Oncol. 2011;22:1736–47.
12. Wirtz RM, Sihto H, Isola J, Heikkilä P, Kellokumpu-Lehtinen PL, Auvinen P, Turpeenniemi-Hujanen T, Jyrkkiö S, Lakis S, Schlombs K, Laible M, Weber S, Eidt S, Sahin U, Joensuu H. Biological subtyping

of early breast cancer: a study comparing RT-qPCR with immunohistochemistry. Breast Cancer Res Treat. 2016;157(3):437–46.

13. Laible M, Schlombs K, Kaiser K, Veltrup E, Herlein S, Lakis S, Stöhr R, Eidt S, Hartmann A, Wirtz RM, Sahin U. Technical validation of an RT-qPCR in vitro diagnostic test system for the determination of breast cancer molecular subtypes by quantification of ERBB2, ESR1, PGR and MKI67 mRNA levels from formalin-fixed paraffin-embedded breast tumor specimens. BMC Cancer. 2016;16:398.

14. Laible M, Hartmann K, Gürtler C, Anzeneder T, Wirtz R, Weber S, Keller T, Sahin U, Rees M, Ramaswamy A. Impact of molecular subtypes on the prediction of distant recurrence in estrogen receptor (ER) positive, human epidermal growth factor receptor 2 (HER2) negative breast cancer upon five years of endocrine therapy. BMC Cancer. 2019;19(1):694.

15. Darb-Esfahani S, Wirtz RM, Sinn BV, Budczies J, Noske A, Weichert W, Faggad A, Scharff S, Sehouli J, Oskay-Ozcelik G, Zamagni C, De Iaco P, Martoni A, Dietel M, Denkert C. Estrogen receptor 1 mRNA is a prognostic factor in ovarian carcinoma: determination by kinetic PCR in formalin-fixed paraffin-embedded tissue. Endocr Relat Cancer. 2009;16(4):1229–39.

16. Zamagni C, Wirtz RM, De Iaco P, Rosati M, Veltrup E, Rosati F, Capizzi E, Cacciari N, Alboni C, Bernardi A, Massari F, Quercia S, D'Errico Grigioni A, Dietel M, Sehouli J, Denkert C, Martoni AA. Oestrogen receptor 1 mRNA is a prognostic factor in ovarian cancer patients treated with neo-adjuvant chemotherapy: determination by array and kinetic PCR in fresh tissue biopsies. Endocr Relat Cancer. 2009;16(4):1241–9.

17. Brueckl WM, Al-Batran SE, Ficker JH, Claas S, Atmaca A, Hartmann A, Rieker RJ, Wirtz RM. Prognostic and predictive value of estrogen receptor 1 expression in completely resected non-small cell lung cancer. Int J Cancer. 2013;133(8):1825–31.

18. Atmaca A, Al-Batran SE, Wirtz RM, Werner D, Zirlik S, Wiest G, Eschbach C, Claas S, Hartmann A, Ficker JH, Jäger E, Brueckl WM. The validation of estrogen receptor 1 mRNA expression as a predictor of outcome in patients with metastatic non-small cell lung cancer. Int J Cancer. 2014;134(10):2314–21.

19. Wirtz RM, Fritz V, Stöhr R, Hartmann A. Molecular classification of bladder cancer possible similarities to breast cancer. Pathologe. 2016;37(1):52–60.

20. Breyer J, Wirtz RM, Otto W, Laible M, Schlombs K, Erben P, Kriegmair MC, Stoehr R, Eidt S, Denzinger S, Burger M, Hartmann A. Predictive value of molecular subtyping in NMIBC by RT-qPCR of ERBB2, ESR1, PGR and MKI67 from formalin fixed TUR biopsies. Oncotarget. 2017;8(40):67684–95.

21. Kriegmair MC, Wirtz RM, Worst TS, Breyer J, Ritter M, Keck B, Boehmer C, Otto W, Eckstein M, Weis CA, Hartmann A, Bolenz C, Erben P. Prognostic value of molecular breast cancer subtypes based on Her2, ESR1, PGR and Ki67 mRNA-expression in muscle invasive bladder cancer. Transl Oncol. 2018;11(2):467–76.

22. Kim C, Tang G, Pogue-Geile KL, Costantino JP, Baehner FL, Baker J, Cronin MT, Watson D, Shak S, Bohn OL, Fumagalli D, Taniyama Y, Lee A, Reilly ML, Vogel VG, McCaskill-Stevens W, Ford LG, Geyer CE Jr, Wickerham DL, Wolmark N, Paik S. Estrogen receptor (ESR1) mRNA expression and benefit from tamoxifen in the treatment and prevention of estrogen receptor-positive breast cancer. J Clin Oncol. 2011;29(31):4160–7.

23. Schneeweiss A, Chia S, Hegg R, Tausch C, Deb R, Ratnayake J, McNally V, Ross G, Kiermaier A, Cortés J. Evaluating the predictive value of biomarkers for efficacy outcomes in response to pertuzumab- and trastuzumab-based therapy: an exploratory analysis of the TRYPHAENA study. Breast Cancer Res. 2014;16(4):R73.

24. Kaemmerer D, Wirtz RM, Fischer EK, Hommann M, Sänger J, Prasad V, Specht E, Baum RP, Schulz S, Lupp A. Analysis of somatostatin receptor 2A immunohistochemistry, RT-qPCR, and in vivo PET/CT data in patients with pancreatic neuroendocrine neoplasm. Pancreas. 2015;44(4):648–54.

25. Rajasekaran SA, Christiansen JJ, Schmid I, Oshima E, Ryazantsev S, Sakamoto K, Weinstein J, Rao NP, Rajasekaran K. Prostate-specific membrane antigen associates with anaphase-promoting complex and induces chromosomal instability. Mol Cancer Ther. 2008;7:2142–51.

26. Chang SS. Overview of prostate-specific membrane antigen. Rev Urol. 2004;6(Suppl. 10):S13–8.

27. Sartor O, de Bono J, Chi KN, Fizazi K, Herrmann K, Rahbar K, Tagawa ST, Nordquist LT, Vaishampayan N, El-Haddad G, Park CH, Beer TM, Armour A, Pérez-Contreras WJ, DeSilvio M, Kpamegan E, Gericke G, Messmann RA, Morris MJ, Krause BJ, VISION investigators. Lutetium-177-PSMA-617 for metastatic castration-resistant prostate cancer. N Engl J Med. 2021;385(12):1091–103.

28. Yadav MP, Ballal S, Sahoo RK, Dwivedi SN, Bal C. Radioligand therapy with (177)Lu-PSMA for metastatic castration-resistant prostate cancer: a systematic review and meta-analysis. Am J Roentgenol. 2019;213:275–85.

29. Kratochwil C, Giesel FL, Heussel CP, Kazdal D, Endris V, Nientiedt C, Bruchertseifer F, Kippenberger M, Rathke H, Leichsenring J, Hohenfellner M, Morgenstern A, Haberkorn U, Duensing S, Stenzinger A. Patients resistant against PSMA-targeting α-radiation therapy often harbor mutations in DNA damage-repair-associated genes. J Nucl Med. 2020;61(5):683–8.

30. Bourton EC, Ahorner PA, Plowman PN, Zahir SA, Al-Ali H, Parris CN. The PARP-1 inhibitor olaparib suppresses BRCA1 protein levels, increases apoptosis and causes radiation hypersensitivity in BRCA1+/− lymphoblastoid cells. J Cancer. 2017;8:4048–56.

31. Ku SY, Gleave ME, Beltran H. Towards precision oncology in advanced prostate cancer. Nat Rev Urol. 2019;16:645–54. https://doi.org/10.1038/s41585-019-0237-8.

32. Brueckl NF, Wirtz RM, Reich FPM, Veltrup E, Zeitler G, Meyer C, Wuerflein D, Ficker JH, Eidt S, Brueckl WM. Predictive value of mRNA expression and dynamic changes from immune related biomarkers in liquid biopsies before and after start of pembrolizumab in stage IV non-small cell lung cancer (NSCLC), Transl Lung Cancer Res. 2021;10:4106; (accepted for publication).

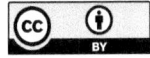

Zhi Yang, Xiangxi Meng, Xiaoyi Guo, and Hua Zhu

Abbreviations

ICPO   International Centers for Precision Oncology
PET   Positron emission tomography
PKUCH   Peking University Cancer Hospital

37.1 Prof. Zhi Yang and His Team

Dr. Yang received his PhD in radiochemistry from China Institute of Atomic Energy (401 Institute) and got his visiting scholar training in the University of Texas MD Anderson Cancer Center. He started his assistant professorship in 1992 and became a professor and the director of Nuclear Medicine Department at Peking University Cancer Hospital in 2014. Dr. Yang focused on the clinical translational research of nuclear medicine. The research interests of the department include nuclear medicine clinical research, as well as the development of multimodality/multiplexed molecular probes for tumor diagnosis and therapy. Dr. Yang's current research interest mainly focuses on the production, labeling, and clinical application of solid target-based nuclides (^{64}Cu, ^{89}Zr, ^{124}I). Dr. Yang has published about 100 research papers and a number of book chapters, conference proceedings, and other publications. Now, 4 postdoctoral scholars, 11 PhD students, and 2 master students are under his supervision. Three students have received master degrees (Figs. 37.1 and 37.2).

Z. Yang (✉)
Chinese Society of Radiopharmaceutical Sciences,
Department of Nuclear Medicine, Peking University
Cancer Hospital and Institute, Beijing, China

X. Meng · X. Guo
Peking University Cancer Hospital and Institute,
Beijing, China
e-mail: mengxiangxi@pku.edu.cn; 1911110575@
bjmu.edu.cn

H. Zhu
Chinese Society of Radiopharmaceutical Sciences,
Nuclear Medicine Department, Molecular Imaging
Teaching and Research Section, Peking University
Cancer Hospital and Institute, Beijing, China

© The Author(s) 2024
V. Prasad (ed.), *Beyond Becquerel and Biology to Precision Radiomolecular Oncology: Festschrift in Honor of Richard P. Baum*, https://doi.org/10.1007/978-3-031-33533-4_37

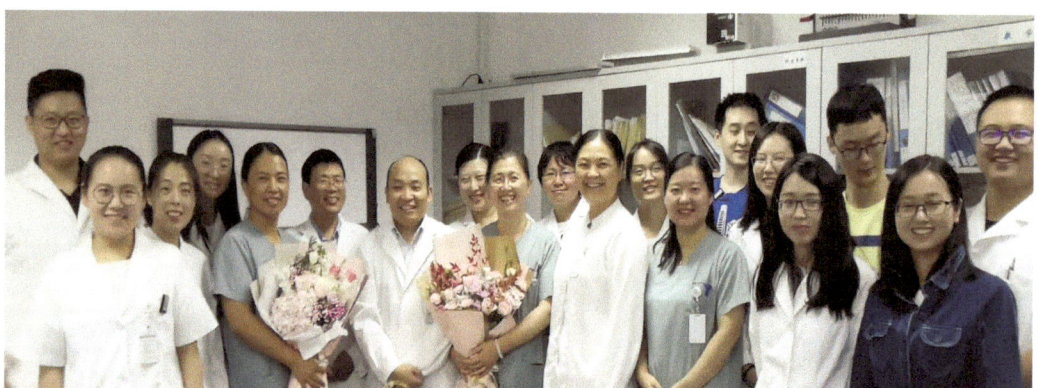

Fig. 37.1 Group photo of Prof. Yang and the students (Sep 10, 2019, teacher's day celebration)

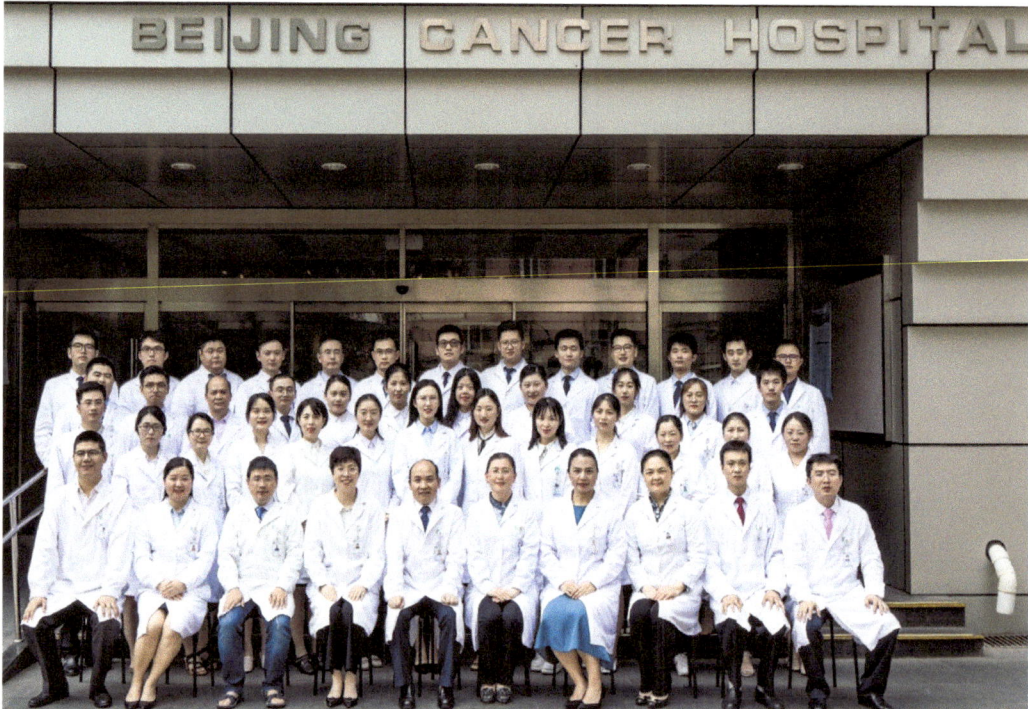

Fig. 37.2 Group photo of Prof. Yang and the faculty and staff at the nuclear medicine department (summer 2019)

37.2 Beijing Cancer Hospital: Nuclear Medicine Department Clinical Translation Platform

37.2.1 Introduction of the Department

Research activities in Nuclear Medicine Department, Beijing Cancer Hospital (BCH-NM) are primary focused on three areas:

1. The translational medical research. The department aims to improve the health of individuals (especially tumor patients) and the community by translating basic scientific findings into radiopharmaceuticals or radiotracers.

2. The development of targeted imaging probes for noninvasive characterization of molecular events associated with tumor progression and regression. Molecular imaging probes which used in nuclear, optical imaging modalities

are developed to enhance the sensitivity and selectivity of early tumor detection, tumor-marker profiling, and the monitoring of early treatment responses.

3. The development of new target, novel drug-delivery systems for selective delivery of diagnostic and therapeutic agents.

Our long-term goal is to apply the "seek and treat" strategy in the development of targeted imaging/therapeutic agents that eventually translate to the clinics to improve the management of cancer through early tumor detection and individualized therapy.

In a word, the overall objective of the laboratory is to develop novel molecular imaging probes for clinical noninvasive detection of tumor.

BCH-NM holds great advantages in clinical translational studies (Table 37.1). Two PET/CT scanners, an HM-20 cyclotron, two SPECT/CT scanners, two ^{68}Ge-^{68}Ga generators, and more than ten hot cells equipped in the NM departments. The department holds the fourth level (highest) of radiopharmaceutical certification approved by China-FDA (CFDA) which allows independent clinical studies (Fig. 37.3).

37.2.2 PKUCH-NM Honored to be the First ICPO Partner

On August 27, 2019, the signing ceremony for the cooperation between Peking University Cancer Hospital (PKUCH) and the International Centers for Precision Oncology (ICPO) was held successfully in the scientific research building of BCH-NM. The cooperation agreement was signed by President Ji Jiafu from PKUCH and President Richard P. Baum from ICPO Academy and Founding ICPO Board Member (Fig. 37.4).

PKUCH is one of the most recognized large specialty hospitals in the field of cancer research and treatment in China. PKUCH is aiming to build a prestigious international cancer center. Initial talks in cooperation between PKUCH and ICPO initiated in December 2018. After half a year of intense preparations, both parties established an official document in June 2019 and signed the agreement on August 27, 2019. As such, PKUCH-NM becomes the first ICPO Cooperation Partner, significantly supporting the large-scale development of PRRT and PRLT in clinical trials. PKUCH-NM is also aiming to establish a Precision Radionuclide Oncology Center for tumor therapy, contributing to cancer

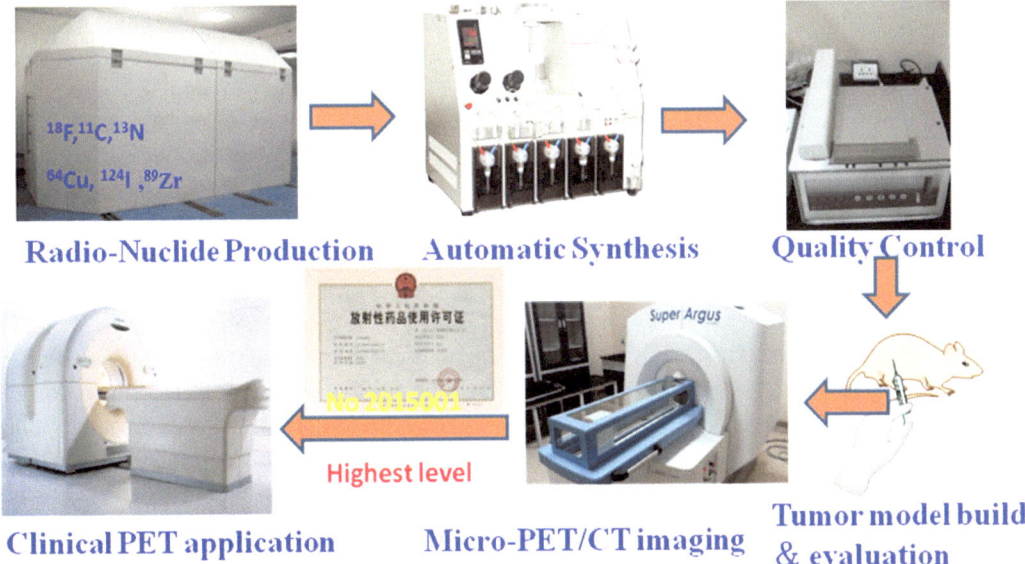

Fig. 37.3 Typical clinical translation study in BCH-NM "from bench to bedside"

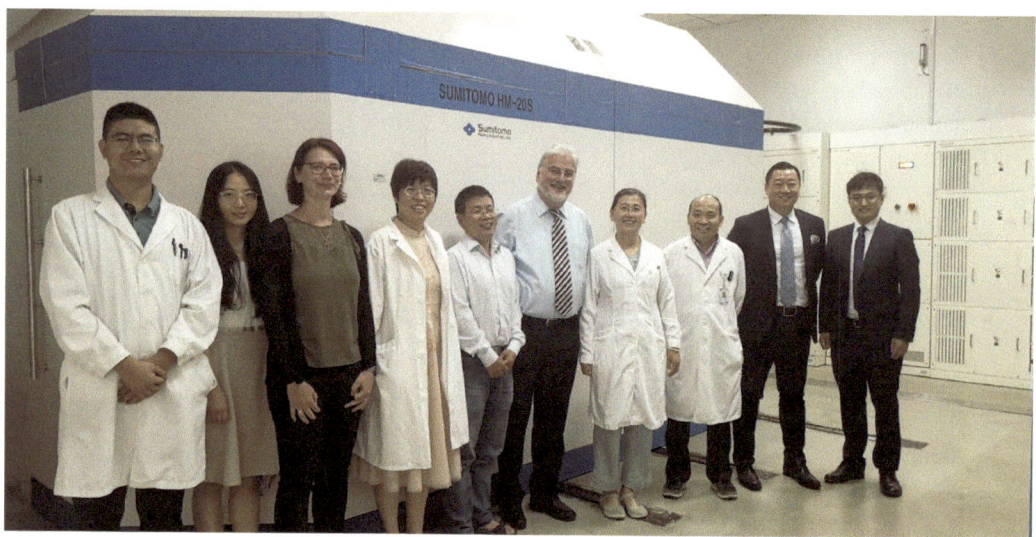

Fig. 37.4 Signing ceremony attendees tour PKUCH-NM facilities

prevention and treatment, and provide a platform for deepening bilateral education/medical cooperation between China, Germany, and other countries.

37.3 Clinical Translational Study

37.3.1 Concise Introduction

Peking University Cancer Hospital's nuclear medicine department holds great advantages in clinical translational studies. More than 1200 clinical PET/CT diagnosis are performed annually, and this guarantees a large spectrum of malignancies to enable clinical translational studies. Approximately 25% of those patients participate in the novel radiopharmaceutical researches (Table 37.1).

37.3.2 Clinical Evaluation of ^{99m}Tc-Rituximab for Sentinel Lymph Node Mapping

Rituximab is a chimeric monoclonal antibody against the CD20 antigen presenting on the membrane of pre-B and mature B lymphocyte.

Considering the large number of B cells presenting in LNs, we hypothesized that radiolabeled rituximab can serve as an effective imaging tool for SLN identification. Therefore, in this work rituximab was directly labeled with the most widely used SPECT radionuclide, ^{99m}Tc. The resulting tracer, ^{99m}Tc-rituxmab, was further evaluated in a large cohort of breast cancer patients (total no. of patients 2317; typical images shown in Fig. 37.5) [1]. This tracer showed great feasibility, safety, and effectiveness for SLN mapping in breast cancer patients. Further clinical research and related evaluation on large cohorts of breast cancer and/or melanoma lymphoscintigraphy are in process.

37.3.3 Tumor Amino Metabolism PET Imaging

Glucose is the most common source of nutrient in normal cells, and glucose generates energy via aerobic metabolism (TCA cycle in the mitochondria). In certain cancer cells, due to various mutations and the unmet needs for high metabolic energy, glucose is consumed via the less efficient anaerobic glycolysis. This phenomenon is common referred as the "Warburg effect." Adaptations

Table 37.1 Present clinical translational studies in BCH-NM department

No.	Name of tracer	Clinical application	Target	IRB code
1	^{99m}Tc-rituximab	SLN detection	CD 20 antigen	–
2	^{99m}Tc-HYNIC-TOC	NET detection	SSTR	2,012,031,313
3	^{68}Ga-DOTA-TATE	NET imaging	SSTR	2,014,011,313
4	^{68}Ga-PMSA-617	Prostate cancer	PSMA	2016YJZ15
5	Radionuclide therapy	Tumor therapy	–	2017XJS15
6	^{177}Lu-DOTA-TATE	NET therapy	SSTR	2018YJZ01
7	^{177}Lu-PSMA-617	Prostate cancer therapy	PSMA	–
8	[18]F-(2S,4R)-glutamine	Tumor metabolism	Glutamine metabolism	2017KT38
9	^{18}F-NOTA-PSMA	Prostate cancer	PSMA	2017KT94
10	^{64}Cu-NOTA-PSMA	Prostate cancer	PSMA	2017KT110
11	^{64}Cu-NOTA-Trastuzumab	Gastric cancer	HER2	2018KT02
12	[124]I-Trastuzumab	Gastric cancer	HER2	2018KT48
13	^{68}Ga-P-15-041	Bone metastasis	Bone phosphate	2018KT50
14	^{18}F-Plaquitide	Plaquitide dysfunctional	Plaquitide	2018KT51
15	^{18}F-FPY	Tumor metabolism	Amino acid	2018KT52
16	^{68}Ga-HK	Pancreatic cancer	Avβ6	–
17	^{68}Ga-HER2 Affibody	Gastric cancer	HER2	2018KT61
18.	PET/CT vs. PET/MR	Tumor	Tumor	2018KT110 2018KT110-GZ01
19.	^{18}F-FHBG	Glioma	HSV1-tk	2018KT112
20	[89]Zr-CTB006	Solid tumor	DR05	2018YJZ64
21	^{68}Ga-P16–093	Prostate cancer	PSMA	2019KT04
22	[124]I-RP215	Solid tumor	Tumor IgG	2019KT58
23	^{68}Ga-RM2	Breast cancer	GRPR	2019KT61
24	^{68}Ga-WL12	Solid tumor	PDL1 expression	2019KT62
25	[68]Ga- P14–032	CAA	Brain blood	2019KT60
26	^{68}Ga-JR11	NET	SSTR agonist	2019KT63
27	[124]I-JS001	Solid tumor	PD1 expression	2019KT67
28	[68]Ga- NOTA-PTDGd	Tumor hypoxia	Gla-1	2019KT82
29	[68]Ga /[18]F- NOTA-PTDGd	Solid tumor	FAPI	2019KT95
30	^{99m}Tc-RGD	Lung cancer	RGD	2019YW134
31	^{18}F-HER2 Affibody	Gastric and breast cancer	HER2	2019KT114
32	[89]Zr-RP215	Solid tumor	Tumor IgG	2019KT115
33	^{18}F-WL12	Solid tumor	PDL1 expression	2019KT116
34	^{99m}Tc-MIRC208	Gastric and breast cancer	HER2	2019KT117

of cancer cells (and sometimes occurring in fast-dividing cells) will switch to use glutamine as a source for energy production. Thus, glutamine plays an important role in proliferation, especially in cancer cells. Changes in cellular metabolic mechanism are essential in order to adapt to glutamine metabolism, which is an important functional adjustment of fast-growing cells. PET imaging with [18]F-(2S,4R)-4- fluoroglutamine (^{18}F-FGln) has been demonstrated as a highly attractive approach for studying glutamine metabolism in cancer patients. ^{18}F-FGln was syn-thesized in PKUCH NM department by using a radio-synthesizer module equipped with a semi-preparation HPLC in 10% radiochemical yield (decay corrected).

Our preliminary studies evaluated ^{18}F-FGln in a small number of different cancer patients suggested that certain tumors (brain metastases, breast cancers, or gliomas) could display high uptake of ^{18}F-FGln [2].

^{18}F-FGln displayed a bio-distribution profile dominated by fast uptake and was excreted via kidneys. ^{18}F-FGln is most likely to have signifi-

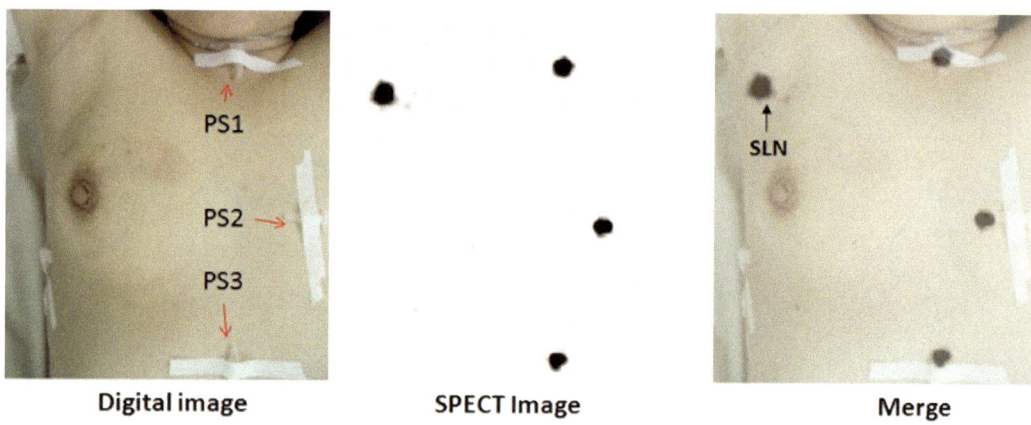

Fig. 37.5 JNM Highlight picture. Lymphoscintigraphy of a patient (2016. J Nucl Med. 57(8), 1214–1220)

cant uptake in the pancreas because of its exocrine function and high rates of amino acid and protein turnover. Additionally, the very low uptake in the brain, breast, lungs, and muscle could represent an advantage in PET imaging. In our most recent study in a cohort of 44 subjects (13 healthy volunteers, 8 lung cancer patients, 17 breast cancer patients, and 6 thyroid cancer patients), ^{18}F-FGln PET demonstrated higher uptake in the trabecular bone of the ribs, vertebrae, and pelvis, which are rich in red marrow [3]. This finding may be because that the proliferation of rapidly dividing bone marrow-derived cells is strongly dependent on the availability of free glutamine, whose uptake might be mediated through different amino acid transporters. With regard to the ^{18}F-FGln dynamic PET/CT imaging in 17 breast cancer patients, two breast tumors, ductal carcinoma in situ, and mucinous carcinoma showed slight ^{18}F-FGln activity (SUVmax <3) at all stages. Nevertheless, two tumors appeared unclear on the ^{18}F-FDG scan but were clear on ^{18}F-FGln images.

Furthermore, we reported that using clinical PET VOI-based quantification analysis, ^{18}F-FGln gradually accumulated in the bone marrow of cervical, thoracic, and lumbar vertebra in three healthy controls, with [SUV(s)mean] from 3.1 to 3.6. Myelosuppression patients (n = 3) showed reduced ^{18}F-FGln uptakes in bone marrow of the corresponding regions. The average SUV(s) mean was 2.0 ± 0.2. Significant difference ($P < 0.001$) in bone marrow uptake was observed

in healthy volunteers (HV) and myelosuppression patients (MP). The skull cortical bone (bone-only) in both healthy volunteers and myelosuppression patients exhibited similar uptake, with the average SUVmean from 0.4 to 1.0. ^{18}F-FGln/PET imaging may be a useful tool for assessing reduced bone marrow activity in cancer patients, who may be at risk of myelosuppression after chemotherapy [4].

One hundred and ten patients have been subjected to ^{18}F-FGln PET scans since 2018, and the results indicate that ^{18}F-FDG was not an ideal tracer for identifying benign and malignant mediastinal lymph nodes, while ^{18}F-FGln appeared to be a suitable agent in these situations. In the future, additional cancer patients will need to be enrolled for ^{18}F-FGln PET imaging studies, and the results will provide sufficient statistical power to differentiate between the different types of tumor metabolism that drives the proliferation. An increased understanding of tumor metabolism could be essential not only for assisting diagnoses but also for better patient management strategies based on their tumor metabolism status.

37.4 Solid Target Radionuclide Production and Labeling Process

The nonstandard positron nuclides copper-64 (^{64}Cu, $T_{1/2}$ = 12.7 h), zirconium-89 (^{89}Zr, $T_{1/2}$ = 78.41 h), and iodine-124 (^{124}I) have become some of the most fascinating PET nuclides because of their long half-lives compared with fluorine-18 (^{18}F, $T_{1/2}$ = 110 min) or carbon-11 (^{11}C, $T_{1/2}$ = 20.4 min). As a result, it is very popular for using labeled pharmaceuticals with these isotopes to carry out some long-term clinical examinations and experiments. For example, ^{64}Cu-labeled monoclonal antibodies or peptides can provide a period of several days to allow PET imaging in vivo which will show the therapeutic effect of monoclonal antibodies in tumors. The combination of PET with mAb is referred to as immunological positron emission tomography (immune-PET).

We presented a routinely and robust method for the preparation of novel next-generation PET radioisotope ^{124}I. Key points for the method are: (1) casting the ^{124}TeO$_2$/Al$_2$O$_3$ mixture by pressing; (2) adhering the layer to Pt-disk by sintering; (3) purifying ^{124}I through dry distillation; (4) reduce ^{123}I contamination by optimizing the decay time between the end of irradiation and purification. The micro-PET/CT imaging indicated that ^{124}I we produced could be used for PET imaging, and as the starting material to synthesize other radioligands [5].

As it known, there are no commercial supplies of such kinds of radionuclides in mainland China. We are the only center in China that provides high-quality ^{124}I for research.

37.5 The Development of New Target, Novel Drug-Delivery Systems

37.5.1 Noninvasive Micro-PET Predicting Tumor Resistance to Radiotherapy

Galectins are members of huge carbohydrate-binding lectins, and characterized by high-affinity binding to β-galactosides through a highly conserved carbohydrate recognition domain. Increasing evidence indicates that the overexpression of galectin-1, a member of the galectin family, is related to tumor progression and inva-

sion, as well as tumor resistance to therapies (e.g., radiotherapy). We investigated whether near-infrared fluorescence (NIRF) imaging and positron emission tomography (PET) were sensitive approaches for detecting and quantitating galectin-1 upregulation in vivo. An anti-galectin-1 antibody was labeled with either an NIRF dye or ^{64}Cu, and NIRF and PET imaging using the resulting probes (Dye-aGal-1 and ^{64}Cu- 1,4,7-triazacyclononane-1,4,7-triacetic acid [NOTA]-aGal-1) were performed in 4 T1 breast cancer-bearing mice treated with several rounds of sorafenib [6].

37.5.2 Synthesis of Site-Specific Radiolabeled Antibodies for RIT Via Genetic Code Expansion

Radio-immunotherapy (RIT) delivers radioisotopes to antigen-expressing cells via monoclonal antibodies for the imaging of lesions or as the therapeutics. Chelators are conjugated to the antibody through cysteine or lysine residues, resulting in heterogeneous chelator-to-antibody ratios and various conjugation sites. To overcome this heterogeneity, we developed an approach for site-specific radiolabeling of antibodies by a combination of genetic code expansion and click chemistry [7]. As a proof-of-concept study, model systems including anti-CD20 antibody rituximab, PET isotope ^{64}Cu, and a newly synthesized bifunctional linker (4-dibenzo-cyclooctynol-1,4,7,10-tetraazacyclotetradecane-1,4,7,10-tetraacetic acid, DIBO-DOTA) were used. We used heavy-chain A122NEAK rituximab and obtained a homogeneous radio-conjugate with precisely two chelators per antibody, incorporated only at the chosen sites. The conjugation did not alter the binding and pharmacokinetics of the rituximab, as indicated by in vitro assays and in vivo PET imaging. We believe this research is a good supplement to the genetic code expansion technique for the development of novel radio-probes.

References

1. Li N, Wang X, Lin B, Zhu H, Liu C, Xiaobao X, Zhang Y, Zhai S, OuYang T, Li J, Yang Z. Clinical evaluation of ^{99m}Tc-rituximab for sentinel lymph node mapping in breast cancer patients. J Nucl Med. 2016;57(8):1214–20.
2. Xiaoxia X, Zhu H, Liu F, Zhang Y, Yang J, Zhang L, Zhu L, Li N, Kung HF, Yang Z. Imaging brain metastasis patients with ^{18}F-(2S,4R)-4-fluoroglutamine. Clin Nucl Med. 2018;43:e392–9.
3. Xiaoxia X, Zhu H, Liu F, Zhang Y, Yang J, Zhang L, Xie Q, Zhu L, Li N, Kung HF, Yang Z. Dynamic PET/CT imaging of ^{18}F-(2S,4R) 4-fluoroglutamine in healthy volunteers and oncological patients. Eur J Nucl Med Mol Imaging. 2020;47:2280. https://doi.org/10.1007/s00259-019-04543-w.
4. Zhu H, Fei L, Zhang Y, Yang J, Xiaoxia X, Guo X, Liu T, Li N, Zhu L, Kung HF, Yang Z. [^{18}F](2S,4R)-4-fluoroglutamine as a PET indicator for bone marrow metabolism dysfunctional: from animal experiments to clinical application. Mol Imaging Biol. 2019;21:945–53.
5. Wang F, Liu T, Li L, Guo X, Duan D, Liu Z, Zhu H, Yang Z. Production, quality control of next-generation PET radioisotope Iodine-124 and its thyroid imaging. J Radioanal Nucl Chem. 2018;318:1999–2006.
6. Lai J, Dehua L, Zhang C, Zhu H, Gao L, Wang Y, Bao R, Zhao Y, Jia B, Wang F, Yang Z, Liu Z. Noninvasive small-animal imaging of galectin-1 upregulation for predicting tumor resistance to radiotherapy. Biomaterials. 2018;158:1–9.
7. YimingWu HZ, Zhang B, Liu F, Chen J, Wang Y, Wang Y, Zhang Z, Ling W, Si L, Huan X, Yao T, Xiao S, Xia Q, Zhang L, Yang Z, Zhou D. Synthesis of site-specific radiolabeled antibodies for radioimmunotherapy via genetic code expansion. Bioconjug Chem. 2016;27(10):2460–8.

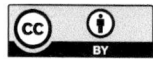

Is It Possible to Target HER2 Using Affibody Receptor Radionuclide Therapy?

38

Hua Zhu, Xiaoyi Guo, Xiangxi Meng, and Zhi Yang

Abbreviations

ARRT — Affibody receptor radionuclide therapy
HER2 — Human epidermal receptor type 2
PRRT — Peptide receptor radionuclide therapies

Human epidermal receptor type 2 (HER2; also known as ErbB2) is a member of the HER family that is encoded by the HER2 gene (also known as HER2/neu or ErbB2 gene). The HER2 pathway promotes cell growth and division when it functions normally; however, when it is overexpressed, cell growth accelerates beyond its normal limits. In cancer cells, HER2 protein can be expressed up to 100 times more than in normal cells (2,000,000 vs. 20,000 per cell). This overexpression leads to strong and constantly proliferative signaling and hence tumor formation. Overexpression of HER2 also causes deactivation of checkpoints, allowing for even greater increases in proliferation.

HER2-targeted treatments with trastuzumab and its derivates or analogues can improve the overall survival of patients with HER2-overexpression tumors. HER2 is overexpressed in about 30% of breast cancer and 7% to 34% of advanced gastric cancer patients, respectively. Researches have contributed great efforts on the development of noninvasive, whole-body HER2-targeted imaging in both HER2 overexpressed mice models and patients, by applying the advanced positron emission tomography (PET) molecular imaging technique.

H. Zhu (✉) · Z. Yang
Key Laboratory of Carcinogenesis and Translational Research (Ministry of Education/Beijing), NMPA Key Laboratory for Research and Evaluation of Radiopharmaceuticals (National Medical Products Administration), Department of Nuclear Medicine; Peking University Cancer Hospital & Institute, Beijing, China

Peking University Cancer Hospital and Institute, Beijing, China

Chinese Society of Radiopharmaceutical Sciences, Department of Nuclear Medicine, Peking University Cancer Hospital and Institute, Beijing, China

X. Guo · X. Meng
Key Laboratory of Carcinogenesis and Translational Research (Ministry of Education/Beijing), NMPA Key Laboratory for Research and Evaluation of Radiopharmaceuticals (National Medical Products Administration), Department of Nuclear Medicine; Peking University Cancer Hospital & Institute, Beijing, China
e-mail: mengxiangxi@pku.edu.cn

38.1 HER2 Overexpression Tumor Model Construction

Currently, cell derivatives xenografts (CDX) models are the most commonly used models in preclinical studies. CDX models are established by injecting human tumor cells, typically from an

V. Prasad (ed.), *Beyond Becquerel and Biology to Precision Radiomolecular Oncology: Festschrift in Honor of Richard P. Baum*, https://doi.org/10.1007/978-3-031-33533-4_38

immortalized cell line, into immunodeficient animals, which are likely to develop the same type of lesions. The high HER2-expressing (BT474 human breast cancer cells, SK-BR3 human breast cancer cells, SK-OV3 human ovarian cancer cells) and low HER2-expressing (MCF7 tumor and MDA-MB-231) cell lines are widely used for developing HER2-targeted drugs and molecular probes. Almost all cell lines have been subcultured many circles and may have lost most of patient's original characteristics. More seriously, the microenvironments of these tumor models were completely different from the in situ scenario, due to the lack of blood vessel supply, tumor-associated stroma, and so on.

Patient-derived tumor xenograft (PDX) models have become much more popular in the last several years and have more advantages than CDX models. Nowadays, most PDX models are established by subcutaneously transplanting tumor tissues of patients into NOD/SCID (Non-obese Diabetic/Severe Combined Immunodeficiency) mice, and PDX models form various tumors have been established, such as non-small-cell lung carcinoma, breast cancer, and gastric cancer. PDX models can not only faithfully preserve the molecular phenotype and genotype changes of the tumor focus of the patient, but also reproduce the heterogeneity of the tumor of the source patient. Therefore, it is gradually applied to the research of tumor drug resistance mechanism and antitumor drug screening, and plays an irreplaceable role in the research of clinical tumor therapy and translational medicine. We previously reported the generation of gastric cancer-based PDX models using gastroscopic biopsies technology. We built HER2-positive (case 176) and HER2-negative (case 168) PDX tumor models based on two gastric cancer patients. The HER2 expression of both patient tumor tissues and PDX mice model tumor tissues were confirmed by H&E, IHC, FISH, DNA amplification, and/or autoradiography [1]. ^{64}Cu-NOTA-Trastuzumab noninvasive PET imaging makes the monitoring of gastric cancer progresses in PDX models feasible. There were barely signals in tumor tissues that could be found using ^{18}F-FDG PET, while brain showed very high uptake. This means ^{18}F-FDG cannot indicate the tumor tissues of case 176 PDX mice models and may get false

negative PET/CT results in this patient. Stronger PET signals in tumor tissues could be detected by ^{64}Cu-NOTA-Trastuzumab in HER2 overexpression PDX models, whereas the weaker uptake could be detected in low HER2-expressing PDX models. According to ROI-based quantification analysis, the ^{64}Cu-NOTA-Trastuzumab tumor accumulation was about 3.5 times higher than the contrast probe ^{64}Cu-NOTA-Trastuzumab at 36 h p.i., further underlining the clinical relevance of these tumor models. In conclusion, we confirmed that ^{64}Cu-NOTA-Trastuzumab could make noninvasive, specific detection of HER2 overexpression lesions in gastric cancer PDX models.

38.2 HER2 Targeting Immune-PET Imaging

High sensitivity, high spatial resolution, and proven quantification ability make PET the modality of choice for applying molecular imaging to the clinical setting. HER2 targeting immune-PET imaging uses radioactive molecular probes to specifically and noninvasively detect and evaluate HER2 expression information of systemic lesions of cancer patients, which enables patient screening, therapeutic monitoring, drug response evaluation, and early warning of recurrence and metastasis in the treatment process of HER2 high-expression tumors.

Many of antibody-based HER2-targeted probes have been used to image HER2-positive breast cancer over the past 20 years. The monoclonal antibody is labeled with long physical half-life isotopes such as ^{124}I ($T_{1/2} = 100.2$ h) or ^{89}Zr ($T_{1/2} = 78$ h), which matches the biological half-life of monoclonal antibody ($T_{1/2}$ about 72 h). For example, Prof. Dijrkes et al. were the first to label clinical-grade trastuzumab with ^{89}Zr and use it for immune-PET imaging in HER2-positive breast cancer patients. This radiotracer can detect HER2 status not just in primary tumor, but in patients with non-accessible metastases. The best imaging time of ^{89}Zr-trastuzumab was 4–5 days after the injection.

Our preliminary researches demonstrated that clinical-grade novel ^{64}Cu-NOTA-Trastuzumab can be formulated with good stability, immune activity, and specificity. The gastric cancer PDX models were successfully established, validated, and evaluated by ^{64}Cu-NOTA-trastuzumab. It was highly consistent with gastric cancer patients regarding the expression of HER2, which made this model a superb tumor model for clinical translational study. He reported that co-injection of nonspecific hIgG1 antibody with ^{64}Cu-NOTATrastuzumab appeared to enhance the tumor uptake in PDX models.

Based on these researches, his team successfully translated ^{64}Cu-NOTA-trastuzumab into clinical gastric cancer patient PET/CT imaging. It exhibited comparable lesion detection ability compared with ^{18}F-FDG, even in liver metastases. All those results guaranteed the further clinical application of ^{64}Cu-NOTA-Trastuzumab in patients.

^{124}I-trastuzumab has been developed by Prof. Zhu et al. as a PET imaging reagent for assessing HER2 expression status preclinically and clinically [2]. ^{124}I-trastuzumab gives higher imaging contrast than ^{64}Cu-NOTA-tratuzumab because of lower nonspecific uptake and better tumor-to-soft tissue ratios. In animal studies, PET imaging of ^{124}I-tratuzumab shows significant higher tumor uptake than that of ^{124}I-IgG1 in HER2-positive PDX mouse models at 24 h. The low tumor uptake of ^{124}I-tratuzumab in HER2-negative PDX models further confirmed the specificity. In human clinical studies, the PET images showed significant difference in tumor uptake between HER2-positive and HER2-negative lesions at 24 h. Quite striking difference in tumor uptake was observed between ^{124}I-trastuzumab and ^{18}F-FDG in HER2-negative lesions, further confirming the specific binding of ^{124}I-trastuzumab in HER2-positive lesions. No toxicities or adverse effects were observed in any of the patients. The PET imaging indicated that the use of ^{124}I-trastuzumab to detect HER2-positive lesions in primary and metastatic gastric cancer patients to differentiate HER2-positive and HER2-negative lesions quantitatively was feasible.

38.3 HER2 Targeting Affibody PET Imaging

However, the clinical application of antibodies is limited because of their high molecular weight (MW = 150 kDa), resulting in low tumor penetration and slow clearance. To improve the imaging performance, alternative ligands have been developed over the past few years, such as F(ab′)2, F(ab′), single-chain Fv, and affibodies. Among them, the HER2 affibody is extensively studied preclinically and clinically. Affibody adapts the short half-life isotopes such as ^{68}Ga ($T_{1/2}$ = 68 min) or ^{18}F ($T_{1/2}$ = 110 min). Medium half-life nuclides such as ^{64}Cu ($T_{1/2}$ = 12.7 h) can also be used to label monoclonal antibodies and affibodies. The first clinical study using radiolabeled affibody was performed by Richard Baum and the team, ^{68}Ga-labeled ABY-002 for molecular imaging in breast cancer patients. The initial attempt established the validity of the strategy, yet further research is need to solve the problem caused by the high background level in surrounding nonmalignant liver tissue that might prevent the detection of liver metastases. Then, Prof. Sörensen and his team produced a ^{68}Ga-labeled ABY-025 for the diagnosis of HER2-positive breast cancer tumors. The results showed that HER2-positive primary and distant metastases were clearly visualized at 4 h after the injection.

Apart from trastuzumab modification, his team also pursued fancier HER2 targeting PET imaging. As we all known, HER2-binding affibody ^{68}Ga-ABY-025 accurately quantified whole-body HER2-receptor status in patients with metastatic breast cancer at 2 to 4 h postinjection. Recent progress has been made on labeling novel HER2 affibody (NOTA-MAL-MZHER2) with ^{18}F for micro-PET scans in nude mice bearing HER2-positive tumors (SKOV-3). Prof. Yang and his team translated this ^{68}Ga-ZHER2 in clinical PET imaging [3]. As shown in Fig. 38.1, the high ^{68}Ga-ZHER2 uptake is compatible with HER2 overexpression of the primary tumor. Compared with ^{18}F-FDG, ^{68}Ga-ZHER2 PET/CT showed better image contrast, especially in the bone lesions (with SUVmax, 66.0).

This novel PET/CT reveals the whole-body lesions at 1 h postinjection in patients with recurrent HER2-positive gastric cancer, which is much earlier than ^{64}Cu-labeled (2 days) or ^{89}Zr-labeled (5–8 days) intact antibody.

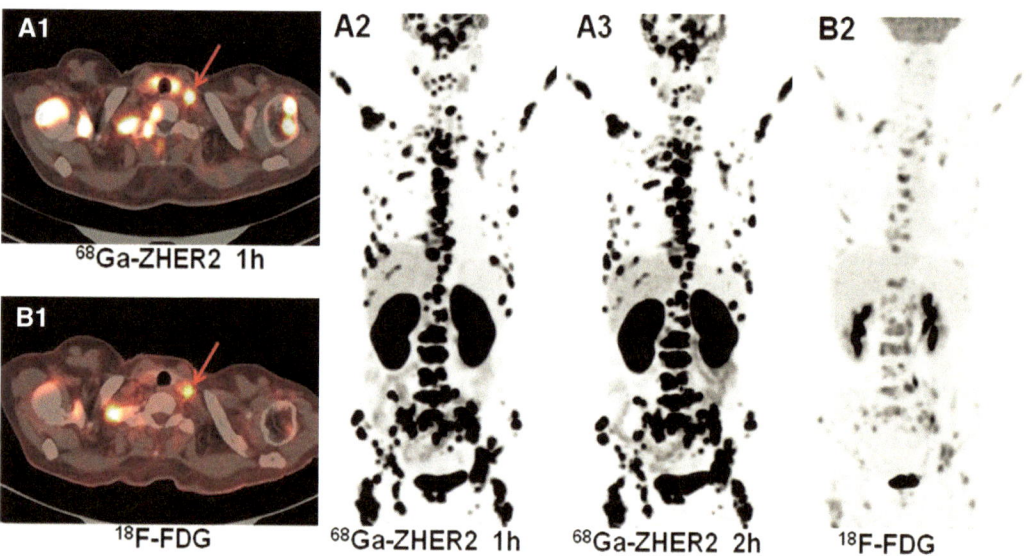

Fig. 38.1 ^{68}Ga-ZHER2 affibody PET/CT was performed 1 h and 2 h after 218 MBq ^{68}Ga-ZHER2 injection. The axial PET/CT image (A1) showed the left supraclavicular lymph node, and maximum intensive projection (MIP)

PET images (A2-A3) showed multiple ^{68}Ga-ZHER2-avid lesions in bones. B1 and B2 exhibit the ^{18}F-FDG PET images in the same patient

38.4 HER2 Targeting Therapy

Continuous low-dose irradiation from a tumor-targeted radiolabeled mAb produces tumoricidal effects. For therapy, α- and β-emitters are of practical relevance. There have been numerous investigations with a number of these radionuclides; however with intact antibodies, the most promising and practical radionuclides are the β-emitters such as ^{90}Y, ^{177}Lu, and ^{225}Ac. Currently, the research on HER2-targeted therapy is still in preclinical stage, and no clinical research report has been published.

Trastuzumab can be labeled with ^{90}Y and ^{177}Lu using DOTA, DTPA, or 3p-C-NETA as the chelator. Clearance of ^{177}Lu-DTPA-Trastuzumab in Swiss mice was predominantly through the hepatobiliary route with minimal bone uptake. Prof. Nasir Abbas et al. compared the bio-distribution, normal tissue toxicity, and therapeutic effect of the α-emitting ^{227}Th-trastuzumab and the β-emitting ^{177}Lu-trastuzumab in mice with HER2-expressing SKBR-3 breast cancer xeno-

grafts. The result showed that the relative biological effect (RBE) was higher for ^{227}Th-trastuzumab than for ^{177}Lu-trastuzumab, while the therapeutic index of ^{177}Lu-trastuzumab was superior to that of ^{227}Th-trastuzumab.

Recently, Prof. Tolmachev V et al. prepared ^{177}Lu-CHX-A''-DTPA-F(ab')$_2$-trastuzumab and ^{177}Lu-CHX-A''-DTPA-trastuzumab for nuclide therapy of HER2-positive SKOV3 models. The findings of this study indicate that both ^{177}Lu-CHX-A''-DTPA-F(ab')$_2$-trastuzumab and ^{177}Lu-CHX-A''-DTPA-trastuzumab are equally effective under in vitro conditions and could be employed with other apoptosis-inducing chemotherapeutic drugs for combinational therapy. The cellular toxicity exhibited by both ^{177}Lu-CHX-A''-DTPA-trastuzumab and ^{177}Lu-CHX-A''-DTPA-F(ab')$_2$-trastuzumab was similar in triggering membrane damage, inducing apoptosis, and causing cell death particularly at high radiation doses of ^{177}Lu-CHX-A''-DTPA-trastuzumab and its ^{177}Lu-CHX-A''-DTPA-F(ab')$_2$-trastuzumab. These in vitro results indicate that ^{177}Lu-CHX-A"-DTPA-F(ab')$_2$-trastuzumab could be a potential theranostic agent; however, its in vivo efficacy needs to be studied extensively.

38.5   HER2 Using Affibody Receptor Radionuclide Therapy

Based on the mentioned molecular imaging technology, especially the HER2-affibody-based PET image, SUVmax reaches to incredible high 66.0. This initial study strongly shows that ^{68}Ga-ZHER2 PET/CT can supply a whole-body vision of tumor load and HER2 expression including the heterogeneous as early as 1 h postinjection.

Inspired by recently most popular peptide receptor radionuclide therapy with lutetium-177 dotatate (^{177}Lu-DOTATATE) for advanced gastroenteropancreatic neuroendocrine tumors (GEP-NETs) and ^{177}Lu-PSMA-617 for metastatic castration resistant prostate cancer therapy (mCRPC), the establishment of affibody receptor radionuclide therapy (ARRT) has the potential to provide an alternative treatment option for HER2 positive resistant patients. As shown in Fig. 38.1, the high uptake of ^{68}Ga-HER2 affibody in systemic bone metastases indicated a high affinity of this probe for the lesions, and it is expected that these patients would benefit from the ^{177}Lu labeled HER2 affibody therapy.

38.6   Clinical Significance of HER2 ARRT

HER2 PET molecular probe can provide a whole-body view of the tumor load and HER2 expression status, and since lesions with very high uptake indicated that the drug had a very high affinity to the lesion, this method also reveals what the response to anti-HER2 drug will be, if de novo resistance occurs. Combined HER2 PET examinations and ctDNA sequencing is promising and may conquer the heterogeneity of HER2-positive cancer. These results of these indicators have a great impact on the overall prognosis of patients. The treatment plan of HER2-positive patients is different from that of HER2-negative patients, which can be intervened from the early stage of patients' treatment and affect the whole course of patients. During the treatment, some of patients may develop trastuzumab resistance; monitoring HER2 expression by PET imaging could help us to adjust the treatment plan in time [4].

Radionuclide-targeted therapy provides a new therapeutic method. These biological missiles can be fired with pinpoint accuracy, more in line with our concept of individualized and precise treatment for patients. When patients have intolerance to chemotherapy, targeted therapy can be used as a supplementary means.

References

1. Guo X, Zhu H, Zhou N, Chen Z, Liu T, Liu F, Xiaoxia X, Jin H, Shen L, Gao J, Yang Z. Non-invasive detection of HER2 expression in gastric cancer by ^{64}Cu-NOTA-trastuzumab in PDX mouse model and in patients. Mol Pharm. 2018;15(11):5174–82.
2. Guo X, Zhou N, Chen Z, Liu T, Xiaoxia X, Lei X, Shen L, Gao J, Yang Z, Zhu H. Construction of ^{124}I-trastuzumab for noninvasive PET imaging of HER2 expression: from patient-derived xenograft models to gastric cancer patients. Gastric Cancer. 2020;23:614. https://doi.org/10.1007/s10120-019-01035-6.
3. Zhou N, Guo X, Yang M, Zhu H, Yang Z. ^{68}Ga-ZHER2 PET/CT reveals HER2-positive metastatic gastric cancer with better image quality than 18F-FDG. Clin Nucl Med. 2020;45:e101. https://doi.org/10.1097/RLU.0000000000002859.
4. Zhou N, Liu C, Guo X, Yuping X, Gong J, Qi C, Zhang X, Yang M, Zhu H, Shen L, Yang Z. ^{68}Ga-NOTA-MAL-MZHER2 PET imaging in advanced gastric cancer patients and therapeutic response monitoring. Eur J Nucl Med Mol Imaging. 2020;48:161. https://doi.org/10.1007/s00259-020-04898-5.

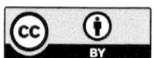